Sex Offenders

SEX OFFENDERS

Identification, Risk Assessment, Treatment, and Legal Issues

Edited by

Fabian M. Saleh, MD
Albert J. Grudzinskas, Jr., JD
John M. Bradford, MD
Daniel J. Brodsky, LLB

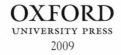

OXFORD
UNIVERSITY PRESS
2009

OXFORD
UNIVERSITY PRESS

Oxford University Press, Inc., publishes works that further
Oxford University's objective of excellence
in research, scholarship, and education.

Oxford New York
Auckland Cape Town Dar es Salaam Hong Kong Karachi
Kuala Lumpur Madrid Melbourne Mexico City Nairobi
New Delhi Shanghai Taipei Toronto

With offices in
Argentina Austria Brazil Chile Czech Republic France Greece
Guatemala Hungary Italy Japan Poland Portugal Singapore
South Korea Switzerland Thailand Turkey Ukraine Vietnam

Published by Oxford University Press, Inc.
198 Madison Avenue, New York, New York 10016
www.oup.com

Oxford is a registered trademark of Oxford University Press

Library of Congress Cataloging-in-Publication Data

Sex offenders : identification, risk assessment, treatment, and legal
issues / edited by Fabian M. Saleh ... [et al.].
p. ; cm.
Includes bibliographical references and index.
ISBN 978-0-19-517704-6
1. Sex offenders—Mental health.   2. Psychosexual disorders—Treatment.
3. Sex offenders.   4. Sex crimes.   5. Paraphilias.   6. Psychosexual disorders.
I. Saleh, Fabian M., 1965-
[DNLM: 1. Sex Offenses. 2. Paraphilias. W 795 S51813 2008]
RC560.S47S483 2008
616.85'836—dc22   2008028745

1 3 5 7 9 8 6 4 2

Printed in the United States of America
on acid-free paper

Foreword

Twenty years ago, it would have been difficult to imagine that the problems created by sex offenders would be high-profile issues on the public policy agenda. The past decade, however, has seen furious legislative activity—at both the state and federal levels—addressing sex offenders, and the controversies created by these initiatives can be found on the front pages of newspapers around the country. Contentious public hearings about these issues have become routine, and professional and lay groups expend considerable time and resources supporting or fighting assorted policy initiatives.

Consider the knotty issues raised by debates about what to do with sex offenders. Should states adopt civil commitment statutes, of the type repeatedly upheld as constitutional by the U.S. Supreme Court, that redefine offenders as mentally ill and subject them to indefinite confinement in secure treatment facilities? Or is this a misuse of the mental health treatment system to deal with a problem better handled by the courts and the correctional system? How much of the data that every state now collects on the whereabouts of released sex offenders should be available to the public? Do we all have a right to know about the former sex offenders in our midst, or do such laws merely provide a patina of reassurance, without making us or our children materially safer? And is their major consequence to make it impossible ever to reintegrate persons who have committed sex offenses into the community?

Why are these issues in the forefront of public consciousness today, when a few decades ago they were largely ignored? The undoubtedly complex answer to this question begins with a seemingly unrelated development: the movement in the last quarter of the twentieth century away from indeterminate sentencing and toward fixed, determinate prison terms for crimes. Indeterminate sentencing, the legacy of an earlier era in corrections during which the mantra was to "punish the offender, not the crime," was geared toward a rehabilitative model of corrections, under which prisoners would be detained as long as necessary to reduce their proclivities for recidivism. Hence, under the indeterminate approach there was no necessary correlation between the severity of an offense and the punishment imposed. Discharge was dependent on whether a parole board or similar entity deemed the prisoner ready to reenter society. Sex offenders in particular, who always evoke primal fears, were susceptible to being held for very long periods, or at least until there was every reason to believe that they would not offend again.

But the results of efforts to rehabilitate offenders, whatever the approach taken, were not impressive, and a countertrend developed—typified by the federal sentencing guidelines adopted in the mid-1980s—to "punish the crime, not the offender." According to this directive, sentences were graded by the severity of the offense, regardless of the characteristics of the offender, and judges' discretion was usually cabined within a fixed range of options. Now the dominant model, determinate sentencing implies that in all but the most extreme circumstances the offender will some day be released, and that day is often much sooner than many members of the general public might think. With an increasing return flow of sex offenders to the community not many years after their conviction and imprisonment, it was inevitable that horrific crimes would occur and that there would be public outcry for a remedy.

Once sex offenders were on the radar screens of reporters and politicians, it took little effort to stir up powerful concerns about the safety of the citizenry, especially children. The first consequence was the adoption of the civil commitment statutes that are denoted sexually violent predator laws or similar appellations. In the public policy aviary, these are odd birds. They are meant to take effect when a prisoner who committed an offense that falls within their scope (usually a crime involving violence, but sometimes with considerable flexibility as to how violence is defined) is about to be released from prison. At that point, the statutes allow the prisoner to be examined for evidence of mental disorder, and to be subject to indefinite confinement in a secure facility if both disordered and deemed likely to offend again. However, the definitions of disorder are substantially circular, resting on impairment in the ability to control sexual impulses, which can be proved largely by the prisoner's conviction of the offense for which he was imprisoned. And the liabilities of concluding that a sexual offender will never repeat his crime make it difficult to avoid committing offenders about whom any doubts exist and even harder to release them once initially confined.

Moreover, by focusing attention on persons about to be released, the statutes ratify the current approach of ignoring the possibility of treatment in prison, when offenders are arguably more amenable to successful intervention. Thus, 10 or 20 years after conviction and incarceration, current policies suddenly manifest a desire to provide treatment to persons who could usefully have been receiving treatment all along. And this is accomplished in a context in which the difficulty of winning release probably diminishes the perceived incentives for offenders to cooperate. It is hard to avoid the conclusion that many of the advocates of the new generation of civil commitment statutes are using the treatment rationale to provide constitutional "cover" for holding on to sex offenders as long as they live. The foreseeable consequence of these statutes is now upon us: states are finding that they have created extremely expensive detention facilities that are rapidly filling with offenders for whose discharge no one is willing to take responsibility. Pressure is already growing to expand existing facilities or to build new ones, and the costs continue to mount. It seems only a matter of time before a pendulum swing brings us to a reconsideration of this costly mistake.

Meanwhile, for those offenders who do return to the community, we have created a system of registration and tracking that essentially involves lifetime oversight. But again, rather than this information being used to provide meaningful rehabilitation and support, it is instead posted on the Internet or taped onto neighborhood lampposts in a manner designed to stir fear even among the most rational citizens. What is one to do, after all, when one is informed by a state agency that a convicted sex offender has moved in next door, down the street, or into an apartment building that one's child passes on the way to school? As if the resulting uproar is not enough to ensure that released sex offenders will find it impossible to reintegrate into almost any community, municipalities are passing ordinances restricting them from living near schools and other facilities, creating offender-free zones that in many cases encompass most or all of the jurisdiction's residential areas. Although homeowners arguably might have an equally strong interest in knowing when a released house breaker has moved into their community, the laws that enable or require disclosure of such information are uniformly limited to sex offenders.

If the phrase "moral panic" has any legitimate application in the early twenty-first century, it is to the rampant fear mongering that has led to consistently counterproductive policies for addressing the difficult problems raised by people who commit sexual offenses. What is needed today is soundly reasoned policy based on real data—and that is where efforts such as those embodied in this book come into play. The escape route from the current policy quagmire wends its way through solid research on the phenomenology, assessment, treatment, and risk assessment of persons who commit sexual offenses. It is worth considering briefly what each of those bodies of work might foreseeably encompass.

There is a tendency to talk about sex offenders and the problems they create as if every person who commits a sexual offense is similar to every other. Yet, offenders differ in ways that may have significant implications for treatment and the risk of recidivism, including the presence of substance abuse and concomitant mental illness, mental retardation, and personality disorders. Juvenile sex offenders, who may still be at an early stage of psychosocial development, often need to be differentiated from older perpetrators of similar crimes. Assessment approaches, addressed by a number of chapters in this book, must be developed so as to permit us to distinguish among groups of offenders with different potentials for treatment and varying likelihoods of reoffense. Until we have a better grasp of the epidemiology of sexual offenses and the motivations of the persons who commit them, along with a clearer understanding of the varying pathways to offending, we will be left with a Procrustean approach to management that holds little hope of advancing the current state of prevention and treatment.

More effective treatments of paraphilias and related phenomena stand at the top of the wish list of anyone involved with this population. Although not all sexual offenses reflect underlying disorders, many do, and the ongoing controversy about treatment effectiveness bespeaks the need for a much stronger evidence base on treatments that are likely to succeed with the offender population. Indeed, in a world of rational policy development, the money now being spent on expensive sex offender commitment facilities would be allocated instead to an intensive program of research on treatments for these problems. Only when clear-cut evidence was at hand of real-world effectiveness population might it make sense to invest in long-term treatment facilities, and then only if treatment could not safely be rendered in the community. And even if states felt the imperative—which it is clear that they do—to confine sex offenders under the guise of providing effective treatment, in that same rational world substantial investments in treatment research would be made alongside the expenditures for new staff and facilities. Yet, not only is this not the case, but the politically sensitive nature of sexual offenses and possible interventions makes it particularly difficult to obtain funding and to conduct such studies, especially in the United States. It is worth saying again: the only hope for escaping the legal, ethical, and political tangle associated with sex offenders is the development of effective treatment, which should be an absolute policy priority.

Along with studies of treatment, of course, must come improved methods of assessing the future risk presented by persons who have committed sexual offenses. In fact, without such measures it may be impossible to know when treatment has been effective. Like most areas of clinical risk assessment, sexual violence risk assessment has been hampered by approaches that rely largely on static variables. Thus, while it is becoming increasingly possible to identify persons in high-risk groups on the basis of their past behavior and fixed characteristics, it remains difficult to adjust risk predictions according to the presumed impact of treatment. For meaningful risk assessment to be paired with effective treatment, it will need to include variables that are subject to modification and that have been shown to affect risk accordingly. Several of the more promising biological measures are discussed in this book, but it is clear that this too needs to be the focus of an assertive research strategy.

The chapters that follow provide a thorough overview of the state of the art in dealing with sexual offenders: from phenomenology to biology, from assessment to treatment, and including a variety of special populations. If we are serious about dealing with the real dilemmas of sexual offenders and their crimes, we will use this work as a launching pad for the development of research and clinical approaches that can undergird rational policy for this extremely challenging population.

Paul S. Appelbaum MD
Elizabeth K. Dollard, Professor of Psychiatry, Medicine, and Law
Department of Psychiatry
Columbia University College of Physicians & Surgeons; and
Director, Division of Law, Ethics, and Psychiatry
New York State Psychiatric Institute

Contents

Part VII—Forensics

Contributors

Gene G. Abel, MD
Professor, Department of Psychiatry, Emory University and Morehouse School
of Medicine; Director, Behavioral Medicine Institute of Atlanta, Atlanta, GA

James C. Beck, MD, PhD
Professor of Psychiatry, Harvard Medical School; Associate Chief, Law and Psychiatry Service,
Massachusetts General Hospital, Boston, MA

Elissa P. Benedek MD
Adjunct Professor, Department of Psychiatry, University of Michigan School
of Medicine, Ann Arbor, MI

Fred S. Berlin, MD, PhD
Associate Professor, Department of Psychiatry and Behavioral Sciences,
The Johns Hopkins University School of Medicine, Baltimore, MD

Wolfgang Berner, MD
Professor and Director, Insititute for Sex Research and Forensic Psychiatry, Center of Psychosocial
Medicine, University Medical Center Hamburg-Eppendorf,Hamburg, Germany

**John M. Bradford, MB ChB, DPM, FFPsych, FRCPsych, DABPN, DABFP, FAPA,
FACPsych, FCPA**
Professor and Head, Division of Forensic Psychiatry, Faculty of Medicine and Professor, School
of Criminology, University of Ottawa, Ottawa, ON; Professor of Psychiatry, Faculty of Medicine,
Queen's University, Kingston, ON; Associate Chief (Forensic), Royal Ottawa Health Care Group,
Ottawa, ON, Canada. Honorary Titles: Fellow of the Royal College of Psychiatrists (UK);
Distinguished Fellow, American Psychiatric Association; Fellow, American College of Psychiatrists

S. Jan Brakel, JD
Adjunct Professor of Law, DePaul University College of Law; Director of Legal Research,
Isaac Ray Center, Inc., Chicago, IL

Peer Briken, MD
Assistant Professor of Pychiatry and Psychotherapy, Institute of Sex Research
and Forensic Psychiatry, University Medical Centre, Hamburg, Germany

Daniel J. Brodsky, LLB
Criminal Defence Lawyer, Toronto, ON, Canada

Alec Buchanan, MD
Associate Professor, Department of Psychiatry, Yale University School
of Medicine, New Haven, CT

Jonathan C. Clayfield, MA, LMHC
Project Director II, Department of Psychiatry, University of Massachusetts
Medical School, Worcester, MA

Frank DiCataldo, PhD
Assistant Professor, Department of Psychology, Roger Williams University, Bristol, RI;
Director, Forensic Evaluation Service, NFI Massachusetts

Liam Ennis, PhD
Assistant Clinical Professor, Department of Psychiatry, Faculty of Medicine and Dentistry,
University of Alberta, Edmonton, AB, Canada

Peter J. Fagan, PhD
Associate Professor of Medical Psychology, Department of Psychiatry and
Behavioral Sciences, The Johns Hopkins University School of Medicine; Director of Research,
Johns Hopkins HealthCare LLC, Baltimore, MD

J. Paul Fedoroff, MD
Associate Professor, Department of Psychiatry, Institute of Mental Health Research,
University of Ottawa; Director, Sexual Behaviors Clinic, Integrated Forensic Program,
Royal Ottawa Mental Health Care Group, Ottawa, ON, Canada

Graham Glancy, MB, ChB, FRCPsych, FRCPC
Assistant Professor, Department of Psychiatry, Faculty of Medicine, University of Toronto,
Toronto, ON, Canada

Carmen L. Z. Gress, PhD
Adjunct Professor, Department of Educational Psychology,
University of Victoria, BC, Canada

Dorothy Griffiths, PhD
Associate Dean, Faculty of Social Sciences, Brock University,
St. Catharines, ON, Canada

Albert J. Grudzinskas, Jr., JD
Clinical Associate Professor and Coordinator of Legal Studies, Department of Psychiatry,
University of Massachusetts Medical School, Worcester, MA

Ronnie B. Harmon, MA, MPhil
Clinical Assistant Professor, Department of Psychiatry, New York University School of Medicine, New York, NY

Stephen D. Hart, PhD
Professor, Department of Psychology, Simon Fraser University, Burnaby, BC, Canada

Andreas Hill, MD
Assistant Professor of Psychiatry and Psychotherapy, Institute of Sex Research and Forensic Psychiatry, University Medical Centre Hamburg-Eppendorf, Hamburg, Germany

Stephen J. Hucker, MB, BS, FRCPC, FRCPsych
Professor of Psychiatry, Law & Mental Health Program, University of Toronto; Consulting Forensic Psychiatrist, Sexual Behavior Clinic, Centre for Addiction and Mental Health, Toronto, ON, Canada

Scott Humphreys, MD
Instructor, Department of Forensic Psychiatry, University of Colorado Denver School of Medicine, Denver, CO

Meg S. Kaplan, PhD
Associate Clinical Professor, Department of Psychiatry, Columbia University College of Physicians and Surgeons; Director, Sexual Behavior Clinic, New York State Psychiatric Institute, New York, NY

Richard B. Krueger, MD
Associate Clinical Professor, Department of Psychiatry, College of Physicians and Surgeons, Columbia University; Associate Attending Psychiatrist, New York-Presbyterian Hospital, New York, NY

Michael Kuban, Msc, MEd
Laboratory Coordinator, Clinical Sexology Services, Center for Addiction and Mental Health, Toronto, ON, Canada

Ron Langevin, PhD
Associate Professor, Department of Psychiatry, Faculty of Medicine, University of Toronto; Director, Juniper Associates, Toronto, ON, Canada

Gregory K. Lehne, PhD
Assistant Professor of Medical Psychology, Department of Psychiatry and Behavioral Sciences, The Johns Hopkins University School of Medicine, Baltimore, MD

Stephen B. Levine, MD
Clinical Professor of Psychiatry, Case Western Reserve University School of Medicine, Beachwood, OH; Co-director, Center for Marital and Sexual Health, University Hospital of Cleveland, Cleveland, OH

H. Martin Malin, PhD, MA, MFT
Professor, Department of Clinical Sexology, Institute for Advanced Study
of Human Sexuality; Research Associate, National Institute for the Study,
Prevention, and Treatment of Sexual Trauma, Benicia, CA

L. Alvin Malesky, Jr., PhD
Assistant Professor, Department of Psychology, Western Carolina University,
Cullowhee, NC

Shannon M. Maney, MA (Clinical Psychology), MA (Forensic Psychology)
Project Manager, Department of Psychiatry, University of Massachusetts Medical School,
Worcester, MA

Liam E. Marshall, MA
Research Director, Rockwood Psychological Services, Kingston, ON, Canada

William Marshall, PhD, OC, FRSC
Emeritus Professor, Department of Psychology, Queen's University; Director,
Rockwood Psychological Services, Kingston, ON, Canada

Jeffrey L. Metzner, MD
Clinical Professor, Department of Psychiatry, University of Colorado Denver School
of Medicine, Denver, CO

Denise L. Mumley, PhD
Assistant Professor, Department of Psychiatry, University of Massachusetts Medical School;
Forensic Psychologist, Forensic Science, Worcester State Hospital, Worcester, MA

Lisa Murphy
Master's of Criminology Applied (MCA) Candidate
Department of Criminology, University of Ottawa, Ottawa, ON, Canada

Christine E. Negendank, MD
Adult and Forensic Psychiatrist, Department of Psychiatry, University Of Michigan School
of Medicine, Ann Arbor, MI; Staff Psychiatrist, Washtenaw County Community Support
and Treatment Center, Ypsilanti, MI

Stewart S. Newman, MD
Assistant Clinical Professor, Department of Psychiatry, Oregon Health & Science University
School of Medicine, Portland, OR

Matt D. O'Brien, BSC (Hons), MA, MSC
Therapist, Rockwood Psychological Services, Kingston, ON, Canada

Roy J. O'Shaughnessy, MD
Clinical Professor and Head of Forensic Program, Department of Psychiatry, Faculty
of Medicine, University of British Columbia, Vancouver, BC, Canada

Michael Petrunik, PhD
Professor (Adjunct), Department of Criminology, University of Ottawa, Ottawa, ON, Canada

Debra A. Pinals, MD
Associate Professor and Director of Forensic Education, Department of Psychiatry,
University of Massachusetts Medical School, Worcester, MA

Ernest Poortinga, MD
Adjunct Clinical Assistant Professor, Department of Psychiatry,
University of Michigan School of Medicine; Forensic Psychiatrist, Michigan Center
for Forensic Psychiatry, Ann Arbor, MI

Rusty Reeves, MD
Clinical Associate Professor, Department of Psychiatry, University of Medicine and
Dentistry of New Jersey, Robert Wood Johnson Medical School, Trenton, NJ

Candace B. Risen, MSW
Assistant Clinical Professor of Social Work, Department of Psychiatry,
Case Western Reserve University School of Medicine, Cleveland, OH; Co-director,
Center for Marital and Sexual Health, Beachwood, OH

Richard Rogers, PhD, ABPP
Professor, Department of Psychology, University of North Texas, Denton, TX

Richard Rosner, MD
Clinical Professor, Department of Psychiatry, New York University School of Medicine;
Medical Director, Forensic Psychiatry Clinic, Department of Psychiatry,
Bellevue Hospital Center, New York, NY

Gail Ryan, MA
Assistant Clinical Professor, Department of Pediatrics, University of Colorado
Denver School of Medicine, Denver, CO

Michael Saini, PhD, MSW, RSW
Assistant Professor, Factor-Inwentash Faculty of Social Work, University of Toronto,
Toronto, ON, Canada

Fabian M. Saleh, MD
Assistant Professor of Psychiatry, Harvard Medical School;
Law & Psychiatry Service, Massachusetts General Hospital, Boston, MA

Charles Scott, MD
Professor of Clinical Psychiatry and Chief, Division of Psychiatry and the Law, Department
of Psychiatry and Behavioral Sciences, University of California, Davis School
of Medicine, Sacramento, CA

Geris A. Serran, PhD, CPsych
Clinical Director, Sex Offenders Treatment Programs, Rockwood Psychological
Services, Kingston, ON, Canada

Chad E. Tillbrook, PhD
Assistant Professor, Department of Psychiatry, University of Massachusetts Medical School;
Forensic Psychologist, Forensic Service, Worcester State Hospital, Worcester, MA

Gina M. Vincent, PhD
Assistant Professor, Department of Psychiatry and Center for Mental Health Services Research, University of Massachusetts Medical School, Worcester, MA

Michael J. Vitacco, PhD
Associate Director of Research, Department of Psychology, Mendota Mental Health Institute, Madison, WI

Michael H. Wechsler, MD
Assistant Professor of Clinical Urology, Department of Urology, College of Physicians & Surgeons, Columbia University; Attending, New York Presbyterian Hospital, New York, NY

Markus Wiegel, PhD
Therapist, Behavioral Medicine Institute of Atlanta, Atlanta, GA

Matt Zaitchik, PhD, ABPP
Associate Professor, Department of Pscyhology, Roger Williams University, Bristol, RI.

Howard Zonana, MD
Professor, Department of Psychiatry, Yale University School of Medicine; Clinical Professor (Adjunct) of Law, Yale University Law School, New Haven, CT

Part 1

Introduction

Chapter 1

Perspectives on Sex and Normality

Peter J. Fagan

In his annual lecture to second year medical students, Dr. Fred Berlin describes an interview he had, early in his career, with a man whom he was evaluating following the man's arrest for child sexual abuse. Halfway through the interview, the arrested man interrupted Dr. Berlin's questions and said,

> You know, Doctor, *your society* takes a newborn baby boy; gathers family and friends, takes a knife and without any anesthesia cuts skin off the tip of his penis. This is accepted as a religious act. I bend over and kiss that same penis, and I am arrested as a child sexual abuser. Can you explain that to me? (Berlin, 2000).

The man in Dr. Berlin's story was a member of the North American Man/Boy Love Association (NAMBLA), an organization whose website describes its goal, "to end the extreme oppression of men and boys in mutually consensual relationships." The "society" referred to was the mainstream culture in

North America, symbolized by the status awarded to the medical profession. The evaluee's society was composed of all those who would espouse the benefits of "consensual" sexual relationships between and among men and boys.

For many individuals, the response to the question posed would involve a reference to "normality": the religious ceremony of circumcision with its infliction of pain on an unconsenting infant is normal (therefore a good act or at least morally neutral act); the act of kissing an unconsenting child's penis for the purpose of sexual gratification is abnormal (therefore wrong). In this type of response, the use of "normal" and "abnormal" is descriptive, not explanatory. It does not, therefore, advance a rational understanding about the behaviors of adults and children, in one case religiously motivated, in the other erotically motivated.

The question of Dr. Berlin's patient reveals not only the dramatic gulf that exists between NAMBLA and the majority culture in the United States, but suggests that there may be similar, if perhaps not as graphically stated, differences about the cultural legitimacy or ethical morality of certain sexual behaviors among individuals and groups, not only in North America, but also throughout the world. The Internet with its instantaneous sharing of sexual fantasies, the migration of peoples across traditional national boundaries, and a growing awareness of cultural diversity forces people to recognize that the evaluation of sexual behaviors by different groups and cultures and by different individuals within the same society is varied, sometimes extremely so.

Frequently the clashing of views about sexual behaviors, including those classified as sexual offenses by a jurisdiction, is framed in terms of normality versus non-normality. "It's just not normal for a person to (reader supply here whatever the sexual behavior is in dispute)." At this point, the discussion usually revolves around what is "normal" sexual behavior. The revolving discussion then becomes a devolving debate because the parties typically cannot agree on what is normality for sexual behaviors.

This chapter enters the discussion/debate by examining the question of normality and sexual behavior. The chapter will not satisfy the reader who wants two lists, one for normal sexual behaviors and one for non-normal or abnormal sexual behaviors. Rather, the chapter will seek to provide a structure within which discussants (presumably all of us) may advance our understanding of normality and sexual behaviors on a mutually agreed on rational basis, identifying the perspective from which we are speaking.

The structure of the chapter is that of the four perspectives of psychiatry first elaborated by McHugh and Slavney (1998) and later applied to sexual disorders by the author (Fagan, 2003). The four perspectives of disease, dimension, behavior, and life story provide a methodological framework for discussing and hopefully advancing the answer to the questions about normality and sexual behaviors.

The chapter, then, will describe briefly the essential features of each perspective and then apply the perspective to the discussion of normality and sexual behaviors. In the conclusion, we shall urge readers to employ all four perspectives in this discussion with the belief that doing so will not only inform their responses to the question about normality and sexual behaviors but also lend an often needed quality of civility to the discussion turned debate about this topic.

SEXUAL NORMALITY AND THE DISEASE PERSPECTIVE

Viewing sexual behaviors through the disease perspective is to inquire whether the behavior is the product of a disease process in the body. The logic of the disease perspective is categorical: the individual either has the disease or not. If the individual is positive for the disease, the question then is whether the sexual behaviors in question are a result of the disease state. For example, the hypersexual behaviors of bipolar disorder are often the result of the affective illness. While the individual may have had a diathesis toward the particular form of the behavior, the actual expression of the sexual behavior is directly caused by the impairment of social judgment and the increased libido in bipolar illness. An individual with moderate bipolar disorder may make seductive or sexually harassing comments to fellow workers. While the behavior may be consistent with his or her sexual orientation, the frequency and intensity of the comments are inconsistent with the behavior of the individual before the onset of the affective illness.

Assessing the normality of sexual behaviors from the disease perspective is a judgment of whether a person has a disease that is an etiologic factor in the expression of that person's behaviors. Normality in the disease perspective will be referred to with terms such as "abnormal" and "disordered." The hypersexual behaviors of the individual with bipolar illness would rightly be labeled "abnormal," not only because they are not normative for the individual, but because they are accurately seen as a behavioral manifestation of the disease. Another term that can be used in the disease perspective is "addictive" sexual behavior when the disease origins of the behavior are elaborated (Goodman, 1992).

On further examination, however, the disease perspective in some cases is not completely categorical in which a simple "yes" or "no" can be given to the question, "Does the individual have the disease?" Many diseases such as hypertension and adult onset diabetes are the result of application of dimensional features. Exceeding certain values (which may change according to practice guidelines) results in the naming of the condition as a disease. Also, the changes in bodily functions that are the result of "normal" aging versus "disease" process also challenge a simple categorical application of the disease perspective.

Applied to sexual normality, the application of a dimensional component to the disease perspective is apparent in questions relating to intelligence and sex hormone levels. Both intelligence and hormonal milieu can affect the expression of sexual behaviors. In general, low intelligence or a dementia may result in poor social judgment and/or disinhibition while androgen levels are associated with sexual drive in men and women. Both are somatic conditions that may independently or in consort cause sexual behaviors to occur. Separately they may not be considered a "disease," for example, an I.Q. of 85 and a serum testosterone level of 850 (250 to 750 range). However, because of the multidetermined nature of the interaction of these somatic conditions and the environmental factors in which the individual may be sexually stimulated, it is not always simple to establish a primarily somatic causal role in the sexual behaviors. But if the interaction of somatic factors producing sexual behaviors can be established with a clinical level of certainty, then the disease perspective would suggest that the sexual behaviors are abnormal.

In summary, the disease perspective addresses the question of normality by assessing whether the sexual behavior in question is a product of a disease state. Many times, this can be accomplished with a high degree of clinical certainty, for example, bipolar disorder in hypersexuality and hypogonadism in hyposexuality. In other situations where there may be an interaction between somatic and environmental factors, the use of the disease perspective may be necessary but not sufficient to address the question of sexual normality. Other perspectives, especially the dimension perspective, are often required to supplement the disease perspective.

SEXUAL NORMALITY AND THE DIMENSION PERSPECTIVE

The dimension perspective addresses sexual normality quantitatively by measuring the behavior in question. The dimension perspective counts the frequency and/or measures the duration and intensity of the sexual behavior. It then compares these measures to sampling of other subjects or population before returning its verdict of normality or non-normality. Whereas the logic of the disease perspective is in the main category (a person has or does not have the disease), the

logic of the dimension perspective is measurement (count, degree, ratio).

With measurement as the logic of the dimension perspective, the discussion of normality versus abnormality is largely about the arbitrary cutoffs on each tail of the distribution curves. For example, with a predetermined two-tail alpha of 0.025, if a behavior is practiced by only 2% of the population, then that behavior might be considered statistically not normal, therefore statistically abnormal. But if it were practiced by 3% of the population, then by that same measurement logic the arbitrary cutoffs would indicate that the sexual behavior in question is normal. Indeed even the term *paraphilic* mirrors this distinction between the extremes and the central normality. Its Greek entomology, *para* "along side of" suggests that it occurs along the side of normal or "normophilic" sexual behaviors.

Employing the dimension perspective to measure a construct and the occurrence of which one assumes to be normally distributed in the population (a false assumption for sexual offenses), one can, by setting a point at the extremes of the normal curve, label the measured construct as "normal" or "abnormal." A blood pressure of 200/120 is abnormal for a 30-year-old man; similarly a daily frequency of 10 orgasms is abnormal for him. But 10 years without an orgasm during wake state would not be abnormal for a 30-year-old man who happens to be an observant celibate monk. Thus, in the dimension perspective the terms "normal" and "abnormal" relate to statistical normality within a specific population. They do not address the questions of value. Value relating to the meaning of the behaviors in the context of the life of the individual requires the life story perspective while further qualitative descriptors of the behavior employ the behavior perspective.

Those who argue for the normality of a selected sexual behavior on the grounds that it is practiced by predetermined percentage of the population are employing the dimension perspective. In recent years, the Internet's sexual oriented websites and western culture's increased permissiveness about discussing sexual behaviors has given sexual minorities fodder for their assertion of sexual normality. Those who would disagree rarely argue about the choice of the measurement's cutoff. They resort to other perspectives, largely the life story perspective with its stress on values, to counter the claims of normality. The debate ends with each side arguing from different perspectives and, without consciously doing so, talking past one another. Normality in the dimension perspective is not a value judgment. It is a statistical measurement.

NORMALITY: FORM VERSUS FUNCTION

The distinction of *form* and *function* is a component of each of the four perspectives but needs to be considered, especially in any discussion of the dimensional measurement of normality of sexual behaviors. The *form* of a behavior consists of the quantifiable descriptors of the behavior. The *form* is the *what* of the behavior: the physical and mental activity as well as its manner of expression in terms of frequency, intensity, and duration. The *function* of a behavior is the *purpose* that the behavior plays in the life of the individual, the *why* of the activity. Function is attributed to the behavior by the individual or by the observers; form is constitutive of the behavior.

An example of the form versus function distinction applied to exhibitionism might clarify the distinction. The *form* of exhibitionism consists of an individual intentionally exposing his or her genitals or erotogenic parts of the body to an unconsenting individual and, at some point, becoming sexually aroused by the experience. The *function* of exhibitionism is often multidetermined: assertion of gender; aggression at object of exposure; enjoyment of risk-taking; attempt to seduce. If they conduct a sufficiently rigorous inquiry, independent observers should be able to have fairly high inter-rater reliability on the *form* of a specific behavior. There will be less agreement on *function*, however, because the observers are attributing to the subject psychological need and motivation regarding the behavior. And as the many schools of psychological theory attest to, there can be many rational, coherent, and, at times, contradictory understandings regarding human motivation.

The issue of discussing normality in terms of form and function has a caveat: there may not be concurrence between form and function in terms of normality. Applied to the exhibitionism described, the form of the behavior in the particular individual is likely abnormal because of its presumed low *prevalence* in the general population. (Its *incidence* may be less abnormal in the population because of the frequency of the behaviors by those with exhibitionism.) The functional attributions are in themselves normal

motivations, albeit perhaps toward the tails of the normal curves for some, for example, aggression.

It is the blurring of normal motivations with abnormal behaviors that can result in an inappropriate conclusion about the normality of sexual behaviors when trying to employ the dimension perspective. An understanding of the function, that is, motivations of the sexual behaviors in the individual, (*verstehen*) as Jaspers (1997) would describe it, is not the measurement of dimensional perspective. It is not sufficient from the dimension perspective to hypothesize confidently why the sexual behavior was done by the individual. This is the work of the life story perspective; it is not the task of the dimension perspective.

The dimension perspective takes the form of the sexual behavior in question and measures its frequency, duration, and intensity. How often does the behavior occur? Is it episodic or is it a constant component in the sexual repertoire of the individual? How long does the activity take to be completed? Is it measured in seconds, minutes, or hours? How intensely is it experienced by the individual? Is there a sense of being on "automatic pilot" once the behavior has begun? Is there a compromise of social judgment or awareness of consequences during the behavior? Is there any dissociative element in the experience for the individual? These measurements of subjective intensity rely somewhat on observation; but ultimately they depend upon the self-report of the individual performing the sexual behaviors.

Once the form of the behaviors has been measured, the task of the dimension perspective is to compare the measurements to some sample of other individuals and their (non)experience of the behavior. While there are some population-based studies that provide a range of normality for some sexual behaviors, most of the sexual behaviors in these studies are limited to childhood experience of sex (including with an adult), adult noncriminal activities, and sexual dysfunction (Laumann, Gagnon, Michael, & Michaels, 1994). There is perhaps no reliable population measurement to establish statistical normality for those behaviors which are categorized as paraphilia in the DSM-TR-IV (American Psychiatric Association, 2000). The same condition exists for sexual offensives, both paraphilic and nonparaphilic.

The problem, then, for judging the normality of sexual behaviors from a dimension perspective is in the question, "Normal as compared to what?" In judging the incidence or prevalence of a disease, the epidemiologists will take care to ensure that the population denominator over which the disease is placed as a numerator is carefully determined (Gordis, 2000). The denominator is the "compared to what" population.

For sexual behaviors, especially those that are illegal, socially censored, or culturally unaccepted, it is extremely difficult to ascertain incidence or prevalence rates. While the numerator is arrested and/or referred for clinical treatment, the denominator is uncertain at best, guesstimated at worst. In general, despite the numerous surveys and samplings of convenience, we do not know the prevalence or incidence of sexual offenses or paraphilic sexual behaviors in the general population.

The question, "So what is normal, anyway?," is from a dimension perspective largely unanswered when it comes to what is currently labeled as sexual offenses or paraphilic sexual behaviors. There are some indications of other sexual behaviors in the population that have been given some preliminary responses, for example, prevalence/incidence of same sex behaviors, the prevalence/prevalence of extramarital sexual activity (Laumann et al., 1994). What is not normal within the general population denominator may be normal within a more stratified sample, for example, the higher educated, urban. According to the sampling frame, the boundaries of normality may shift.

In summary, the dimension perspective addresses normality by measuring the frequency, duration, and intensity of the form of the sexual behavior in question. It selects an arbitrary and hopefully acceptable cutoff in the measurement for what will be considered normal and abnormal on each side of the cutoff. The dimension perspective is currently limited by the lack of information about the incidence and prevalence of sexual behaviors and so is limited in addressing the question, "Normal as compared to what?" It should, however, be a perspective that can be a meeting ground for discussion about sexual behaviors because, like science, its logic is measurement, not evaluation of probity. The evaluation of probity is the work of the behavior and life story perspectives in their approach to the question of the normality of sexual behaviors.

SEXUAL NORMALITY AND THE BEHAVIOR PERSPECTIVE

Like the dimension perspective, the behavior perspective examines what the individual *does*. But unlike the dimension perspective, it examines the individual's human behavior as a series of unique goal-directed, or teleological, activities that have both antecedents that set the behavior in motion and consequences that result from the commission of the behavior. The terms for "normality" employed in the behavior perspective are those such as "disordered," "maladaptive," "compulsive," "addictive," and "(self) harmful." These, and similar terms are used to indicate that the behavior results in consequences that are not positive either for the individual or for others.

Between the antecedents and the consequences, the individual chooses to perform the behavior. If there is no element of choice, the behavior is not a human act (*actus humanus*) but simply an act of a (wo)man (*actus hominis*). If choice is absent, as it certainly may be compromised if not absent in bipolar disorder, then the behavior perspective is not the appropriate perspective to employ in discussing the normality of the sexual behavior. The behavior perspective *assumes* that the individual has some component of choice in the sexual behavior he or she has engaged in.

Given the assumption of choice and with the unique behavior as the object of observation, what does the behavior perspective contribute to the discussion of the normality of sexual behaviors? Put in simple terms, the behavior perspective is the perspective of a culture's normative institutions: religious, civil, and social. The norms are taught, legislated, decreed, and agreed upon by these institutions and consented to in varying degrees by the individuals within the institution. When applied to sexual behaviors, the norms are typically restrictive although occasionally may be proscriptive, for example, the duty to have intercourse to bear progeny or fulfill spousal obligations. The norms may be justified based on the behavior itself, for example, ecclesial prohibitions against masturbation, or based on the consequences of the behavior, for example, the putative harm to a child whose trust in adults/parents has been compromised by sexual abuse. The behavior perspective judges a sexual behavior to be normal based on its observation of and conformity to the prevailing norms.

There are two immediate problems. The first is that the norms are prevailing—some for centuries, some only for decades. Institutional norms, even those of religious institutions, change. If the sexual behavior is being judged normal in a period of institutional normative transition, it is difficult to reach consensus based on the prevailing norm under pressure to change. Certainly homosexual behaviors have been subject, in the past century, to many changes in the prevailing civil, ecclesial, and societal laws and norms. Yet today there is no consensus about the normality of homosexual behavior.

The second problem in judging sexual behaviors as normal based on prevailing norms is that there are discrepancies among the intersecting institutions about the normative probity of specified sexual behaviors. The civil jurisdiction may say a behavior is not normative, for example, the State of Georgia's anti-sodomy law, while an ecclesial body, for example, the Metropolitan Community Church, may teach that it is normal and not against the church teachings. In such situations of normative conflict, individuals may have to determine their ultimate normative institution and, of course, individuals will differ in their choices.

When the question of the normality of a behavior is discussed using the behavior perspective, the first answer usually comes rather quickly, but then on further examination (or rebuttal), comes up against its inherent limitation: it is relative. Despite quests of most institutions for absolute norms, the fact is that the norms legislated are prevailing and relative. Institutions, even autocratic ones, ultimately depend upon the consent of their populations for their norms to be normative. The Soviet Union has collapsed and the antiusury and toleration of slavery norms of the Roman Catholic Church have changed (Noonan, 2005). Consensus will shift and consent of the populations will always be tentative—even if held constant for centuries.

The behavior perspective is teleological, that is, that behaviors are goal seeking and purposeful. Beyond the concurrence with institutional norms, the behavior perspective can address the normality of sexual behavior by using the theoretical construct of Antecedents→Behaviors→Consequences involved in teleology. To the extent that the intensity, duration, or frequency of certain sexual behaviors effect negative consequences for the individual or those whom they may involve as objects or partners, terms such as "dysfunctional," "maladaptive," "fixated," "compulsive," and "disordered" may apply. The logic of the judgment is consequential: negative results mean the action was negative. In ethical terms, if the "bad" results are present, the action is considered "bad" in itself. This is basic consequentialist ethics. The strength of the consequentialist argument lies in two further determinants: (1) the causal connection

between the behavior and the consequences; and (2) the evaluation of the positive versus negative ratio of the consequences.

Another limitation of the behavior perspective is that while it examines the antecedents and consequences of the behavior, discourse about what the individual does, his or her sexual behavior, is not on the level of the values that are being supported by the norm that is being applied. Thoughtful discussion of norms and laws should drill into the institutional values that gave birth to the norm. This requires, however, another perspective, the fourth and final one, the life story perspective.

In summary of the behavior perspective, the normality of sexual behavior is deceptively simple to determine. Is the sexual behavior prohibited by prevailing institutional norms? If so, it is not normal to choose to commit the behavior. Is the sexual behavior prescribed by prevailing institutional norms? Then the behavior is normal. To omit a prescribed sexual behavior or to commit a prohibited sexual behavior is to incur the judgment of abnormal, illicit, illegal, or unacceptable sexual behavior.

In addition to its concurrence with institutional norms, the behavior perspective can address the question of normality by using a consequentialist ethic. Good results mean good behavior and the converse. The behavior perspective is limited by the historical relativity of institutional norms and its dependence upon a supplemental perspective to examine the institutional values that the norm protects. It is also limited by the weaknesses of a consequentialist ethic. While the behavior perspective is a necessary component in the discussion of the normality of sexual behavior, it requires the addition of the life story perspective for advancing the question of sexual normality.

SEXUAL NORMALITY AND THE LIFE STORY PERSPECTIVE

Enter, finally, the life story perspective. To address the question of the normality of sexual behavior, the life story perspective asks what meaning and values are attributed to sexual behaviors. What is the purpose of sexual intercourse? Why is there sexual pleasure? And ultimately, why is the human person sexual? The questions and therefore the responses are teleological, philosophical, psychological, and, for the religious communities, theological. The terms for "normal" using the life story perspective are those such as "developmental," "adaptive," "natural," "ethical," and "good."

At this point in history, there are as many theoretical systems responding to these questions as there are philosophical and theological traditions. But before any tradition offering responses, we encounter the current challenge to the assumption of philosophical or theological "truth." Some deny its possibility; others hold that truth is objective and absolute (even if not knowable). That debate is epitomized by the fundamental differences between those who have been described as *social constructionists* and those as *essentialists*. The debate between these two camps has been especially rancorous when human sexuality is the topic of discussion (DeLamater & Hyde, 1998).

Social constructionists assert that communities construct meaning out of the social context of the behavior. The central assertion of social constructionists is that "reality is socially constructed by language" (Berger & Luckman, 1966). With the passage of time and tempering in social attitude constructs that had a pejorative connotation transmute into more socially acceptable or neutral words. "Prostitutes" becomes "sex workers." "Perversion" becomes "paraphilia," which then becomes "sexual variations." According to this school of thought, even our understanding of body and gender has been socially constructed (Laquer, 1990). Sexual normality for a specific behavior can and will be constructed by the social communities because normality itself is a social construct that is entirely plastic, entirely relative. Social constructionists freely employ the life story perspective, albeit giving the social community more than the individual, the salient role in constructing meaning.

Essentialists hold that there is a given order in nature that can be discovered by reason and/or, in the religious traditions, revealed by God. The normality of any behavior is whether the behavior is consistent with the order or teleology for which the individual performing the behavior exists and for which the behavior is intended. The essentialist position relies on both philosophy (for the secular humanist and intellectual theist) and theology (for the theists) to address such profound questions as the nature of the human person and the purpose that he or she has in life. Sexual behaviors tend to be judged as having a specific purpose in the history of the human race. For example, the purpose of sexual intercourse has

been seen as intended for procreation and, in recent centuries, also for the expression of love and intimacy. Essentialists posit natural laws or a Natural Law that governs the purposes of all human behavior, the normality—or the morality—of sexual behaviors is not relative. Employing a confident Aristotelian epistemology that says that reality is "out there" and knowable, essentialists assert that normality may be perceived differently by different cultures or in difference epochs, but the normality of all behaviors—including sexual behaviors—can be discovered (not constructed) by the human community.

The debate between the social constructionists and the essentialists has been seen by many as the debate between moral relativists and moral absolutists. For our purposes, it is the debate between the relativity of normality and the absolute fixedness of normality. While this view of the two camps, social constructionists and essentialists, may be stereotypical, it contains more than a grain of accuracy. Both camps when speaking theoretically tend to confirm the stereotype. When the discussion becomes applied to a specific behavior in a specific situation, one witnesses a healthy stretching of the basic assumptions of each school. Social constructionists would by and large reject the forcing of sex upon an unconsenting individual. Essentialists would, by and large, admit a development (therefore a change) of what might be judged as "good" sexual behavior. For example, in the Roman Catholic tradition, engaging in marital intercourse for the purpose of experiencing the pleasure of orgasm is no longer seen as sinful as it was by St. Augustine in the fourth century.

The future of the social constructionist versus essentialist debate about sexual normality may lie therefore, in continued discussion about applied sexuality behavior. At the present, there is, in general, a lack of mutual respect. Progress will be made in reaching a fuller understanding from the life story perspective when each school listens carefully and thoughtfully to the positions of the other. There may be, in the end, no agreement. The assumptions of each school appear to preclude this. But societies will be enlightened by the rationality of both social contructionists and essentialists if each can be heard.

There is one other approach to understanding sexual normality that is an examination of specific behaviors using the life story perspective. The agenda of the Communitarian movement is to elaborate the rights and responsibilities of individuals within their communities. Based on the seminal writings of sociologist Amitai Etzione (1993), Communitarian thought is a reaction to rugged individualism with its stress on the rights of the individual in western culture, typified by the Libertarian movement. The Communitarian mantra is *"rights and responsibilities."* Individuals not only have rights; they also have responsibilities to the communities in which they exist and to the communities which will follow them. The morality, or the normality, of behaviors will be achieved in the successful and proper balancing of individual rights and community responsibilities in human behavior.

In the Communitarian agenda, the entire discussion of the nature and parameters of the rights of individuals and the individual's communitarian responsibilities is applied to specific situations. The foundation of the rights of the individual are examined and the corresponding communitarian responsibilities are acknowledged and justified. There is ground here for both social constructionists and essentialist to contribute to the discussion of rights and responsibilities. The discussion can obviously be about sexual behaviors, about its normality, about the rights of the individual to be sexual and behave sexually. In the Communitarian framework the discussion will be about the responsibilities that the individual has toward the community in which he or she chooses to act sexually. For example, according to Communitarian thought, sexual offenses are likely to be abnormal behaviors not because they break societal laws or taboos, but because they fail to exercise the responsibility that individuals have to honor and respect the physical and psychological boundaries of others. Obviously the philosophical basis of the individual's right to physical and psychological integrity will need to be elaborated in establishing the corresponding responsibility.

In summary of the life story perspective's contribution to an understanding of sexual normality, there is a basic disagreement between those who would argue for the relativity of sexual normality and those who would assert a foundational normality for human sexuality. Between these two basic schools, often referred to as social constructionist and essentialist, there exists a wide chasm in the public debate. An approach which may provide a common ground for the application of sexual behaviors to specific situations is found in the Communitarian movement. Employing Communitarian structure, the public

discussion of the normality of sexual behavior will be had by examining both the individual's rights to be sexual and the responsibility that the individual has to the partner with whom and the community in which his or her sexual behavior occurs.

THE QUESTION OF NORMALITY OF SEXUAL BEHAVIORS

Is then the question of normality of sexual behaviors ever to remain a quest to which there will be no satisfying answer? Returning to the confrontation of Dr. Berlin and the man he was evaluating for a sexual offense, will there ever be common ground for discussion? While complete unanimity may never be achieved—certainly not in the case described—there are steps that can be taken to make the quest more satisfying and more informative for those who are asking such questions.

The disease perspective calls for continued research into the neurological and physiological determinants of sexual behavior. The past two decades of the biological bases of sexual behavior have been productive in animal research. We are beginning to see reflections of this in human sexual research. We look for more findings that are robust and replicated. The dimension perspective requires more valid and reliable measures of sexual behaviors as they are practiced in varied cultures. Normality cannot be addressed in the dimension perspective unless we have valid measurement of the behavior in the population. The behavior perspective challenges researchers in the psychology of human behavior to examine the multiple causes of sexual behavior. What are the causal components, both of ordered sexual behavior and sexual behavior that causes harm to self or other? A growing identification of these factors is contributing to our use of the term "normality" in sexual behaviors.

Lastly, those who would move the discussion of normality into the life story perspective are doing their societies a service if they engage in this discussion of meaning and values using both rational arguments and respectful listening to conflicting opinions. Not to include the disciplines of ethics, philosophy, and theology into the discussion of sexual normality is to reduce the question to skills of the scientific disciplines. Many will be content, even praise that limitation. However, this author believes that the fullest exploration of human sexuality requires not only science, but also wisdom. For this we must turn to our wisdom traditions for assistance. The behavioral and basic sciences must continue their work to help us explain sexual behavior; the wisdom traditions must continue their work to help us understand sexual normality.

CONCLUSION

In summary, each of the four perspectives calls for more disciplined research to respond to the question of normality of sexual behaviors. Each of the four perspectives will potentially deepen the discussion of normality if employed consciously by the discussants. The following chapters in this volume are examples of researchers and clinicians who applied their disciplines to this question as pertaining to sexual offenders. They promise to deepen our understanding and our discussion of sexual normality.

References

American Psychiatric Association. (2000). *Diagnostic and Statistical Manual of Mental Disorders, Fourth Edition*, Text Revision ed. Washington, D C.: American Psychiatric Association.

Berger, P. & Luckman, T. (1966). *The Social Construction of Reality; A Treatise in the Sociology of Knowledge.* Garden City, NY: Doubleday.

Berlin, F. S. (2002). Medical Student Lecture. Lecture by Berlin F. S. John Hopkins University School of Medicine, Baltimore, Maryland. January 11.

DeLamater, J. D. & Hyde, J. S. (1998). Essentialism Versus Social Constructionism in the Study of Human Sexuality. *Journal of Sex Research*, 35(1), 10–18.

Etzioni, A. (1993). *The Spirit of Community: Rights, Responsibilities and the Communitarian Agenda.* New York: Crown.

Fagan, P. J. (2003). *Sexual Disorders: Perspectives on Evaluation and Treatment* Baltimore, MD: Johns Hopkins University Press.

Goodman, A. (1992). "Sexual Addiction: Designation and Treatment," *Journal of Sex and Marital Therapy*, 18(4), 303–314.

Gordis, L. (2000). *Epidemiology, 2nd Edition.* Philadelphia: W.B. Saunders.

Jaspers, K. (1997). *General Psychopathology*, Vol. 1. Baltimore, Maryland: The Johns Hopkins University Press.

Laquer, T. (1990). *Making Sex: Body and Gender from the Greeks to Freud.* Cambridge, MA: Harvard University Press, p. 313.

Laumann, E. O., Gagnon, J. H., Michael, R. T., & Michaels, S. (1994). *The Social Organization of Sexuality: Sexual Practices in the United States.* Chicago, IL: The University of Chicago Press.

McHugh, P. R. & Slavney, P. R. (1998). *The Perspectives in Psychiatry, 2nd.* Baltimore and London: The Johns Hopkins University Press.

Noonan, J. T. (2005). *The Church that Can and Cannot Change: The Development of Catholic Moral Teaching.* Notre Dame, Ind: University of Notre Dame Press.

Chapter 2

Phenomenology of Paraphilia: Lovemap Theory

Gregory K. Lehne

Understanding the psychological experience of individuals who have unusual sexual interests and behavior has fascinated professionals and the public since the first publication, in the last quarter of the nineteenth century, of the twelve editions of *Psychopathia Sexualis* by Krafft-Ebing (1903–1965). Many of his 237 clinical and forensic cases describe individuals with paraphilia. Until the last quarter of the twentieth century, most sexuality that significantly differed from potentially procreative behavior in a marital context was considered sexually disordered. Contemporary diagnostic standards, represented by DSM-IV-TR (APA, 2000), offer a more ambiguous perspective on what is a sexual disorder or paraphilia. The diagnostically specified paraphilias have been defined in terms of their focus on behaviors which are frequently illegal or cause distress, usually for others: exhibitionism and its complements voyeurism and frotteurism; pedophilia, sexual sadism, and its complement sexual masochism; and fetishism and its complement transvestic fetishism. The content of the sexually arousing fantasies or sexual urges is what is considered to make these conditions mental disorders, so they are clinically diagnosed from fantasy rather than behavior (for a more clinical discussion, see Fagan, Lehne, Strand, & Berlin, 2005; Plaut & Lehne, 2000). DSM-IV-TR adds the proviso for diagnosis that the individual is significantly distressed or there is associated impairment in functioning. Traditionally, however, the paraphilias have been conceptualized in terms of their divergence from what was believed to be normative heterosexual sexual interests, and popularly in terms of the bizarreness or kinkiness of their sexual content.

Human sexual interests and practices, however, are now known to be very diverse. Aspects of many types of paraphilic imagery are found in individuals who are not considered to have sexual psychopathology. Sexual looking and showing are commonplace. Touching is the most typical invitatory sexual activity of couples. A sexual interest in children is normative among children. Sadomasochism is a widespread sexually variant play activity among married couples. A very large nonsexual commercial fashion market thrives merchandizing clothing that is similar to fetishistic items.

The Internet has exposed the fact that interest in a variety of sexual content, previously thought of as paraphilias not otherwise specified, may be more widespread than ever imagined. The diversity of paraphilic sexual interests almost defies categorization or even enumeration (see, for example, Francoeur, Cornog, Perper, & Scherzer, 1995; Love, 1992). Alphabetically, it starts with sexual interests in abduction, abuse, accidents (automobile & others); acousticophilia (arousal by sounds); acrophilia (heights); acrotomophilia and apotemnophilia (amputee partner or self); adolescents (ephebophilia); autonepiophilia or infantalism (adult babies); agalmatophilia (statues); age play, agoraphilia (sex in public place); aidoiomania (nymphomania, satyriasis); algolagnia (sadism & masochism); anal fetishism, anasteemaphilia (difference in heights of sex partners); andromimetophilia (attraction to a lady with a penis), animals (zoophilia); anthromorphism (role play as an animal); apodysophilia (appearing naked in public); asphyxiophilia (strangulation, self or other); augmentation (various body parts, including penile vacuum pumps); autoerotic activities beyond enumeration, autofellatio, autogynophilia (self as woman); autonephiophilia (aischrolatreia, love of filth or obscenities); autogonistophilia (being observed in sexual activity); autoassassinatophilia (staging masochistic death of self, complement of lust murder); autofetishism, and there is no end in sight. Being abstinent may not yet be a paraphilia, but asexualization, as for example, castration or becoming a eunuch, may be. Possibly new paraphilias seem to arise frequently, based on the criteria of bizarre sexual content, while other paraphilias, such as a sexual interest in statues, seem to have disappeared (although perhaps the modern equivalent is life-size sex dolls). Clearly we have reached, if not exceeded, the limit in defining paraphilias in terms of the bizarre content of sexual interests.

Defining paraphilias in terms of illegal behavior is societally and temporally limiting. The definitions of mental conditions should not change with national boundaries and historical practices. Defining paraphilia in terms of bizarre sexual content is similarly limiting, particularly when it is limited by professional knowledge about what people actually think about and do sexually. Even the criteria of distress or impairment are inadequate for characterizing paraphilia, now that the Internet has reduced the guilt and isolation of many individuals with paraphilia, so that their sexualities are no longer ego-dystonic.

I propose that the phenomenology of paraphilia is characterized by the *specificity of the sexual content* combined with the *intensity of the sexual arousal/ motivation*. An analogy can be made to the phobias (as McConaghy, 1993, has mentioned) or obsessive-compulsive disorders (see Bradford, 1999). Phobias (like paraphilia) are all highly specific in content, previously enumerated by a long list of Greco-Latinate names that specified the content. Their content may be a type that arouses some fear or anxiety in many people, but also could be individualistic or bizarre (usually related to a childhood origin). Phobias (like paraphilia) are all intensely arousing, which affected individuals recognize as excessive or unreasonable. Phobias are derived from the body's underlying autonomic or vasovagal arousal process experienced as anxiety and associated with a very strong avoidance motivation. For paraphilias, the underlying autonomic arousal is experienced as sexual, and there is a very strong approach motivation. Phobias (like paraphilia) differ in factors that contribute to their etiology, such as childhood experience, physiological, and familial factors.

In the sections that follow, I first discuss normative sexual content in terms of lovemaps. Then I apply the concept of lovemaps to the phenomenology of highly specific paraphilic content. Next I discuss sexual arousal/motivation related to paraphilia. Then I look at the developmental manifestation of paraphilia in terms of origin and expression, followed by the phenomenology of some paraphilia case histories. Finally I discuss the implications of this approach. The approach that I take is developed from my work over the last 25 years with Dr. John Money of the Psychohormonal Research Unit and Dr. Fred Berlin of the Sexual Disorders Clinic, both at the Johns Hopkins University School of Medicine, and the many hundreds of men with paraphilia who shared their stories with me. Please note that I discuss primarily males in this chapter.

LOVEMAPS

Human sexuality is characterized by diversity in the content of sexual urges, fantasies, and behavior.

Human sexuality is thus different from animal sexuality, which is not diverse in any specific species, but instead focuses on an exclusive goal of reproduction. Most animals are hormonal or physiological robots in terms of sexuality, responding to highly specific signals for reproductive breeding. The sexuality of human beings functions for pleasure and bonding, infinitely more frequently than just for reproduction. People, unlike animals, vary greatly in the types of partners they are aroused by and attracted to, and the types of sexual and affectional activities they find arousing and engage in. The diversity of sexuality extends to issues of gender (Roughgarden, 2004).

Dr. John Money (1986, 1999) first proposed the concept of *lovemaps* to describe the diversity of human sexuality and the paraphilias. He defined lovemap as the developmental representation or template in the mind and brain depicting the idealized partner and program of sexuoerotic imagery or behavior (1986, p. 290). Every person has an individualized lovemap which represents the variety of characteristics of partners and activities that are sexually arousing and erotically (in the sense of love) appealing. Money published several lovemap autobiographies of men with paraphilias (Keyes & Money, 1993; Money, Wainwright, & Hingsburger, 1991). Human lovemaps are diverse because people are diverse—there is no one ideal type of partner, sexual behavior is not a standardized ritual, and sexual activity is not limited to one type of act.

The diversity of lovemaps comes from many sources. Some of it may result from genetic, hormonal, or prenatal influences. But the specificity of the partners that are attractive or the many scenarios that are sexually arousing, for example, has to come through the senses—there are no genes or hormones that could determine whether an individual is attracted to people of specific ethnic backgrounds or body types, or personality styles, for example. Thus aspects of lovemap diversity have to come from input through the senses related to experiences that occur during early development and later input or learning from life experiences. For reasons that are not yet understood, certain aspects of sensory input are eroticized and encoded in the lovemap, perhaps because of associations with random or provoked changes in hormonal levels or autonomic arousal. The lovemap cartographic system may operate like a multisensory camera that episodically takes photos of the immediate environment and stores them as depictions of the sexual terrain.

Lovemaps depict a variety of activities and partners that are potentially sexually and erotically exciting for a specific individual. Lovemaps can be thought of like a mental map composed of many different terrains and political/social territories. Some individuals' lovemaps include vast areas, while others are more limited in scope—some people have a world of possibilities while others have a small village of choices to explore.

But the geography of the lovemap is not automatically known to the individual. The individual may not be aware when parts of the lovemap are encoded through development and experience. Individuals learn about their own lovemaps from reflection upon their fantasies, actual experiences, and vicarious experiences (such as reading, looking at pictures, hearing stories). They discover what attracts or arouses them and what does not. Some individuals explore much of the territory of their lovemap, while others are equally content to live only in a small but satisfying part of their lovemap realm. In the end, most people settle down to a limited number of partners and sexual activities. The challenge of relationships is to find a partner and associated erotic and sexual activities that correspond to a highly charged area of your lovemap, while you correspond to reciprocal highly charged parts of your partner's lovemap.

Lovemaps allow for choices about which areas to explore or not explore. Just because an area exists in a lovemap does not mean that an individual must explore it. Generally people explore those parts of their lovemaps that are either more highly sexually/erotically charged or are more socially available (which may also mean more socially acceptable). These areas of an individual's lovemap may be similar or dissimilar, or may conflict. Areas of the lovemap that an individual explores become more familiar, and thus may be more likely to be revisited. In experiencing a familiar area, other associated aspects of the terrain that were not initially important may become more erotically charged with experience. Thus people tend to settle into delimited areas that correspond to their lovemap.

The commonalities of lovemaps are related to the commonalities of human experience. Typical developmental experiences in a shared social environment tend to produce lovemaps with large areas in common. Atypical experiences may contribute to diversity in lovemap content. And then there is a certain random factor. There are two aspects to experience—the experience in reality, and the representation of the experience in the mind and brain. Like all maps, the lovemap is only a depiction that represents or corresponds to reality. Parts of experience that are unfamiliar or not understood may not be accurately represented in the mind's lovemap, while experiences that are associated with different types of arousal may be encoded differently in the brain's lovemap.

In a similar way, the content or territory of the lovemap may have different valences. One is positive or "present" while the other is negative or "absent," or there may be no valence specified. This is like a figure/ground distinction. The figure may define the outline of what is appealing or the ground may define it. For example, a person may be attracted only to people who share their ethnic background (positive), or they may be attracted only to people who do not share their ethnic background (negative), or ethnic background may not matter (no valence). Similarly, lovemap characteristics may apply to the self or to the other, corresponding to a learning process of identification or complementation. The self may be represented in the lovemap with reference to the partner (other) both in terms of erotic attraction as well as sexual activity. This is why many lovemaps and paraphilias have complements.

LOVEMAPS AND PARAPHILIA

Paraphilic lovemaps can be considered vandalized lovemaps (Money & Lamacz, 1989). Instead of the individual developing an extensive lovemap with a diversity of areas to explore, the lovemap territory is very limited. Or the individual may have a more extensive lovemap, but is trapped in repetitively exploring only a very limited and dysfunctional territory.

In their book, *Vandalized Lovemaps*, Money and Lamacz (1989) describe seven cases of paraphilic outcomes in children born with different congenital sexological disorders. The cases include a male with a history of hypothyroidism who developed pedophilia, different types of sadomasochism in males with micropenis or genital ambiguity, masochism in a 46, XY female with the androgen-insensitivity syndrome, and bondage and discipline paraphilias in females with two different syndromes of birth defects of the sex organs. In these cases, congenital factors contributed vulnerability for the development of paraphilia, although the specific contribution varied in the

cases. More important were also socially induced vulnerabilities and experiences that contributed to the specific content of the paraphilia. All these children had problems with stigmatization, and limited participation or negative experiences in sexual rehearsal play. It is not likely a coincidence that the sadomasochistic types of paraphilia were so prevalent in this sample. Difficulties in coping with their anomalies led to difficulties in social learning experiences and identity development. However, there are also many other children with similar sexological disorders who did not develop vandalized lovemaps, although the incidence would seem to be higher in this vulnerable population.

Lovemaps may be vandalized by traumatic experiences. Sometimes these experiences may be sexual victimization. For example, a boy who is sexually abused may develop paraphilic fantasies involving sexual activity with a boy (Dhawan & Marshall, 1996; Hanson & Slater, 1988). Nonsexual punishments or humiliations may have inadvertent sexual consequences for lovemap development. For example, paraphilic arousal associated with spanking may be more prevalent in boys who were spanked with a paddle (and perhaps inadvertently became sexually aroused during the experience). Similarly, being punished or embarrassed by being cross-dressed as a young boy may lead to some boys eroticizing the experience, which later is expressed as transvestism. Medical procedures or administration of enemas may lead to paraphilic eroticization of those procedures in lovemap development. Punishing children unfairly for sexual rehearsal play experiences may contribute to heightened eroticization of those activities in lovemaps.

Several principles seem to be operating for the creation of vandalized lovemaps. First, the individual may have some vulnerability, which might not be associated with dysfunction or hyperfunction in the sexual system but could instead be developmental, cognitive, or brain based. For example, individuals with brain dysfunction including brain damage seem more likely to manifest paraphilias (Lehne, 1986; Mendez, Chow, Ringman, Twitchell, & Hinkin, 2000; Simpson, Blazcynski, & Hodgkinson, 1999). Second, there may be experiences typically before the age of 8 that involve potential sexual content associated with high autonomic or sexual arousal (Money, 1999, pp. 94–99). The sexual arousal may be a result of direct sexual stimulation, as in juvenile sexual experiences which might be consensual with peers or associated with molestation, or force. Or the sexual stimulation may occur as a result of physical or genital stimulation, for example during a physical activity or medical procedure. Or the sexual stimulation may occur spontaneously associated with other stimuli, perhaps related to testosterone surges or just episodes of erection which young boys experience. Nonsexual autonomic arousal may also play a role, such as that which occurs during some situations of punishment or humiliation. Sometimes the experience may be something which is not understood, and thus stored in a literal way in memory, which somehow becomes associated with other sexual imagery. Third, other areas of the lovemap may not be as well elaborated. This may be because the higher arousal associated with the potentially paraphilic content diverts formative energy from the other areas, or distracts from exploring them. Thus the elaborated paraphilic area becomes expanded and explored, while other potential areas are never developed. The result can be an area of atypical sexual imagery that is associated with a large amount of sexual arousal.

Individuals can have areas of their lovemaps that they never discover, explore, or express in fantasy or behavior. Thus a vandalized lovemap also requires other experiences which lead to its recognition and possible expression. Little is known about these releaser factors, but some individuals do report that awareness of the paraphilic imagery emerged full-blown in fantasy (or in rarer cases behavior), or was triggered by an actual experience or a vicarious experience through reading or viewing media including pornography. In other cases, a paraphilic lovemap may not emerge until late in life, perhaps associated with the physical deterioration of the brain.

Sexual Arousal/Motivation of Paraphilia

Paraphilias are typically associated with high levels of sexual arousal or motivation. It is not unusual for some men with a paraphilia to report long periods of hypersexuality, to the extent that some of them maintain erections for hours and may masturbate to orgasm six or eight times a day or be constantly preoccupied with paraphilic fantasy and imagery. There is an obsessional aspect to paraphilic imagery that is even more obsessive than typical sexual and falling-in-love imagery, and less time limited. This may be associated with high levels of testosterone in some

cases, but whether this is a cause of the high sexual arousal or an effect has not been determined. But in most cases, the levels of testosterone are not elevated.

In some cases, the acting-out of a paraphilia is also associated with high levels of autonomic arousal, more than what is typically associated with sexual activity. Some men report sweating profusely or stomach upset. Fugue-like states are common, where extraneous stimuli are blocked by the extreme focus on the paraphilic scenario, and behavior seems almost automatic (like a psychomotor fugue). Tunneling in vision and selective hearing is often reported. Thus there can be a dissociative aspect to paraphilic enactment.

While acting-out a paraphilia may include an elaborate and well-practiced ritual, younger men report highly specific fantasies but less commonly report planning or practicing this behavior. Instead they describe their behavior unfolding like a chain of behaviors triggered by an external stimulus or an internal drive state, rather than consciously motivated or determined. Men frequently talk about the paraphilia controlling them rather than them controlling the paraphilia. Some talk about behavioral enactment or orgasm primarily as a way to get relief from the sexual pressure or urge rather than as an achievement of a positive goal, as would be the case for more typical sexual activity.

It is tempting to use a hydraulic model to explain this high energy force of arousal or motivation. If a typical lovemap includes a larger territory to explore and act upon in sexual situations, like water flowing over a broad plateau, the energy is spread out and there are many options for run off. However, if the territory is very limited, like water flowing through a small valley, the force of the sexual energy is much greater.

Developmental Phenomenology of Paraphilia

Individuals with paraphilias often report developmental vulnerabilities and early experiences that were eroticized and seem to be closely related to the content of the paraphilic imagery or fantasy. Once established, the paraphilic lovemap may lay dormant until it is energized by the hormones of puberty. In retrospect, some individuals with paraphilia report a special fascination with content related to the paraphilia in childhood, although this was not recognized as sexual. For example, men with a paraphilia involving bondage might recall being particularly interested in playing games such as cowboys and Indians as children, where they or another child might be tied to a tree. In another case, the mother of a man with a shoe fetish recalled that as a child he would hide under the card table when her friends would come for bridge games and seemed fascinated by their shoes. Of course this led to an uproar, as the women assumed he was looking up their skirts, and he was traumatically banished. A transvestite might recall some experiences cross-dressing as a child, and perhaps even a special feeling associated with those activities. In most cases, these experiences were not interpreted as being sexual, or sometimes not even unusual or significant. However, many men with paraphilias recall no such childhood experiences. Others can recall one significant experience which may be related to the origin of the paraphilia, but no other subsequent experiences until adolescence.

After puberty, the paraphilic lovemap becomes progressively characterized by obsessional thoughts and fantasies. In many cases, these may present themselves uninvited and unwanted to the individual. The individual may struggle to reduce or eliminate this imagery, or there may be hypersexual masturbation or associated sexual behavior. There is a questioning and eventually realization that the individual may not be like others in his private sexual thoughts or interests.

Sexual thoughts and fantasies may soon lead to compulsive acting-out of sexual behavior. Control of sexual behavior becomes even more difficult if the lovemap does not include many nonparaphilic options. The paraphilic imagery and behavior by its nature is very ritualistic and limited. It may be expressed by obsessive collecting of items associated with the paraphilia, including viewing and collecting pornography.

The course of adolescent and young adult development may become altered depending upon the nature of the paraphilic interests (see Lehne, 1990). There may be reduced sexual motivation to pursue more socially conventional paths of heterosexual or homosexual relationships. Or there may be increased pursuit of more conventional erotic and sexual activities in an attempt to overcome the paraphilic interests. The individual may find that he has to rely upon the paraphilic imagery or practices for sexual arousal or ejaculation, and may experience sexual dysfunction when he does not.

The paraphilic lovemap content has to be integrated into the self-concept. How this occurs depends greatly on the specific paraphilia. Awareness of a primary sexual interest in boys, for example, may not be apparent until the individual is out of adolescence. Then as the individual develops a lifestyle that allows more contact with boys, he is not involved in activities with adults who might be potential sexual partners or at least help broaden his interests in typical adult activities. As he realizes the stigmatized nature of his sexual interest, he may develop a negative self-concept and a secretive style to avoid getting into trouble. He begins to develop cognitive distortions and justifications of his behavior, which may further increase his social alienation or feelings of being different. A man with a lovemap involving cross-dressing might experience confusion about gender identity or sexual orientation, or unusual social beliefs about clothing or the importance of men expressing their feminine side. An exhibitionist with a history of frequent arrests but otherwise no criminal interests may find himself a social outcast unable to pursue his otherwise conventional social and work interests.

The paraphilia interferes with pair bonding, since the process of sexual arousal may be focused on something other than an available partner. The paraphilic sexual fantasy comes between the man and his partner. Sex with a partner is much less exciting than paraphilic sexual activities. The man is likely to continue to explore paraphilic sexual outlets, which diverts sexual energy away from a relationship. Aspects of his life become secretive, and he becomes more emotionally walled off from a partner. A relationship is likely to become more based on companionship rather than erotically bonded. There may not even be sufficient nonparaphilic territory in the lovemap to lead to attempts to find a romantic or sexual partner.

In the end, depending upon the specific paraphilia, there may be characteristic distortions in the path of typical psychosocial development. Instead there is development of a lifestyle that centers around the paraphilia. More typical patterns of heterosexual or homosexual relationships and lifestyles may be eschewed in favor of lifestyles that support the justification and expression of the paraphilia.

Multiplex Paraphilia

When paraphilias are defined according to a single behavioral focus (such as DSM-IV-TR criteria), an individual may be diagnosed with several different paraphilias. When paraphilias are conceptualized in terms of lovemaps, all these multiple paraphilias may be seen to be manifestations of one multiplex paraphilia that is the embodiment of an earlier life experience which was sexually imprinted in the lovemap. A man with a multiplex paraphilia who was followed for more than 40 years provides an illustrative case example of the phenomenology of paraphilia (Lehne & Money, 2000, 2003). The history is particularly interesting because much of it was recorded prospectively instead of retrospectively.

Jack was punished for rowdy behavior in the first grade by being made to wear a girl's dress and stand in the corner; he was humiliated by the other children. At age 7, when he was still frequently wetting the bed, his mother gave him a similar corrective punishment of dressing him in a diaper and girl's skirt and parading him around their housing project telling him, "If you are going to act like a sissy baby, you are going to be treated like one." When Jack was 9, his mother once used him as a dressmaker dummy, forcing him to wear a skirt while she hemmed it. Although he protested that he was embarrassed, he found that he enjoyed this experience. He began secretly wearing his mother's skirts when he had a chance, and although prepubescent, he reported that he had an erection and a good sexual feeling at those times.

Jack's social presentation was very macho, and he had extensive heterosexual experience. He cross-dressed at times for masturbation (transvestic fetishism), and at other times for relaxation, except while he was in the Army. He married soon after his discharge. He had an active sexual relationship with his wife, but often would also have from two to eight orgasms a day through masturbation. Although he had not intended to resume cross-dressing after his marriage, he had an increasing "urgency" to wear women's clothing. Soon Jack was involved secretly with transvestite groups and writing TV erotic stories for publication. His wife was upset by his cross-dressing, and said that she could tell from his demeanor when he had done it while she was gone. She also said that she could tell when he had cross-dressing fantasies during sexual relations, because intercourse was like he was masturbating in her vagina.

When his son was 6 years old, Jack started playing "TV games" with him. He cross-dressed his son in girl's clothes and at some of those times he sexually aroused the boy (pedophilia). This led to his treatment

with Depo-Provera, and all sexual activity with his son stopped and his cross-dressing stopped. Jack had long periods of time without cross-dressing after he stopped the Depo-Provera, and also had episodes of relapses into cross-dressing. He never engaged in any other sexual activities with children.

In his forties, Jack had stopped cross-dressing for years, but appeared to have developed a new sexual preoccupation with being an adult baby (infantilism). Messy play with diapers, urination and defecation, was part of his sexual scenario (urophilia & coprophilia), which was not associated with erection or ejaculation. However, he would recall his behavior and write stories about it, which was accompanied by masturbation. This remained his primary sexual interest for the next 20 years, although he also continued to have a regular sexual relationship with his wife.

Using traditional diagnostic criteria, Jack would be diagnosed at different times in his life as having the five paraphilias of transvestic fetishism, pedophilia, infantilism, urophilia, and coprophilia. However, all of these manifestations of paraphilias can be thought of as one multiplex paraphilia related to his experience at age 6 of being dressed in a diaper and skirt as a punishment for bedwetting. At different times in his life he sexually enacted different parts of this multiplex paraphilic scenario that was most likely, sexually imprinted at the time of his juvenile punishment.

There is a complementarity in Jack's multiplex paraphilia. The core experience is being cross-dressed (as a girl and a baby) when he was a 6-year-old boy. Part of the paraphilic enactment involved cross-dressing himself and also being a baby himself. But the complementary enactment of this paraphilia was cross-dressing his son when he was 6, about the same age as Jack's critical experience. Thus multiple perspectives of the same experience may be literally imprinted as the paraphilia.

Complementary Paraphilias: Sadomasochism

The story of Ron is reported in his lovemap autobiography called *The Armed Robbery Orgasm* (Keyes & Money, 1993). His story became notorious when he committed a series of 20 armed robberies over a 6-week period, with no prior criminal history. He used an insanity defense that he was a sexual masochist and his dominatrix girlfriend ordered him to commit the robberies as part of their sexual activities.

This defense based on paraphilia (and bipolar disorder) was not successful.

Ron's parents separated when he was 5 years old. However, his father continued to return to the house for visits until he was age 9. During those visits his father would administer unjustified beatings with a belt on the children's bare buttocks, according to the order of his mother who said the children had to be punished for misbehavior. At about the age of 8 or 9, Ron experienced an erection during a beating, which shocked his father. His mother continued to spank him into his teens, and he would have erections during many of those times from age 12 on. It is possible that his father was a masochist and his mother was a sadist.

When Ron began to masturbate, he would spank himself to achieve erection and orgasm. His sexual fantasies were of women dominating him in various ways, and punishing him especially by spanking for his misbehavior. He did not have fantasies of romantic or affectionate relationships with women. His sexual outlet in fantasy, and later usually in reality, was self-masturbation rather than intercourse or other sexual interactions. Ron did briefly marry, but could only become aroused for intercourse by having fantasies of being dominated and punished by women. He never had a love affair, but has had obsessional relationships with prostitutes, who would dominate him.

Ron always had a very high degree of sexual arousal and obsession with masochistic fantasies. When in a paraphilic state, he could continuously masturbate for up to 10 to 12 hours with a constant erection, ejaculating up to 12 separate times in a day. Although he could be highly successful in his work as a salesman, he was never able to accumulate money or be consistently successful because of the time and money he spent seeking out dominatrix prostitutes.

He met a stripper in a bar, on the Block in Baltimore, and dominating men seemed to be her sexual interest, not just her act. Physically she resembled his mother. He did not talk with her at their initial meeting, but he sexually fantasized about her continuously for about 8 hours afterwards. They commenced a weekly paid sexual relationship, where she dominated him and punished him, but there was no genital sexual contact for the first 6 months. He would masturbate thinking about their encounters for 10 to 12 hours later. Then he persuaded her to move in with him, and they were able to engage in intercourse for about a month until they both needed to resume their sadomasochistic relationship for sexual arousal. She ordered him to do an armed robbery with her pistol, then they would use the money to buy lingerie and an expensive dinner. They would spend 12 or more hours in a sexual episode, describing the robbery and punishing him for his bad behavior. He would have a constant erection from the time they set out to do the robbery and frequent ejaculations, and she would also be very sexually turned on and orgasmic. They did this several times a week for more than a month.

Feeling totally out of control, Ron finally told her that she had to move out. She then turned him in to the police, and later she testified against him for his final punishment of several concurrent 10-year sentences of incarceration.

This is an example of two complementary paraphilias in sexual partners, a paraphilic *folie a deaux*. Complementary matching of paraphilias between two partners is more likely to occur for sadism and masochism than any other paraphilia. It is also more likely to occur for same-sex couples than for opposite-sex couples. However, although Ron and his dominatrix partner had an extremely strong bond based on shared complementary sexual fantasies, the couple was not erotically bonded—they were bonded by sex activity, not sexual love. The intensity of the paraphilic sexuality was too strong for either partner, and their relationship exploded from the intensity.

A number of paraphilias are complements of each other, and some may coexist within the same person. Sadism and masochism occur together so frequently that they are often lumped together as sadomasochism. The roles of victim and perpetrator can be switched in sexual fantasies and behaviors. Even Ron and his partner in crime occasionally switched roles in their later sexual play. Fetishism and transvestic fetishism can be complimentary. In these cases, the fetishistic items may be erotic on the self (transvestic) and also erotic off the self (as objects) or on the other.

EXHIBITIONISM AND VOYEURISM

Exhibitionism (showing) and voyeurism (looking) are complementary in the sense that they are different sides of the same coin related to the forbidden or shock value of sexual nudity, but they do not usually coexist within the same person. They do not flourish in situations where nudity is expected instead of prohibited, like nudist camps or nude beaches. The acceptance of nudity among people of the same sex generally means that exhibitionists typically are heterosexual. Exhibitionism usually focuses on the response of the viewer, be it surprise, or disgust, or shock, or interest. Each exhibitionist is usually looking for one particular type of reaction, and is not satisfied with other types of reactions. In this sense exhibitionism shares a commonality with obscene telephone calls, where the reaction of the caller is tantamount for sexual excitement. In rare cases, exhibitionists show photos of their penis to elicit a response from a targeted female. Thus what is sexually arousing for exhibitionists is the response of the target, not the act of exposing. In this sense it is not the compliment of voyeurism, where the turn on is seeing what you are not supposed to see, without being seen so there is no response from the target.

For voyeurism, the looking must be illicit, forbidden, for it to be exciting. In this sense looking at pornography is not characteristic of voyeurism, because pornography is a sexual media made to be seen. But looking at webcams or secret photographs (i.e., up-skirting, down-blousing, bathroom shots) of unsuspecting women may be voyeuristic. Since this is a prevalent heterosexual male interest, we can see how conventional sexual lovemaps begin to shade into paraphilic lovemaps in content. What is missing is the ritualistic, repetitive driving quality of the motivation that is characteristic of paraphilia.

INTERNET, LOVEMAPS, AND PARAPHILIA

The Internet offers a lovemap library that illustrates both the diversity of human sexuality and the specificity of paraphilic sexuality. The Internet has quickly become a primary source of sex education for individuals to learn about their lovemaps. Individuals can check out stories, photographs and videos to learn about what turns them on and what does not. The range of content is staggering.

One commercial website that primarily sells mainstream adult DVDs offers more than 500 keyword descriptor terms for heterosexual DVDs and more than 250 for gay DVDs. The descriptors specify the characteristics of the people, the sexual activities, and the settings and themes. Potential buyers can search for DVDs using any term(s) they choose. The site will also suggest related DVDs purchased by other customers who bought the DVD under consideration for purchase. The range of choices reflects the diversity of normative human sexuality—this type of site, selling mass market DVDs, is not catering to highly specialized or potentially illegal sexual interests. Individuals tend to explore a limited number of fantasy themes present in their own lovemaps. Customers must purchase a DVD to see the content, so customers tend to buy what they know they like. This allows the individuals to explore in depth a relatively delimitated area of their lovemaps. In the process of exploration, this area of the lovemap may become more highly erotically charged. However, any specific item of pornography tends to lose its highly arousing erotic charge after repeated viewing. So the suggestion of other DVDs, based not on keywords but on other customers' purchasing patterns, allows customers to explore possibly related areas of their lovemaps which they might not have explored before.

Individuals do not develop new sexual interests simply as a result of being exposed to pornography with a content that is new to them. They become interested and aroused primarily by sexual content that is already represented in their lovemaps. However, in some cases they may not be aware of all of the types of content in their lovemaps. Exciting new content has to be related to a territory previously delineated in their lovemaps, but perhaps not explored. Exploration creates the excitement of a first-time visit, and with familiarity there may be some expansion of the sexual content which they find arousing. If something is absolutely not present in the lovemap of an individual, it may be potentially interesting to look at but will not be revisited. Or it may not be appealing, or even be disgusting and avoided.

However, certain types of lovemap content commonly go together. For example, there are certain characteristics of men or women that are more commonly associated with certain themes and certain sexual activities. For example, sexual domination is more often associated with an older partner, certain activities like spanking, and certain outfits like leather, and perhaps specific settings. Other content may not be included or excluded, and sometimes even basic sex acts like intercourse or acts of affection like kissing are not included. The practiced sex act of the viewer is typically masturbation. So the types of lovemap content that are explored and which commonly go together in conjunction with sexual arousal and orgasm may become associated in the lovemap. Thus a person may initially explore a lovemap area for the mountain scenery and end up developing an associated love of the cuisine. In this sense exploration of a lovemap may change the terrain of the lovemap, as a person may come to eroticize sexual content which could be associated with the lovemap territory but was not initially eroticized. This eroticization can become paraphilic.

Viewing sexual depictions of children is one dangerous example of developing somewhat paraphilic interests. Since all adults were once children, they may have represented in their brains affectionate and erotic imagery of children. Many people still have imagery in their lovemaps, infrequently reviewed, of a boy or girl who was their first love when they were age 8 to 12. Perhaps they were frustrated or limited in their opportunities for adolescent exploration of sexuality or relationships. In coming across child pornography on the Internet, they may become interested in seeing if the imagery is sexually arousing for them. Or they may become interested in looking at what they feel that they missed out on, or revisiting experiences that they found highly erotic in childhood. Thus an individual who may not be aware of pedophilic sexual interests may become caught up in looking at child pornography on the Internet. This exploration, while initially not paraphilic, can lead to dangerous (and illegal) developments in lovemap exploration.

The development of a long-term bonded sexual relationship can illustrate this process of lovemap elaboration in a positive sense. Erotically and sexually bonded love relationships may indeed be a specific, normative case of paraphilia. Individuals are initially attracted to each other because of certain characteristics in their lovemaps. In the course of their relationship, other associated characteristics of the partner and the activities they engage in together become more eroticized. The partners themselves change over time, and their new characteristics also may become eroticized (or at least less de-eroticized than they may have been). For example, with the aging of partners their more mature physical characteristics may become more sexualized in their lovemaps. A tragic situation is where the lovemap does not change, and the sexual relationship stops at a certain point or the partner is abandoned for a perhaps younger or different looking partner who better matches the characteristics specified in the lovemap. This is always the case with paraphilic lovemaps, because they are highly resistant to change.

But when lovemaps are explored not with a partner but on the Internet, the situation is potentially different. While the Internet offers sexual diversity as a learning choice, it also offers specificity as an alternative. Thus a person can explore hundreds of variant scenarios, or hundreds of variants of one sexual scenario. A lovemap becomes paraphilic when the content that is explored as the primary source of arousal is highly limited and specific and also highly sexually charged or motivated. Because of the massive amount of highly specific sexual content available on the Internet, some individuals focus all of their sexual energy on increasingly small amounts of territory. It may be that this is the only territory available to them as a product of their physiological status and life history. Or it may be that this is the only territory they choose to explore, and which therefore becomes highly erotically charged for them. While the Internet does make available access to partners for sexual exploration, the primary sexual activity associated with pornography on the Internet is masturbation. On the Internet, the individual can always find more of the same for masturbation. Some individuals develop sexual arousal patterns that function only for masturbation, and do not allow a role for a partner in sexual activity, which could become characteristic of a paraphilia.

The activity of looking at pornography or sexual images and stories on the Internet itself can become paraphilic for some individuals. They are able to tailor the sexual content they look at to their own highly specific interests. In some cases these specific interests are themes—like the forbidden or the desire to see something new. They go into trance-like states, transfixed by the multitude of images and losing track of time and their surroundings. They become obsessed with their sexual looking. Their time on the Internet becomes so compulsive that it crowds out other activities from their lives, limiting their sleep, interfering with work. They collect and catalogue huge inventories of images. Masturbation to Internet imagery diverts their sexual energy away from sexual relations with a partner, or seeking to find a partner. It interferes with pair-bonding and relationships.

Individuals with paraphilia are often drawn to the Internet. Much truly paraphilic imagery cannot be consistently expressed in reality. It is best represented in fantasy, in the same way that pictures or movies of beautiful vacation places are often more attractive than the reality. The Internet offers both breadth and depth of paraphilic depictions. It also offers contact with other individuals who share aspects of their paraphilic interests, regardless of how bizarre or unusual or specific. Newsgroups, with paraphilic focus, offer an opportunity to exchange information, imagery, and perhaps even meet others with the same interest. Usually when people share a paraphilic interest they are more like friends with an interest in common, rather than people who are interested in each other as sexual or erotic partners. These Internet contacts encourage individuals to define their paraphilic interests as being acceptable, to at least some social group. Ego-dystonic paraphilias may thus become ego-syntonic.

Many paraphilias are better expressed on the Internet than in reality. For example, consider pedophilia. Pedophiles are typically interested in a highly specific age, sex, and type of child. In reality it can be difficult to develop a connection with such a child. The child may be an object of sexual fantasizing. But actual sexual activity with a child is both wrong and illegal. Furthermore, the child is unlikely to have any reciprocal sexual interest or engage in any type of satisfying sexual behavior with the paraphilic adult. Even if all these obstacles are overcome, the child will soon age out of desirability. Many pedophiles do not even have sexual fantasies of a mutual sexual activity with a child that would bring the pedophile to orgasm. Their fantasies are more akin to masturbating themselves to some recalled or viewed image of the child. So child pornography is actually a more viable and reliable sexual outlet than involvement with children. It allows pedophiles to masturbate to a depiction preserved in time of their idealized imagery. Therefore, many pedophiles become obsessive consumers and collectors of child pornography, which is primarily available through the Internet.

PEDOPHILIA

Pedophilia embodies the complexities of lovemaps and paraphilia. To some extent, all individuals have an erotic and sexual attraction to children previously encoded in their lovemaps. Because of the developmental nature of human sexuality, when individuals are young and in association with other youth, there are sexual and romantic attractions. These attractions are preserved in the lovemap, although they may not be often reviewed or rehearsed years later for masturbation. Similarly, most youth do not have erotic images of significantly older people in their lovemaps. But as they get older, their progressive experiences eroticize more aspects of people their age and older. They may or may not find their attraction to younger people waning. Also societies tend to eroticize certain ages as an ideal, so there is additional input into the lovemap that might, for example, make 25-year-olds appear attractive to 50-year-old men, although they would not find 15-year-olds attractive. At the same time, they now find 50-year-old women attractive as a result of progressive erotic experience, although they might not have found them sexually appealing when they were 15 or 25 years old (or perhaps they did). The presence of residual imagery in the lovemap, even if it remains in areas not explored since youth, is what makes some men vulnerable to sexual involvement with youth in certain situations even though they may not have a paraphilia of pedophilia or ephebophilia. For example, a man might have fallen in love with his wife when she was 16 and he was 18. Many years later he may experience a revitalization of that part of his lovemap in a situation involving a daughter or granddaughter who bears a resemblance to what he found attractive so many years ago in his young wife.

There are two general types of pedophilic lovemaps. One type is most frequently encountered as "boylovers," where the primary pedophilic lovemap specifies the age range and types of boys that the man finds erotically appealing, in the sense of falling in love with them. The pedophile loves the specific qualities of boys (often including their smell), and sexual activities may not be so important. What is important is spending time with boys, almost in the role of another boy, and taking shared pleasure in boy things. This lovemap may correspond to the lovemap the man had at the time he was a boy, and it never changed or was elaborated as he grew up. If those activities include boy-types of sexuality such as show-me play or masturbation, then sexual arousal and ejaculation with boys may also be included in the lovemap of their interactions with boys. These lovemaps focus on developing a relationship with a specific boy or group of boys. Boylovers often do not have any other type of partner that they can fall in love with, and thus do not have a romantic or sexual interest in adults of either sex. For many of this type of boylover, their only sexual outlet is masturbation in private to child pornography or recall of their nonsexual experience. The depiction of boys in erotica may emphasize their physical qualities, often with more focus on the face and involvement in boyish activities rather than showing overt sexual activity with another person. Their sex drive may be low although their obsession in being with boys is high, so these are paraphilias in consideration of the fact that their lovemap is so highly specific in specifying the type of partner for bonding.

Another type of pedophilic lovemap is more specifically sexual, in terms of having a highly specific sexual content and a high intensity of sex drive. This type of pedophilic lovemap may be related to childhood traumatization. Sometimes the imagery incorporates themes of punishment, humiliation, or shame. Sexual activity rather than a relationship with a boy is the focus, and thus the boy can be a stranger. This type of pedophile's interest in child pornography may include depictions of boys in sexual situations or interpersonal sexual activity.

Men whose lovemaps primarily focus on teenagers (ephebophilia) are similar, but some may also have more potential sexual interest in adults. Men whose lovemaps focus on girls are also more likely to have potential sexual interest in adult women.

LOVEMAP PHENOMENOLOGY AND DIAGNOSIS OF SEX OFFENDERS

Lovemap phenomenology is a theoretical approach to describe and explain diversity in the content of human erotosexuality, not to diagnose pathology. Sex offenders engage in illegal sexual activity for a variety of reasons, some of which may be elucidated in the process of differential diagnosis (see, for example, Berlin et al., 1997). The diagnosis of paraphilia may be related to sex offending behavior in many repeat or incarcerated sex offenders, but perhaps not many more than a simple majority depending upon the sample and diagnostic criteria (see, for example, McElroy et al., 1999). Many sex offenses are committed by men who have no sexual diagnosis, and do not have a diagnosis of a major mental illness. Situational factors, personality disorders, such as antisocial personality disorder, and alcohol and substance intoxication also play a large role in sex offending.

Although paraphilias are diagnosed in terms of the content of sexual desire, the reason they contribute to sex offenses is usually because of the intensity of the sexual urges which the affected person cannot or does not control. Individuals with paraphilias may have the largest number of different victims or offenses, but they may not commit the majority of many types of sex offenses. For example, pedophiles are likely to have more child victims per offender, but most sex offenses involving children are not perpetrated by pedophiles. Similarly, paraphilic rapists (who are serial rapists) have the largest number of different victims per offender, but most rapes are not committed by serial rapists. What a diagnosis of paraphilia influences is the likelihood of reoffending. For example, a pedophile is more likely to engage in additional offenses in the future than a nonpedophilic child sex offender, such as an incest offender (Lehne, 1994).

In a similar vein, there are individuals who repeat their inappropriate sexual behavior because they have the high level of sex drive characteristic of paraphilias, although they do not have the distinctively unusual content of sexual interests which are often used to define the paraphilias. Kafka and Hennen (1999) refer to these as paraphilia-related disorders.

The phenomenology of lovemaps provides an additional approach to understanding the sex offenses of nonparaphilic sex offenders. People sometimes engage in exploratory sexual behavior to learn about their own lovemaps, which can particularly be a factor in adolescent sex offending. Otherwise, people usually do not engage in sexual behavior that is not somehow related to their lovemap. What an understanding of lovemaps contributes in the assessment of offenders is what the related content of sexual behavior might be, and what other options there are for sexual behavior.

CONCLUSION

Every person has a highly individualized lovemap that represents the variety of characteristics of partners and activities that are sexually arousing and erotically (in the sense of love) appealing. Lovemaps are diverse because human sexuality is the diverse product of physiological and life history events. Individuals spend their lives learning about and exploring their lovemaps, sometimes elaborating their geography while at other times living in a small territory. Lovemap theory provides a way for thinking about the content and approach motivation of human sexuality and paraphilic sexual disorders. This can be analogous to the way anxiety theory relates to the content and process of human avoidance behavior and phobias.

Sex offenses can be related to the exploration or expression of part of the content of an individual's lovemap. Paraphilias are specific types of vandalized lovemaps characterized by very high specificity of sexual content and high sexual drive or motivation. Paraphilias can be mental disorders which may or may not be related to sex offenses, although the historically named and popularized paraphilias tended to be associated with sex offenses.

References

American Psychiatric Association. (2000). *Diagnostic and statistical manual of mental disorders, 4th (text revision) Edition*. Washington, D.C.: American Psychiatric Association.

Berlin, F. S., Lehne, G., Malin, H. M., Hunt, W. P., Thomas, K. & Furmaneck, J. (1997). The eroticized violent crime: A psychiatric perspective with six clinical examples. *Sexual Addiction & Compulsivity*, 4(1), 9–31.

Bradford, J. M. (1999). The paraphilias, obsessive compulsive spectrum disorder and the treatment of sexually deviant behaviour. *Psychiatric Quarterly*, 70, 209–219.

Dhawan, S. & Marshall, W. L. (1996). Sexual abuse histories of sexual offenders. *Sexual Abuse*, 8, 7–15.

Fagan, P. J., Lehne, G., Strand, J. G. & Berlin, F. (2005). Paraphilias. In Gabbard, G. O., Beck, J. S. & Holmes, J (Eds.), *Oxford textbook of psychotherapy*, (pp. 215–227). Oxford: Oxford University Press.

Francoeur, R. T., Cornog, M., Perper, T. & Scherzer, N. A. (1995). *The complete dictionary of sexology*. NY: Continuum.

Hanson, R. K. & Slater, S. (1988). Sexual victimization in the history of child sexual abusers: A review. *Annals of Sex Research*, 1, 485–499.

Kafka, M. & Hennen, J. (1999). The paraphilia-related disorders: An empirical investigation of nonparaphilic hypersexuality disorders in outpatient males. *Journal of Sex & Marital Therapy*, 25, 305–319.

Keyes, R. & Money, J. (1993). *The armed robbery orgasm: A lovemap autobiography of masochism*. Buffalo, NY: Prometheus Books.

Krafft-Ebing, R. von (1903/1965). *Psychopathia sexualis* (12th Edition, transl: F. Klaf). NY: Bell Publishing Company.

Lehne, G. (1986). Brain damage and paraphilia: Treated with medroxyprogesterone acetate. *Sexuality and Disability*, 7(3/4), 145–158.

Lehne, G. (1990). Adolescent paraphilias. In Perry, M. E. (Ed.), *Handbook of sexology: Childhood and adolescent sexology*, Vol. vii, (pp. 381–394). Amsterdam: Elsevier.

Lehne, G. (1994). Case management and prognosis of the sex offender. In Krivacska, J. & Money, J. (Eds.), *Handbook of forensic sexology*, (pp. 348–363). NY: Prometheus Books.

Lehne, G. & Money, J. (2000). The first case of paraphilia treated with Depo-Provera: 40-year outcome. *Journal of Sex Education and Therapy*, 25(4), 213–220.

Lehne, G. & Money, J. (2003). Multiplex versus multiple taxonomy of paraphilia: Case example. *Sexual Abuse*, 15(1), 61–72.

Love, B. (1992). *Encyclopedia of unusual sex practices*. NY: Barricade Books.

McConaghy, N. (1993). *Sexual behavior: Problems and management*. NY: Plenum.

McElroy, S., Soutullo, C., Taylor, P., Nelson, E., Beckman, D., Brusman, L., et al. (1999). Psychiatric features of 36 men convicted of sexual offenses. *Journal of Clinical Psychiatry*, 60(6), 414–420.

Mendez, M. F., Chow, T., Ringman, J., Twitchell, G., & Hinkin, C. H. (2000). Pedophilia and temporal lobe disturbance. *Journal of Neuropsychiatry and Clinical Neurosciences*, 12, 71–76.

Money, J. (1986). *Lovemaps: Clinical concepts of sexual/erotic health and pathology, paraphilia, and gender transposition in childhood, adolescence, and maturity*. NY: Irvington Publishers.

Money, J. (1999). *The lovemap guidebook: A definitive statement*. NY: Continuum.

Money, J. & Lamacz, M. (1989). *Vandalized lovemaps*. Buffalo, NY: Prometheus Books.

Money, J., Wainwright, G., & Hingsburger, D. (1991). *The breathless orgasm: A lovemap biography of asphyxiophilia*. Buffalo, NY: Prometheus Books.

Plaut, S. M. & Lehne, G. (2000). Sexual dysfunction, gender identity disorders & paraphilias. In Goldman, H. H. (Ed.), *Review of general psychiatry, 5th Edition*, (pp. 354–376). Norwalk, TT: Appleton & Lange.

Roughgarden, J. (2004). *Evolution's rainbow: Diversity, gender, and sexuality in nature and people*. Berkeley, CA: University of California Press.

Simpson, G., Blazcynski, A. & Hodgkinson, A. (1999). Sex offending as a psychosocial sequela of traumatic brain injury. *Journal of Head Trauma Rehabilitation*, 14, 567–580.

Part II

Neurobiology/Neuropsychology

Chapter 3

Neuropsychological Findings in Sex Offenders

Ron Langevin

This chapter explores the brain structures and neuropsychological dysfunction associated with sexual disorders. Evidence is reviewed that shows substantial numbers of sex offenders and men with sexual disorders (paraphilias) have learning disabilities and neuropsychological impairment, which manifest early as significant difficulties in school. For instance, more than half have failed a grade in school and more than a third were in special education classes for children with learning disabilities. A theory that different sexual disorders are associated with pathology in different brain structures is examined. Implications for education and therapy of sex offenders are discussed.

Paraphilias appear to come in a variety of types, from pedophiles, who erotically prefer children; to exhibitionists, who expose their genitals to unsuspecting strangers; and fetishists, who are drawn to inanimate objects for sexual gratification. However, paraphilias can be classified into two broad categories: stimulus preferences and activity or response preferences (see Langevin, 1983). Stimulus preferences can be described as the properties of persons or things that lead to sexual arousal. Typical stimulus preferences involve the age and gender characteristics in the desired sex partner. Pedophiles who erotically prefer children are among the most common stimulus preference group seen in forensic clinics at present. Response or activity preferences can be described as the sexual behaviors an individual wishes to carry out with their preferred person or object. Sexual intercourse or oral–genital sex are the most common conventional activities preferred, but courtship disorders or combinations of voyeurism, exhibitionism, frottage, sexual aggression, rape, and/or sadism, are common sexual disorders seen clinically. Freund et al. (1983) theorized that these sexual behaviors represent abnormalities of normal courtship, which they labelled searching, pretactile interaction, tactile interaction, and genital union with a partner.

Paraphilias make their initial appearance around the time of puberty and, for the most part, persist a lifetime (see Langevin, 2004a). About half of the men who are sexual offenders or who present at forensic clinics have multiple paraphilias, making the study of pure groups such as pedophiles more difficult (Paitich, Langevin, Freeman, Mann, & Handy, 1977). Thus, it is not uncommon to see a pedophile (stimulus preference) in combination with exhibitionism (an activity preference). Why are these aberrant sexual behaviors so strong and enduring and how do these different paraphilias arise?

In case studies in the 1950s and 1960s, neurologists reported unusual sexual behavior associated with brain injury or dysfunction (see Purins & Langevin, 1985 for review). The areas of the brain most associated with the sexually anomalous behavior were the temporal lobes, believed to be a projection area in the more developed brain from the primitive deep limbic brain sites associated with sexual arousal and release. A series of controlled computer tomography (CT) studies by the author and his colleagues in the 1980s found support for these case studies and the involvement of the temporal lobes especially, in that there was significant dilitation of the temporal horns of the brain among pedophiles and sexually aggressive men. It was interesting that the pedophiles more often showed left hemispheric temporal horn dilitation, whereas the sexual aggressives (a generic term for men who sexually assault and rape adult females) showed right temporal horn dilitation. This led to the hypothesis that the two different sexual behaviors may be associated with brain pathology or dysfunction in different hemispheres, the stimulus preference of pedophilia in the left language/classificatory side of the brain and the activity preference of sexual aggression in the right or visual spatial/emotive side of the brain. A study with Percy Wright, Jose Nobrega, and Geroge Wortzmanin. (1990) found that the brain was predominantly smaller on the left side of pedophiles' brains and smaller on the right side of sexual aggressives'. Aigner et al. (2000) provided additional support for these CT findings, using magnetic resonance imaging (MRI) and they suggested that such abnormalities may be associated with violent behavior in general.

Flor-Henry (1980) proposed a theory of normal brain functioning related to sexual behavior. He argued that sexual ideation develops in the dominant (typically left) brain hemisphere and normally triggers an orgasmic response represented in the nondominant (usually right) brain hemisphere. He proposed that, in men with paraphilias, there is damage or pathology in the dominant hemisphere and conventional (nonparaphilic) sexual behavior is not elicited. Flor-Henry et al. (1988) found some support for the theory measuring electroencephalogram (EEG) in exhibitionists.

This chapter reviews evidence that there are functional differences in the brains of sexually disordered men, which are associated with their behavior and may provide possible developmental and causal explanations for the unusual sexual behaviors. School difficulties in learning as children, intelligence, and neuropsychological findings among sex offenders are examined in order.

GRADE FAILURES AND SCHOOL DROPOUTS

When educational attainment is reported in studies of sex offenders, it is usually incidental to some other aspect of the study, such as treatment effectiveness. Grade failures or repeats and placement in special education are rarely mentioned and the mentally retarded are often excluded from studies. Men with sexual disorders, in a variety of studies, typically present as high school dropouts. One may postulate many reasons for individuals leaving school prematurely, such as family problems or lower social class and poverty, rather than learning difficulties per se. Cohen et al. (2002) examined 22 heterosexual nonexclusive pedophiles and 24 controls and concluded that early childhood sexual abuse led to neurodevelopmental abnormalities in the temporal region mediating sexual arousal and erotic discrimination and in the frontal regions mediating the cognitive aspect of sexual desire and behavioral inhibition. However, such conclusions remain highly speculative. As Anderson et al. (2001) indicated, when there is neurocognitive impairment in a child, it may be difficult to determine whether factors such as family problems exacerbate the impairment or result from it. It is beyond the scope of this chapter to report on acknowledged family problems in men with sexual disorders and the present focus is on the neuropsychological findings.

A few studies indicate that not only do sex offenders and paraphilic men leave school prematurely, but about half fail a grade before leaving school for good.

In 1993 our research group (see Langevin & Pope, 1993) reported on 76 cases and found that 63% failed and repeated at least one grade in public or high school. It was interesting that, whereas 48% of the 25 pedophilic men repeated a grade, 85% of the 26 sexually aggressive men did so, suggesting greater learning problems in the latter. It should be noted that the last grade the offender attended was not included in the failures, if the offender had left school before completing his final year in school. A more recent report (Langevin, 2004b) on 1339 cases found similar results and 51.7% of the total sample had failed a grade before leaving public or high school. Results were also similar for pedophilic groups with 51.5% of the 404 cases failing a grade and 60.8% of the 171 sexually aggressive men failing at least one grade. It seems the learning problems appeared at an early age in many cases, with 38.3% of the failures occurring before grade three. The school system in Ontario, Canada, from which these data are drawn, apparently does not keep data on grade failures or repeats because officials, to whom I have spoken, said that it is extremely rare. Children are kept with their age peers and moved up a grade, even if they have not mastered the material in their current grade. However, in this same school system, there are special education classes for children with special needs and learning problems. When they cannot function in the regular grade, they may be moved to a special education class. Data from the province indicate that between 2% and 3% of children in the school system generally were in special education classes. Of the 1359 sex offenders we studied, 38.2% were in such classes. Thus, more than 12 times as many sex offenders, than expected by chance in the Ontario population at large, were in special education classes and were identified as having learning problems. Pattern of grade failures for specific sex offender subgroups was repeated in the findings on attending special education classes. A total of 38.5% of pedophiles versus 52.7% of sexual aggressives were in such classes. One reason for the disparity in these two groups in our sample was the higher incidence of attention-deficit/hyperactivity disorder (ADHD) among sexual aggressives than pedophiles. It is well known that about half of ADHD children also have accompanying learning disabilities. Little attention has been paid by Forensic professionals in the past to ADHD diagnoses among sex offenders, but 20% of the sexual aggressives studies

here did receive a childhood ADHD diagnosis, as did 11.7% of pedophilic men. Vaih-koch et al. (2001) examined 175 sex offenders using DSM diagnoses and found a somewhat higher rate of 28% with an ADHD diagnosis, indicating that ADHD should be more thoroughly and carefully examined among sex offenders. Daderman et al. (2004) reported on 10 rapists and found that 6 suffered from ADHD and 7 were dyslexic. Ponseti et al. (2001) examined 44 violent and sex offenders and 81 nonsex offenders in a German prison and found a similar but noteworthy incidence of ADHD in both groups, suggesting that ADHD is not peculiar to sex offenders, but it is a problem that merits attention in forensic cases generally.

One also may ask if learning disabilities are as common in the criminal population at large or in nonsex offenders as they are in sex offenders, but there is surprisingly little published on the question. Our own findings suggest that grade failures and learning problems are common in the general criminal population seen for psychological assessment, but they are more common among sex offenders. Of the 127 nonsex offenders in the study, 43.5% failed a grade in school, significantly less than the sex offenders, but there were no significant differences in special education placements.

When sex offenders with predominantly stimulus preferences versus activity preferences are examined separately, it is the latter who fail grades significantly more (59.0% vs. 51.2%) and are placed in special education significantly more often (49.0% vs. 36.2%). A possible reason for greater placement of response preference cases is the higher incidence of ADHD in that group. There was a trend ($p < .10$) for response preference cases to be diagnosed more often with ADHD than stimulus preference cases (18.6% vs. 11.3%). Results reported by Vaih-Koch et al. (2001) showed a similar pattern, with 42% of sexual aggressives showing an ADHD diagnosis versus 29% of pedophiles.

These results are not to imply that all learning disabled men or men who have been in special education classes are sex offenders or criminals, but only that sex offenders are overrepresented among individuals with learning problems. It is unknown how many learning disabled individuals end up in a life of crime or with a paraphilia. However, it has been claimed that the mentally retarded are more common among sex offenders, the next topic.

INTELLIGENCE

Griffiths and Marini (2000) have noted that the mentally retarded are often faced with court proceedings and may not be properly represented. This may be especially true in the case of sex offenses. Hawk et al. (1993) examined 2536 cases of offenders seen in the state of Virginia for DSM diagnosis of mental retardation and found that this diagnosis was overrepresented among sex offenders, but not in other criminal groups. Wormith and McKeague (1996), on the other hand, examined Canadian criminal justice statistics on a random sample of 2500 incarcerated offenders and found that mental retardation occurred at an expected chance level for the population at large, with 1.7% of inmates in the federal correctional system being mentally retarded. However, no association of sex offenses and mental retardation was reported. Hawke et al's report. suggests an association of mental retardation with sexual disorders, but no actual intelligence test results were reported and over 400 examiners provided diagnoses with no indication of reliability of diagnosis or that an intelligence quotient (IQ) test had been administered. Some jurisdictions may have a different attitude to mentally retarded or brain injured offenders and may mete out harsher sentences to protect the public. In other cases, the mentally retarded sex offender may not go to trial at all, but is detained indefinitely in institution nonetheless. Studies of intelligence scores among sex offenders have provided different results.

When IQ scores have been reported on sex offenders, they tend to fall in the average or low average range (see Cantor et al., 2005, for a review of these studies). Mentally retarded individuals appear with a chance frequency of about 2.3% when standard tests are used. However, the few available studies indicate that the distribution of IQ scores tends to be skewed to the lower end of normal with an overrepresentation of sex offenders in the borderline retarded or low average range. These results were first reported in a series of studies on small samples of sex offenders, completed with my colleagues in 1985 using a variety of IQ measures. Blanchard et al. in 1999 examined 678 pedophilic and 313 sex offenders against adults for mental retardation, using global estimates of intelligence based on available IQ test results, whether the offender was living in a group home for the mentally retarded, and whether they required accompaniment to the interview. The pedophilic group was not more often retarded than expected by chance.

Cantor et al. (2004) followed up on this study by examining six scales (Information, Similarities, Digit Span, Arithmetic, Picture Completion, and Block Design) of the Wechsler Adult Intelligence Scale-Revised (WAIS-R) in 304 pedophilic and hebephilic (preference for pubertal females) men. They found estimated full IQs in the low average range (80 to 90) to average range (90 to 110).

Recently, the author, Langevin (2004) examined 932 sex offenders from a variety of sex offender groups, who were Canadian born and whose only language was English. Full WAIS-R IQ scores were average overall with an overrepresentation of scores in the 70 to 80 or borderline retarded range and an underrepresentation in the superior IQ range of 120 and higher. Mental retardation occurred with a frequency of 2.4%; close to chance expected at 2.6%. The borderline retarded group (IQ 70 to 80) were slightly, but significantly overrepresented with 9.5% of cases in that range versus 6.9% expected by chance. Mentally retarded and borderline retarded individuals were not overrepresented among any sex offender subgroup, such as pedophiles, but appeared among them on a chance basis. These results collectively indicate that when standard IQ tests are used, sex offenders are not mentally retarded, more than one would expect on a chance basis, but their IQ scores tend to be in the borderline or low average range, offering one reason they may have some learning difficulties in school and hence may experience similar difficulties in sex offender therapy programs, which are typically carried out in groups. The borderline retarded IQ scores are a composite of verbal and performance measures that may reflect large disparities in the two and indicate a learning disability rather than mental retardation or global cognitive impairment.

Full IQ scores may be divided into verbal IQ (VIQ) and performance IQ (PIQ). The former taps language-based abilities, such as vocabulary and language comprehension, whereas the latter taps nonverbal and visual–spatial abilities, represented by block design and picture arrangement. In a gross sense, language abilities tend to be associated more with left brain hemispheric functioning and performance and nonverbal abilities are associated more with the right hemisphere. Significant differences between VIQ and PIQ are used as indices of minimal brain dysfunction or learning disabilities, associated with one brain hemisphere/locus or the other. If VIQ is significantly different from PIQ it suggests that one hemisphere of the brain is not functioning as well as the other. A lower VIQ than PIQ suggests left hemispheric deficits, whereas a lower PIQ than VIQ suggests right hemispheric deficits. The Wechsler Adult Intelligence Scale (WAIS-R) (Wechsler, 1981) is one of the most widely used IQ tests in the history of Psychology. The WAIS-R manual indicates that a VIQ–PIQ difference of 10 points is statistically significant and can be used as an index of a learning disability or brain dysfunction, but, in practice it recommends using 15 points as a clinically significant difference.

Data from the 932 cases noted previously indicates that 38% showed at least a 10-point difference in VIQ and PIQ, when less than 5% would be expected by chance, and 22.5% of the sex offenders showed at least a 15 point VIQ–PIQ difference. A total of 13.1% showed lower verbal than performance scores (using the 15 point criterion), whereas 9.4% showed the opposite. The significant VIQ–PIQ differences were more common in the average and higher IQ range. Thus, both lower IQ and VIQ–PIQ differences appear to contribute to the compromised cognitive functioning of sex offenders. These results were supported in studies employing small mixed samples of sex offenders. Murray et al. (2001) suggested that the VIQ–PIQ difference is significant in sex offenders, but not nonsex offenders. Unique to their study, they examined 42 sex offenders with learning disabilities and 42 nonoffenders with learning disabilities, matched on WAIS-R Full IQ score. The sex offenders, but not the nonoffenders, had significantly lower VIQ than PIQ. On WAIS-R subtests, sex offenders had significantly lower Vocabulary scores, but higher Object Assembly scores. Supporting the latter findings, Ponseti et al. (2001) found poorer spatial abilities in sex offenders than in nonsex offender controls.

When examining the hypothesis that stimulus preferences, such as pedophilia, would show deficits in the left hemisphere, it is expected that more of them would show a lower VIQ than a PIQ score. On the other hand, activity or response preferences seen in sexually aggressive men should show more right hemispheric or nonlanguage based deficits and a lower PIQ score compared to VIQ. Only a few studies have examined this question and results are complicated by incomplete information on sexual history; primarily because of the lack of candor of the offenders. The author (Langevin, 2004) found that, when men are faced with criminal charges, only 69%

acknowledge committing the offense for which they are mostly ultimately convicted and even fewer, 35.5% acknowledge having a sexually deviant preference. Thus, findings are tentative. In the sample of 932 sex offenders noted previously, expected differences in VIQ–PIQ among Stimulus and Response Preference groups was contradicted and showed opposite to expected results, but supported Flor-Henry's theory of left hemispheric deficits in sex offenders. However differences were small and a range effect of means was noted.

Overall results of intelligence testing on sex offenders suggests that the majority of sex offenders' IQs will fall in the average range, but the distribution of scores will be skewed to the lower end of normal. The mentally retarded are not overrepresented, but one can expect to see somewhat more than expected IQs in the borderline retarded range and fewer in the superior range, when standard IQ tests are used. In addition, one might expect to see more learning disabilities and disparities in VIQ and PIQ. These results suggest that other neuropsychological testing may be informative.

NEUROPSYCHOLOGICAL TEST RESULTS

Handedness

The majority of individuals in general are right hand dominant with a 10% to 15% showing mixed hand or left hand dominance. When an individual is nonright-handed, it suggests that brain organization of functions may be the reverse of right handed individuals or may be unusual or mixed. For example, the movement of the right hand side of the body is associated with intact functioning in the left parietal/motor area of the brain, that is, brain function is contralateral to the side of the body it regulates. Some functions are typically specialized in the left hemisphere, for example, Broca's Area is associated with language functioning and typically it is in the left hemisphere. This also may be true of the left-handed person or it may be on the right side of the brain. Thus overall, nonright-handedness suggests a different brain organization and if there are more non–right-handed individuals among sex offenders, it suggests their brains may be organized in a different way and be associated with the development of their paraphilia. Left-handedness is also more common among the learning disabled, adding to their difficulties in learning.

Very few studies have examined handedness among sex offenders and paraphilic individuals. Work by Hucker et al. (1988), Hucker et al. (1986), Langevin et al. (1989), Langevin et al. (1989) on a variety of sex offender cases did not find differences in handedness from chance expectation. Bogaert and Blanchard (1996) reviewed studies suggesting that homosexual men show more non–right-handedness, but they failed to find a greater than chance rate of 10% to 12% non–right-handedness in 1004 homosexual and 4579 heterosexual men from the Kinsey Institute sample. Cantor et al. (2004) examined handedness in 473 pedophiles using the Edinburgh Handedness Inventory and employing a complex scoring scheme with analysis of covariance. They found a significantly higher incidence of non–right-handedness among the pedophiles, but percentages with right versus non–right-handedness were not reported.

The author's data using the Reitan scale for handedness on 766 sex offenders and controls, did not find a statistically significant difference and 90.2% of the sex offenders were found to be exclusively right handed. There were no subgroup differences. These results collectively suggest that if handedness is a factor in the development of paraphilias, it plays a very minor role.

Neuropsychological Test Batteries

There are very few studies of neuropsychological test results for sex offenders. Studies by the author and his colleagues in the 1980s found that pedophiles especially showed significantly more impairment on the HalsteadReitan Neuropsychological Test Battery than controls, with approximately one-in-four showing an overall significant impairment index. Particular deficits were noted in executive (frontal lobe) functioning and inflexibility in changing mental set, that is, the Categories Subtest and Trails Making B Subtest (see Hucker et al., 1986; Hucker et al., 1988; Langevin et al., 1989; Langevin et al., 1989). Hucker et al. (1986) also examined the Luria-Nebraska Neuropsychological Test Battery, but did not find the test to have satisfactory norms. This is a common problem using neuropsychological tests, that is, test validation is often lacking.

More recent work on 766 sex offenders, using the better normed Halstead–Reitan Battery showed results in a number of sex offender groups, similar to our earlier findings with 35.1% failing the Categories Subtest and 29.3% the Trail Making B Subtest.

We also looked at hemispheric transfer more specifically on the Tactual Performance Subtest. In this task, there are ten blocks to be placed in specifically made holes on a board. The subject must place the blocks correctly while blindfolded and initially using only the dominant hand. Time to complete the task is recorded. The task is repeated using the nondominant hand and again time is recorded. It is expected that the subject will be 20% to 40% quicker on the second trial as learning should have taken place and information should have transferred to the nondominant side of the brain via the corpus callosum, the connecting body between the two hemispheres of the brain. A third trial allows the subject to use both hands and again there should be a 20% to 40% decrease in time to complete the task, assuming functioning is intact in each hemisphere and in the corpus callosum. Results showed that 27.0% of the sex offenders took significantly longer using the nondominant hand on the second trial and 8.5% took longer on the third trial using both hands, when they would be expected to be quicker on both second and third trials than they were on the first trial. There were no significant subgroup differences on this task, but results support findings of intelligence scores that there are disparities in brain hemispheric functioning and transfer of information between the brain hemispheres among sex offenders and paraphilics.

BRAIN INJURIES

If neuropsychological deficits are found in sex offenders, the question arises whether the deficits are secondary to a brain injury and/or coincidental to the sexual behavior. Thus, one may ask if the sexual disorder predated the brain injury or any neural insult the brain may have endured (see Delbella et al., 1999; Regenstein & Reich, 1978; Weinstein, 1974, for example).

Simpson et al. (1999) studied 445 clients at a brain injury rehabilitation center and found that 29 (6.5%) had committed sexual offenses after the brain injury. The offenses involved mainly touching, followed by exhibiting and sexual aggression. In the absence of a history of prior sexual offense and alcohol abuse in the majority of cases, the authors concluded that the traumatic brain injury may have been a significant etiological factor underlying the sexual offenses. Luiselli et al. (2000) examined 69 children and adolescents with traumatic brain injuries and found that one third had criminal violations, including sexual assaults, but there was no difference in the pattern of injuries in those who offended and those who did not.

Blanchard and his colleagues (2002 & 2003) examined two samples of pedophiles. In 685 cases, they found that pedophiles had more head injuries before age 13 than controls, but did not differ in the incidence after age 13. In another 413 pedophiles and 793 nonpedophilic forensic cases, they found that childhood accidents before age 6, but not after age 6, were associated with a higher incidence of pedophilia, lower intelligence, and less education. These authors concluded that early childhood head injuries may either increase the risk for pedophilia and/or make the individual more accident prone.

I also examined 513 sex offenders seen at a university psychiatric hospital and in private practice for forensic assessment related to sex offense charges or convictions (Langevin, 2004). A total of 49% had sustained head injuries that led to unconsciousness and 22.5% sustained significant neurological insults. A major causative factor was motor vehicle accidents, but lifestyle factors such as alcohol and drug abuse contributed. The brain injured committed a wide range of sexual offenses, but more often offended against adults and showed somewhat more exhibiting and polymorphous sexual behavior.

The possible origin of the learning disabilities and cognitive deficits among sex offenders has recently been examined (Langevin, 2004) and results suggest that prenatal and perinatal factors may be linked to the cognitive impairment seen in sex offenders. Both maternal and paternal abuse of alcohol were associated with at least two-thirds of the 1526 sex offenders examined and were seen on more than a chance basis. Older maternal age at the birth of the sex offender and later birth order were also significant factors. Noteworthy was the association of alcohol abuse by the parents especially with sex offenders having lower IQs, more grade failures, more placement in special education, and more ADHD diagnoses and symptoms. Results suggest that brain abnormalities and cognitive impairment in sex offenders may have prenatal roots.

CONCLUSION

There have been relatively few studies in the mental health literature on the neurocognitive functioning of sex offenders. Available results indicate that the brain functioning of sex offenders is impaired from an early age and they have problems learning at school with many developing an attitude about learning situations such as therapy (see Langevin, Marentette, & Rosati, 1996). The learning disabled sex offender may be considered uncooperative, may not function in groups, for example, the silent member, or cannot follow the group proceedings, and little account is taken of his disability. The typical sex offender is of average intelligence, but more cases have low average or borderline retarded intelligence, that predominantly reflects the presence of learning disabilities. One can expect to see a small, but significant, minority of sex offenders who have overall neuropsychological impairment. One can expect to see one-in-three or more who show impairment in executive functioning and associated poor judgment and impulsiveness. Cognitive impairment also may interact with other factors, such as abuse of alcohol or drugs, and serve as important disinhibiting and risk factors for acting out in sexually deviant ways. Results of neuropsychological testing suggest that sex offenders as a group have significant deficits that may be related to the etiology of the sexual disorders they suffer.

There was mixed support of the theory of hemispheric differentiation of dysfunction among subgroups of sex offenders and those with predominantly stimulus or response preferences. Candor of sex offenders about their sexual history and limited validation of neuropsychological tests played some role in hampering conclusions in this respect. One may expect to see more language and left hemispheric deficits overall in sex offenders, regardless of group membership, supporting Flor-Henry's (1980) theory although there have been few studies on cognitive functioning in sex offenders, available studies have large samples and the findings are impelling, with implications for treatment, indicating that further work on the topic is warranted. The importance of brain damage and dysfunction cannot be ignored if we are to make progress in understanding and treating individuals with sexually anomalous behavior.

References

Aigner, M., Eher, R., Fruehwald, S., Frottier, P., Gutierrez-Lobos, K., & Dwyer, S. M. (2000). Brain abnormalities and violent behavior. *Journal of Psychology and Human Sexuality*, 11(3), 57–64.

Anderson, V., Northam, E., Hendry, J., & Wrennall, J. (2001). *Developmental Neuropsychology: A Clinical Approach.* (pp. 170–172). East Sussex, Britain: Psychology Press.

Blanchard, R., Watson, M. S., Choy, A., Dickey, R., Klassen, P., Kuban, M., et al. (1999). Pedophiles: mental retardation, maternal age, and sexual orientation. *Archives of Sexual Behavior,* 28(2), 111–127.

Blanchard, R., Christensen, B. K., Strong, S. M., Cantor, J. M., Kuban, M. E., Klassen, et al. (2002). Retrospective self-reports of childhood accidents causing unconsciousness in phallometrically diagnosed pedophiles. *Archives of Sexual Behavior,* 31(6), 511–526.

Blanchard, R., Kuban, M. E., Klassen, P., Dickey, R., Christensen, B. K., Cantor, J. M., et al. (2003). Self-reported head injuries before and after age 13 in pedophilic and nonpedophilic men referred for clinical assessment. *Archives of Sexual Behavior,* 32(6), 573–581.

Bogaert, A. F. & Blanchard, R. (1996). Handedness in homosexual and heterosexual men in the Kinsey interview data. *Archives of Sexual Behavior,* 25(4), 373–378.

Cantor, J. M., Blanchard, R., Christensen, B. K., Dickey, R., Klassen, P. E., Beckstead, A. L., et al. (2004). Intelligence, memory, and handedness in pedophilia. *Neuropsychology,* 18(1), 3–14.

Cantor, J. M., Blanchard, R., Robichaud, L. K., & christensen, B. K. (2005). Quantitative reanalysis of aggregate data on IQ in sex offenders. *Psychological Bulletin,* 131(4), 555–568.

Cohen, L. J., Nikiforov, K., Gans, S., Poznansky, O., McGeoch, P., Weaver, C., et al. (2002). Heterosexual male perpetrators of childhood sexual abuse: a preliminary neuropsychiatric model. *Psychiatric Quarterly,* 73(4), 313–336.

Daderman, A. M., Lindgren, M. L., & Ledberg, L. (2004). The prevalence of dyslexia and AD/HD in a sample of forensic psychiatric rapists. *Nordic Journal of Psychiatry,* 58(5), 371–381.

DelBello, M. P., Soutello, C. A., Zimmerman, M. E., Sax, K. W., Williams, J. R., McElroy, S. L., et al. (1999). Traumatic brain injury in individuals convicted of sexual offenses with and without bipolar disorder. *Psychiatry Research,* 89(3), 281–286.

Flor-Henry, P. (1980). Cerebral aspects of the orgasmic response: normal and deviational. In R. Forleo, & W. Pasini (Ed.), *Medical Sexology,* (pp. 256–262). Amsterdam: Elsevier.

Flor-Henry, P., Lang, R. A., Koles, Z. J., & Frenzel, R. R. (1988). Quantitative EEG investigations of genital exhibitionism. *Annals of Sex Research,* 1, 49–62.

Freund, K., Scher, H., & Hucker, S. (1983). The courtship disorders. *Archives of Sexual Behavior,* 12, 369–379.

Griffiths, D., & Marini, Z. (2000). Interacting with the legal system regarding a sexual offence: social and cognitive considerations for persons with developmental disabilities. *Journal of Developmental Disabilities,* 7(1), 76–121.

Hawk, G. L., Rosenfeld, B. D., & Warren, J. I. (1993). Prevalence of sexual offenses among mentally retarded criminal defendants. *Hospital and Community Psychiatry,* 44(8), 784–786.

Hucker, S., Langevin, R., Wortzman, G., Bain, J., Handy, L., Chambers, J., et al. (1986). Neuropsychological impairment in pedophiles. *Canadian Journal of Behavioural Science,* 18(4), 440–448.

Hucker, S., Langevin, R., Dickey, R., Handy, L., Chambers, J., & Wright, S. (1988). Cerebral damage and dysfunction in sexually aggressive men. *Annals of Sex Research,* 1(1), 32–48.

Langevin, R. (1983). *Sexual Strands: Understanding and Treating Sexual Anomalies in Men.* Hillsdale, NJ: Erlbaum Associates.

Langevin, R. (2004). Who engages in sexual behaviour with children? Are clergy who commit sexual offences different from other sex offenders? In R.K. Hanson, F. Pfafflin, & M. Lutz, (Eds.), *Sexual Abuse in the Catholic Church: Scientific and Legal Perspectives* (pp. 24–43). Vatican City: Libreria editrice Vaticana.

Langevin, R. (2004). New directions in treating sex offenders: have we neglected the obvious? Paper presented at the Eighth Biennial Conference of the International Association for the Treatment of Sex Offenders (IATSO), Athens, Greece, 6–9.

Langevin, R. (2005). An examination of school grade failures and attendance in special education classes among sex offenders (in press).

Langevin, R. & Pope, S. (1993). Working with learning disabled sex offenders. *Annals of Sex Research,* 6, 149–160.

Langevin, R., Lang, R. A., Wright, P., Handy, L., & Majpruz, V. (1989). An examination of brain damage and dysfunction in genital exhibitionists. *Annals of Sex Research,* 2(1), 77–88.

Langevin, R., Wortzman, G., Wright, P., & Handy, L. (1989). Studies of brain damage and dysfunction in sex offenders. *Annals of Sex Research,* 2(2), 163–179.

Langevin, R., Marentette, D., & Rosati, B. (1996). Why Therapy fails with some sex offenders: learning difficulties examined empirically. *Journal of Offender Rehabilitation: Sex Offender Treatment,* 23(3/4), 143–155.

Luiselli, J. K., Aron, M., Marchese, N., Potoczny-Gray, A., & Rossi, E. (2000). Incidence of law-violation behavior in a community sample of children and adolescents with traumatic brain injury. *International Journal of Offender Therapy and Comparative Criminology,* 44(6), 647–656.

Murray, G. C., McKenzie, K., Quigley, A., Matheson, E., Michie, A. M., & Lindsay, W. R. (2001). A comparison of the neuropsychological profiles of adult male sex offenders and non-offenders with a learning disability. *Journal of Sexual Aggression,* 7(2), 57–64.

Paitich, D., Langevin, R., Freeman, R., Mann, K., & Handy, L. (1977). The Clarke SHQ: a clinically sex history questionnaire for males. *Archives of Sexual Behavior*, 6, 421–426.

Ponseti, J., Vaih-Koch, S. R., & Bosinski, H. A. G. (2001). On the etiology of sexual offenses: neuropsychological parameters and comorbidity. *Sexuologie*, 8(2), 65–77.

Purins, J. E. & Langevin, R. (1985). Brain correlates of penile erection. In Langevin, R. (Ed.), *Erotic preference, gender identity, and aggression in men*, (pp. 113–133). Hillsdale, NJ: Erlbaum Associates.

Regenstein, Q. R. & Reich, P. (1978). Pedophilia occurring after onset of cognitive impairment. *Journal of Nervous and Mental Disease*, 166(11), 794–798.

Simpson, G., Blaszczynski, A., & Hodgkinson, A. (1999). Sex offending as a psychosocial sequella of traumatic brain injury. *Journal of Head Trauma Rehabilitation*, 14(6), 567–580.

Vaih-Koch, S. R., Ponseti, J., & Bosinski, H. A. G. (2001). ADHD und storung des sozialverhaltens im kindesalter als pradiktoren aggressiver sexualdelinquenz? *Sexuologie*, 8(1), 1–18.

Wechsler, D. (1981). The Wechsler Adult Intelligence Scale-Revised. San Antonio,TX: Hartcourt Brace.

Weinstein, E. A. (1974). Sexual disturbances after brain injury. *Medical Aspects of Human Sexuality*, 8(10), 10–31.

Wormith, J. S. & Mckeague, F. (1996). A mental health survey of community correctional clients in Canada. *Criminal Behaviour and Mental Health*, 6, 49–72.

Wright, P., Nobrega, J., Langevin, R., & Wortzman, G. (1990). Brain density and symmetry in pedophilic and sexually aggressive men. *Annals of Sex Research*, 3(3), 319–328.

Chapter 4

The Neurobiology of Sexual Behavior and the Paraphilias

John M. Bradford and J. Paul Fedoroff

Recent advances in neurobiological research have improved the understanding of how sexual behavior is influenced by neuroendocrine and neurobiochemical systems. It would be premature to make a statement that the neurobiology of sexual behavior is understood. Major advances have been made in neurobiochemical research particularly with serotonin (5-HT) and specifically with research on serotonin receptors. The role of neuropeptides, as well as other cerebral monoamines has also enhanced this understanding. Much of the research examining the roles of cerebral hormones, monoamines, and neuropeptides has been based on animal research. Research in human sexual behavior has been primarily based on research about the effects of pharmacological agents as well as the effects of hormones The hormone research has a pharmacological basis to it, but in addition there has been research in the brain directly on the actions of cerebral hormones as well as the endocrine system in general. Many of the pharmacological agents used in general psychiatry influence neurotransmitters, such as serotonin (5-HT) and have contributed to the understanding of the role of serotonin (5-HT) and other neurotransmitters on human sexual behavior. Studies on hormones, either influenced by pharmacological agents or studied in vitro have also provided valuable information (Sjoerdsma & Palfreyman, 1990). This chapter is a broad review of the neuroendocrine and neurobiochemical research. As the focus is on the paraphilias, which are typically a male problem, the neuroendocrinology of male sexual behavior as well as the neurobiochemical influences on male sexual behavior will be the principal focus of this chapter.

Fundamental to the understanding of human sexual behavior is the sexual differentiation of the brain and the influences on male and female sexual behavior derived from genetic influences, hormonal influences on the fetus, hormonal influences during puberty, hormonal influences during adulthood, and the influence of declining hormone levels with aging. For many years, there has been an understanding of the role of sex hormones in human sexual behavior (Bancroft, 1989). Hormonal effects on the brain can be divided into organizing effects of hormones on the sexual differentiation of the brain and the activating effects of hormones affecting behavior, particularly in the mature individual (Bancroft, 1984, 1989, 2002). The organizing effects of hormones in the prenatal period influence the sexual differentiation of the fetus into male or female phenotypes as well as the gender identity. Fetal androgenization is responsible for the sexual differentiation of the brain. This will not be covered in detail, as it is the activating component of sex hormones that is more closely related to sexual behavior as is seen in the paraphilias. Sexual drive, and sexual behavior in general, is dependent on the levels of these sex hormones. In general terms, androgens are important for the maintenance of sexual behavior in males. Many studies have shown that from animals (including subprimates) to humans that surgical castration has a significant impact on male sexual behavior. Following surgical castration sexual behavior declines in a predictable manner with ejaculation going first, followed by intromission and then mounting behavior (Bancroft, 1989). The time frame for the decline in male sexual behavior varies according to different species. Many studies have shown that replacement androgen restores the sexual behavior usually in the reverse order (Bancroft, 1989). Studies on hormonal replacement in hypogonadal men, 25 years ago, showed conclusively that androgen withdrawal causing a decline in sexual interest over a 3- to 4-week timeframe that could be reversed with androgen replacement in about 2 weeks (Bancroft, 1989). Erections, either nocturnal or in response to erotic stimuli, although diminished, may not disappear completely (Bancroft, 1989). Research over the past quarter of the last century has supported these earlier findings.

HORMONES, NEUROHORMONES, AND NEUROTRANSMITTERS

Behavioral endocrinology is the study of the influence of hormones on an animal's behavior (Becker, Breedlove, Crews, & McCarthy, 2002). The work in this field has resulted in substantial progress in understanding the neuroanatomical, neuroendocrine, and neurobiochemical aspects of sexual behavior (Pfaus, 1999). All cells in an organism are engaged in the synthesis of proteins. These proteins become intercellular chemical messengers and are known as hormones, neurohormones, and neurotransmitters. Hormones are produced by endocrine cells and released into the general circulation; neurotransmitters are produced by neurons and released at the synapses; and the neurohormones are produced by specialized neurons known as *neurosecretory cells* (Becker et al., 2002). There are distinct differences in terms of where the chemical messengers are produced and where they are released and the effect on various receptors. Cells produce proteins based on their genetic code and generally they are secreted in vesicles. Transmission across the synapses is through neurotransmitters. Neurotransmitters are monoamines, amino acids, purines, and peptides. The neurotransmitters of most significance in sexual behavior are the monoamines, serotonin, and dopamine. The peptide hormone of most significance is gonadotropin releasing hormone (GnRH). Prolactin (PRL), a peptide hormone, is also very significant in relation to sexual behavior and is a common factor in the pharmacological action of many drugs that cause sexual dysfunction. Steroid hormones, such as estradiol and testosterone are very important in the maintenance of sexual behavior.

A neurotransmitter is synthesized and packaged in a synaptic vesicle in the presynaptic terminal. When this package is released, it attaches on the post synaptic receptor. When the neurotransmitter binds to the postsynaptic receptor, changes in the electrical potential of the membrane occurs proportional to the amount of neurotransmitter released. The neurotransmitter can produce either inhibition or excitation depending on the effects on the membrane. If the neurotransmitter does not bind to the postsynaptic receptor it is deactivated through enzymes in the synaptic cleft or by reuptake into the presynaptic terminal (Becker, 2002; Becker et al., 2002).

Peptide hormones and steroid hormones are closely related to the hypothalamic pituitary axis. Steroid hormones are produced in different parts of the body but in addition, are stored partially in the blood where they are bound to plasma proteins. Testosterone is found in three different forms in the plasma, bound to sex hormone binding globulin; bound loosely to albumin; and also as free testosterone. The active portions are the testosterone loosely bound to albumin and the free testosterone. Steroid hormones act on distant receptors in the body and also in the brain. For example, there are testosterone receptors in the testes; the spinal cord; the skin, and the brain. Peptide hormones are stored in the cells that produce them and then are released in a pulsatile fashion. This means their blood levels fluctuate considerably or they may only be present in the plasma for brief periods of time after release. It is these peptide hormones that play an intermediate role as a neurotransmitter and a hormone. This has been recognised by calling them releasing factors as opposed to releasing hormones in some areas. As releasing factors or releasing hormones they are principally responsible for the release of other peptides from their cells of origin. Gonadotropin releasing factor for example, is responsible for the release of lutenising hormone. The complex interaction of neurotransmitters, peptide hormones, and steroid hormones is centred in the hypothalamic pituitary system. In terms of behavioral neuroendocrinology, the hypothalamus is the most important part of the brain. The hypothalamus is part of the diencephalon and has a profound influence on all hormones in the body. The hypothalamus is the center of the relationship between the brain and the endocrine system. It has specialized nuclei that are involved in the regulation of the endocrine system. Within the hypothalamus, the medial preoptic area (POA) and the ventromedial hypothalamic nuclei are involved in sexual behavior. These nuclei have special neuronal cells known as neurosecretory cells which release their chemical messages directly into the blood vessels and are therefore known as neurohormones. These are peptide hormones, luteinising hormone releasing hormone (LHRH), and prolactin inhibiting factor (PIF). The hypothalamus is directly above pituitary gland or hypophysis. The neurosecretory cells of the hypothalamus release neurohormones (LHRH and PIF) into blood vessels that supply the anterior pituitary. These are known as releasing factors and stimulate or inhibit the release of hormones (luteinising hormone [LH], follicle stimulating hormone [FSH] and PRL) from the anterior pituitary, or adenohypophysis. The other neurosecretory cells release neurohormones directly into the general circulation by the posterior pituitary or neurohypophysis. The pituitary hormones act on peripheral endocrine glands to stimulate or inhibit their release of hormones. There is a feedback loop where the circulating levels of these hormones feedback on the hypothalamus to exert feedback control on the levels of releasing factors (LHRH and PIF) from the hypothalamus. Depending on the levels, there is either an increase or decrease in the release of hypothalamic releasing factors (LHRH and PIF). The levels of circulating steroid hormones (plasma testosterone, T) control the release of hypothalamic releasing factors (LHRH and PIF), which in turn affects the release of LH and FSH from the pituitary gland (Becker et al., 2002).

Other peptide hormones or releasing factors that are important for understanding sexual behavior at the hypothalamic pituitary level are oxytocin; PRL; gonadotropin releasing hormone or LHRH, LH, and FSH. Oxytocin is a neurohormone released from the posterior pituitary or neurohypophysis. When oxytocin is released into the bloodstream, it triggers milk ejection as well as uterine contractions during childbirth (Becker, et al., 2002). LH and FSH are peptide hormones known as gonadotropins. Other peptide hormones or neuropeptide transmitters are of less direct significance to sexual behavior, corticotropin releasing factor; endorphins; growth hormone releasing hormone; neurotensin; thyrotropin releasing hormone; vasopressin, and a number of other neuropeptide hormones or neuropeptide transmitters.

The gonads release steroid hormones, in males this is testosterone (T) and dihydrotestosterone (DHT). In females these steroid hormones are estradiol and progesterone. In males T and DHT are produced by the testes, where 95% of the production of testosterone occurs, and by the adrenals where the remaining 5% is produced (Becker et al., 2002). Estradiol is also produced by the testes and the adrenal glands in males.

Hormones exert influences by the expression of various genes. There are differences in the way this manifests in steroid hormones versus peptide hormones (Becker et al., 2002) (see Chapter 2). There are also different receptors for peptide hormones and steroid hormones. The receptors for peptide hormones are found on the surface of the cells. Following this hormone receptor interaction there are changes in intracellular molecules which may result, in some cases, in second messengers (Becker et al., 2002) (see Chapter 2). The most commonly found receptors are G-protein coupled receptors. When a peptide hormone binds to a receptor, a G-protein complex is activated and this results in the production of second messengers. The second messengers are cyclic AMP (cAMP) and inositol phospholipids (ISP). This is the mechanism where by many peptide hormones including oxytocin, LH, FSH, and LHRH exert their influence (Becker et al., 2002) (Chapter 2).

Steroid hormone receptors are known as transcription factors. They interact directly with DNA and either increase or decrease the transcription of particular genes (Becker et al., 2002) (Chapter 2). These receptors are intracellular and are individual proteins and when the steroid molecule enters the cell it binds with the receptor protein. The activated receptor interacts with DNA. Before this occurs the steroid receptor may bind to other proteins. This interaction may involve the binding to other proteins forming what is known as a transcriptional complex. This makes the interaction with DNA highly specific, forming a hormone response element. These hormone response elements are different for each steroid receptor (Becker et al., 2002) (Chapter 2). This is known as a *genomic action* and is regarded as the classic steroid action.

Sexual Differentiation

In the fetus the gonads are initially not differentiated into male or female gonads. The sex chromosomes and particularly the Y chromosome are responsible for the differentiation. Once this has occurred further sexual differentiation is driven by sex hormones. In the presence of the Y chromosome the gonads form into a primitive testis which secretes androgen hormones and a male phenotype develops (Becker et al., 2002) (Chapter 3). In the males there were two hormones responsible for male development, testosterone and a peptide hormone known as antimullerian hormone. This hormone specifically acts to cause a regression of the mullerian ducts. The mullerian ducts in females develop into the vagina, fallopian tubes, and the uterus. The secretion of testosterone results in the masculinization of the body and the brain. These testicular steroids, at a very early point, masculinize the brain as well as future behavior. This process has been studied by Charles Phoenix and colleagues and in 1959 this resulted in the organizational hypothesis. This hypothesis is that the early androgen secretion has a permanent effect on the brain, which leads to masculine behavior during adolescence and in adulthood. This is therefore a permanent sexual differentiation of the central nervous system (Becker et al., 2002) (Chapter 3). These organizational effects on

the central nervous system leading to permanent changes in the developing central nervous system can be seen in contrast to the activational effects of steroid hormones occurring at other times of the life of the organism, for example, puberty, which has transient effects on the brain. It is also clear that steroid hormones particularly T and DHT have a masculinizing effect on the body early in development including the first trimester of pregnancy, and then as the organism grows older these steroid hormones have little structural effect on the central nervous system (Becker et al., 2002). It is not surprising that these organizational affects of androgens would have an effect on adult sexual behavior. The assumption was clearly that early androgenization would have an effect of masculinizing adult behavior and in contrast the absence of androgenization would lead to a feminization effect on adult sexual behavior. Further, the introduction of androgen at specific or sensitive periods could have a specific effect depending on the species. These behaviors were measured in animal research using typical male behaviors such as aggressive play and mounting behavior. To summarize, the organizational hypothesis means that the same hormonal influences that led to the sexual differentiation of the genitalia also leads to the sexual differentiation of the brain (Becker et al., 2002).

The sex differences in central nervous system structures were discovered in the 1970s. Prior to that there was general scientific agreement that steroid hormone exposure early on caused structural changes and had affects on subsequent behavior but this had not been documented in a structural way. Darwin is regarded as the originator of the term sexual dimorphism (Becker et al., 2002). This refers to most species having clearly defined differences in body shape or size depending on sex. In some species the brain differentiation can be observed by the naked eye (Toran-Allerand, 1978). The full exploration of anatomical studies of the sex differences between males and females in the brain is beyond the scope of this chapter. Overall research from the late 1950s up until today has clearly shown male-female differences in various parts of the brain. One of the first areas of male-female differentiation identified was the preoptic area (POA) of the hypothalamus in animal studies. Gorski and colleagues found that there was an area within the POA of the hypothalamus that was five times larger in males compared to the females and they called this the sexually dimorphic nucleus of the

POA (Becker et al., 2002; Gorski, 1973, 1985). The same area in human males has been found to be larger than in human females (Swaab, 2003). In the 1970s, Maclean documented that the limbic system is associated with sexuality (MacLean, 1974, 1978). The mapping of the areas in the brain associated with sexuality has resulted from stimulation studies in animals including implanted electrodes, and then lesion studies. Across a number of mammalian species lesions of the medial preoptic anterior (MPOA) hypothalamic area has a very strong impact on sexual behavior to the point of eliminating it (Bancroft, 1989; 2002). Studies of implanted electrodes in anaesthetized mammals have identified sites that result in ejaculation or an erection. Much of this work was done in the 1960s and 1970s and showed that the areas that have sexual effects when stimulated are, the POA; the lateral hypothalamus; the tegmentum, and the anterior part of the cingulate gyrus (Bancroft, 1989; 2002). There are also excitatory and inhibitory mechanisms affecting the peripheral response to an erection. There appears to be a normal level of inhibition from the higher cerebral centres inhibiting erections by setting an inhibitory cerebral tone. This is supported in spinal injury where the threshold for local reflex erections is decreased. This supports the removal of inhibitory tone from the cerebral centers (Bancroft, 1989; 1999; 2002). In 1979, Perachio and colleagues completed a study of implanted electrodes in the brain of rhesus monkeys that were freely moving and were awake. Stimulation of the lateral hypothalamus and dorsomedial nucleus of the hypothalamus led to coital behavior and ejaculation, which exactly simulated the typical mounting behavior of rhesus monkeys. Stimulation of the POA also resulted in mounting behavior but no ejaculation. They concluded that these areas were responsible for copulatory behavior with the POA being most specific (Perachio & Alexander, 1979).

In humans, various pathological states with specific neuroanatomical lesions has helped understand the cerebral representation of sexuality. This is complicated in the sense that some lesions cause disinhibited of behavior that may include hypersexuality. This can be extrapolated to assume that lesions in various brain areas are specifically related to different types of sexual behavior.

Besides the neuroanatomical structure of the central nervous system, the autonomic nervous system has two parts, the sympathetic and parasympathetic nervous systems which are closely related to sexuality.

The sympathetic nervous system originates in the upper part of the spinal cord from the cervical section to the L4 section of the lumbar spine. The parasympathetic nervous system emerges from the brain through cranial nerves and especially the vagus nerve and in a lower section which originates from the sacral section of the spinal cord. The sympathetic and parasympathetic nervous systems balance each other out. Further, each has their own neurotransmitters, noradrenaline in the sympathetic nervous system, and acetylcholine in the parasympathetic nervous system. The sympathetic nervous system is referred to as adrenergic transmission and the parasympathetic nervous system as the cholinergic system. Adrenergic transmission has two types of receptors, α and β. These are further subdivided into α_1 and α_2 and β_1 and β_2. β receptors are generally inhibitory and α receptors are excitatory. β_1 receptors are mainly in cardiac muscle with β_2 in smooth muscle in the intestine, the bronchi as well as vascular smooth muscle. α_1 receptors constrict smooth muscle and α_2 receptors when stimulated inhibit the release of noradrenaline at the synapses in presynaptic or a regulation role (Bancroft, 1989; 1999). These receptors play an important role in the affects of sexual arousal on the genitals of both males and females. In terms of neurotransmitters in the central nervous system a number of other neurochemical agents are involved including gamma-aminobutyric acid (GABA). They have excitatory and inhibitory effects in the central nervous system which can have an impact on sexuality. A full review is beyond the scope of this chapter.

Sexual Arousal

The central nervous system response to external stimuli is also important in sexual arousal. In nonhuman mammals olfactory stimuli are very important, particularly through pheromones. Vaginal secretions when a female is in oestrus provide olfactory stimulation to males, which leads to sexual interest and sexual arousal. Olfactory stimuli are most likely less important in humans compared to visual stimuli, although there is a current debate about the affects of pheromones in humans. Tactile stimuli are clearly important in the stimulation of the genital region leading to tumescence of the penis and the clitoris. The human male and human female has been shown to become sexually aroused to visual stimuli in the laboratory.

Sexual arousal is a concept that has both psychological and physiological components to it. Sexual arousal can be measured in the laboratory through tumescence in the genitals of both males and females. Sexual arousal can be the result of a subjective sense of sexual interest or sexual appetite, similar to hunger or thirst as other basic biological drives. This sexual appetite function causes the organism to seek out sexual relief by finding a sexual partner to interact with. An intermediate step is clearly sexual arousal which contributes to the motivating function to seek out the sexual partner. As simple as this description of sexual arousal appears to be, it is an extremely complex interacting system of stimulation of the central nervous system by external stimuli such as visual stimuli, internal stimuli such a sexual fantasy; leading to sexually motivated behavior; and then a sexual interaction leading to orgasm. It is extremely complicated in terms of concepts of sexual preference and sexual orientation. This includes sexual orientation and can also include age orientation when seeking out a suitable partner. The underlying neurobiological components of sexual arousal as already outlined involve a complicated interaction between neurotransmitters, neurohormones, and steroid hormones.

erections were impaired by infusions of an oxytocin receptor antagonist or a competitive inhibitor of nitric oxide (NO) administered to the lateral ventricle of the brain.

Infusions of L-arginine or morphine to the paraventricular nucleus of the hypothalamus reduced these types of erections, by reducing concentrations of nitrous oxide (N_2O) in the nucleus. This suggested a central mechanism for NO in noncontact erections. A competitive inhibitor of NO was infused into the medial POA and this increased the number of seminal emissions in a test of the reflex emissions (Cantor et al., 1999; Moses & Hull, 1999; Pfaus, 1999). Testosterone administered to castrated male rats increases the number of NO labeled neurons in the medial POA indicating an increase in the synthesis of NO (Du & Hull, 1999; Melis, Spano, Succu, & Argiolas, 1999; Melis, Succu, Spano, & Argiolas, 1999; Pfaus, 1999). Certain drugs and hormones have an effect on copulation and sexual stimulation. Ejaculation can be facilitated by an agonist of the 5-HT1a receptor. Dopamine interaction with the serotonin system, both in the POA and systematically, has also been examined in terms of the stimulation of sexual behavior (Matuszewich et al., 1999).

Sexual Dysfunction

Animal models of human sexual dysfunction have been studied more recently. Specifically, fluoxetine has been studied in sexually active male and female rats from the standpoint of subchronic effects and chronic effects of treatment. In male rats 6 weeks of daily treatment produced a progressive decline in the number of ejaculations which was both dose and time dependent. There was also a decline in anticipatory sexual excitement. There were no effects on the latency period to initiate copulation or the number or rates of intromissions meaning that fluoxetine did not actually cause specific sexual dysfunction such as impotence or erectile dysfunction. A single dose of oxytocin reduced the decline in ejaculation (Cantor, Binik, & Pfaus, 1999; Pfaus, 1999). Studies on the stimulation of sexual arousal in rats have also helped to elicit underlying neurobiological mechanisms. This research looked at noncontact erections in male rats, which can be compared to erections secondary to sexual fantasies in humans. In sexually experienced but castrated male rats noncontact erections occurred when stimulated by implants of the testosterone and DHT but not estradiol. The noncontact

HUMAN SEXUAL BEHAVIOR

Much of the understanding of the neurobiology of human sexual behavior has been based on pathological studies of endrocrine disorders; as well as the observations of the effects of pharmacological agents on sexual behavior. The neuropharmacology of serotonin has been a very important component of this understanding. By 1953 it was known that serotonin was in three locations in the body, specifically platelets, the gastrointestinal system, and the brain, based on research in animals (Sjoerdsma & Palfreyman, 1990). Methods for the extraction and assays of serotonin were developed and initially its work in humans related to its possible involvement in hypertension (Sjoerdsma & Palfreyman, 1990). This work evolved with the study of carcinoid syndrome and eventually the role of serotonin in mental disorder in the 1950s and 1960s (Sjoerdsma & Palfreyman, 1990). In the 1970s important observations occurred, specifically that serotonin precursors L-tryptophan and 5-hydroxy tryptophan had antidepressant properties; the norepinephrine precursor L-3, 4-dihydroxyphenylalanine (L-dopa) did not have antidepressant properties, coupled with other neuro-chemical work, led to the development of selective inhibitors of serotonin uptake (SSRIs), which proved to be antidepressants (Sjoerdsma & Palfreyman, 1990). This led to the development of the SSRIs as pharmacological agents, following a classic paper by Peroutka and Snyder in 1979 which defined *multiple serotonin receptors*. They provided the classification of 5-HT1 and 5-HT2 receptors. (Peroutka & Snyder, 1979). Further work at the Merrell Dow Research Institute in Strasbourg, France led to the development of SSRIs for use in human pharmacological treatment. (Sjoerdsma & Palfreyman, 1990). Further research of serotonin receptors has led to sub receptors systems 5-HT1a; 5-HT1b; 5-HT1c; 5-HT1d; 5-HT1e; 5-HT1f; 5-HT2a; 5-HT2b; 5-HT-2c; 5-HT3; 5-HT4; 5-HT5; 5-HT6; 5-HT7 as well as other new work some other receptors, based on research work using receptor binding protocols; common second messenger coupling, and research using various ligands. All of the receptors for serotonin belong to a family of G protein–coupled receptors (Kennett, 2000). Serotonin is a sophisticated neurotransmitter involving different receptor classes. These classes of receptors are not only differentiated by their neuropharmacological properties but also by their distribution in various brain systems. Therefore serotonin acts on different brain systems through different receptor subtypes. The serotonin receptors and subtypes of receptors are found principally in the limbic system. The actual distribution and function of the subtypes of receptors is beyond the scope of this chapter. As the limbic system is mostly involved with the modulation of emotion, it is not surprising that drugs that potentiate the action of serotonin would have an effect on mood, aggression, sex, as well as other biological drives such as sleep and appetite. When a SSRI is administered, serotonin concentrations in the synaptic cleft increases as it cannot be removed by the reuptake carrier or serotonin transporter. There is also a decrease in serotonin turnover. This is supported by animal model studies in behavioral pharmacology. There is also evidence that serotonin may be implicated in the regulation of anterior pituitary hormones in particular PRL but also corticotropin and growth hormone (Cowen, Anderson, & Gartside, 1990 a; Cowen & Sargent, 1997). Some time ago it was clear that temperature and endocrine responses could be used to study the functional sensitivity of different serotonin receptor subtypes

(Cowen, Cohen, McCance, & Friston, 1990b). The evidence is that PRL is mediated through 5-HT1 receptors and specifically the 5-HT1a receptor (Cowen, 2000).

There is also an interesting finding that over time the level of reported sexual dysfunction caused by SSRIs has increased in different studies. Stark and Hardison in 1985 reviewed multicenter studies of fluoxetine compared to placebo and imipramine, and overall they reported the incidence of sexual dysfunction in fluoxetine treated patients as 2.7%. Herman et al., (1990) studied 60 patients treated with fluoxetine and reported sexual dysfunction usually anorgasmia or delayed orgasm as 8.3%. This was followed by Zajecka et al. (1991) in the study of 77 patients where the reported incidence of sexual dysfunction was 7.8%. Jacobsen (1992) looked at outpatients over 2 years treated with fluoxetine for major depression and found that 34% of 160 outpatients reported the onset of sexual dysfunction after the successful treatment of major depression. This was broken down into 10% of patients who reported decreased libido; 13% reported decreased sexual responsiveness, and 11% reported declines in both areas. Balon et al. (1993) found that the incidence of sexual dysfunction was 43.3% during antidepressant treatment with fluoxetine. Paterson (1993) reported the incidence to be 75%. (See Table 4.1.) This clearly showed that over time the incidence of sexual dysfunction after treatment with fluoxetine hydrochloride increased dramatically in self-reported surveys. Although it is not clear why this trend occurred, the high levels of sexual dysfunction reported in the latter studies is in keeping with what would be expected on the basis of what is known from animal studies on serotonin. As serotonin levels increase, sexual drive and other aspects of sexual behavior decreases. Further, it is quite clear

TABLE 4.1 Studies of Sexual Dysfunction Associated with Fluoxetine Hydrochloride from 1985 to 1993

Study	Incidence of Sexual Dysfunction (%)
Stark & Hardison, 1985	2.7
Herman et al., 1990	8.3
Zajecka et al., 1991	7.8
Jacobsen 1992	34.0
Balon et al., 1993	42.9
Patterson, 1993	75.0

that different drugs such as fluoxetine and fluvoxamine most likely have different actions at different receptors. Iatrogenically induced sexual dysfunction has been seen in many pharmacological agents and specifically the pharmacological agents used in psychiatry. Drug-induced sexual dysfunction has become an important factor in understanding the neurobiological aspects of human sexuality.

The study of the neurobiology of hypersexuality although limited can also help in understanding the neurobiology of the paraphilias. Although extensive animal research has been conducted in this area, this is beyond the scope of this chapter and only the research in relation to human sexuality will be briefly reviewed. In general terms, research has shown that various brain lesions can lead to disinhibited sexual behavior. The neurological and neuropsychiatric literature has considerable references with regard to disinhibited behavior, including sexual behavior, as a result of frontal lobe lesions. The main issues here are that this is a general disinhibition of behavior and not specific to sexual behavior. What has been described as "presenting clinically in dementia patients with frontal lobe lesions" is paraphilic behavior for the first time in their history. This is clearly contrary to the natural history of the paraphilias and therefore secondary to the dementia and disinhibited behavior. A wide spectrum of disinhibited sexual behavior has been reported including exhibitionism-like, pedophilic-like, and what can be described broadly as hypersexuality. Further paraphilic-like behavior has been reported secondary to a wide variety of neuropsychiatric disorders. These include temporal lobe epilepsy; post encephalitic neuropsychiatric syndrome; septal lesions; frontal lobe lesions; bilateral temporal lobe lesions; cerebral tumors in various brain areas, and multiple sclerosis (Chow, 1999). Nonparaphilic hypersexuality and hyposexuality have been reported in relation to various brain lesions. There has also been some evidence of obsessive-compulsive disorder (OCD)-type behavior reported in association with various brain lesions (Chow, 1999). There are also interesting relationships that have been described with OCD and Tourette's disorder. This points toward the corticostriatal neurocircuits being involved as well as there being various types of behavior that overlap between the two conditions (Comings, 1987; Comings & Comings, 1987a, 1987b; Stein, 1996; Stein, Hugo, Oosthuizen, Hawkridge, & van Heerden, 2000). The types of behavior that

have been described in Tourette's disorder includes a spectrum of paraphilic-like and nonparaphilic-like sexual behaviors and even the classic Tourette's disorder symptoms of coprolalia and copropraxia have a sexual component to them (Kerbeshian & Burd 1991). There is also some evidence that in males, tic-related disorders, including Tourette's disorder may be involved with fetal androgenization (Alexander & Peterson, 2004). There is also an hypothesis that Tourette's disorder has an underlying dopamine abnormality (Minzer, Lee, Hong, & Singer, 2004). In neurobiological terms, Tourette's disorder, obsessive-compulsive disorder, and various manifestations of paraphilic and nonparaphilic behavior are related to dopamine abnormalities and possibly linked to fetal androgenization. Again there is a significant volume of literature that covers this area that supports these connections but only a small fraction of the literature is referenced in this chapter. There is also the literature on treatment that shows the symptoms of OCD as well as Tourette's disorder respond to serotonin reuptake inhibitors as well as pharmacological agents that affect dopamine levels such as conventional and atypical antipsychotic agents.

Hypersexuality is poorly defined in the sexual literature and is not defined in DSM-IV. An attempt by Kinsey to define hypersexuality included the use of the Total Sexual Outlet which was the number of orgasm measured every 7 days. Kafka has also attempted to better define hypersexuality, looking at compulsive sexual behavior and paraphilias and related disorders (Kafka, 1994a, 1994b; Kafka & Hennen, 2003). Individuals with paraphilia-related disorders in a small study were defined as having greater than 5 orgasms per week as well as other measures of sexual behavior (Kafka, 2003). The problem, however, is that large population prevalence studies are needed to clearly define hypersexuality. It is clear, however, that hypersexuality may be paraphilic or nonparaphilic although the absolute measures of orgasm rates are not clearly defined. What is certain is that some individuals report high levels of sexual drive and exhibit compulsive sexual behaviors that cause them significant personal distress and dysfunction. These behaviors may be paraphilic or if they are nonparaphilic include compulsive use of masturbation compulsive use of pornography, and may lead to high risk sexual behaviors such as of promiscuous sexual behavior with prostitutes or anonymous sexual partners.

The actual incidence and prevalence of the paraphilias and paraphilia-related disorders is unknown (Bradford, Boulet, & Pawlak, 1992). The most comprehensive information to assist with the understanding of the neurobiology of the paraphilias comes from the pharmacological treatment studies of sexual offenders and sexually deviant men. The studies have their origins in those involving surgical castration, principally coming out of Europe in the middle part of the last century, followed by antiandrogen treatment studies using cyproterone acetate medroxyprogesterone acetate and to a lesser extent oestrogen treatments. This was followed by the use of SSRIs and LHRH agonists. These treatments now form a significant part of the treatment of sex offenders worldwide. Bradford, (2000), published an algorithm for the treatment of the paraphilias. The first part of the algorithm is a classification of the severity of the paraphilias into four categories:

1. Mild
2. Moderate
3. Severe
4. Catastrophic

These followed the scheme originally outlined in DSM-III-R (American Psychiatric Association & American Psychiatric Association Work Group to Revise DSM-III, 1987). The last category of Catastrophic was added to deal with individuals with sexual sadism and the risk of severe sexual violence or a sexually motivated homicide being the type of sexual behavior they presented with. The actual algorithm consists of six levels of treatment for the four categories of paraphilias:

Level 1: Regardless of the severity of the paraphilia, all paraphilias are treated with some form of cognitive behavioral treatment preferably a relapse prevention program.

Level 2: Pharmacological treatment starts with the use of SSRIs. The common pharmacological treatments are the use of sertraline and fluoxetine. These are the most suitable as they reduce sexual drive and sexual fantasies without causing sexual dysfunction such as erectile difficulties or delayed ejaculation. The usual dosage would be 150 mg to 250 mg of sertraline per day or 40 mg to 60 mg of fluoxetine per day.

Level 3: If the SSRIs are not effective in 6 to 12 weeks of treatment, meaning no reduction in sexual fantasy or significant reduction in sexual drive, using adequate dosages, a small dose of an oral antiandrogen, either cyproterone acetate 50 mg per day or medroxyprogesterone acetate 50 mg per day would be added to the SSRI. This would be the treatment approach most likely used in moderate cases of paraphilias.

Level 4: If control was not adequate (as outlined above in relation to sexual fantasies and sexual drive) at level three men oral antiandrogen treatment would commence. This would generally involve 50 mg to 300 mg of cyproterone acetate per day or 50 mg to 300 mg of medroxyprogesterone acetate per day. This would be used in moderate and in some severe cases of paraphilias.

Level 5: This would be full intramuscular antiandrogen treatment, either cyproterone acetate or medroxyprogesterone acetate. Cyproterone acetate would be given at dosage levels of 100 mg to 200 mg usually biweekly. Medroxyprogesterone acetate would be given starting at 400 mg per week and gradually going to 400 mg every 4 weeks during a maintenance phase.

Level 6: This would be the use of LHRH agonists to create a state of pharmacological castration. The usual medications with the leuprolide acetate, or goserelin acetate given monthly at 7.5 mg per month. With goserelin acetate an optional 3-monthly injection can be given.

The three main categories of pharmacological treatment for the paraphilias are as follows:

- specific serotonin reuptake inhibitors
- antiandrogen and hormonal treatments
- LHRH agonists

The various studies of pharmacological treatment can be found covered in detail in another chapter in this book and in other publications on the subject (Bradford, 1999, 2000, 2001; Bradford & Pawlak, 1993a, 1993b).

CONCLUSION

There is considerable knowledge of the neurobiological underpinnings of the paraphilias and non-paraphilic hypersexuality. Considerable advances have been made in understanding the monoamine neurotransmitters and how they affect sexual behavior. The effects of hormones on sexual behavior are mainly seen in the pharmacological treatment studies. The addition of LHRH agonists has provided a powerful pharmacological castration for the management of difficult and high risk paraphilias. As drugs develop, that have actions on serotonin receptors subtypes this should considerably add to our understanding of the contribution of monoamine neurotransmitters to the neurobiology of sexual behavior. Research on sex hormone and specifically on various types of hormonal receptors and hormone sensitive neurons should also contribute significantly to our understanding of the neurobiology of the paraphilias.

References

Alexander, G. M. & Peterson, B. S. (2004). Testing the prenatal hormone hypothesis of tic-related disorders: gender identity and gender role behavior. *Development and Psychopathology*, 16(2), 407–420.

American Psychiatric Association. & American Psychiatric Association. Work Group to Revise DSM-III. (1987). *Diagnostic and Statistical Manual of Mental Disorders: DSM-III-R*, 3rd Edition. Washington, D.C.: American Psychiatric Association.

Balon, R., Yeragani, V. K., Pohl, R., & Ramesh, C. (1993). Sexual dysfunction during antidepressant treatment. *The Journal of Clinical Psychiatry*, 54(6), 209–212.

Bancroft, J. (1984). Hormones and human sexual behavior. *Journal of Sex & Marital Therapy*, 10(1), 3–21.

Bancroft, J. (1989). *Human Sexuality and its Problems*, 2nd Edition. Edinburgh; New York: Churchill Livingstone.

Bancroft, J. (1999). Central inhibition of sexual response in the male: A theoretical perspective. *Neuroscience and Biobehavioral Reviews*, 23(6), 763–784.

Bancroft, J. (2002). Biological factors in human sexuality. *Journal of Sex Research*, 39(1), 15–21.

Becker, J. B. (Ed.). (2002). *Behavioral Endocrinology, 2nd Edition*. Cambridge, Mass: MIT Press.

Becker, J. B., Breedlove, S. M., Crews, D., & McCarthy, M. M. (2002). *Behavioral Endocrinology*. Cambridge, MA: Massuchusetts Institute of Technology Press.

Bradford, J. (2000). The treatment of sexual deviation using a pharmacological approach. *Journal of Sex Research*, 37, 248–257.

Bradford, J. M. (1999). The paraphilias, obsessive compulsive spectrum disorder, and the treatment of sexually deviant behaviour. *The Psychiatric Quarterly*, 70(3), 209–219.

Bradford, J. M. (2001). The neurobiology, neuropharmacology, and pharmacological treatment of the paraphilias and compulsive sexual behaviour. *Canadian Journal of Psychiatry. Revue Canadienne De Psychiatrie*, 46(1), 26–34.

Bradford, J. M., Boulet, J., & Pawlak, A. (1992). The paraphilias: a multiplicity of deviant behaviours. *Canadian Journal of Psychiatry. Revue Canadienne De Psychiatrie*, 37(2), 104–108.

Bradford, J. M. & Pawlak, A. (1993a). Double-blind placebo crossover study of cyproterone acetate in the treatment of the paraphilias. *Archives of Sexual Behavior*, 22(5), 383–402.

Bradford, J. M. & Pawlak, A. (1993b). Effects of cyproterone acetate on sexual arousal patterns of pedophiles. *Archives of Sexual Behavior*, 22(6), 629–641.

Cantor, J. M., Binik, Y. M., & Pfaus, J. G. (1999). Chronic fluoxetine inhibits sexual behavior in the male rat: Reversal with oxytocin. *Psychopharmacology (Berl)*, 144(4), 355–362.

Chow T. W. C. J. (1999). *Neuropsychiatry: Clinical Assessment and Approach to Diagnosis*, 7th Edition. Philadelphia: Lippincott Williams and Wilkins.

Comings, D. E. (1987). A controlled study of Tourette syndrome. VII. Summary: A common genetic disorder causing disinhibition of the limbic system. *American Journal of Human Genetics*, 41(5), 839–866.

Comings, D. E. & Comings, B. G. (1987a). A controlled study of Tourette syndrome. II. Conduct. *American Journal of Human Genetics*, 41(5), 742–760.

Comings, D. E. & Comings, B. G. (1987b). A controlled study of Tourette syndrome. IV. Obsessions, compulsions, and schizoid behaviors. *American Journal of Human Genetics*, 41(5), 782–803.

Cowen, P. J. (2000). Psychopharmacology of 5-HT(1A) receptors. *Nuclear Medicine and Biology*, 27(5), 437–439.

Cowen, P. J., Anderson, I. M., & Gartside, S. E. (1990a). Endocrinological responses to 5-HT. *Annals of the New York Academy of Sciences*, 600, 250–257; discussion 257–259.

Cowen, P. J., Cohen, P. R., McCance, S. L., & Friston, K. J. (1990b). 5-HT neuroendocrine responses during psychotropic drug treatment: An investigation of the effects of lithium. *Journal of Neuroscience Methods*, 34(1–3), 201–205.

Cowen, P. J. & Sargent, P. A. (1997). Changes in plasma prolactin during SSRI treatment: Evidence for a delayed increase in 5-HT neurotransmission. *Journal of Psychopharmacology (Oxford, England)*, 11(4), 345–348.

Du, J. & Hull, E. M. (1999). Effects of testosterone on neuronal nitric oxide synthase and tyrosine hydroxylase. *Brain Research*, 836(1–2), 90–98.

Gorski, R. A. (1973). *Mechanisms of Androgen Induced Masculine Differentiation of the Rat Brain*. New York,: Plenum Press.

Gorski, R. A. (1985). Sexual dimorphisms of the brain. *Journal of Animal Science*, 61(Suppl 3), 38–61.

Herman, J. B., Brotman, A. W., Pollack, M. H., Falk, W. E., Biederman, J., & Rosenbaum, J. F. (1990). Fluoxetine-induced sexual dysfunction. *The Journal of Clinical Psychiatry*, 51(1), 25–27.

Jacobsen, F. M. (1992). Fluoxetine-induced sexual dysfunction and an open trial of yohimbine. *The Journal of Clinical Psychiatry*, 53(4), 119–122.

Kafka, M. P. (1994a). Paraphilia-related disorders—common, neglected, and misunderstood. *Harvard Review of Psychiatry*, 2(1), 39–40; discussion 41–32.

Kafka, M. P. (1994b). Sertraline pharmacotherapy for paraphilias and paraphilia-related disorders: An open trial. *Annals of Clinical Psychiatry*, 6(3), 189–195.

Kafka, M. P. (2003). Sex offending and sexual appetite: The clinical and theoretical relevance of hypersexual desire. *International Journal of Offender Therapy and Comparative Criminology*, 47(4), 439–451.

Kafka, M. P. & Hennen, J. (2003). Hypersexual desire in males: Are males with paraphilias different from males with paraphilia-related disorders? *Sexual Abuse*, 15(4), 307–321.

Kennett, G. (2000). *Serotonin Receptors and Their Function*. Bristol (UK): Tocris.

Kerbeshian, J. & Burd, L. (1991). Tourette syndrome and her current paraphilic masturbatory fantasy. *Canadian Journal of Psychiatry*, 36, 155–157.

MacLean, P. D. (1974). *Influence of Limbic Cortex on Hypothalamus. New Anatomic and Microelectrode Findings.* Basel, New York: Karger.

MacLean, P. D. (1978). *Challenges of the Papez Heritage.* New York: Plenum Press.

Matuszewich, L., Lorrain, D. S., Trujillo, R., Dominguez, J., Putnam, S. K., & Hull, E. M. (1999). Partial antagonism of 8-OH-DPAT'S effects on male rat sexual behavior with a D2, but not a 5-HT1A, antagonist. *Brain Research*, 820(1–2), 55–62.

Melis, M. R., Spano, M. S., Succu, S., & Argiolas, A. (1999). The oxytocin antagonist d(CH2)5Tyr(Me)2-Orn8-vasotocin reduces non-contact penile erections in male rats. *Neuroscience Letters*, 265(3), 171–174.

Melis, M. R., Succu, S., Spano, M. S., & Argiolas, A. (1999). Morphine injected into the paraventricular nucleus of the hypothalamus prevents noncontact penile erections and impairs copulation: involvement of nitric oxide. *The European Journal of Neuroscience*, 11(6), 1857–1864.

Minzer, K., Lee, O., Hong, J. J., & Singer, H. S. (2004). Increased prefrontal D2 protein in Tourette syndrome: A postmortem analysis of frontal cortex and striatum. *Journal of the Neurological Sciences*, 219(1–2), 55–61.

Moses, J. & Hull, E. M. (1999). A nitric oxide synthesis inhibitor administered into the medial preoptic area increases seminal emissions in an ex copula reflex test. *Pharmacology, Biochemistry, and Behavior*, 63(3), 345–348.

Patterson, W. M. (1993). Fluoxetine-induced sexual dysfunction. *The Journal of Clinical Psychiatry*, 54(2), 71.

Perachio, A. A, Marr, L. D, & Alexander, M. (1979). Sexual behaviour in male rhesus monkeys elicited by electrical stimulation of the preoptic and hypothalamic areas. *Brain Research*, 177, 523–525.

Peroutka, S. & Snyder, S. H. (1979). Multiple serotonin receptors: Differential binding of [3H] 5-hydroxy tryptamine,[3H] lysergic acid diethylamide and [3H] spiroperidol. *Molecular Pharmacology*, 16, 687–699.

Pfaus, J. G. (1999). Neurobiology of sexual behavior. *Current Opinion in Neurobiology*, 9(6), 751–758.

Sjoerdsma, A. & Palfreyman, M. G. (1990). History of serotonin and serotinin disorders. *Annals of the New York Academy of Sciences*, 600, 1–7; discussion 7–8.

Stark, P. & Hardison, C. D. (1985). A review of multicenter controlled studies of fluoxetine vs. imipramine and placebo in outpatients with major depressive disorder. *The Journal of Clinical Psychiatry*, 46(3 Pt 2), 53–58.

Stein, D. (1996). The neurobiology of obsessive-compulsive disorder. *The Neuroscientist*, 2, 300–305.

Stein, D., Hugo, F., Oosthuizen, P., Hawkridge, S. M., & van Heerden, B. (2000). Neuropsychiatry of hypersexuality. *CNS Spectrums*, 5, 36–46.

Swaab, D. F. (2003). *The Human Hypothalamus : Basic and Clinical Aspects, 1st Edition.* Amsterdam; Boston: Elsevier.

Toran-Allerand, C. (1978). Gonadal hormones and brain development: Cellular aspects of sexual differentiation. *American Zoologist*, 18(3), 553–566.

Zajecka, J., Fawcett, J., Schaff, M., Jeffriess, H., & Guy, C. (1991). The role of serotonin in sexual dysfunction: fluoxetine-associated orgasm dysfunction. *The Journal of Clinical Psychiatry*, 52(2), 66–68.

Part III

Assessment and Diagnosis

Chapter 5

Violence Risk Assessment

Debra A. Pinals, Chad E. Tillbrook, and Denise L. Mumley

Risk assessment is a broad concept with many meanings that vary depending on the context. Sex offender and violence risk assessments have common features but have emerged with some distinct approaches. Clinical interviews may focus on different aspects of a person's history, and actuarial tools have emerged that are unique to these distinct types of assessments. The involvement of psychiatric and other mental health professionals in violence risk assessment most appropriately encompasses those situations involving questions related to diagnostic assessments, treatment needs, and risk management. Mental health expertise is often sought in clinical and medicolegal contexts, as a means of assisting decision makers involved in commitment and release contexts.

Overlap often exists between the need to assess risk factors related to harmful sexual behaviors and the need to assess risk of future violence. As the two lines of research in sex offender risk assessment and violence risk assessment continue to expand, clinicians in the position of assessing risk among sex offenders will also need to maintain an awareness of the literature related to general violence risk assessment. The purpose of this chapter is to review research and current knowledge related to general violence risk assessment and its overlap with mental illness, and to delineate approaches to violence risk assessments on the basis of current understanding of risk factors. The impact of a clinician providing an assessment of an individual's risk of violence, just like assessment of risk of sexual reoffending, can be great, influencing determinations that may result in loss of liberty and even death (e.g., Estelle vs. Smith, 1980). Thus, it behooves professionals involved to have up to date knowledge of assessment approaches and potential consequences, both intended and unintended, in any given context.

CONTEXTUAL BASIS FOR VIOLENCE RISK ASSESSMENTS

Mental health professionals have long been aware of the need to assess their patients for risk of suicide.

Historically, however, patients were not consistently assessed for homicidal thoughts (Sanders, Milne, Brown, & Bell, 2000). Several factors have converged that have resulted in an increased awareness, on the part of mental health professionals, of the importance of incorporating evidence-based violence risk assessment into routine clinical management and clinical assessment. Evolving laws related to civil commitment in nonsex offender contexts (Allbright, Levy, & Wagle, 2002; Lessard vs. Schmidt, 1972; Pinals & Hoge, 2003), release decisions for forensic and correctional populations (Baxstrom vs. Herold, 1966; Foucha vs. Louisiana, 1992; R. vs. Demers, 2004; Winko vs. British Columbia [Forensic Psychiatric Institute], 1999), liability concerns related to public safety (Smith vs. Jones, 1999; Tarasoff vs. Regents of the University of California, 1976), and management of violence risk among out-patients and persons moving to less restrictive settings (Douglas, Ogloff, & Hart 2003; R. vs. Tulikorpi, 2004; Swartz et al., 1999), for example, have influenced this trend. As clinicians have found themselves increasingly in positions where violence risk assessments are conducted, examples of overzealous predictions of future violence, and trepidation about jeopardizing public safety have heightened the need to better understand the potential impact of and best approaches to violence risk analyses. Though a detailed review of risk management strategies is beyond the scope of this chapter, Borum et al. (1996), identified four important areas in understanding the assessment and management of violence risk: The relationship between violence and various mental disorders, the rates of violence among clinical populations, the ability of mental health professionals to "predict" violence, and specific risk factors related to violence. Aspects of these topic areas as they relate to violence risk assessment are reviewed subsequently.

VIOLENCE AND MENTAL ILLNESS: AN EVOLVING LITERATURE

The assumption that persons with mental illness are dangerous is not new, and the disadvantage that has historically faced persons with mental disabilities as a result of that assumption has been acknowledged many times over in many contexts. For example, the Supreme Court of Canada observed that mental illness is one of the least understood and least accepted of all illnesses. Further, the

Court said it creates fear and stereotypical responses that may lead to discrimination and labeling (Battlesfords and District Co-operatives Ltd. vs. Gibbs 1995; R. vs. Swain, 1991). As well, images of persons with mental illness engendering fear because of their perceived great risk of violence have been popularized in the modern media but are longstanding perceptions (Monahan, 1992) that continue to be investigated (Van Dorn, Swanson, Elbogen, & Swartz, 2005). Early research of the twentieth century, however, indicated that persons with mental illness did not present a greater risk of violence than persons in the general population. Although this notion took hold and predominated for many years, the relationship between mental disorders and violence continued to command research attention. Over time, a new generation of scientific thought regarding the relationship between mental illness and violence evolved. Specifically, several studies emerged leading to conclusions that there is a significant association between mental illness and the likelihood of engaging in violence, though the relationship is felt to be small (Appelbaum, 1994; Monahan, 1992; Mulvey, 1994).

Several studies from the late 1980s to early 1990s demonstrated increased rates of violence among persons who were hospitalized (Hodgins, 1992; Steadman et al., 1994). Further solidifying the research related to violence and mental illness were several studies examining large community samples. The first of such studies, often cited, is the report by Swanson and colleagues (1990). In their study, they reviewed data derived from the Epidemiological Catchment Area (ECA) Surveys, one of the largest American studies of the prevalence of psychiatric disorders in the community at the time. The ECA study involved structured diagnostic interviews, and respondents were assessed to see whether they met criteria for psychiatric disorders within the 12 months preceding the interviews. Embedded in the diagnostic items were five questions related to violence (e.g., whether subjects had ever hit or thrown things at their spouse or partner and whether subjects had been in more than one fight since age 18 that came to swapping blows, etc.). Additionally, questions were asked regarding how recently any reported violence occurred.

Out of approximately 10,000 respondents, Swanson and colleagues (1990) identified a base rate of reported violence of 2% among persons with no diagnosable disorder. A 5-fold increased risk (approximately 11%) of reported violence was observed among persons with a diagnosable mental illness. Interestingly, this pattern appeared similar for those with schizophrenia, bipolar disorder, and major depressive disorders. Alcohol-related disorders accounted for approximately a 12-fold increase (24.6%) in violence risk, while other drug-related disorders accounted for approximately a 15-fold increased risk (34.7%). Moreover, the combination of diagnoses increased violence risk, especially when a substance use disorder was one of the diagnoses involved.

Subsequent community studies supported and expanded the findings of Swanson and colleagues. Link et al. (1992) found that community patient groups (where no diagnoses were reported) had significantly higher rates of arrest, hitting, weapon use, and hurting someone in a fight, compared to the community sample of nonpatient groups, even when socioeconomic factors were considered. Furthermore, they found that psychotic symptoms contributed to the violence risk among all subjects.

A follow-up study by Link and Stueve (1994) examined whether specific types of psychotic symptoms accounted for the increased rates of violence in the earlier study by Link and colleagues. Violence examined, included hitting, fighting, and weapon use. Symptoms of particular interest included those referred to as "threat/control-override," or TCO, delusions, such as beliefs that subjects were being threatened, that thoughts were being inserted into subjects' minds, or that their minds were controlled by outside forces. Looking at 232 patients and approximately 521 community residents, these authors found that the greater the degree of TCO symptoms, the greater the likelihood of violence. A subsequent reexamination of data by Swanson and colleagues (1996) similarly found an association between TCO symptoms and reports of violent behavior, and an even greater risk of violence when TCO symptoms were combined with substance abuse. The association between TCO symptoms and increased violence risk has since been called into some doubt (Monahan et al., 2001). Still, robust findings regarding the relationship between substance use and risk of violence among persons with mental disorders continue to be replicated, with one author suggesting that very early onset of substance use followed by the emergence of mental illness may be associated with the highest risk of violence in the community (Fulwiler, Grossman, Forbes, &

Ruthazer, 1997). Additional studies examining other symptoms of mental illness and their relationship to violence risk are described in the following text.

As the number of studies related to the relationship of violence and mental illness grew, increasing attention was paid to the methodology behind the science. The MacArthur Violence Risk Assessment Study sought to examine the issue of the prevalence of violence among persons with mental illness using methods that addressed many of the limitations of prior studies. Several studies have emerged from their data. The crux of the study design involved repeated follow-up of 1136 patients who had been recently discharged from civil psychiatric hospitals across three sites. In a major publication of their findings, Steadman and colleagues (1998) identified several critical factors that bear on violence risk assessment and the relationship to mental illness. First, they noted that one data source alone will not provide all the information related to a person's violence risk, and that utilizing self-report (which still provides the most robust information), in combination with records of arrest and hospitalization, and a collateral contact can each incrementally provide additional information. Second, their findings highlighted the importance of defining outcome; in their study "violence" was divided into acts that resulted in physical injury (which included sexual assault, use of a weapon, and threat with a weapon in hand) and other aggressive acts that did not result in injury. Third, they distinguished between persons with more serious mental disorders and those with "other" mental disorders, such as personality disorders and adjustment reactions.

In their study, Steadman and colleagues (1998) reported a 1-year aggregate prevalence of violence as being highest for those persons with "other" mental disorders and substance use disorders (43%). Patients with major mental disorders and substance use demonstrated a 1-year aggregate rate of violence of 31.1%, but when no substance use was involved, patients' 1-year aggregate rate of violence was much lower (17.9%). Furthermore, rates of violence among patients without substance use appeared statistically indistinguishable from rates of violence among the community sample that also did not engage in substance abuse. The findings of the MacArthur study have been discussed widely (Torrey, Stanley, Monahan, & Steadman, 2008) and have highlighted to role of substance use in increasing violence risk and the importance of ongoing research in this area.

In a separate study looking at violence and mental disorders from a birth cohort of young adults in New Zealand, Arsenault and colleagues (2000) reported that individuals with alcohol dependence, marijuana dependence, and disorders of the schizophrenia spectrum were more likely to be violent than controls. This study specifically attempted to explore rates of violence among individuals at an age that is correlated with increased violence (i.e., young adulthood). Further, the study examined substance use in the hours before the violent offense in an effort to examine the effects of acute intoxication on violence, along with issues related to conduct disorder and threat perception. Findings from the study highlighted that persons with mental disorders accounted for significant violence particularly when substance abuse was involved, but that different mental disorders were linked to violence in different ways. The findings suggested that that a variety of contextual and historical variables should also be explored in violence prevention strategies.

A more recent study looking at the prevalence of violence and its correlates among persons with schizophrenia who were residing in the community found that certain symptoms, such as ideas of being persecuted, labeled as "positive" psychotic symptoms, increased the risk of both serious violence and more minor violence (Swanson et al., 2006). In this study looking at approximately 1400 persons with schizophrenia across numerous communities, social withdrawal and other "negative" symptoms seemed to lower risk of serious violence. In general, more serious violence was associated with a history of victimization and childhood misconduct, as well as with psychotic and depressive symptoms. The authors noted that the risk of minor violence seemed to be increased by nonclinical variables such as age, sex, housing environment, and degree of vocational involvement, among other factors. Substance abuse was found to be related to minor violence, but its association with serious violence disappeared once age, recent victimization, positive symptoms of schizophrenia, and childhood conduct problems were controlled for.

Summarizing the findings of these types of studies, it appears that mental disorders (especially personality disorders and adjustment disorders) increase the risk of violence to an extent that is important to track, but that substance abuse specifically, as well as contextual, demographic, and historical variables contribute more significantly to overall violence risk.

PREDICTION OF VIOLENCE BY MENTAL HEALTH PROFESSIONALS

Given the prevailing view at the time that there was little relationship between mental illness and violence, Monahan (1981) reviewed five studies, as of the late 1970s, on the accuracy of clinical prediction of violent behavior. Monahan concluded in a now-often-repeated reference that

> Psychiatrists and psychologists are accurate in no more than one out of three predictions of violent behavior over a several-year period among institutionalized populations that had both committed violence in the past (and thus had higher base rates of violence) and who were diagnosed as mentally ill (Monahan, 1981, p. 47).

In making this statement at the time, Monahan had been relying upon findings based on "first-generation" prediction studies, which were cast in a sociopolitical climate focused on controlling the lives of persons with mental disorders (Melton, Petrila, Poythress, & Slobogin, 1997). Melton and colleagues noted that clinical decisions erred toward making erroneous findings that these persons were dangerous (e.g., many studies were discovering false–positive percentage rates exceeding 50%). These findings are not surprising given the numerous problems that plagued first-generation research, some of which could be fixed and some of which have proven to be inherently difficult to address when studying the prediction of violent behavior (Otto, 1992).

Citing methodological and research design flaws, Monahan called for the "second-generation" of studies described earlier. Given that much of the earlier assessment research was characterized by restricted predictors and simplistic outcome criteria, researchers began paying greater attention to the conceptualization and measurement of risk factors and of violence. Coinciding with the appeal by Monahan, the field began to move away from studying the accuracy of categorical predictions of "dangerous" or "not dangerous," and instead promoting research that focused on risk assessment. The aim has been to begin providing more empirically supported information that is not only clinically meaningful but, importantly, could also inform legal judgments and risk management interventions (Melton et al., 1997).

Four methods to assessing violence risk

Both Douglas and Kropp (2002) and Melton et al. (1997) reviewed the advantages and shortcomings of several methods to assess risk of violence, including clinical, actuarial, anamnestic, and structured professional judgment. Unstructured clinical assessment is a method that relies on unsystematic and potentially dissimilar approaches to case formulations (Melton et al., 1997). The process involves no guidelines for the evaluator, although presumably the clinician would have some familiarity with literature related to violence risk assessment. Decisions are made with considerable clinical discretion and are usually justified according to the qualifications and experience of the person making them (Douglas & Kropp, 2002). An advantage of this unstructured clinical approach is that it allows for an individualistic analysis of the person's problematic behavior. Clinicians who employ this method indicate that they are able to attend to a large number of variables. However, because this method maximizes professional discretion, it is vulnerable to evaluator bias and missing important factors (Douglas & Kropp), and the clinical accuracy and utility of combining and weighing of relevant factors by clinicians yielding findings of "dangerous" or "not dangerous" is unknown (Dawes, Faust, & Meehl, 1989; Melton et al., 1997). This clinical method has been criticized for its lack of reliability, validity, and accountability (Harris, Rice, & Cormier, 2002; Quinsey, Harris, Rice, & Cormier, 1998b).

Actuarial methods predict an individual's likelihood of future violence by mathematically comparing the person to a norm-based reference group using a specific violence risk assessment tool. In contrast to unstructured clinical prediction, an actuarial approach to risk assessment is designed to estimate, in a relative sense, the risk posed by an individual within a specific timeframe, according to the time parameters identified by the research that formed the basis of the actuarial instrument. Grove and Meehl (1996, p. 294) described this approach as a formal "mechanical and algorithmic" method. A mathematical combination of variables is used to generate a prediction that is very rigid; once the specific predictors in an actuarial technique are set, all other information is irrelevant. The advantage lies in the ability to offer predictions and risk assessments with minimal bias, solely on the basis of an examination of empirically supported risk factors. However, its apparent advantages can be viewed as disadvantageous in clinical and forensic settings. For example, an offender who has unique violence-reducing characteristics (e.g., quadriplegic) or situations (e.g., previously targeted victim immigrated to another country) that are not recognized in the literature may still be classified as "dangerous" by an actuarial procedure (Melton et al., 1997). Additional shortcomings include difficulty in generalizing findings to persons outside of the normative group and a tendency on the part of decision makers, such as judges, to favor clinical data and, at times, even ignore highly relevant actuarial data (Melton et al., 1997). Douglas and Kropp (2002) further suggest that actuarial assessments are limited since they only inform us about one's overall level of risk, without information related to risk management.

A third method is referred to as the anamnestic approach to risk assessment (e.g., Melton et al., 1997; Otto, 2000). In this approach, evaluators must "identify violence risk factors through a detailed examination of the individual's history of violent and threatening behavior" (Otto, 2000, p. 1241). Clinicians attempt to identify violent patterns or themes as well as any unique risk factors particular to the individual. By reviewing historical information, clinicians attempt to examine past episodes of violence to ascertain whether there are recurrent themes or patterns related to victims or situations that lead to aggression or violence (Melton et al., 1997). Unlike methods previously discussed, this approach informs risk management strategies and can be applied to violence prevention efforts. As such, the treatment literature supports identifying violence patterns so that plans can be created to recognize an offender's early signs of escalation to break that pattern (Douglas & Kropp, 2002). This method, however, does not lend itself easily to procedural or empirical evaluation, given that individual clinical judgment and data gathering are utilized to form the assessment. Belfrage and Douglas (2002) commented that this model assumes a behavioral chain that will repeat itself and thus be predictable. It does not recognize the complex nature of violence and its multifaceted contributing factors (Douglas & Kropp, 2002).

Finally, the fourth method of violence risk assessment, known as the guided clinical approach (Hanson, 1998) or structured clinical decision making (Hart, 1998), employs structured professional judgment. Tools incorporating this approach offer guidelines that "reflect current theoretical, clinical, and empirical knowledge about violence" (Douglas & Kropp, 2002, p. 626). Typically, relevant clinical data are gathered from multiple sources, reviewed and compared against operationally defined criteria to determine whether a specific risk factor is present. One measure described subsequently that can be used to help with this type of clinical risk assessment, the HCR-20 (Webster, Douglas, Eaves, & Hart, 1997), offers recommendations about how to implement risk management strategies, utilizing a guided clinical type of approach. Additionally, this assessment approach systematically informs clinicians of those risk factors that are most relevant for a given population and linked empirically to violence. Methods using structured professional judgment are more flexible than actuarial techniques because they do not impose restrictions on how to combine and weigh risk factors, and they are more flexible than anamnestic approaches because clinicians are not bound by the need to identify violent themes. The guided clinical approach relies on professional judgment and discretion in the final step, when combining and weighing the importance of risk variables and making the overall judgment of relative risk (Douglas & Kropp, 2002; Douglas et al., 2003). Clinicians also may account for idiosyncratic variables that may have critical importance to an individual's violence risk (e.g., direct, specific homicidal threats). Moreover, treatment providers can capitalize on this systematic approach when creating interventions to manage an offender's risk of violence. This method not only assesses relative risk but also can link pertinent risk factors (e.g., dynamic) to theoretically and/or empirically supported treatment strategies.

Clinician-Based Versus Actuarial Violence Risk Prediction

We refer to clinician-based prediction as assessment without the use of any structured aids. In comparison to instrument-aided prediction, only a few studies on clinicians' predictions of violence have been published since Monahan's (1981) proclamation that only one out of three predictions of violent behavior is accurate. In a large study, Mossman (1994) examined clinicians' predictive accuracy by reexamining 58 data sets from 44 published studies dating from 1972 to 1993. Although all focused on violence risk prediction, the studies included a broad range of subjects, settings, population sizes, and clinical criteria for assessing violence. On the basis of this review,

Mossman suggested that clinicians were able to distinguish violent from nonviolent patients with a "modest, better than chance level of accuracy" (Mossman, 1994, p. 790).

Lidz et al. (1993) studied a large sample of patients examined in a psychiatric emergency room setting and found that clinicians' accuracy in predicting male violence exceeded chance, regardless of whether the patient had a history of violence. However, clinicians' predictions of female violence did not differ from chance, even though the actual rate of violent incidents among discharged female patients (46%) was higher than the rate among discharged male patients (42%). Lidz et al. noted that this discrepancy at predicting violence appeared to be a function of the clinicians' serious underestimation of the base rate of violence among mentally disordered women. Moving away from predicting violence in the community, McNiel and Binder (1991) focused on clinical predictions of inpatient violence. They had nurses estimate the probability (low: 0% to 33%, medium: 34% to 66%, and high: 67% to 100%) that patients would become violent within the first week of hospitalization. Of the patients estimated to have a low and medium probability, 10% and 24%, respectively, committed a violent act. Among those estimated to have a high likelihood (i.e., 67% to 100%) of becoming violent, only 40% were later found to have acted violently.

As seen earlier, a number of studies have indicated that clinical decisions can be made at above-chance levels in some contexts (e.g., Lidz et al., 1993) and that they can be consistently accurate regarding short-term risk of violent behavior (Binder, 1999). Such findings are infrequently represented in the literature, however.

Many studies comparing actuarial and clinical decision making have concluded that actuarial techniques typically outperform unstructured clinical approaches (Dawes et al., 1989; Faust & Ziskin, 1988; Lidz et al., 1993; Mossman, 1994) and that this alone is an argument for the sole use of actuarial methods (Grove, Zald, Lebow, Snitz, & Nelson, 2000; Quinsey et al., 1998b). Proponents of the actuarial measures note that clinicians typically have too much information, with hundreds if not thousands of facts about each patient, to consider before reaching a decision (Harris, Rice, & Quinsey, 1993), and that actuarial methods offer the advantage of being transparent, systematic, and thorough in their approach (Mossman, 2004).

Although Monahan et al. (2001) asserted that the demonstrated superiority of actuarial methods over clinical approaches is a "dead horse," there are those who suggest the debate between the accuracy of clinical and actuarial predictions will continue. Buchanan (2008) commented that the accuracy of actuarial predictions of violence among persons with mental illness exceeds chance, but also noted that with very low base rates of violence, predictions are more error-prone, such that when making hospitalization decisions, to prevent a few acts of violence one might end up hospitalizing many who would not have become violent if relying on actuarial predictions. In a notable exchange with Harris and her Violence Risk Appraisal Guide (VRAG; Harris et al., 1993) colleagues over the years, Litwack (2001) argued that actuarial versus clinical prediction methods have never been tested head-to head. Others (see Campbell, 2000) also argue that the superiority of actuarial methods has not been established in "real world" (Dvoskin & Heilbrun, 2001) forensic and clinical settings.

Critics of the purported superiority of actuarial methods have argued that risk factors and outcomes materialize in a complex interaction between human behavior and environment (Sturidsson, Haggard-Grann, Lotterberg, Dernevik, & Grann, 2004), and that clinical risk assessments are often conducted by multidisciplinary teams rather than individuals, as is the case with actuarial approaches. This methodological distinction raises questions about the validity of actuarial instruments, given that multiple clinical assessments of violence have been shown to be much more accurate than those generated by individual clinicians (Huss & Zeiss, 2004; McNiel, Lam, & Binder, 2000). Furthermore, risk assessment measures (even with recent advances) have not consistently been able to address the multifaceted nature of risk (Douglas & Ogloff, 2003a). Huss and Zeiss (2004) note that violence risk assessment measures do not consider the severity and imminence of violence and fail to capture anything about the risk assessment process.

Comparison studies on the predictive validity of clinical judgment narrowly focus on risk factors rather than on protective factors (Rogers, 2000). Also, the focus has been on individual risk factors (e.g., substance use, psychiatric symptoms) rather than contextual (e.g., housing, employment, support) risk management factors. Clinicians have the *potential* to consider, on the other hand, protective and contextual factors as well as aggravating clinical and risk

factors known to be associated with increased violence potential. Given these facts, Monahan (2003) also has since posited that clinically adjusted actuarial approaches are probably best.

That said, the literature in this area is growing rapidly, and over time we will gain a more informed perspective on actuarial instruments, clinical judgment, and mechanisms for maximizing our ability to assess and manage violence risk.

SELECT VIOLENCE RISK ASSESSMENT INSTRUMENTS

As noted earlier, over the years several more structured risk assessment instruments have been developed. Early risk assessment scales were nonempirically based, idiosyncratic lists of items that varied from clinician to clinician on the basis of their training, background, and experience as to what they believed was linked to increased risk of violence (Witt, 2000). These unstructured professional opinions, or first-generation assessments, had at best marginal predictive validity for general and violent recidivism (Andrews, Bonta, & Wormith, 2006). With the advent of tools and measures, empirically based item selection, improved methodology (e.g., samples, and predictor and outcome variables), and more rigorous validation research, researchers have continued to build momentum.

One of the early tools, the Violence Screening Checklist (VSC; McNeil & Binder, 1991), was developed with the aim of predicting inpatient violence. Other measures have focused on predicting risk of more specific types of violent behavior, such as domestic violence (Spousal Assault Risk Assessment Guide—SARA; Kropp, Hart, Webster, & Eaves, 1999), fire setting (Rice & Harris, 1996), and male institutional violence (Rice, Harris, Varney, & Quinsey, 1989), but many of these tools are still early in their development within research contexts and have produced only mixed results.

An alternative way of classifying risk assessment tools is to sort them from an evolutionary point of view. Following the unstructured professional assessments came second-generation risk assessment instruments that employed historical or static predictors such as criminological variables. The VRAG (Quinsey, Harris, Rice, & Cormier, 1998a), for example, has demonstrated good predictive validity and outperformed first-generation measures

(Andrews et al., 2006), but second-generation measures are limited as they cannot generally assess changes in risk. Wong and Gordon (2006) argue that such tools are not treatment-friendly as they provide little information about "the client's problem areas, treatment potential, criminogenic needs, strengths, current functioning, and so on" (p. 280).

Measures such as the Level of Service Inventory—Revised (LSI-R; Andrews & Bonta, 1995) are representative of third-generation tools. They may be based in theory (e.g., Andrews & Bonta, 1995) and account for dynamic variables such as social, lifestyle, and attitudinal variables, mental illness and substance use, and community supports. While dynamic variables have been shown to predict risk as well as static variables, the efforts of third-generation measures are still limited because, as Wong and Gordon (2006) state, predicting risk should not be the end product. Violence reduction and prevention should be the ultimate goal of risk assessment (Hart, 1998). In response to the perceived need for tools that address these issues, two fourth-generation measures have recently appeared in the literature: Level of Service/Case Management Inventory (LS/CMI; Andrews, Bonta, & Wormith, 2004) and Violence Risk Scale (VRS; Wong & Gordon 1998–2003). These tools have been designed to guide services that monitor and manage offenders and provide treatment services.

The VRS (Wong & Gordon, 1998–2003) assists treatment providers in integrating risk assessments with treatment services among high-risk, high-need nonsexual offenders (Wong & Gordon, 2006). The VRS not only identifies who is at high-risk, but also what variables are linked to violence and what therapeutic approaches may be effective in reducing this risk. This tool is also designed to monitor changes in a client's risk profile by allowing clinicians to periodically measure the effectiveness of treatment as it is linked to a quantitative reduction in violence risk (Wong & Gordon, 2006). The VRS, and its companions the VRS—Sex Offender Version and VRS—Youth Version, holds much promise as a psychometrically sound risk assessment tool and has the advantage of providing clinicians with information on how to design and deliver risk reduction interventions. Future research will likely shed more light on this instrument and may place it among the more useful models for tools to assess violence risk and management.

As noted in Chapter 6, there has also been a proliferation of tools designed to assess the risk of future sexual offending behavior. With regard to general violence risk assessment, prototypical empirically-researched measures include the HCR-20: Assessing Risk for Violence (HCR-20), the VRAG, and the MacArthur Violence Risk Assessment Study's Iterative Classification Tree (ICT), currently being marketed as the Classification of Violence Risk (COVR). The following sections will review each of these in turn.

HCR-20: Assessing Risk for Violence (Version 2)

The HCR-20 (version 2; Webster, Douglas, Eaves, & Hart, 1997) comprises three domains (Historical, Clinical, and Risk Management) and 20 risk items, which are listed in Table 5.1. Technically not

TABLE 5.1 Variables on the Historical, Clinical, and Risk Management-20 (HCR-20) Violence Risk Scheme

Historical scale

Previous violence

Young age at first violent incident

Relationship instability

Employment problems

Substance use problems

Major mental illness

Psychopathy

Early maladjustment

Personality disorder

Previous supervision failure

Clinical scale

Lack of insight

Negative attitudes

Active symptoms of major mental illness

Impulsivity

Unresponsive to total treatment

Risk management scale

Plans lack feasibility

Exposure to destabilizers

Lack of personal support

Noncompliance with remediation attempts

Stress

Webster, C. D., Douglas, K. S., Eaves, D., & Hart, S. D. (1997). HCR-20: Assessing Risk for Violence (version 2). Burnaby, BC, Canada: Mental Health Law, and Policy Institute, Simon Fraser University.

considered an actuarial instrument, it is an example of the structured professional judgment approach for assessing risk of violence, and referred to as an aide-mémoire. The 10 Historical items are primarily static risk factors, as they reflect the "temporal stability" of past conduct, mental illness and substance use, and social adjustment (Webster et al., 1997, p. 27). The five Clinical items measure changeable or dynamic risk information, allowing risk levels to be modified or adjusted on the basis of relevant clinical factors. The last five items make up the Risk Management domain. With dynamic content, they focus on how individuals will manage and adjust to future circumstances. Temporally, the three scales emphasize past, present, and future (Witt, 2000). The items were chosen following a review of the literature and selection of those 20 factors that had consistent empirical support. When designing the HCR-20 the authors also wanted a measure that could be integrated easily into clinical practice but, primarily, was empirically sound.

Clinicians rate the extent (0—absent, 1—partially present, or 2—definitely present) to which each risk factor is present. A total score is not particularly meaningful, as it is not compared to a normative reference group. Generally, higher scores on the HCR-20 relate to a greater incidence and frequency of violence than lower scores. This measure allows for the possibility that just the presence of a small number of risk factors may be substantial enough to determine that a person is likely to behave violently. Rather than relying on cut scores, clinicians are encouraged to come to a clinical decision about a person's risk for violence using terms outlined in the instrument (low, moderate, or high) relative to other persons in comparable settings. This risk level is associated with the degree of intervention or management that is required to prevent violence (Douglas & Kropp, 2002). Given the problems with rigid actuarial approaches, low, moderate, and high-risk levels are purposefully not associated with specific scores. Even so, scholars (e.g., Heilbrun, Dvoskin, Hart, & McNiel, 1999; Monahan & Steadman, 1996; Otto, 2000) contend that these general categories are clinically meaningful and can yield reasonable reliability and validity estimates (Douglas & Ogloff, 2003a, 2003b).

There have been many studies with diverse criminal and civil populations involving the HCR-20. In a retrospective study with prisoners, Douglas and Webster (1999) found that offenders with scores above the median on the HCR-20 increased the odds of past violence and antisocial behavior by an average of four times. Within a civilly committed population, Douglas et al. (1999) found that over a 2-year community follow-up, patients scoring above the median were 6 to 13 times more likely to be violent than those scoring below the median. In an unpublished study cited by Belfrage and Douglas (2002), the measure predicted incidents of onward aggression and postdischarge violence over a 6-month period among psychiatric patients on an acute care unit.

In some studies of the HCR-20, Clinical and Risk Management factors contributed more to the predictive accuracy than the Historical factors (Strand, Belfrage, Fransson, & Levander, 1998). In a study of inmates receiving mental health services (Grann, Belfrage, & Tengstrom, 2000), the HCR-20's historical variables demonstrated better predictive accuracy regarding future violence among personality-disordered offenders and those diagnosed with schizophrenia, compared to variables on an actuarial measure (i.e., VRAG [see subsequent text]). However, the authors noted that clinical and risk management factors, as compared to the historical items, may have greater predictive accuracy for offenders with major mental illness. In a pseudo-prospective study of male forensic psychiatric patients discharged from medium secure units, the HCR-20 total score, and the historical and risk subscale scores but not the clinical subscale scores, were good predictors of violent and other offenses after discharge (Gray, Taylor, & Snowden, 2008). Given its structured professional judgment approach, the HCR-20 uniquely considers empirically-based clinical and risk management matters, thus permitting an ongoing assessment of changes made in these areas. Although historical variables have been shown to be significantly correlated with risk of future violence, the aforementioned studies have demonstrated that the Clinical and Risk Management domains can also be significantly related to violence (Belfrage, 1998). Further, these scales, unlike the historical items, are sensitive to changes related to individuals' participation in psychiatric treatment and the development and modification of release plans (e.g., Douglas, Webster, Eaves, Hart, & Ogloff, 2001). This suggests that psychiatric treatment, as well as situational variables and suitable risk planning can play a significant role in postdischarge violence. For instance, some authors report that scores on the Clinical and Risk scales declined in the context of forensic and civil psychiatric inpatient treatment (Belfrage & Douglas, 2002; Douglas & Belfrage, 2001; Webster, Douglas, Belfrage, & Link, 2000).

Accompanying the HCR-20 is the Violence Risk Management Companion Guide (Douglas et al., 2001). Distinguishing itself from many other risk assessment measures and embracing the goal of violence reduction and prevention, this guide provides assistance to clinicians making recommendations to care providers for managing a client's violence risk. Ongoing research related to the HCR-20 and possible future revisions of this measure will continue to shed light on what appears to be the promising effectiveness of this tool for risk assessment and management.

Violence Risk Appraisal Guide

The Violence Risk Appraisal Guide (VRAG; Harris et al., 1993) was developed using a sample of over 600 men from a maximum-security forensic hospital in Canada, all of whom were charged with a serious criminal offense. After assembling a wide variety of predictor variables from institutional files, the authors defined the criterion variable as any new criminal charge for a violent offense or return to that institution for an act that would have resulted in such a charge. A series of regression models were computed, and the authors identified 12 variables for inclusion in the final actuarial instrument (see Table 5.2). As noted in the table, the most heavily weighted risk factor is the individual's score on the Psychopathy Checklist—Revised (PCL-R; Hare, 1991). Additionally, four variables relate negatively to risk of violent behavior. According to the foundational VRAG studies, male offenders who were older, who chose a female victim, who injured a victim in the index offense, or who were diagnosed with schizophrenia were significantly less likely to be violent recidivists than other male offenders in the comparison sample (Banks et al., 2004). A complete description of the development of the VRAG as well as scoring instructions has been published (Quinsey et al., 1998a).

When Harris and colleagues (1993) dichotomized the VRAG scores into high and low, the results indicated that 55% of the high scoring participants committed a new violent offense, compared with 19% of those participants scoring low. Rice and Harris (1995) found that the VRAG predicted violent recidivism reasonably well in studies of 3.5, 6, and 10 years. Later studies conducted by Rice and Harris (1997) found

TABLE 5.2 Violence Risk Appraisal Guide (VRAG) Predictor Variables[a]

Psychopathy Checklist—Revised (PCL-R) Score

Elementary school maladjustment

DSM-III diagnosis of any personality disorder

Age at time of the index offense[b]

Separation from either natural parent (except death) under age 16

Failure on prior conditional release

Cormier–Lang scale score for extent and severity of nonviolent criminal behavior

Never married

DSM-III diagnosis of schizophrenia[b]

Severity of physical injury suffered by the victim of the index offense[b]

Severity of alcohol abuse history

Female victim in the index offense[b]

[a]Predictor variables are listed in descending order of weight or relation to future violence.
[b]These variables are inversely (negatively) related to future violence.
Harris, G. T., Rice, M. E., & Quinsey, V. L. (1993). Violent recidivism of mentally disordered offenders: the development of a statistical prediction instrument. *criminal Justice and Behavior*, 20, 315–335.

that the VRAG's predictive performance was less successful when used to predict violence in sex offender populations. Initially, Webster et al. (1994) held the position that after the VRAG score was obtained, there may be some instances where clinicians might find it appropriate to vary the VRAG probability estimate using clinical judgment, but no more than 10% in either direction. This clearly violates the assumptions postulated by the actuarial approach, and 4 years later, Quinsey et al. (1998a) changed their position, stating that any clinical adjustment reduced the VRAG's predictive accuracy.

As an actuarial risk assessment instrument, the VRAG is an advancement from the first-generation efforts, and it has been especially influential in the prediction of violence among serious offenders who are released into the community. However, similar to other subsequent instruments, these actuarial measures are only applicable to the specific groups on which they have been normed. Therefore, populations of civil committees on acute psychiatric units, women, and adolescents, for example, may not be appropriate for assessment with the VRAG or other actuarial instruments. There are two other critiques of the VRAG. With so few items, it has been criticized for being overly simplistic (Grann et al., 2000) and overly reliant on historical and static factors (Dolan & Doyle, 2000). After first permitting clinical adjustment to VRAG estimates and then changing their stance that the predictions should not be altered, the authors subsequently recommended that the actuarial predictions be supplemented by a checklist of clinical factors to produce the Violence Prediction Scheme (Dolan & Doyle, 2000; Webster et al., 1994).

MacArthur Violence Risk Assessment Study's Classification of Violence Risk

Most recently, the MacArthur Risk Assessment Project developed an actuarial risk assessment tool that is founded in what the researchers refer to as an ICT scheme. This approach to violence risk assessment is based on interactive and contingency models, allowing clinicians to consider many different combinations of risk factors in classifying a person as being at high or low risk of engaging in violent behavior (Monahan et al., 2000; Steadman et al., 2000). The classification tree begins with a question asked of all persons being evaluated. On the basis of the answer to that question, one of two more questions is posed, the answer to which determines the next question asked. This continues until each person is classified into a category based on violence risk (Banks et al., 2004; Steadman et al., 2000; Monahan et al., 2006). This method contrasts with the usual approach to actuarial risk assessment, in which a common set of questions is asked of everyone being assessed and every answer is weighted and summed to produce a score that can be used for the purposes of categorization (Monahan et al., 2001).

The principle results of the MacArthur Violence Risk Assessment Study are reported in Steadman et al. (2000) and in Monahan et al. (2000). The ICT decision tree approach selects an optimal predictor of violence from a pool of over 100 risk factors. Monahan et al. (2001) sought to maximize the ICT's utility for real-world clinical decision making by applying it to a set of violence risk factors commonly available in clinical records or those capable of being routinely assessed in clinical practice. Results showed that the prototype-ICT partitioned three-quarters of a sample of psychiatric patients into one of two categories with regard to their risk of violence toward others during the first 20 weeks after discharge. One category consisted of groups whose rates of violence were no more than half the base rate of the total patient sample (i.e., equal to or less than 9% of violence). The other category consisted of groups whose rates of violence were at least twice the base rate of the total patient sample (i.e., equal to or greater than 37% violent). The actual prevalence of violence within individual risk groups varied from 3% to 53% (Banks et al., 2004; Monahan et al., 2001).

After the initial development and evaluation of the prototype-ICT model, the MacArthur group opted to adopt an approach that integrates the predictions of many different risk assessment classification trees, each of which may capture a different but important facet of the interactive relationship between the measured risk factors and violence (Banks et al., 2004). Table 5.3 illustrates the 10 ICT models they identified. Using a multiple ICT approach, these researchers ultimately combined the results of five decision trees, or prediction models, generated by this methodology. Each of the five trees features a different risk factor as the starting point for the development of the tree. Using computer technology and taking only 10 minutes for a brief chart review and instrument administration, the COVR, as it became known, holds promise for those clinicians conducting violence risk assessments on civilly committed psychiatric patients before discharge to the

TABLE 5.3 MacArthur Violence Risk Assessment Study's Classification of Violence Risk (COVR)[a]

Model[b]	First Variable	Variables	ROC-AUC[*]
1	Seriousness of arrest[c]	12	0.803
2	Drug abuse diagnosis	9	0.738
3	Alcohol abuse diagnosis	13	0.764
4	Primary diagnosis	8	0.753
5	Anger reaction[c]	11	0.778
6	Schedule of imagined violence	10	0.769
7	Child abuse[c]	14	0.791
8	Prior violence	10	0.766
9	Age[c]	16	0.784
10	Gender[c]	14	0.806

[a]Adapted from Banks et al. (2004).
[b]Characteristics of the multiple iterative classification tree models.
[c]The five models retained for the multiple-model risk classification.
[*]ROC-AUC = Receiver Operating Characteristics—Area Under the Curve—a measure of violence risk that allows for assessment without confounds related to base rate. Numbers closest to 1.0 reflect best predictive accuracy.

community. The COVR software can generate a report that contains an estimate of the patient's violence risk (ranging from 1% to 76% likelihood), though, as the authors note, this estimate of violence risk should not be the equivalent of a determination of whether a patient should be discharged (Monahan et al., 2006). However, it is recommended that clinicians could utilize the information that the COVR provides to aid in risk assessment and risk management planning (Monahan et al., 2006). Monahan and colleagues (2005, 2006) emphasized that the multiple ICT model was constructed and validated, to date, only on samples of psychiatric inpatients in acute facilities in the United States who would be discharged into the community. Until additional research is conducted, the use of the COVR should be restricted to circumstances that meet those parameters.

CLINICAL APPROACH TO VIOLENCE RISK ASSESSMENT

Violence risk assessments typically involve gathering data from a number of sources, including relevant records (e.g., police reports, criminal record, victim/witness statements, hospital records), third parties (e.g., family members, police officers, mental health treatment providers), and often most importantly, the individual being evaluated. In addition to providing useful data, collateral sources such as records, contact with third parties, and laboratory tests (e.g., toxicology screens) can offer information regarding the reliability of the examinee's self-report. The purpose and time frame of the risk assessment, as well as the type and amount of data available will vary depending on the setting (Borum et al., 1996). Therefore, an important first step is to focus and shape the parameters of the assessment process and question. Regardless of the specific reason(s) for referral, however, any risk assessment should ideally involve a clinical interview addressing the examinee's history and mental status. Given its notable predictive power regarding violence risk, an examinee's history of violence must be thoroughly assessed in the clinical interview. Borum and colleagues (1996) and Otto (2000), for example, recommend beginning with screening questions aimed at determining the presence of potential risk, followed by conducting an anamnestic analysis of the examinee's violence history that addresses the nature and precipitants of past aggressive behavior and any

discernible patterns across violent episodes (regarding factors such as motivation, targets, and the examinee's mental state at the time).

In conducting an interview aimed at violence risk assessment, the complex interplay of appropriate probing, respect for the examinee, and attention to safety is important to bear in mind. Clinicians less experienced with violence risk assessment interviews should be mindful to avoid common pitfalls, including the failure to probe because of a concern that it may be best to "let sleeping dogs lie" or a fear that the person will target the clinician when next violent. Clinicians sometimes fail to elicit data because of an erroneous assumption that treatment providers already know that aspect of the patient's history. Also, clinicians conducting violence risk assessments should strike a balance between asking structured questions that may be based on known violence risk factors and open-ended questions that allow for a more individualistic and anamnestic history.

RISK FACTORS FOR VIOLENCE

As noted earlier, guided clinical assessments involve gathering data about factors shown to be empirically related to violence risk and using clinical judgment to integrate this and other relevant information in formulating opinions about risk, possibly including the use of a structured tool to help in the assessment, such as the HCR-20 (Webster et al., 1997). As noted by Monahan et al. (2001), research delineating particular risk factors for violence has focused on variables identified in both the criminological and clinical literatures. These factors cluster into two primary domains: static (i.e., variables that do not change or are not readily changed) and dynamic (i.e., variables that can change). Identification of both types of factors is important in terms of assessing an examinee's absolute level of risk and planning appropriate risk management interventions (Otto, 2000). Table 5.4 presents a nonexhaustive list of variables identified in the literature as most relevant to violence risk. Following is a summary of the factors shown to be associated with violence potential, as well as a brief discussion of the relevant research. Although many of the studies cited focus on samples of psychiatric patients, some involve persons not diagnosed with mental disorders. For detailed reviews of the research in this area, the reader is referred to Borum et al.

TABLE 5.4 Select Factors Associated with Increased Violence Risk

Static Variables

Age

Sex

Intelligence/neurological impairment

History of violence/criminal behavior

History of childhood physical abuse/Domestic violence

Psychopathy

Dynamic Variables

Neighborhood context

Stress/Social support

Victim availability and specificity

Substance abuse/dependence

Comorbid mental disorder (with substance abuse)

Threat/control-override (TCO) symptoms[a]

Command hallucinations[a]

Violent thoughts

Anger

[a] Although the available data regarding these factors are equivocal, some studies have found support for their association with increased violence risk.

(1996), Melton et al. (1997), Monahan et al. (2001), and Otto (2000).

Select Static Risk Factors

Studies in both the clinical and criminological arenas have identified *age* as a risk factor for violence, with late adolescence to early adulthood (i.e., ages 18 to 25) representing the period of greatest risk for violent or threatening behavior (Bonta, Law, & Hanson, 1998). For the most part, research has noted the association between age and violence among persons in the general population as well as those with mental illness. In his examination of violent behavior among psychotic patients, however, McNeil (1997) suggested that age may have less predictive utility with respect to violence among more symptomatic persons because clinical risk factors are likely to assume prominence in the analysis of violence potential.

The criminological literature has long reported sex as a risk factor for violence in the general population, with men exhibiting a much greater likelihood of engaging in violent behavior than women (e.g., Reiss & Roth, 1993). Research on persons with mental illness, however, suggests minimal or no differences in rates of violence between men and women (Estroff & Zimmer, 1994; Lidz et al., 1993; McNiel & Binder, 1995; Monahan et al., 2001; Tardiff, Marzuk, Leon, Portera, & Weiner, 1997). Despite similar prevalence rates of violent behavior among mentally disordered men and women, some recent studies have noted gender differences in the severity and/or context of the violence committed. For example, Hiday et al. (1998) found similar rates of self-reported, prehospitalization violence among male and female patients but noted that men engaged in more serious forms of violent behavior (i.e., resulting in injuries or involving weapons) than women. In an examination of posthospitalization violence, the MacArthur Violence Risk Assessment Study yielded similar data, as well as findings that men were more likely than women to have been using substances and failing to comply with psychiatric medications before committing violent acts (Monahan et al., 2001). The MacArthur group also found that women were more likely than men to assault family members and to engage in violent behavior in the home. Similar findings were reported by Swanson et al. (1999), who noted that male psychiatric patients were more likely to engage in violent behavior with acquaintances and strangers in public places, while females were more likely to fight with family members in the home.

Data from a number of studies have indicated a relationship between *low intelligence/neurological impairment* and violence (see review by Krakowski, 1997). Among clinical and nonclinical populations, a *history of violence or criminal behavior* is a particularly robust predictor of future violence (Bonta et al., 1998; Klassen & O'Connor, 1994; McNiel, Binder, & Greenfield, 1988; Mossman, 1994). A related relevant factor is the age at which the first serious offense occurred and the versatility of prior criminal behavior (Borum, 1996; Patterson & Yoerger, 1993). In his review of the variables relevant to violence risk assessment in outpatient settings, Otto (2000) noted that persons with histories of serious illegal acts before the age of 12 have been shown to be at increased risk of engaging in violent and more serious criminal behavior over the course of their lives.

A *history of physical abuse or having witnessed domestic violence as a child* is also predictive of later violence (Klassen & O'Connor, 1994). The MacArthur Study reported an association between childhood physical abuse and posthospitalization violence but not between childhood sexual abuse and violence (Monahan et al., 2001). Data from the study also indicate a relationship between excessive substance use by a parent and increased rates of later patient violence, although the strength of this association varied as a function of gender and race.

Over the past several years, there has been an increasing focus on the utility of the construct of *psychopathy* to predict violence. According to Hare (1998), psychopathy may be understood as a fixed array of affective, interpersonal, and behavioral characteristics, including egocentricity, deceitfulness, impulsivity, irresponsibility, superficiality, manipulativeness, and a lack of remorse or empathy, as well as a history of rule violations. Psychopathy is typically assessed using the Hare Psychopathy Checklist—Revised (PCL-R; Hare, 1991) or the Hare Psychopathy Checklist—Screening Version (PCL-SV; Hart, Cox, & Hare, 1995), each of which, contains items representing the aforementioned domains and allows for ratings on each criterion. Chapter 10 in the text provides a more detailed description of this. Related to violence risk, as reviewed by Hare (1998), research has shown that persons scoring in the "psychopathic" range on these measures are at increased risk of engaging in violent and threatening behavior as well as criminal acts in general. The three violence risk assessment instruments discussed earlier in the chapter incorporate the Psychopathy Checklists to some extent. Not surprisingly, one of the most robust risk factors on the HCR-20 and other measures is the presence of psychopathy (Dolan & Doyle, 2000). The MacArthur Study findings (Monahan et al., 2001) indicated that scores on the PCL-SV among civil psychiatric patients were strongly associated with future violent behavior. Of note, Monahan and colleagues (2001) found that most of the PCL-SV's basic and unique predictive power was related to the "antisocial behavior" factor, not the "emotional detachment" factor.

Select Dynamic Risk Factors

Data from the MacArthur Study (Monahan et al., 2001) indicate that the *contexts* into which, hospitalized patients are discharged is relevant to predicting their risk of subsequent violent behavior. In interpreting associations between individual-level predictors (such as race) and violence, for example, it appears especially important to consider contextual variables. In the MacArthur Study sample, the significant relationship between race and violence disappeared when neighborhood crime rate was statistically controlled. Another key contextual variable is "neighborhood disadvantage," defined by the MacArthur group as encompassing a number of factors, including neighborhood poverty, income, employment rates, and residential stability. They found no differences between the violence rates of African Americans and whites living in similarly disadvantaged neighborhoods, despite the overall relationship between race and violence. These data appear consistent with the findings of Swanson (1994) that higher rates of violence among African Americans than whites may be attributable to differences in socioeconomic status (SES).

As noted by Otto (2000), there has long been theoretical support for the idea that perceived *stress* is a risk factor for violence, and this notion has also received some indirect empirical support. In addition to studies reporting an association between frustration/stress and violent or threatening behavior (e.g., Berkowitz, 1998), the aforementioned findings of increased rates of violence among populations with higher stress levels, such as low SES or a high-crime neighborhood, seems to support this notion. Although it may be reasonable to assume that *social support* is associated with decreased violence rates, the available data suggest that the relationship between these two variables may be mediated by level of functional impairment related to severe mental illness (Swanson et al., 1998). According to the findings of Swanson and colleagues, it may be that persons with significant functional impairment are more likely to be violent in the context of increased contact with family and friends, while higher-functioning persons are less likely to engage in violent behavior in the context of frequent social contact.

Important contextual variables to consider in any violence risk assessment are *victim specificity* (e.g., is the target one particular person or a broader group of people?) and *victim availability*. A number of studies of aggression committed by persons with mental disorders have found that family members are especially likely to be targets of patients' violent behavior (Steadman et al., 1998; Straznickas, McNiel, & Binder, 1993). Estroff et al. (1998) found that mothers residing with adult children diagnosed with schizophrenia and comorbid substance abuse were at significant risk of being assaulted by their children. This line of research seems to suggest that for some persons with mental illness, contexts involving intensive contact with family members may be a risk factor for violence. A number of other variables may increase or mitigate this risk, however, including the patient's functional level, as noted earlier (Swanson et al., 1998).

A diagnosis of *substance abuse or dependence* has been shown to be a robust risk factor for violence, and the presence of a *coexisting major mental illness or other psychiatric disorder* appears to increase this risk (Arsenault et al., 2000; Monahan et al., 2001; Swanson et al., 1990; Swanson et al., 1996). Data reported by Swartz and colleagues (1998) indicate that subjects with severe mental illness who failed to comply with their psychotropic medications and suffered from a comorbid substance abuse disorder were at significantly increased risk for engaging in violent behavior. As noted earlier in the chapter, however, a diagnosis of a major mental disorder alone has been shown to be a protective factor, that is, associated with lower rates of violence than a diagnosis of other types of psychiatric disorders, such as adjustment or personality disorders (Lidz et al., 1993; Monahan et al., 2001; Quinsey et al., 1998a). The MacArthur group found that among major mental disorders, a schizophrenia diagnosis was associated with lower rates of violence than a diagnosis of depression or bipolar disorder, which is consistent with data from other studies (e.g., Gardner, Lidz, Mulvey, & Shaw, 1996; Quinsey et al., 1998a). Related findings suggest that persons experiencing a manic episode are at increased risk for violent behavior (Beck & Bonnar, 1988; Binder & McNiel, 1988). That is not to say, however, that a patient who is actively symptomatic may not be at greater risk, and one would not want to rely on diagnosis alone to make a risk determination. One study, for example, demonstrated the association of treatment noncompliance and substance use as a predictor of violent behavior among persons with serious mental illness (Swartz et al., 1998).

Studies examining the relationship between schizophrenia and violence during the 1990s noted the relevance of particular types of delusions involving perceptions of threat and beliefs that one's thoughts and actions are being controlled by others. As noted previously, Link and Steuve (1994) described these *TCO symptoms* as a risk factor for violence, as did others (Swanson et al., 1996). Similarly, McNeil and Binder (1995) reported that acute hospital patients who exhibited suspiciousness were more likely to engage in aggressive behavior than patients who

were not suspicious. In contrast to prior findings related to TCO and other delusional symptoms, the MacArthur group reported no significant relationship between delusions (regardless of content) and violence among recently discharged psychiatric patients (Monahan et al., 2001). Of particular note is their finding that TCO delusions failed to predict higher rates of violence. A related result may offer an explanation for the discrepancy between these data and previous research regarding TCO symptoms. However, nondelusional suspiciousness (i.e., possibly in the form of a hostile attributional bias) was found to be associated with subsequent violence in the MacArthur sample. Monahan and colleagues (2001) caution that despite the MacArthur Study findings regarding delusions, these symptoms may be salient predictors of violence in particular cases and thus should not be ignored as potential risk factors. This is likely to be especially true in cases of individuals who have a history of acting violently in response to delusions (Appelbaum, Robbins, & Monahan, 2000).

Although conventional clinical wisdom suggests a strong link between *command hallucinations* and violent behavior, empirical findings have been more equivocal. In a review of seven studies, Rudnick (1999) reported that none found a positive association between command hallucinations and violence. Rudnick noted that when violent behavior did occur in response to command hallucinations, it appeared positively associated with the familiarity of the hallucinated voice and negatively related to the severity of the violent behavior ordered. Subsequently, Braham et al. (2004) posited that methodological limitations of prior studies confounded the ability to draw conclusions from them. In their review of the literature, they indicated that the weight of the evidence indicated that some individuals who hear commands will act on them, but that there is a complex interplay of individualized factors that account for who might act on such commands . In their review, Hersh and Borum (1998) concluded that compliance with command hallucinations was more likely if the voice was familiar and if the nature of the command was consistent with a coexisting delusion. Similarly, others identified compliance with commands to be associated with congruent delusions, a positive view of the command hallucination, as well as increasing age and low maternal control in childhood (Shawyer et al., 2008). The findings of the MacArthur Study indicated no relationship between command hallucinations in general and violence, but they did suggest an association between command hallucinations with violent content and subsequent violence. In particular, subjects who reported hearing voices ordering them to commit acts of violence against others were significantly more likely to engage in violence following hospital discharge than subjects who did not experience violent command hallucinations. Thus, as McNeil and colleagues (2000) noted, there is clinical utility in asking about command hallucinations in conducting risk assessments in patients with major mental illness, though command hallucinations should not be considered in isolation, as the risk assessment formulation should examine them in light of the total clinical picture.

Consistent with the clinical practice of inquiring about homicidal ideation as a means of assessing violence risk, the MacArthur data indicate a positive relationship between *imagined violence* during hospitalization and violence following discharge (Grisso, Davis, Vesselinov, Appelbaum, & Monahan, 2000; Monahan et al., 2001). This risk was increased among subjects who continued to experience violent thoughts after leaving the hospital. A much earlier study by McNiel and Binder (1989) also reported an association between verbal threats and subsequent violence among acute psychiatric patients. The authors noted, however, that patients' ultimate victims were not necessarily the same persons they had threatened.

Common sense suggests that *anger* is a risk factor for violence, and the results of empirical work (much of it done by Raymond Novaco) support this notion. For example, among samples of psychiatric inpatients, anger has been shown to be positively correlated with prior criminal convictions, use of seclusion and restraint while hospitalized, and hospital assaults (Novaco, 1994). Anger was linked to a risk of assaultiveness during forensic hospitalization (Novaco & Taylor, 2004; Doyle & Dolan, 2006). Similarly, data from the MacArthur Study indicate that patients with elevated scores on the Novaco Anger Scale (Novaco, 1994) during hospitalization were twice as likely as those with low scores to commit violent acts following discharge. In a study involving psychiatric inpatients who had reportedly engaged in violent behavior before hospitalization, Swanson et al. (1999) found that according to subjects' reports, their aggressive acts were most often accompanied by feelings of intense anger. Further, exposure to parental anger and violence was associated with anger and

inpatient assaults for male forensic patients with developmental disabilities (Novaco & Taylor, 2008).

INTEGRATING INFORMATION FOR CLINICAL RISK ASSESSMENTS

Once the relevant information is obtained from the various sources, the clinician may begin to integrate it to generate hypotheses about the examinee's risk of violent behavior. In some cases, the examinee may not be willing or available to be interviewed, but that may not necessarily preclude conducting a risk assessment. Clinicians should generally indicate the data sources utilized and any limitations in the information available. Opinions then should be qualified accordingly. Approaches such as those utilizing the VRAG, COVR and HCR-20 provide formulas and/ or algorithms that outline relevant variables and produce a quantitative or qualitative risk estimates. Clinicians utilizing the actuarial tools must remain mindful of the debate in the literature regarding pure and adjusted actuarial estimates and the populations with which, the actuarial measures have been studied.

It has been suggested that risk assessment opinions often require some mention of the type of violence in question, the time frame for which risk is being predicted, and an understanding of the base rate of violence for the population from which, an examinee is drawn (Borum et al., 1996). Once these factors have been taken into account, precipitants and circumstances of violent behavior and patterns across incidents of aggression warrant consideration, as in an anamnestic approach. Using all available data, the clinician should then be able to specify the conditions under which the examinee may be more or less likely to commit violence. It can be helpful to identify known aggravating and mitigating factors for potential future violence.

After determining the salience of these conditions during the time frame in question, the clinician in some cases may wish to formulate an opinion about the examinee's level of risk for violent behavior during the specified time period in the identified context in which the examinee will be situated. However, identifying levels of risk, especially if utilized in the absence of a structured professional tool that offers some mechanism for anchoring such classifications, should be explained so that the reasoning behind the identified level of risk is clear. When indicated, it may also be important to incorporate recommendations in one's formulation that aim to reduce risk related to risk factors that are amenable to intervention. It should be understood that risk assessments and risk management recommendations can inform clinical decisionmaking, but that decisions regarding privileges, discharge, appropriate community placements and the like involve a host of additional factors (e.g., available resources, a person's willingness to participate in recommended programming, legal requirements, etc.) that may come into play as such decisions are being formulated.

For clinicians conducting risk assessments, the challenge lies in linking the data available to what is understood about the individual's violence risk potential. For other professionals who utilize clinical risk assessments in arenas such as legal cases, it is important to recognize the importance and limitations of undividualized assessments as they relate to prediction and management. With the ongoing evolution of actuarial and clinical methodologies, understanding empirically driven approaches to violence risk assessment and risk management and incorporating them when indicated will continue to be important for optimizing the standard of practice in this complex clinical endeavor.

References

All bright, A., Levy, F., & Wagle, N. C. (2002). Outpatient civil commitment laws: an overview. *Mental and Physical Disability Law Reporter*, 26, 179–182.

Andrews, D. A. & Bonta, J. (1995). *LSI-R: The Level of Service Inventory—Revised*. Toronto, Ontario, Canada: Multi-Health Systems.

Andrews, D. A., Bonta, J., & Wormith, J. S. (2004). *LS/CMI: The Level of Service/Case Management Inventory*. Toronto, Ontario, Canada: Multi-Health Systems.

Andrews, D. A., Bonta, J., & Wormith, J. S. (2006). The recent past and near future of risk and/or need assessment. *Crime and Delinquency*, 52, 7–22.

Appelbaum, P. S. (1994). New directions in the assessment of the dangerousness of mentally ill. *Japanese Journal of Psychiatry and Neurology*, 48, 77–83.

Appelbaum, P. S., Robbins, P. C., & Monahan, J. (2000). Violence and delusions: Data from the MacArthur Violence Risk Assessment Study. *American Journal of Psychiatry*, 157, 566–572.

Arseneault, L., Moffitt, T. E., Caspi, A., Taylor, P. J., & Silva, P. A. (2000). Mental disorders and violence in a total birth cohort: Results from the Dunedin Study. *Archives of General Psychiatry*, 57, 979–986.

Banks, S., Robbins, P. C., Silver, E., Vesselinov, R., Steadman, H. J., Monahan, J., et al. (2004). A multiple-models approach to violence risk assessment among people with mental disorder. *Criminal Justice and Behavior*, 31, 324–340.

Battlesfords and District Co-operatives Ltd. v. Gibbs 3 S.C.R. 566 (1995).

Baxstrom v. Herold, 383 U.S. 107 (1966).

Beck, J. C. & Bonnar, J. (1988). Emergency civil commitment: Predicting hospital violence from behavior in the community. *Journal of Psychiatry & Law*, 16, 379–388.

Belfrage, H. (1998). Implementing the HCR-20 scheme for risk assessment in a forensic psychiatric hospital: Integrating research and clinical practice. *Journal of Forensic Psychiatry*, 9, 328–338.

Belfrage, H. & Douglas, K. S. (2002). Treatment effects on forensic psychiatric patients measured with the HCR-20 violence risk assessment scheme. *International Journal of Forensic Mental Health*, 1, 25–36.

Berkowitz, L. (1998). Affective aggression: The role of stress, pain, and negative affect. In R. G. Geen & E. Donnerstein (Eds.), *Human aggression: Theories, research, and Implications for Social Policy*, (pp. 49–72). San Diego, CA: Academic Press.

Binder, R. L. (1999). Are the mentally ill dangerous? *Journal of the American Academy of Psychiatry and the Law*, 27, 189–201.

Binder, R. L. & McNiel, D. E. (1988). Effects of diagnosis and context on dangerousness. *American Journal of Psychiatry*, 145, 728–732.

Bonta, J., Law, M., & Hanson, K. (1998). The prediction of criminal and violent recidivism among mentally disordered offenders: A meta-analysis. *Psychological Bulletin*, 123, 123–142.

Borum, R. (1996). Improving the clinical practice of violence risk assessment: Technology, guidelines, and training. *American Psychologist*, 51, 945–956.

Borum, R., Swartz, M., & Swanson, J. (1996). Assessing and managing violence risk in clinical practice. *Journal of Practical Psychiatry and Behavioral Health*, 2, 205–215.

Braham, L. G., Trower, P., & Birchwood, M. (2004). Acting on command hallucinations and dangerous behavior: a critique of the major findings of the last decade. *Clinical Psychology Review*, 24, 513–528.

Buchanan, A. (2008). Risk of violence by psychiatric patients: Beyond the "actuarial vs. clinical" assessment debate. *Psychiatric Services*, 59, 184–190.

Campbell, T. W. (2000). Sexual predator evaluations and phrenology: Considering issues of evidentiary reliability. *Behavioral Sciences and the Law*, 18, 111–130.

Dawes, R. M., Faust, D., & Meehl, P. E. (1989). Clinical versus actuarial judgment. *Science*, 243, 1668–1674.

Dolan, M. & Doyle, M. (2000). Violence risk prediction: Clinical and actuarial measures and the role of the Psychopathy Checklist. *British Journal of Psychiatry*, 177, 303–311.

Douglas, K. S., Ogloff, J. R. P., Nicholls, T. L., & Grant, I. (1999). Assessing risk for violence among psychiatric patients: The HCR-20 violence risk assessment scheme and the Psychopathy Checklist: Screening Version. *Journal of Consulting and Clinical Psychology*, 67, 917–930.

Douglas, K. S. & Webster, C. D. (1999). The HCR-20 violence risk assessment scheme: Concurrent validity in a sample of incarcerated offenders. *Criminal Justice and Behavior*, 26, 3–19.

Douglas, K. S., Webster, C. D., Eaves, D., Hart, S. D., & Ogloff, J. R. P. (Eds.) (2001). *The HCR-20 Violence Risk Management Companion Manual*. Burnaby, BC, Canada: Mental Health, Law, and Policy Institute, Simon Fraser University.

Douglas, K. S. & Belfrage, H. (2001). Use of the HCR-20 in violence risk management: Implementation and clinical practice. In K. S. Douglas, C. D. Webster, D. Eaves, S. D. Hart, & J. R. P. Ogloff (Eds.), *The HCR-20 violence risk management companion manual*. Burnaby, BC, Canada: Mental Health, Law, and Policy Institute, Simon Fraser University.

Douglas, K. S. & Kropp, P. R. (2002). A prevention-based paradigm for violence risk assessment: Clinical and research applications. *Criminal Justice and Behavior*, 29, 617–658.

Douglas, K. S., Ogloff, J. R. P., & Hart, S. D. (2003). Evaluation of a model of violence risk assessment among forensic psychiatric patients. *Psychiatric Services*, 54, 1372–1379.

Douglas, K. S. & Ogloff, J. R. P. (2003a). Multiple facets of risk for violence: The impact of judgmental specificity on structured decisions about violence risk. *International Journal of Forensic Mental Health*, 2, 19–34.

Douglas, K. S. & Ogloff, J. R. P. (2003b). The impact of confidence on the accuracy of structured professional and actuarial violence risk judgments in a sample of forensic psychiatric patients. *Law and Human Behavior*, 27, 573–587.

Doyle, M. & Dolan, M. (2006). Evaluating the validity of anger regulation problems, interpersonal style, and disturbed mental state for predicting inpatient violence. *Behavioral Sciences and the Law*, 24, 783–798.

Dvoskin, J. A. & Heilbrun, K. (2001). Risk assessment and release decision-making: Toward resolving the great debate. *Journal of the American Academy of Psychiatry and the Law*, 29, 6–10.

Estelle v. Smith, 451 U.S. 454 (1980).

Estroff, S. E. & Zimmer, C. (1994). Social networks, social support, and violence among persons with severe, persistent mental illness. In J. Monahan & H. J. Steadman (Eds.), *Violence and Mental Disorder: Developments in Risk Assessment* (pp. 259–295). Chicago, IL: University of Chicago Press.

Estroff, S. E., Swanson, J. W., Lachicotte, W. S., Swartz, M., & Bolduc, M. (1998). Risk reconsidered: Targets of violence in the social networks of people with serious psychiatric disorders. *Social Psychiatry and Psychiatric Epidemiology*, 33, 95–101.

Faust, D. & Ziskin, J. (1988). The expert witness in psychology and psychiatry. *Science*, 241, 31–35.

Foucha v. Louisiana, 112 S.Ct. 1780 (1992).

Fulwiler, C., Grossman, H., Forbes, C., & Ruthazer, R. (1997). Early-onset substance abuse and community violence by outpatients with chronic mental illness. *Psychiatric Services*, 48, 1181–1185.

Gardner, W., Lidz, C. W., Mulvey, E. P., & Shaw, E. C. (1996). A comparison of actuarial methods for identifying repetitively violent patients with mental illnesses. *Law and Human Behavior*, 20, 35–48.

Grann, M., Belfrage, H., & Tengstrom, A. (2000). Actuarial assessment of risk for violence: Predictive validity of the VRAG and the historical part of the HCR-20. *Criminal Justice and Behavior*, 27, 97–114.

Gray, N. S., Taylor, J., & Snowden, R. J. (2008). Predicting violent reconvictions using the HCR-20. *British Journal of Psychiatry*, 192, 384–387.

Grisso, T., Davis, J., Vesselinov, R., Appelbaum, P. S., & Monahan, J. (2000). Violent thoughts and violent behavior following hospitalization for mental disorder. *Journal of Consulting and Clinical Psychology*, 68, 388–398.

Grove, W. M. & Meehl, P. E. (1996). Comparative efficiency of informal (subjective, impressionistic) and formal (mechanical, algorithmic) prediction procedures: The clinical-statistical controversy. *Psychology, Public Policy, and Law*, 2, 293–323.

Grove, W. M., Zald, D. H., Lebow, B. S., Snitz, B. E., & Nelson, C. (2000). Clinical versus mechanical prediction: A meta-analysis. *Psychological Assessment*, 12, 19–30.

Hanson, R. K. (1998). What do we know about sex offender risk assessment? *Psychology, Public Policy, and Law*, 4, 50–72.

Hare, R. D. (1991). *The Hare Psychopathy Checklist-Revised*. Toronto, ON, Canada: Multi-Health Systems.

Hare, R. D. (1998). Psychopaths and their nature: Implications for the mental health and criminal justice systems. In T. Millon, E. Simonsen, M. Birket-Smith, & R. D. Davis (Eds.), *Psychopathy: Antisocial, Criminal, and Violent Behavior.* (pp. 188–212). New York: Guilford Press.

Harris, G. T., Rice, M. E., & Quinsey, V. L. (1993). Violent recidivism of mentally disordered offenders: The development of a statistical prediction instrument. *Criminal Justice and Behavior*, 20, 315–335.

Harris, G. T., Rice, M. E., & Cormier, C. A. (2002). Prospective replication of the Violence Risk Appraisal Guide in predicting violent recidivism among forensic patients. *Law and Human Behavior*, 26, 377–394.

Hart, S. D. (1998). The role of psychopathy in assessing risk for violence: Conceptual and methodological issues. *Legal and Criminological Psychology*, 3, 121–137.

Hart, S., Cox, D., & Hare, R. (1995). *The Hare Psychopathy Checklist: Screening Version.* Toronto: Multi-Health Systems.

Heilbrun, K., Dvoskin, J., Hart, S., & McNeil, D. (1999). Violence risk communication: Implications for research, policy, and practice. *Health, Risk and Society,* 1, 91–106.

Hersh, K. & Borum, R. (1998). Command hallucinations, compliance, and risk assessment. *Journal of the American Academy of Psychiatry and the Law,* 26, 353–359.

Hiday, V. A., Swartz, M. S., Swanson, J. W., Borum, R., & Wagner, H. R. (1998). Male-female differences in the setting and construction of violence among people with severe mental illness. *Social Psychiatry and Psychiatric Epidemiology,* 33, 68–74.

Hodgins, S. (1992). Mental disorder, intellectual deficiency, and crime: Evidence from a birth cohort. *Archives of General Psychiatry,* 49, 476–483.

Huss, M. T. & Zeiss, R. A. (2004). Clinical assessment of violence from inpatient records: A comparison of individual and aggregate decision making across risk strategies. *International Journal of Forensic Mental Health,* 3, 139–147.

Klassen, D. & O'Connor, W. A. (1994). Demographic and case history variables in risk assessment. In J. Monahan & H. J. Steadman (Eds.), *Violence and Mental Disorder: Developments in Risk Assessment* (pp. 229–257). Chicago, IL: University of Chicago Press.

Krakowski, M. (1997). Neurologic and neuropsychologic correlates of violence. *Psychiatric Annals,* 27, 674–678.

Kropp, P. R., Hart, S. D., Webster, C. W., & Eaves, D. (1999). *Spousal Assault Risk Assessment Guide (SARA).* Vancouver, BC: Canada: Multi-health Systems, Inc.

Lessard v. Schmidt, 349 F. Supp. 1078 (1972).

Lidz, C., Mulvey, E., & Gardner, W. (1993). The accuracy of predictions of violence to others. *Journal of the American Medical Association,* 269, 1007–1011.

Link, B. G., Andrews, H., & Cullen, F. T. (1992). The violent and illegal behavior of mental patients reconsidered. *American Sociological Review,* 57, 275–292.

Link, B. G. & Stueve, A. (1994). Psychotic symptoms and the violent/illegal behavior of mental patients compared to community controls. In J. Monahan & H. J. Steadman (Eds.), *Violence and Mental Disorder: Developments in Risk Assessment* (pp. 137–159). Chicago, IL: University of Chicago Press.

Litwack, T. R. (2001). Actuarial versus clinical assessments of dangerousness. *Psychology, Public Policy, and Law,* 7, 409–443.

McNeil, D. E. (1997). Correlates of violence in psychotic patients. *Psychiatric Annals,* 27, 683–690.

McNeil, D. E., Binder, R. L., & Greenfield, T. K. (1988). Predictors of violence in civilly committed acute psychiatric patients. *American Journal of Psychiatry,* 145, 965–970.

McNiel, D. E. & Binder, R. L. (1989). Relationship between preadmission threats and later violent behavior by acute psychiatric inpatients. *Hospital & Community Psychiatry,* 40, 605–608.

McNiel, D. E. & Binder, R. L. (1991). Clinical assessment of the risk of violence among psychiatric inpatients. *American Journal of Psychiatry,* 148, 1317–1321.

McNiel, D. E. & Binder, R. L. (1995). Correlates of accuracy in the assessment of psychiatric inpatients' risk of violence. *American Journal of Psychiatry,* 152, 901–906.

McNiel, D. E., Eisner, J. P., & Binder, R. L. (2000). The relationship between command hallucinations and violence. *Psychiatric Services,* 51, 1288–1292.

McNiel, D. E., Lam, J. N., & Binder, R. L. (2000). Relevance of interrater agreement to violence risk assessment. *Journal of Consulting and Clinical Psychology,* 68, 1111–1115.

Melton, G. B., Petrila, J., Poythress, N. G., & Slobogin, C. (1997). *Psychological Evaluations for the Courts: A Handbook for Mental Health Professionals and Lawyers.* New York: Guilford Press.

Monahan, J. (1981). *The Clinical Prediction of Violent Behavior.* Washington, DC: U.S. Government Printing Office.

Monahan, J. (1992). Mental disorder and violent behavior: Perceptions and evidence. *American Psychologist,* 47, 511–521.

Monahan, J. (2003). Violence risk assessment. In A. M. Goldstein (Ed.), *Handbook of Psychology: Forensic Psychology, Vol. 11* (pp. 527–540). Hoboken, NJ: John Wiley & Sons, Inc.

Monahan, J. & Steadman, H. J. (1996). Violent storms and violent people: How meteorology can inform risk communication in mental health law. *American Psychologist,* 51, 931–938.

Monahan, J., Steadman, H. J., Appelbaum, P. S., Grisso, T., Mulvey, E. P., Roth, L. H., et al. (2006). The Classification of violence risk. *Behavioral Sciences and the Law,* 24, 721–730.

Monahan, J., Steadman, H. J., Appelbaum, P. S., Robbins, P. C., Mulvey, E. P., Silver, E., et al. (2000). Developing a clinically useful actuarial tool for assessing violence risk. *British Journal of Psychiatry,* 176, 312–319.

Monahan, J., Steadman, H.J., Silver, E., Appelbaum, A., Robbins, P., Mulvey, E., et al., (2001). *Rethinking Risk Assessment: The MacArthur Study of Mental Disorder and Violence.* New York: Oxford University Press.

Monahan, J., Steadman, H. J., Robbins, P. C., Appelbaum, P., Banks, S., Grisso, T., et al. (2005). An actuarial model of violence risk assessment for persons with mental disorders. *Psychiatric Services,* 56, 810–815.

Mossman, D. (1994). Assessing predictions of violence: Being accurate about accuracy. *Journal of Consulting and Clinical Psychology,* 62, 783–792.

Mossman, D. (2004). Understanding prediction instruments. In R. I. Simon, & L. H. Gold (Eds.), *The

American Psychiatric Publishing Textbook of Forensic Psychiatry (pp. 501–523). Washington, DC: American Psychiatric Publishing, Inc.

Mulvey, E. P. (1994). Assessing the evidence of a link between mental illness and violence. *Hospital & Community Psychiatry*, 45, 663–668.

Novaco, R. W. (1994). Anger as a risk factor for violence among the mentally disordered. In J. Monahan & H. J. Steadman (Eds.), *Violence and Mental Disorder: Developments in Risk Assessment* (pp. 21–59). Chicago, IL: University of Chicago Press.

Novaco, R. W. & Taylor, J. L. (2004). Assessment of anger and aggression in male offenders with developmental disabilities. *Psychological Assessment*, 16, 42–50.

Novaco, R. W. &Taylor, J. L. (2008). Anger and assaultiveness of male forensic patients with developmental disabilities: links to volatile parents. *Aggressive Behavior*, 34, 380–393.

Otto, R. K. (1992). Prediction of dangerous behavior: A review and analysis of "second-generation" research. *Forensic Reports*, 5, 103–133.

Otto, R. K. (2000). Assessing and managing violence risk in outpatient settings. *Journal of Clinical Psychology*, 56, 1239–1262.

Patterson, G. R. & Yoerger, K. (1993). Developmental models for delinquent behavior. In S. Hodgins (Ed.), *Mental Disorder and Crime* (pp. 140–172). Thousand Oaks, CA: Sage Publications, Inc.

Pinals, D. A. & Hoge, S. K. (2003). Treatment refusal in psychiatric practice. In R. Rosner (Ed.), *Principles and Practice of Forensic Psychiatry, 2nd Edition* (pp. 129–136). London: Arnold Press.

Quinsey, V. L., Harris, G. T., Rice, M. E., & Cormier, C. A. (1998a). *Violent Offenders: Appraising and Managing Risk.* Washington, DC: American Psychological Association.

Quinsey, V. L., Harris, G. T., Rice, M. E., & Cormier, C. A. (1998b). Clinical judgment. In V. L. Quinsey, G. T. Harris, M. E. Rice, & C. A. Cormier (Eds.), *Violent Offenders: Appraising and Managing Risk* (pp. 55–72). Washington, DC: American Psychological Association.

R. v. Demers, 185 C.C.C. (3d) 257 (S.C.C.) (2004).

R. v. Swain, 1 S.C.R. 933 (1991).

R. v. Tulikorpi, 1 S.C.R. 498 (2004).

Reiss, A. & Roth, J. (1993). *Understanding and Preventing Violence.* Washington, DC: National Academy Press.

Rice, M. E., Harris, G. T., Varney, G. W., & Quinsey, V. L. (1989). *Violence in Institutions: Understanding, Prevention, and Control.* Ashland, OH: Hogrefe & Huber Publishers.

Rice, M. E. & Harris, G. T. (1995). Violent recidivism: Assessing predictive validity. *Journal of Consulting and Clinical Psychology*, 63, 737–748.

Rice, M. E. & Harris, G. T. (1996). Predicting the recidivism of mentally disordered firesetters. *Journal of Interpersonal Violence*, 11, 364–375.

Rice, M. E. & Harris, G. T. (1997). Cross-validation and extension of the Violence Risk Appraisal Guide for child molesters and rapists. *Law and Human Behavior*, 21, 231–241.

Rogers, R. (2000). The uncritical acceptance of risk assessment in forensic practice. *Law and Human Behavior*, 24, 595–605.

Rudnick, A. (1999). Relation between command hallucinations and dangerous behavior. *Journal of the American Academy of Psychiatry and the Law*, 27, 253–257.

Sanders, J., Milne, S., Brown, P., & Bell, A. J. (2000). Assessment of aggression in psychiatric admissions: Semistructured interview and case note survey. *British Medical Journal*, 320, 1112.

Shawyer, F., Mackinnon, A., Farhall, J., Sims, E., Blaney, S., Yardley, P., et al. (2008). Acting on harmful command hallucinations in psychotic disorders: An integrative approach. *The Journal of Nervous and Mental Disease*, 196, 390–398.

Smith v. Jones, 1 S.C.R. 455 (1999).

Steadman, H. J., Monahan, J., Appelbaum, P. S., Grisso, T., Mulvey, E. P., Roth, L. H., et al. (1994). Designing a new generation of risk assessment research. In J. Monahan & H. J. Steadman (Eds.), *Violence and Mental Disorder: Developments in Risk Assessment* (pp. 297–318). Chicago, IL: University of Chicago Press.

Steadman, H. J., Mulvey, E. P., Monahan, J., Robbins, P. C., Appelbaum, P. S., Grisso, T., et al. (1998). Violence by people discharged from acute psychiatric inpatient facilities and by others in the same neighbourhoods. *Archives of General Psychiatry*, 55, 393–401.

Steadman, H. J., Silver, E., Monahan, J., Appelbaum, P. S., Robbins, P. C., Mulvey, E. P., et al. (2000). A classification tree approach to the development of actuarial violence risk assessment tools. *Law and Human Behavior*, 24, 83–100.

Strand, S., Belfrage, H., Fransson, G., & Levander, S. (1998). Clinical and risk management factors in risk prediction of mentally disordered offenders— more important than actuarial data? A retrospective study of 40 mentally disordered offenders assessed with the HCR-20 violence risk assessment scheme. *Legal and Criminological Psychology*, 4, 67–76.

Straznickas, K. A., McNiel, D. E., & Binder, R. L. (1993). Violence toward family caregivers by mentally ill relatives. *Hospital & Community Psychiatry*, 44, 385–387.

Sturidsson, K., Haggard-Grann, U., Lotterberg, M., Dernevik, M., & Grann, M. (2004). Clinicians' perceptions of which factors increase or decrease the risk of violence among forensic out-patients. *International Journal of Forensic Mental Health*, 3, 23–36.

Swanson, J. W., Holzer, C. E., Ganju, V. K., & Jono, R. T. (1990). Violence and psychiatric disorder in the community: Evidence from the Epidemiologic

Catchment Area surveys. *Hospital & Community Psychiatry*, 41, 761–770.

Swanson, J. W. (1994). Mental disorder, substance abuse, and community violence: An epidemiological approach. In J. Monahan & H. J. Steadman (Eds.), *Violence and Mental Disorder: Developments in risk assessment* (pp. 101–136). Chicago, IL: University of Chicago Press.

Swanson, J. W., Borum, R., Swartz, M. S., & Monahan, J. (1996). Psychotic symptoms and disorders and the risk of violent behaviour in the community. *Criminal Behaviour and Mental Health*, 6, 309–329.

Swanson, J. W., Swartz, M. S., Estroff, S., Borum, R., Wagner, R., & Hiday, V. (1998). Psychiatric impairment, social contact, and violent behavior: Evidence from a study of outpatient-committed persons with severe mental disorder. *Social Psychiatry and Psychiatric Epidemiology*, 33, 86–94.

Swanson, J. W., Borum, R., Swartz, M., & Hiday, V. (1999). Violent behavior preceding hospitalization among persons with severe mental illness. *Law and Human Behavior*, 23, 185–204.

Swanson, J. W., Swartz, M. S., Van Dorn, R. A., Elbogen, E. B., Wagner, H. R., Rosenheck, R. A., et al. (2006). A national study of violent behavior in persons with schizophrenia. *Archives General Psychiatry*, 63, 490–499.

Swartz, M. S., Swanson, J. W., Hiday, V. A., Borum, R., Wagner, H., Ryan, B., et al. (1998). Violence and severe mental illness: The effects of substance abuse and nonadherence to medication. *American Journal of Psychiatry*, 155, 226–231.

Swartz, M. S., Swanson, J. W., Wagner, H., Ryan, B., Barbara J., Hiday, V. A., et al. (1999). Can involuntary outpatient commitment reduce hospital recidivism? Findings from a randomized trial with severely mentally ill individuals. *American Journal of Psychiatry*, 156, 1968–1975.

Tarasoff v. Regents of the University of California, 551 P.2d 334 (1976).

Tardiff, K., Marzuk, P. M., Leon, A. C., Portera, L., & Wiener, C. (1997). Violence by patients admitted to a private psychiatric hospital. *American Journal of Psychiatry*, 154, 88–93.

Torrey, E. F., Stanley, J. D., Monahan, J., Steadman, H. J., & the MacArthur Study Group. (2008). The MacArthur Violence Risk Assessment Study revisited: Two views ten years after its initial publication. *Psychiatric Services*, 59, 147–152.

Van Dorn, R.A., Swanson, J.W., Elbogen, E.B., & Swartz, M.S. (2005). A comparison of stigmatizing attitudes toward persons with schizophrenia in four stakeholder groups: perceived likelihood of violence and desire for social distance. *Psychiatry*, 68, 152–63.

Webster, C. D., Harris, G. T., Rice, M. E., Cormier, C., & Quinsey, V. L. (1994). *The Violence Prediction Scheme: Assessing Dangerousness in High Risk Men*. Toronto, Canada: University of Toronto Centre of Criminology.

Webster, C. D., Douglas, K. S., Eaves, D., & Hart, S. D. (1997). *HCR-20: Assessing Risk for Violence* (version 2). Burnaby, BC, Canada: Mental Health, Law, and Policy Institute, Simon Fraser University.

Webster, C. D., Douglas K., Belfrage, H., & Link, B. (2000). Capturing change. An approach to managing violence and improving mental health. In S. Hodgins (Ed.), *Effective Prevention of Crime and Violence Among the Mentally Ill* (pp. 119–144). Dordrecht, the Netherlands: Kluwer Academic.

Winko v. British Columbia (Forensic Psychiatric Institute), 2 S.C.R. 625 (1999).

Witt, P. H. (2000). A practitioner's view of risk assessment: The HCR-20 and SVR-20. *Behavioral Sciences and the Law*, 18, 791–798.

Wong, S. C. P. & Gordon, A. (1998–2003). *Violence Risk Scale*. (Available from the authors, Department of Psychology, University of Saskatchewan, Saskatoon, Saskatchewan, Canada S7N 5A5, or online at http://www.psynergy.ca).

Wong, S. C. P. & Gordon, A. (2006). The validity and reliability of the Violence Risk Scale: A treatment-friendly violence risk assessment tool. *Psychology, Public Policy, and Law*, 12, 279–309.

Chapter 6

The Use of Actuarial Risk Assessment Instruments in Sex Offenders

Gina M. Vincent, Shannon M. Maney, and Stephen D. Hart

Sexual offending is increasingly seen as a major public health concern (Matson & Lieb, 1997). By virtue of this increased concern about sexual violence, sexual offenders are more likely than any other type of offenders to undergo psychological evaluations of their risk for reoffending. Canada has legislated dangerous offender and long-term offender sentences in the Criminal Code of Canada (1985) for the control of the risks presented by sex offenders at the community interface. Provinces may also resort to civil mental health enactments (Starnaman vs. Penetanguishene Mental Health Centre, 1995) to incapacitate the risk to the public sex offenders present after the expiration of their criminal sentences. In the United States, many states have enacted Sexually Violent Predator (SVP) statutes to extend the confinement of sex offenders under civil commitment laws (Janus & Meehl, 1997). These preventive detention hearings frequently call on psychological or psychiatric experts to assess whether a person is at elevated risk for engaging in future sexual violence, the primary condition for commitment. The initiation of SVP/DO laws challenged the profession to increase the specificity of *general violence* risk assessments to estimate the likelihood of future *sexually violent* recidivism.

Risk assessment schemes traditionally have taken one of two forms, *clinical* or *actuarial* decision making. *Clinical* decision making involves unstructured, subjective predictions made by a decision-maker after combining all the available data. *Actuarial* prediction is more mechanical and "involves a formal, algorithmic, objective procedure (e.g., equation) to reach the decision" (Grove & Meehl, 1996, p. 293). Because of the consistency and predictive validity of actuarial tools, several researchers have argued persuasively for the superiority of actuarial decision making to estimate the likelihood of future violence.

In the past decade, many risk assessment tools have been designed on the basis of the actuarial approach to estimate the probability that a given sex offender will commit an illegal sexual act in the future. Researchers have demonstrated that many of these tools have sound inter-rater reliability and predictive validity within restricted samples, and authors of a few of these tools have made revisions to the instruments to improve their predictive accuracy. These actuarial tools increasingly are being used to make decisions about whether a person should be incapacitated to prevent future violence.

Though the accuracy of many of these tests has been demonstrated under controlled conditions, there is still insufficient justification for heavy reliance on these tests in legal and clinical decision making (Grisso, 2000). Comprehensive reliability studies of measures of risk for sexual recidivism are nonexistent and have yet to be conducted systematically across various settings and populations. There is some evidence that the accuracy of these tools is variable across populations, the quantity of historical information, and the length of time at risk (Harris, Rice, Quinsey, Lalumiare, Boer, & Lang, 2003b). The instruments do not provide any information relevant to a person's treatment or management needs and there is no evidence that the risk for sexual recidivism tools have the ability to detect improvement or deterioration in risk nor is good management of risk reflected in the actuarial score. This undertaking is complicated because little is known about actual base rates of sexually violent recidivism after treatment and the validity of methods for measuring change. Finally, the largest concern is that many of these tools are interpreted as prescribing estimates of the probability of future sexual offending to individuals, which, as this chapter will explain, cannot be done with known precision (Hart, Michie, & Cooke, 2007).

This chapter will begin with a brief review of the purpose of risk assessments for sexual reoffending and will describe the nature of tools using the actuarial approach. The next section provides a detailed summary of the characteristics and psychometric properties of the most prominent actuarial tools available for assessing risk for sexual recidivism. We focused on information that would be essential for making informed decisions about selecting and evaluating these psychological tools for clinical use. Finally, we provide a critique of these risk instruments for sexual offenders and actuarial approaches in general and conclude with recommendations for current practice, alternative approaches (i.e., structured professional judgment) and guidelines for future research.

PURPOSE OF RISK FOR SEXUAL RECIDIVISM ASSESSMENTS

Sexual violence can be defined as *"actual, attempted, or threatened sexual contact with a person who is nonconsenting or unable to give consent"* (Boer, Hart, Kropp, & Webster, 1998, p. 9). Sexual violence has become a major public health concern because of its high prevalence and perceptions of its resistance to treatment. According to reported victimization data, one in five American females above the age of 16 has been the victim of a completed rape (Furby, Weinrott, & Blackshaw, 1989). According to a more recent survey by the National Institute of Justice (2000), 17.6% of all women surveyed had been victims of a completed or attempted rape at some point in their lives, 21.6% of which were under the age of 12 at the time of the event. Mendel (1995) reviewed the studies of prevalence of sexual abuse among males. In general, the consensus was that between one in five and one in eight males have been abused in childhood. Among sex offenders, according to the meta-analysis by Hanson and Morton-Bourgon (2005), the observed sexual recidivism rate was 13.7% after an average 76 month follow-up. Given reporting rates of sex crimes, 13.7% is probably a gross underestimation of actual recidivism rates over the long-term. Doren (1998) estimated the actual long-term base rate to be around 52% for child molesters and 39% for rapists.

Sexual offenders comprise a group of criminals who have been singled out and subjected to special statutes for commitment and detention to an extent unparalleled by any other group of criminal offenders (Becker & Murphy, 1998). Between 1988 and 1990, the number of incarcerated sex offenders in the United States increased by 48%, and by 1998, approximately one-third of the incarcerated population in some states were sex offenders (Grubin & Wingate, 1996; Prentky, Lee, & Knight, 1997; Quinsey, Harris, Rice, & Cormier, 1998). In addition to mandatory chemical castration, sex offender registries, dangerous offender, and "three strikes legislation" enacted in some states and Canada, SVP laws have been enacted or are developing in at least 35 states since the constitutionality of SVP statutes was upheld by the U.S. Supreme Court (Kansas v. Hendricks, 1997).

SVP laws permit continued preventative detention of sex offenders after completion of a criminal sentence if there is a high likelihood of their engaging in future acts of sexual violence on account of mental disorder. SVP statutes generally require four conditions for commitment: (1) a history of sexual violence, (2) a current mental abnormality, (3) an elevated risk for future sexual violence, and (4) a causal link between the mental illness and the risk. There is some evidence to suggest that many states with SVP laws have been civilly committing sex offenders that do not even reach, on average, a 50% probability of reoffending (Janus & Meehl, 1997). As Janus and Meehl argue, this is likely a result of the use of static measures that have not been validated as being able to accurately capture reoffense within an acceptable level among civilly committed patients.

Often these civil hearings call for forensic evaluator's opinions as to whether or not an offender is at elevated risk for future acts of sexual violence (Hanson, 1998; Hart, 2003). After one is determined to be SVP, the question for forensic evaluators becomes whether the confined SVP has responded to treatment well enough to warrant release. Forensic evaluators have been assigned with the task of (1) making reliable and valid decisions about an examinee's level of risk and the influence of a mental abnormality on that risk, and (2) reassessing risk in a manner that will detect improvement or deterioration.

Nature of Actuarial Decision Making

For the past 20 years, research into the risk factors and recidivism rates for sex offenders has grown steadily in the psychological literature. Previous to this, reviews indicated that mental health professionals had no special skills for determining risk and often were performing, at levels of accuracy that barely exceeded chance (Borum, 1996; Grisso & Tomkins, 1996). With the contributions of the second generation of risk research in the past two decades, it has become generally recognized that forensic evaluators have some modest ability to predict violent behavior. This improvement reflects not only a growing foundation of knowledge about the factors related to violence and violent reoffending, but also increasing knowledge of the methods and analyses that are best suited to the study of violence risk assessment (Mossman, 1994). One problem in the past was reliance on unstructured clinical decisions which do not necessarily make risk variables explicit, may not be empirically validated, and have demonstrated little value in the prediction of recidivism (Grisso & Tomkins, 1996; Monahan, 1996; Quinsey et al., 1998).

Risk assessment tools applying actuarial decision-making schemes have demonstrated superior predictive validity, relative to unstructured clinical decision making (Grove & Meehl, 1996). What defines actuarial decision making is applying a formal procedure, generally an algorithm, to make a judgment, in this case a judgment as to a sex offender's level of risk for engaging in sexual offending in the future. Actuarial instruments were designed to *predict the future*. The majority of these instruments purport to calculate the probability that a given examinee will sexually reoffend. Typically, the items of these tools are selected empirically on the basis of their association with a given outcome (reoccurrence of sexual violence) and are scored and combined according to some algorithm to aid in producing a decision about the likelihood of recidivism. The Sex Offender Risk Appraisal Guide (SORAG; Quinsey et al., 1998), for example, contains items selected on the basis of the strength of each variable's prediction for sexual recidivism based on retrospective studies of sexual recidivism in male offenders from a single setting. The objectivity and predictive accuracy of actuarial tools has led some to advocate for their sole usage without contamination from clinical judgment (Grove & Meehl, 1996; Quinsey et al., 1998).

REVIEW OF ACTUARIAL RISK ASSESSMENT TOOLS FOR SEXUAL REOFFENDING

Over the past decade we have seen the advent of a number of psychological actuarial tools designed for assessing risk for sexual violence or recidivism. This section reviews the most prominent actuarial instruments and covers basic information that would be essential for clinicians to evaluate the usefulness and applicability of the test to their needs. We included nine tools in this chapter because each tool fits two main criteria. First, we only included tools designed for actuarial decision making or, in the case of the Psychopathy Checklist-Revised, tools that may not have been designed for actuarial use but have been used actuarially with sex offender samples. Instruments like the Sexual Violence Risk-20 (SVR-20) are not included in this chapter because these tools use structured professional judgment as opposed to actuarial decision making. Second, we only included tools that had been published or at least were in widespread distribution for clinical use (as opposed to research use) at the time of this review.

Each instrument summary that follows includes information about the intended examinee population (e.g., adult male sex offenders), purpose of the instrument (e.g., to predict sexual recidivism), design (number of items and scales), administration procedures (e.g., requires an interview with the offender), scoring procedures, how the instrument was developed, and a summary of research findings on the psychometric properties. Before reading these reviews, readers should be familiar with a few issues. One issue pertains to the nature of *risk factors*—circumstances or life events that increase the likelihood of engaging in criminal activity. Risk factors (items in risk assessment tools), can be either *static* (e.g., past sexual abuse) or *dynamic* (e.g., negative mood, substance use, attitudes that support rape). Dynamic factors are variable and can be used to guide rehabilitative efforts by targeting influences on sexually offending behavior and guiding interventions aimed at changing those factors. Static factors on the other hand, are generally historical and difficult if not impossible to change.

A second issue pertains to how one evaluates whether a tool has demonstrated adequate predictive validity. In other words, since these actuarial tools were designed to *predict sexual reoffending*, the quality of the research used to demonstrate each tool's predictive validity is of utmost importance. Here it is important to be familiar with some of the methods of longitudinal research. The longitudinal studies can vary in the length of follow-up periods, operational definition of "time at risk" (the length of time one has an opportunity to reoffend), method, and definition of outcomes. The method can be *prospective*, studying trends by recording data at one point in time and again during several points in time in the future (e.g., risk factors at Time 1 and recidivism at Time 2), or *retrospective*, studying trends by recording data from various time periods simultaneously.

Recidivism studies vary widely in the operationalization of outcomes. Most recidivism studies employ a single method for measuring recidivism, generally official criminal records, but a minority supplement official records with self-report and/or collateral information. Added variability is found in the metric used to quantify recidivism . This may include mere occurrence of a reoffense (any vs. no recidivism), frequency (number of reoffenses during follow-up), or imminence (time to reoffending). Among the sex offender studies, some made a clean distinction between *generally violent* and *sexual recidivism*, but more commonly, violent recidivism outcomes include both sexual reoffenses and generally violent reoffenses. This is important to note because, in these cases, the violent recidivism category always will have higher base rates than the sexual recidivism category, making it easier to predict for statistical reasons.

As summarized by Hart (1998) and Douglas et al. (2006), in general, *broader definitions of violence* and *longer follow-up periods* will lead to higher base rates and more powerful statistical predictions. Further, *self-report measures* of violence will generate significantly greater and ostensibly more accurate reports of violent incidents. Unless the follow-up period is fixed, it is particularly crucial that outcome measures *incorporate time at risk* before reoffending, using survival or Cox proportional hazards regression analyses, because of the wide variability within samples. Generally, statistics using dichotomous outcomes will underestimate predictive accuracy because these ignore the complexity of the data.

In the summaries that follow, when dichotomous outcomes were used, we reported findings from the recommended test of predictive accuracy, the receiver operating characteristic (ROC) analysis (Mossman, 1994). ROC curves plot the association between sensitivity (the true positive rate) and 1—specificity (the false positive rate) for all possible cutoff scores on the measure of interest. The area under the ROC curve (AUC) is an index of the measure's overall classification accuracy. The AUC can range from 0 to 1.0 where 0.5 indicates chance-level accuracy, greater than 0.5 indicates above-chance accuracy, and less than 0.5 indicates below-chance accuracy. For example, an AUC of 0.68 would imply that there is a 68% chance that a sex offender who was charged with a sexual reoffense obtained a higher score on the specific tool (e.g., SORAG) than a randomly chosen individual who did not commit a sexual reoffense. This figure does *not* tell us that an offender with a certain test score has a 68% probability of recidivism (Mossman, 2006), a common misinterpretation. According to Swets (1988), AUCs for an acceptable screening tool would be between 0.70 and 0.90.

Sex Offender Risk Appraisal Guide

The *Sex Offender Risk Appraisal Guide* (SORAG) is a 14-item rating scale designed to predict violent and sexually violent recidivism in men known to have committed a sexual offense involving physical contact. The SORAG is a derivative of the VRAG developed to predict violent recidivism, including sexual recidivism in sex offenders (Rice & Harris, 1997). The SORAG includes all 10 items of the Violence Risk Appraisal Guide (VRAG; Quinsey et al., 1998); for example, the *Psychopathy Checklist-Revised* (PCL-R; Hare, 2003) score, Elementary School Maladjustment, Cormier–Lang criminal history, and alcohol abuse history; plus an additional four items specifically related to sexual reoffending (e.g., phallometric deviance). Each item can be scored on the sole basis of solely institutional file information, with the exception of the PCL-R. Ostensibly, the SORAG needs to be completed by a psychologist or other qualified examiner since the PCL-R is one of its items. Like the VRAG, the SORAG items have varying low to high risk scale ranges (from negative to positive integer weights), and these item scores are summed into an overall risk score. Overall risk scores are translated into one of nine categories ("bins") that give the individual's probability of recidivism using the risk score table. The probability of recidivism ranges from 9% for Bin 1 (scores ≤11) to >99% for Bin 9 (scores ≥32). It is important to note that the bins are intended to estimate only the likelihood of another sex offense occurring. Like most of the actuarial tools described in this chapter, the risk categories of the SORAG say nothing about the likely severity of the sex offense—ostensibly, the reoffense could be an act like indecent exposure, which involves no physical harm to a victim.

The items of the SORAG were selected using stepwise multivariate methods with samples of sex offenders institutionalized in a maximum security psychiatric hospital (Quinsey et al., 1998). The interrater reliability of the SORAG appears to be quite high, ranging from 0.90 (Bartosh et al., 2003) to 0.96 (Harris et al., 2003b), and has been calculated between research assistant raters and masters level clinicians (Barbaree et al., 2001). Several studies reported the SORAG's concurrent validity with other tools known to predict violent recidivism or sexual recidivism specifically. Correlations with measures known to predict general violence, like the PCL-R ($r = 0.72$) or VRAG ($r = 0.90$ to 0.93), are higher than those with measures designed to predict sexual recidivism specifically, such as the Rapid Risk Assessment for Sexual Offense Recidivism (RRASOR) ($r = 0.45$ or

lower), Static-99 (around $r = 0.65$), and MnSOST-R ($r = 0.41$) (Barbaree et al., 2001; Harris et al., 2003b).

The predictive validity of the SORAG has been tested on fairly heterogeneous samples by independent researchers with significant findings in the prediction of recidivism. The samples under study have included incarcerated sex offenders, sex offenders housed in a sex offender treatment program, and nonincarcerated offenders referred to an outpatient treatment program (Barbaree et al., 2001; Bartosh et al., 2003; Harris et al., 2003b; Nunes, Firestone, Bradford, Greenberg, & Broom, 2002). All of these studies involved retrospective file-based scoring of the SORAG and an average follow-up period ranging from 3 years to more than 7 years. Most studies have found the SORAG to be a significant predictor of sexual recidivism, with the highest AUC only around 0.69 (Looman, 2006). The SORAG seems to be a better predictor of sexual recidivism for child molesters than rapists (AUC = 0.70 vs. 0.62, respectively, Harris et al., 2003b), and is better at predicting violent recidivism generally than sexual recidivism specifically (Ducro & Pham, 2006).

Rapid Risk Assessment for Sexual Offense Recidivism

The Rapid Risk Assessment for Sexual Offense Recidivism (RRASOR; Hanson, 1997) is the shortest tool available for predicting sexual reoffending. The RRASOR is a 4-item rating scale designed specifically to predict sexual recidivism among men who have been convicted of a sexual offense. The items are based on one's age and details of their sex offense history and are scored easily by using file information. Total scores range from 0 to 6 with higher scores indicating higher risk. No other guidance is given about how to use total scores. Presumably, little to no training is necessary for scoring the RRASOR but authors have not formally addressed rater qualifications.

The items used for the RRASOR were derived from a sample of seven risk predictors taken from the meta-analysis of sexual offense recidivism by Hanson and Bussiere (1996). Intercorrelations were computed for the seven data sets and the correlations were averaged into a single correlation matrix (Hanson, 1997). The best predictor variables were identified on the basis of their high β in a stepwise regression (Hanson & Thornton, 1999). Thus, the RRASOR's items were selected on the basis of the best predictors of sexual recidivism found across a wide range of samples and studies. Inter-rater reliability of the RRASOR has been reported to range between $r = 0.90$ (Bartosh, Garby, Lewis, & Gray, 2003) to 0.95 (Harris et al., 2003b) amongst research assistant raters and has been reported at $r = 0.94$ (Barbaree, Seto, Langton, & Peacock, 2001) between master level clinicians. Several studies have reported the RRASOR's concurrent validity with other tools known to predict violent recidivism or sexual recidivism specifically. Correlations with the Static-99 ($r = 0.69$ to 0.87) are higher than those with the SORAG ($r = 0.45$ or lower) and MnSOST-R ($r = 0.32$ or lower), and correlations with the PCL-R have been reported as nonsignificant (Barbaree et al., 2001; Harris et al., 2003b; Roberts, Doren, & Thornton, 2002).

Studies have tested the RRASOR's ability to predict recidivism primarily using some type of prison sample comprising individuals convicted of a sex offense (Långström, 2004). Like the SORAG, studies of the RRASOR have used retrospective follow-up designs and file-based ratings and have spanned an average follow-up from 3 to 5.5 years. Studies have identified the RRASOR to be a better predictor of sexual recidivism than violent recidivism with fair consistency, with the highest AUCs for sexual recidivism at 0.77 (Barbaree et al., 2001; Långström, 2004). In a study combining the samples from 10 studies, there was little difference in the RRASOR's predictive accuracy for child molesters (AUC = 0.67) versus rapists (AUC = 0.69) (Hanson & Thornton, 2003), albeit individual studies have found larger differences in the test's predictive accuracy between these groups (see Harris et al., 2003b; Sjostedt & Langstrom, 2001).

Static-99/Static-2002

According to a recent survey, the Static-99 is the most widely used sex offender risk assessment instrument among forensic evaluators in North America (Archer, Buffington-Vollum, Stredny, & Handel, 2006). The Static-99 was designed to assess the long-term potential of risk for recidivism of violent and sexual offenses among adult males who have been convicted of at least one sexual offense against a child or nonconsenting adult (Hanson & Thornton, 2003). The Static-99 is a 10-item tool that was created by combining items from the RRASOR and Thornton's Structured Anchored Clinical Judgment

Scale (SACJ). Its revision, the Static-2002, is a 13-item tool that added and refined items to the Static-99 to improve the ease and consistency of scoring. The authors selected and weighted items for the Static-2002 from the meta-analysis by Hanson and Bussiere (1998) on the basis of the strength of the prediction for sexual recidivism, simplicity, and relevance. So, like the RRASOR, the items for the Static-99 or Static-2002 were selected on the basis of the strongest predictors of sexual recidivism across a wide range of samples and studies. Although this review discusses both the Static-99 and Static-2002, it is important to note that it is still the Static-99 that should be used in practice until the Static-2002 has a comprehensive test manual and more extensive cross-validation (Hanson, 2006; Langton, Barbaree, Hansen, Harkins, & Peacock, 2007).

All items on these tools are static and scored on the basis of file information. The coding is meant to be straight-forward for an experienced evaluator, which includes researchers, police, psychologists, and parole and probation officers. There is a detailed test manual that describes the scoring rules for each item. The Static-99 provides estimates of risk on the basis of the raw score. For example, a score of 0 to 1 indicates "low risk," a score of 2 to 3 indicates "low to medium" risk, and so forth. There is also a probability of recidivism table based on these categories that is separated by 5, 10, and 15 year probabilities for both violent and sexual recidivism (Harris, Phenix, Hanson, & Thornton, 2003a). The 2003 manual for the Static-2002 does not contain such categories so the prescribed use of scores is unclear at this time.

Inter-rater reliability for the Static-99 has been reported around $r = .90$ between researchers (e.g., Barbaree, Seto, Langton, & Peacock, 2001; Harris et al., 2003b) and an intra-class correlation coefficient (ICC) of 0.80. Interrater reliability for the Static-2002 ranges from 0.72 to 0.92 (Langton, Barbaree, Hansen, Harkins, & Peacock, 2007a). The Static-99 is significantly, but only moderately correlated with other measures of risk for sexual and violent recidivism, having the highest correlation reported with the SORAG. The Static-2002 correlates with other tools reasonably well, starting with 0.71 with the SORAG, 0.69 with the RRASOR, and 0.58 with the MnSOST-R (Langton et al., 2007a).

As far as its relation to recidivism, the Static-99 probably has been tested more than any other risk assessment for sexual recidivism tool. Samples include prisoners convicted of a sex offense, individuals evaluated at an outpatient sexual behavior clinic, and forensic psychiatric patients in Swedish, Canadian, and Dutch populations. These have been retrospective follow-up studies, of periods ranging from 3 to more than 9 years that have used the Static-99 code based on archival information. Hanson and Thornton (2003) coded both the Static-99 and Static-2002 using archival information from the combined sex offender datasets of 10 recidivism studies, making a sample of more than 4000 cases. Across studies, the Static-99 appeared to predict sexual recidivism and serious and violent recidivism equally well with an average AUC around 0.68. The Static-2002 showed a slight improvement over the Static-99, resulting in an AUC of 0.72 for sexual recidivism and 0.71 for violent recidivism. The Static-2002's predictive accuracy differed between child molesters (AUC = 0.68) and rapists (AUC = 0.73) by 5% points. A cross-validation study of the Static-2002 recently reported similar findings using an archival sample of 468 sex offenders that were followed for an average of 5.9 years (Langton et al., 2007b).

In a 9-year follow-up study, Stadtland et al. (2005) compared the predictive validity of the Static-99 to other risk assessment measures using three heterogeneous samples of sex offenders in Germany. The Static-99 predicted contact sexual recidivism (AUC = 0.66) with relatively the same accuracy as the other instruments (e.g., PCL-R, HCR-20, SVR-20), which was lower than its predictive accuracy for noncontact sexual recidivism and violent recidivism. Survival analyses indicated that the groups of sex offenders falling into the higher risk categories on the Static-99 had significantly earlier relapses than the low risk category groups.

Violence Risk Scale—Sexual Offender Version

The Violence Risk Scale—Sex Offender Version (VRS-SO) (Wong, Olver, Nicholaichuck, & Gordon, 2003) was designed to assess the risk for sexual recidivism in forensic populations before and following treatment. The VRS-SO uses 24 items, seven static and 17 dynamic, rated on a 4-point scale (0–3) with 0 reflecting "less risk" and 3 reflecting "higher risk." These items were chosen based on empirical or conceptual links to sexual recidivism. The Total PreTreatment Risk score (range from 0 to 72)

combines the static and dynamic risk items, and is representative of current risk for sexual recidivism. The VRS-SO also helps to identify treatment targets (based on dynamic factors), readiness for treatment, and can measure pre- and posttreatment risk to identify changes in risk. The Total Post-Treatment Risk score combines the static and dynamic risk scores and subtracts a change score based on the stage of change of the individual before and following treatment (e.g., precontemplation/contemplation stage, preparation stage, action stage, and maintenance stage). Both Total Risk Scores can be divided into static or dynamic risk scores. A clinical override is provided in order to allow the rater to change the risk level based on idiosyncratic factors. To score the VRS-SO, a file review and semistructured interview are required, and if available, other collateral information can be used to assist in scoring. The scoring of the VRS-SO requires only a couple days of training and the tool can be used by front-line criminal justice staff; no professional qualifications are required.

The VRS-SO is one of the newer risk assessment tools, so there has only been one psychometric study reported to date (Olver, Wong, Nicholaichuck, & Gordon, 2007). The study used a sample of 321 male federal offenders who participated in a sex offender treatment program in a maximum-security Canadian mental health facility. In this study, four risk categories were created: low risk (0–20), moderate-low (21–30), moderate high (31–40), and high (41–72). Three factors were identified within the dynamic risk items (sexual deviance, criminality, and treatment responsivity). The VRS-SO demonstrated acceptable internal consistency and interrater reliability (pretreatment dynamic risk score ICC = 0.74 and posttreatment dynamic risk score ICC = 0.79). The VRS-SO total scores positively correlated with the Static-99 (pretreatment risk score, r = 0.55 and posttreatment risk score, r = 0.54). The predictive accuracy of the VRS-SO over an average period of 10 years was better for the static score (AUC = 0.74) than for the dynamic pretreatment (AUC = 0.66) or dynamic posttreatment (AUC = 0.67) scores.

Minnesota Sex Offender Screening Tool-Revised

The Minnesota Sex Offender Screening Tool-Revised (MnSOST-R) (Epperson, Kaul, Huot, Hesselton, Alexander, & Goldman, 2000) is a 16-item rating scale designed to predict sexual recidivism among rapists and extrafamilial child molesters. The authors excluded intrafamilial sex offenders because they were thought to be different than other offenders. Twelve items of the MnSOST-R are Historical/Static and four items are Institutional/Dynamic in nature. The total score is then used to assign an overall risk level of low, moderate, or high risk for sexual recidivism. Items are scored by trained examiners on the basis of institutional file information and well-defined scoring criteria. An advantage of the MnSOST-R is its ability to produce different cut scores for different decisions to reduce the likelihood of false positives and negatives.

The original version of the MnSOST was created around 1995 (Epperson, Kaul, Huot, Hesselton, Alexander, & Goldman, 1995). Based on a review of the literature, 14 items were identified, and the authors assigned weights to these items based on clinical judgment. Preliminary studies found fair reliability and validity but the MnSOST was still criticized for its clinical versus statistical formulation of the relative weights within the items (Doren, 1999). The revision of the MnSOST began in 1996 to apply an empirical approach to the clinically based item selection and scoring. Its revision, the MnSOST-R, was published in 2000 with risk prediction and scoring based on a 6-year follow-up of the development sample (Epperson et al., 2000). In 2003, the authors extended the follow-up of the development sample, updated the validity data, and suggested risk level cut scores (Epperson, Kaul, Huot, Goldman, & Alexander, 2003).

The MnSOST-R's inter-rater reliability based on the development sample was reported in the test manual to be $ICC_2 = 0.76$. The authors also reported an ICC = 0.86 from a reliability study conducted in the field, which better reflects the conditions where the MnSOST-R is usually scored. A few studies have reported the concurrent validity between the MnSOST-R and other measures of risk for violent or sexual recidivism. Although the MnSOST-R has been significantly correlated with other measures, the strength of these correlations has been quite inconsistent. For example, Roberts et al. (2002) found the correlation between the PCL-R and MnSOST-R to be 0.61, whereas Barbaree et al. (2001) reported the correlation at only 0.30. Only a couple published studies have examined the predictive validity of the MnSOST-R on independent samples. Earlier studies

found that the MnSOST-R did not significantly predict violent or sexual recidivism (Barbaree et al., 2001; Bartosh et al., 2003). However, a more recent study found that it performed about as well as other risk instruments in predicting risk for sexual (AUC = 0.70) and serious (AUC = 0.64) recidivism (Langton et al., 2007b) in a 5.9 year follow-up study of an archival sample of sex offenders.

Sex Offender Need Assessment Rating

The Sex Offender Need Assessment Rating (SONAR; Hanson & Harris, 2000) is a 9-item tool designed to assess change in risk for sexual recidivism among sex offenders, and to aid in developing responsive interventions and management plans. Currently, this is the only actuarial instrument among those in widespread distribution which was designed to be dynamic and capable of measuring actual changes in risk. As the authors of this tool noted, most items on the extant scales are historical in nature and consequently, are of little use when it comes to evaluating long-term risk.

The items of the SONAR were identified as relevant to recidivism among sex offenders as informed by theory, previous research, and observation. To identify dynamic predictors of recidivism, the authors compared a group of sexual offenders who recidivated ($n = 208$) sexually or violently while on community supervision to a matched group of sexual offenders who did not recidivate ($n = 201$; Hanson & Harris, 2001). The authors recorded variables based on the offenders' background, scores on the Static-99 and VRAG, and structured interviews with probation and parole officers who supervised the offenders in the community. The officers were asked whether certain problems were of a concern during the time they supervised the offenders and whether each problem was worse 6 months before recidivism (for the recidivist group only) or 1 month before recidivism (the past month of supervision for the nonrecidivist group). The dynamic risk factors that differed between the groups were included in the SONAR.

The SONAR contains five relatively stable factors (intimacy deficits, negative social influences, attitudes tolerant of sex offending, sexual self-regulation, and general self-regulation) scored on a three-point scale (0 to 2) with scores corresponding to the 12-month time period preceding the assessment. It also contains four acute factors (substance abuse, negative mood, anger, and victim access) that were designed to help identify *when* sex offenders are most likely to reoffend, rather than identify long-term recidivism potential. These items are scored on a scale ranging from −1 to +1, which were designed to capture whether an examinee's specific behavior improved, stayed the same, or worsened over the previous month or since the last assessment. The sum of the stable and acute factors results in a total score of −4 to 14. Total scores are summed and translated into one of five risk categories (low, low moderate, moderate, high moderate, and moderate).

The examiner qualifications and necessary assessment procedures for the SONAR are not entirely clear but it appears that the test can be administered by probation officers and requires a combination of a structured interview and review of case information. To date, the psychometric properties for the SONAR are based on only the development sample. Hanson and Harris (2001) calculated the inter-rater reliability of the SONAR from a sample of sex offenders on community supervision. Inter-rater agreement on the scale was high for file codings (95% average agreement) and interview codings (97%) and internal consistency was fairly low ($\alpha = 0.43$). Concurrent validity appears low in terms of its relation to the Static-99 ($r = 0.14$) and moderate in its relation to the VRAG ($r = 0.39$). Based on the development sample the SONAR seems to have adequate predictive accuracy (AUC = 0.74) with regards to sexual recidivism, and incremental predictive validity over the VRAG and Static-99; however, its ability to predict recidivism has yet to be validated on other samples.

Sexually Violent Predator Assessment Screening Instrument

The *Sexually Violent Predator Assessment Screening Instrument* (SVPASI) was designed by the Colorado Division of Criminal Justice (DCJ) and the Colorado Sex Offender Management Board (SOMB) in 1999 for use with convicted adult sex offenders or juveniles tried as adults in the Colorado criminal justice system. The SVPASI is separated into 4 parts plus the SOMB checklist. Part 1 consists of demographic and index offense information, Part 2 regards the relationship to the victim, Part 3 consists of 10 yes/no items known as the DCJ Sex Offender Risk Scales (SORS), and Part 4—Mental Abnormality, contains results from the PCL-R or the Millon Clinical Multiaxial Inventory—III (MCMI-III). The SOMB checklist

contains seven categories (motivation, denial, readiness to change, social skills, positive social support, deviant sexual practices, and taking care of business) with 56 items rated on a scale from 0 "Not at All" to 5 "Very Much." Some Parts of the SVPASI are completed by probation officers and some require SOMB evaluators.

The development sample consisted of 494 adult male sex offenders involved in probation corrections, or parole in Colorado during the time spanning December 1, 1996 to November 30, 1997. The study investigated the relation between both static and dynamic variables to recidivism during a 12-month and a 30-month follow-up period. The SORS was developed using a stepwise regression model. Ten risk factors were identified, including, for example, juvenile felony adjudications, prior adult felony convictions, drug or alcohol use at the time of offense, and employment. Internal consistency for the SOMB checklist scale range from 0.74 to 0.94. Odds ratios demonstrate that individuals scoring 4 or more on the SORS are at increased risk of failure at 12-months and at 30-months after release.

Each Part of the SVPASI has a specified procedure to determine whether criteria have been met. For example, criteria is met for Part 4 when an offender scores 18 or higher on the Psychopathy Checklist: Screening Version (PCL:SV), 30 or higher on the PCL-R, or scores 85 or more on the narcissistic, antisocial, and paranoid scales of the MCMI-III. If an offender meets criteria for Parts 1 and 2 plus criteria for Part 3 or Part 4, then the offender will be referred to the court as a SVP (however, the court makes the final determination for designation as a SVP). There is a detailed manual for the SVPASI but this tool has yet to be validated on independent samples outside of the development sample.

Registrant Risk Assessment Scale

The Registrant Risk Assessment Scale (RRAS; Whitman & Farmer, 2000) was created for use with convicted sex offenders in New Jersey to provide prosecutors with a method for making community sex offender notification decisions mandated by statute. The intent of the RRAS was to allow prosecutors to apply the notification law uniformly throughout the state. The RRAS has 13-items organized into four general areas: (1) seriousness of the offense, (2) offense history, (3) characteristics of the offender, and

(4) community support (e.g., therapeutic support, residential support, employment/educational stability). Each item is scored on a 3-point scale and each of the four areas is weighted on the basis of the relevance of their relation to recidivism. Total scores are translated into categories of low, moderate, or high risk, which are used to place offenders into tiers for levels of notification. Prosecutors can only override these tiers in specific situations.

Development of the RRAS began in 1995 when New Jersey's attorney general commissioned a panel of forensic experts to design an objective measure for making notification decisions for sex offenders. Items were selected on the basis of empirical support but they were weighted on the basis of the judgment of this expert panel. The RRAS can be completed by "trained personnel" on the basis of file information alone using detailed scoring criteria in the manual (Ferguson, Eidelson, & Witt, 1998). The RRAS has been published and is available for widespread use. The RRAS' factor structure and ability to classify groups of offenders was cross-validated on half of the development sample, but the structure and predictive validity has yet to be replicated in independent samples. To date its inter-rater reliability has not been reported.

Vermont Assessment of Sex Offender Risk

The Vermont Assessment of Sex Offender Risk (VASOR; McGrath & Hoke, 2001) is a 19-item scale designed for use with adult male sex offenders to assist probation and parole officers in making placement and supervision decisions. The VASOR was designed to be scored by probation officers and correctional caseworkers who have completed some practice scoring and have some familiarity with risk factors and psychological assessment. The items are coded on the basis of scoring criteria in the test manual using information from case files and offender interviews. The authors claim it is best used as a decision-making aid along with professional judgment and other tools until more research has been conducted.

The VASOR items were chosen on the basis of an exhaustive literature review, clinical experience, and ease of scoring. Items were weighted on the basis of "empirically guided clinical judgment" (McGrath & Hoke, 2001). Most items are historical and static in nature, but a few pertain to more dynamic factors

such as amenability to treatment and lifestyle stability. The VASOR contains two scales, a 13-item scale that assesses reoffense risk and a 6-item scale that assesses violence. Scores on the two scales are plotted on a scoring grid that places the offender into a category of low, moderate, or high risk. Low risk suggests one can be considered for community supervision and treatment, moderate risk suggests one may or may not be appropriate for community placement, and high risk suggests the offender is not appropriate for community supervision and treatment. The tool correctly classified 92.6% of offenders in the development sample as being in one of these three levels of supervision.

The VASOR has undergone rigorous tests of its inter-rater reliability, finding good agreement with an ICC = 0.83 for the reoffense risk scale, ICC = 0.89 for violence, and an ICC = 0.87 for total scores (Langton, Barbaree, Harkins, Seto, & Peacock, 2002; McGrath, Hoke, Livingston, & Cumming, 2001). The VASOR scales and total scores are significantly related to other measures of sexual violence and general violence risk, including the MnSOST-R, RRASOR, and PCL-R (Packard & Gordon, 1999). Finally, the VASOR's predictive validity has been tested with independent samples. In terms of its 3-year prediction of sexual recidivism it performs as well as, or better than other instruments listed in this chapter (Langton et al., 2002) with an AUC = 0.75. To date, no studies on the VASOR's reliability or validity have been published.

LIMITATIONS WITH ACTUARIAL RISK ASSESSMENT TOOLS FOR SEXUAL REOFFENDING

Several critics have pointed out the limitations of actuarial assessments and the dangers of reliance on actuarial decision making (Berlin, Galbreath, Geary, & McGlone, 2003; Dvoskin & Heilbrun, 2001; Grisso, 2000; Hart, 2003; Hart, Kropp, Laws, Klaver, Logan, & Watt, 2003). We will discuss several of these issues in light of the tools and their research findings covered in this chapter.

Questionable Inter-rater Reliability

Few studies of the actuarial risk tools for sexual recidivism have reported indices of inter-rater reliability.

Grisso (2000) stated, "I see a field that does not know much about the inter-examiner reliability of its measures." Grisso went on to note that, despite the ostensible objectivity, evidence that the actuarial risk assessments for sexual offending are impervious to rater error and variability is lacking. One should expect some rater variability because many instruments do not have detailed technical manuals that would prevent examiner error when coding difficulties arise.

The precision of ratings across raters is particularly important with these actuarial risk tools given even very small differences (+/−1 point) can lead to very different estimates of risk. Though inter-rater reliability estimates that have been reported are promising, the majority of these estimates were based on the ratings of two research assistants and small subsets (10 to 30 cases) of fairly homogeneous samples of male sex offenders from prison settings. The generalizability of these parameters across populations, raters, and in real world settings remains uncertain. Most studies have been retrospective file reviews conducted by research assistants despite the fact that some of these tools were intended to be administered in an interview setting by probation/parole officers, correctional case managers, or mental health professionals.

LIMITED CLINICAL UTILITY

Actuarial tools have limited clinical utility. A product of empirical test construction methods is that, many risk factors in these tests make little sense theoretically or clinically. Consequently, assessment procedures are not tied to intervention strategies in a prescriptive manner. Actuarial measures are also of little value when it comes to understanding the etiology of sexual offending because of the undue focus on the effect of a variable, rather than its meaning (Grubin & Wingate, 1996). Most of the factors included in actuarial schemes are static variables that are difficult if not impossible to change, and thus provide little guidance with respect to risk management (Grisso, 2000; Hanson, 1998; Hart et al., 2003). For example, Hanson and Thornton (1999) stated in the Static-99's test manual that this tool was not to be used to measure changes in risk.

Grisso (2000) referred to this problem as the "tyranny of static variables," arguing that if actuarial instruments are the sole clinical criterion for release decisions, "examinees will be doomed to perpetual commitment because they will always achieve the same score." The measurement of change in risk for sexual reoffending is a crucial issue because once civilly committed as a SVP, or criminally as a dangerous offender, an offender's risk level has to decrease sufficiently before they will be released. The problem is that the majority of these sex offender risk assessment tools were based almost entirely on static risk factors that, by definition, do not change.

Although we may infer that change in risk can be measured during the course of treatment or institutionalization by focusing on dynamic variables supported in the literature, no risk assessment measure has been tested rigorously for its ability to measure change. The validation study for the SONAR (Hanson & Harris, 2000) provides some limited support for its ability to measure changes in risk, reporting that a one point increase in SONAR scores corresponded to a 38% increase in the likelihood of sexual recidivism. However, this was only one study and the decrease in an individual's risk for future sexual offending, which is difficult to operationalize, was measured by only official reports of reoffending. The VRS-SO appears promising for the purpose of measuring change, but we will need to see future research with this tool.

LIMITED LEGAL RELEVANCE

Another issue worth noting is the limited legal relevance of actuarial risk assessment tools designed for sexual violence or sexual recidivism. Note that in SVP cases evaluators must determine whether the individual's elevated risk for sexual violence is due to a mental abnormality. If the risk is not due to disorder, then civil commitment is not possible. But the actuarial tools do not allow one to determine the quantum of risk attributable to mental abnormality. In fact, most of them ignore mental disorder as a risk factor altogether. So, they do not address the fundamental legal questions. The existence of a mental disorder or personality disorder can be established easily using other clinical assessment tools (e.g., PCL-R, SCID); but this depends on how the court has defined mental abnormality, which is not clear in the legislation. Some would argue that psychopathy and other personality disorders should not qualify (Prentky, Janus, Barbaree, Schwartz, & Kafka, 2006). Nonetheless, as it stands, actuarial tools do nothing to provide direction for forensic evaluators as to how to establish a causal link between the disorder and the criminal activity.

ABILITY TO PREDICT RECIDIVISM HAS UNKNOWN GENERALIZABILITY

Studies have demonstrated the reasonable predictive validity of actuarial tools for sexual and nonsexual violence both within single samples from various settings (i.e., male prisoners and male forensic psychiatric patients) in different countries (i.e., Sweden, Germany, United States, Canada, and Wales), and across multiple samples (Hanson & Thornton, 2000; Roberts et al., 2002). Nonetheless, the research on which this evidence has been based has substantial limitations that threaten the generalizability and validity of these results.

First, validity in the "laboratory" does not necessarily translate to validity in the field. Evidence of the accuracy of these tools in the field is limited because all of the research has been based on small construction samples, use of archival information to code the measures, and retrospective designs, all of which increase the chance of making false positives in the real world (e.g., Berlin, 2003; Dvoskin & Heilbrun, 2001; Hart et al., 2003). None of the studies reviewed in this chapter used outcome measures other than official records of reoffending and few if any studies used statistics that accounted for within-sample variability in the actual time at risk.

Another issue that limits the generalizability of actuarial tools is the representativeness of the samples on which they were created. The more representative the development sample is of the population on which the test will be used, the more generalizable the test's predictive power. As Gottfredson and Moriarty (2006) explained, the problem is that there is no way to tell in the development sample how much of the observed relation between the variables and recidivism is due to underlying associations that will be shared in new samples and how much is due to unique characteristics of the development sample. We see one consequence of the lack of representative development samples in the evidence that parameter estimates of several of the actuarial SVR tools vary on the basis of the setting of participants and some participant-characteristics. For example, the Harris et al. study

indicated that the predictive accuracy of actuarial tools (i.e., SORAG, RRASOR, and Static-99) varied as a function of setting, availability of file information, and length of follow-up period.

Further, sex offenders are an extremely heterogeneous group. The most obvious area of variability is in the type of sex crime. There is some evidence that tests are better at predicting recidivism among child molesters and incest offenders than rapists (see Bartosh et al., 2003). Aside from the obvious variance in crimes, there are several other factors that separate groups of sex offenders. Some actually suffer from a paraphilia (e.g., pedophilia, sadism) while others do not. Some will have a major mental illness while others will not. Say a given tool is developed on the basis of the most powerful predictors of sexual recidivism within a prisoner sample, which consisted primarily of child molesters and rapists. Can we assume this tool would have the same predictive accuracy for a forensic psychiatric patient who may be more likely to have a paraphilia with a comorbid major mental illness? More importantly, can we assume that the cutoff scores for any of these tools generalize to the case of deciding whether to release a SVP into the community? To date, no violent recidivism studies have been published using a sample of SVPs released from civil confinement. Finally, the relevance of any of these tools to the case of a civil psychiatric patient demonstrating inappropriate sexual behavior, yet who may never have been convicted of a sex offense, is unknown.

Another issue is that many of these tools have been "cross-validated" using independent samples in other studies—however, these studies have cross-validated actuarial tools as measures of *relative risk* for sexual violence, not *absolute risk*. In other words, assigning a probability of recidivism for particular test scores on the basis of the percentage of individuals from the development sample who recidivated and had the same score is not a valid practice. Doren (2004) indicated that this was a valid practice in a recent study. In a persuasive secondary analysis, Doren demonstrated that the 5-year recidivism percentages for the RRASOR remained stable for every risk percentage category using multiple datasets from other studies resulting in a sample of more than 4000 sex offenders. He also concluded that the 5-year risk percentages for the Static-99 were stable across multiple datasets of real cases for every risk category except category 4 ("moderate risk"). In the development study, 25.8%

of the sample fell into the moderate risk category; whereas 12.9% of the aggregate sample from seven studies fell into this category.

However, Doren's (2004) work is overly optimistic. Mossman (2006) provided an excellent critique of Doren's work indicating that he erred in his analyses of the problem. Basically, most categories did not cross-validate within individual samples, but some appeared to after collapsing across samples. So, it wasn't evidence of good cross-validation. Mossman (2006, p. 59) demonstrated that the recidivism rate associated with each category of the RRASOR or Static-99 is a "function of the scale's sorting properties and the base rate of reoffending in the population being evaluated." He went on to conclude that the discriminative properties of an actuarial tool (e.g., predictive accuracy) can stay constant across samples if the development sample was representative but the probability of recidivating associated with a particular score definitely does not. However, a score on one of these tools can *only* tell us "where an evaluee ranks within his population" (Mossman, 2006, p. 60). It *cannot* tell us the evaluee's probability of recidivating.

Another issue that limits the generalizability of the predictive validity and accuracy of these tools is that, since only a few factors can be included in any one actuarial measure, factors that are idiosyncratic to an examinee do not enter assessments of risk regardless of their relevance to a specific case (Campbell, 2003; Gottfredson & Moriarty, 2006). To give an extreme example, say a high risk sex offender was in an accident that left him quadriplegic. This offender would continue to be identified as high risk for sexual recidivism on the basis of these actuarial tools despite the substantial decrease in risk resulting from severe physical disability. Thus, the emphasis on empiricism that went into the creation of each of these tools, can lead to the exclusion of factors that are undeniably related to risk but have unknown validity (e.g., homicidal ideation, physical ability). As summarized by Campbell, this limitation of actuarial tools has led some to suggest use of *adjusted actuarial estimates*. The adjusted actuarial approach involves modification of an instrument-derived actuarial estimate of risk based on other factors that may be related to recidivism risk. However, this has been criticized because it is an unstandardized method that lacks research evidence as to its accuracy (Campbell, 2003; DeClue, 2005). In the words of Prentky et al. (2006),

this approach "provides little more than empirical window dressing for clinical judgment" (p. 380).

PROBABILITY ESTIMATES HAVE SUBSTANTIAL MARGINS OF ERROR

Possibly the most important limitation in the use of actuarial risk assessment tools are the substantial margins of error in the risk estimates made using test scores, particularly when it comes to individual predictions (Hart et al 2007). According to actuarial tools, "violence risk" is defined as the "probability of committing future violence." As Hart et al. explained, actuarial tools apply the following logic to estimate the probability that an individual will reoffend. For a given test, the first line of reasoning is that in the sample used to construct the test, 68% of people with scores in the high risk category were known to have committed violence during the follow-up period. Say a particular examinee scores in this high risk category. The conclusion then is that the risk of this examinee committing violence in the future is similar to the risk of people in the construction sample—68%. This is how actuarial tools generally operate.

As Hart et al. (2007) explains, the problem is that moving the focus of analysis from groups to individuals changes the way in which risk is conceptualized (see Hajek & Hall, 2002). Say we have a bag of 100 marbles, 75% of which are black and 25% are white. Each time we draw a marble, we return the marble to the basket and then draw a marble again. I say an individual does this 1000 times. The person should expect to draw a black marble 750 times (or 75% of the time), but the 95% confidence interval is 720 to 780 times. In other words, the person can be 95% certain that they will draw a black marble between 720 and 780 times (or 72% to 78% of the time). Decrease the number of draws to 100 and the confidence interval gets wider—now the 95% CI is 66 to 82 (or 66% to 82%). So, although the estimated probability that the individual will draw a black marble is still 75 times out of 100—the margin of error in this estimate is larger.

Now, take this down to the individual level—if a person draws a marble only one time—although the best guess is that it will be black, because this is what it should be 75 times out of 100—we cannot say this with any degree of precision. We do not have 95%

confidence intervals for individual cases at this point in our science.

When we bring this issue to violence risk assessment—any probability estimates are also hindered by the fact that the individual we are assessing would need to be like the individuals in the test's validation sample for the probability estimates to generalize at all. It is often unclear what it means to be "like the people in the development sample." One issue is that the average probability for the validation sample does not necessarily reflect any individual case in that sample. A second issue is that examinees do not come to us with characteristics that are random. In the case of sex offenders—even the type of sex offender could impact our confidence in the probability estimates of a given test. Studies have shown that the predictive accuracy of many of these tests differ by 2% to 5% points between child molesters and rapists. A rapist comes to us with a characteristic that is not random—they are already at decreased probability of recidivating sexually (at least according to studies using official records for recidivism) and, in many cases, obtain test scores with a decreased predictive accuracy. To give a different example, say we know that 60% of majors in psychology are female. Should we predict that J. Smith has a 60% chance of being female?

Aside from the problems with the individual case, Hart et al. (2007) demonstrated that, because of the nature of the scale construction of even those tools with the most rigorous developmental and validation studies, the margin of error in the probability estimates even at the group level are substantial. The authors used probability theory and a method for estimating the precision of group estimates using the Static-99 as an example. Group estimates for the 6 risk categories of the Static-99 showed that the confidence intervals for these groups of recidivists overlapped substantially, indicating that the Static-99 actually has only two distinct group estimates of risk: Low (Categories 0–3) and High (Categories 4–6+).

The latter issue; namely, the group estimate problem, could be rectified by using a significantly larger development sample (see Hart et al., 2007, for a discussion of this). The problem with individual estimates and generalizing from group data to the individual, however, is not unique to violence risk assessment. This is a limitation with any aspect of medical or social science and although it can be improved—by improving our prediction models so they explain more of the variance in violence risk assessment, by increasing

and diversifying our samples, and by conducting more tests of individual differences within these samples—it will not go away.

CONCLUSIONS AND RECOMMENDATIONS

Though some support this use of risk measures in commitment hearings unequivocally, Grisso (2000) warned forensic evaluators that the practice of solely relying on these tools for such high-stake decisions is ethically questionable until more research has been conducted. In 2001, Litwack pronounced that the complete replacement of clinical decisions with actuarial instruments would be premature.

It must be underscored that preventative detention legislation targets the reasonable possibility of controlling an offender's risk in the community. It is not the same as segregating the offender from society until s/he gets control of his or her lawlessness thereby entirely eradicating risk. Rather, the court must be satisfied that the risk can be controlled in the community. Can we as a society justify the indeterminate internment of citizens on the basis of actuarial predictions that involve a fair amount of error—especially when the prisoner has behaved perfectly while incarcerated and when the detainee has been permitted to cascade to low security facilities without getting into trouble?

RECOMMENDATIONS FOR RESEARCH

The actuarial tools and, thus, actuarial decision making can be improved with more research. The problems described in this chapter may be seen as an outline for a much needed research agenda. Most notably, these tools should be tested systematically for inter-rater reliability, particularly for examiners working in the field (Grisso, 2000; Hart et al., 2003). Many of the tools lack test manuals that are comprehensive enough to meet the requirements of psychological tests. For example, few specify rater qualifications or the essential rater training and few if any include comparative norms aside from those obtained in the development samples.

We need more validation studies, on more diverse samples (SVPs being released from confinement), with large enough sample sizes to examine systematic differences in the accuracy of these tools on the basis of demographic differences. This would at least allow the field to provide known estimates of the generalizability of these tools. Another big issue here is the definition of "cross-validation." Actuarial SVR assessment tools have been cross-validated as measures of relative risk—high scores are associated with more recidivism, as revealed by ROC analyses. However, they have not been validated as measures of absolute risk—that is, their ability to make specific probability predictions is unknown. There is also the problem of probability estimates based on group data. Hart et al. (2007) suggested that, when designing actuarial tools, test developers need samples in the several thousands to derive accurate estimates and they should identify score categories with extreme estimates of violence risk.

Further, enhancing both the clinical and legal relevance of actuarial SVR assessment tools would be a worthwhile endeavor. First, the prediction models themselves can be improved. The problem is very few of these tools take dynamic or contextual variables into account. The few tools that were designed to detect changes in risk should be seen as a step in the right direction but these have yet to be properly validated. Second and particularly in SVP cases, we also need legally relevant instruments—those that attempt to estimate the degree of risk attributable to mental disorder, such as sexual deviation or personality disorder.

RECOMMENDATIONS FOR CURRENT PRACTICE

The restrictions of actuarial tools cannot be discounted and are great enough that sole reliance on these tools for making detention decisions are unwarranted. Indeed, it could be argued that "any" reliance on actuarial tools is unwarranted. Currently, a given sexual recidivism risk actuarial tool, like the Static-99, may be one of the best single predictors that our science has to offer in the area of sex offender risk assessment. It is evident from recidivism studies that this tool does not account for much of the variance in recidivism and, even at the group level, performs at only 70% accuracy. Thus, it would be careless to expect this tool to do the forensic evaluator's jobs for them. It is impossible for one of these actuarial-derived tools to cover the universe of relevant risk factors to an individual case. Not to mention the Static-99/

Static-2002, like most all of the tools described in this chapter, does little to assist us in decreasing a person's risk. In this sense, a well-trained forensic examiner should consider the prominent and clinically-useful risk factors identified from meta-analyses in addition to the Static-99 score (Hanson, 2006). The training of the clinician in this sense is crucial given the notion that when left to clinicians to adjust actuarial scores upwards or downwards, they generally decrease the validity of the actuarial tool.

There are some serious cautions to the use of this approach. Given the high stakes of SVR assessment, particularly in the context of an SVP or dangerous offender hearing, forensic mental health professionals have an ethical responsibility to familiarize themselves with the limitations of actuarial risk assessment instruments (Heilbrun, 1992). Examiners should be extremely cautious when using actuarial instruments. As is the case with all areas of assessment, the examiners must educate the consumers of test information (i.e., the courts) about the limits of the data. They should understand that it is impossible to make accurate estimates about the probability of an individual reoffending using these tests (Hart et al., 2007). This is particularly important in high stakes cases where prediction errors at the individual level have a high cost. It also is important to remember that actuarial tools should only be one part of a comprehensive clinical assessment of an individual's risk. This needs to be supplemented with contextual information (e.g., risks present in the environment in which an offender would likely be released) and clinical information (e.g., amenability to treatment).

An alternative to the use of actuarial tools is risk assessment tools developed on the basis of the SPJ framework. SPJ risk assessment tools were developed in response to the limited clinical utility and the rigidity that may limit the generalizability of actuarial tools. These tools are informed by the state of the discipline in clinical theory and empirical research to provide guidance for clinical decision making and treatment planning (Borum, 1996). The intent of this model was to improve clinical judgment by adding structure, and improve actuarial decision making by adding clinical discretion. These instruments are not designed to provide absolute determinations of risk. They emphasize "prevention" as opposed to "prediction." Thus, these tools contain both static and dynamic risk factors because they assume that risk is not entirely stable and can change as a result of various factors, such as, treatment quality and quantity, treatment adherence, protective factors, and context. Structured professional judgment risk assessment tools are designed to guide forensic evaluators to determine what level of risk management is needed, in which contexts and at what points in time.

The *Risk for Sexual Violence Protocol* (RSVP; Hart et al., 2003), previously known as the SVR-20, is a SPJ risk assessment for sexual violence instrument that allows evaluators to characterize the risks in terms of the nature, imminence, severity, and frequency while determining what steps should be taken to minimize the risk. Although RSVP items can be summed into a total test score for research purposes, the RSVP *does not* use an algorithm to make determinations about an examinee's risk level. Instead, it guides the examiner to make a judgment as to an examinee's risk level (high, medium, or low) for engaging in future sexual violence. Framing decisions in terms of relative risk may be preferable to giving probability estimates; unfortunately, research of clinicians indicates that there is limited agreement as to how to categorize low, medium, or high risk (Hilton, Carter, Harris, & Sharpe, 2008).

Though few studies have been conducted in this area, there is evidence that these structured clinical summary risk ratings have incremental predictive validity over actuarial risk ratings (Dempster, 1998; Kropp & Hart, 2000). In fact, de Vogel et al. (2004) recently reported that the SVR-20 outperformed the Static-99 at predicting sexual recidivism in their Dutch sample of sex offenders followed over an average of 11.6 years. The AUCs for the SVR-20 and Static-99 were 0.80 and 0.66 respectively. This is not to say that tools like the RSVP do not suffer some of the same limitations as the actuarial instruments covered in this chapter, at least in terms of the need to demonstrate inter-rater reliability and the ability to assess changes in risk. As critics have noted, the limitation with any SPJ approach is that the sensitivity, specificity, and error rates are unknown. However, these factors are largely unknown for the actuarial tools as well when faced with the problem of the individual case.

References

Archer, R. P., Buffington-Vollum, J. K., Stredny, R. V., & Handel, R. W. (2006). A survey of psychological test use patterns among forensic psychologists. *Journal of Personality Assessment*, 87(1), 84–94.

Barbaree, H. E., Seto, M. C., Langton, C. M., & Peacock, E. J. (2001). Evaluating the predictive accuracy of six risk assessment instruments for adult sex offenders. *Criminal Justice and Behavior*, 28(4), 490.

Bartosh, D. L., Garby, T., Lewis, D., & Gray, S. (2003). Differences in the predictive validity of actuarial risk assessments in relation to sex offender type. *International Journal of Offender Therapy and Comparative Criminology*, 47(4), 422–438.

Becker, J. V. & Murphy, W. D. (1998). What we know and do not know about assessing and treating sex offenders. *Psychology, Public Policy, and Law*, 4(1–2), 116–137.

Berlin, F. S., Galbreath, N. W., Geary, B., & McGlone, G. (2003). The use of actuarials at civil commitment hearings to predict the likelihood of future sexual violence. *Sexual Abuse: A Journal of Research and Treatment*, 15(4), 377–382.

Boer, D. P., Hart, S. D., Kropp, P. R., & Webster, C. D. (1998). *Manual for the Sexual Violence Risk – 20: Professional guidelines for assessing risk of sexual violence*. Vancouver, B.C.: British Columbia Institute Against Family Violence and the Mental Health, Law, and Policy Institute, Simon Fraser University.

Borum, R. (1996). Improving the clinical practice of violence risk assessment: Technology, guidelines, and training. *American Psychologist*, 51, 945–956.

Campbell, T. W. (2003). Sex offenders and actuarial risk assessment: ethical considerations. *Behavioral Sciences and the Law*, 21, 269–279.

Criminal Code, R. S. 1985, c. C-46.

DeClue, G. (2005). Avoiding garbage 2: Assessment of risk for sexual violence after long-term treatment. *Journal of Psychiatry & Law*, 33(2), 179–206.

Dempster, R. J. (1998). *Prediction of sexually violent recidivism: A comparison of risk assessment instruments*: Unpublished master's thesis, Simon Fraser University, Burnaby, British Columbia, Canada.

de Vogel, V., Ruiter, C., Beek, D., & Mead, G. (2004). Predictive validity of the SVR-20 and Static-99 in a Dutch sample of treated sex offenders. *Law and Human Behavior*, 28(3), 235–251.

Doren, D. M. (1998). Recidivism base rates, predictions of sex offender recidivism, and the "sexual predator" commitment laws. *Behavioral Sciences and the Law*, 16, 97–114.

Doren, D. M. (1999). *Using and testifying about sex offender risk assessment instrumentation*. Unpublished manuscript.

Doren, D. M. (2004). Stability of the interpretive risk percentages for the RRASOR and Static-99. *Sexual Abuse: A Journal of Research and Treatment*, 16(1), 25–36.

Douglas, K., Vincent, G. M., & Edens, J. (2006). Risk for criminal recidivism: the role of psychopathy. In C. Patrick (Ed.), *Handbook of psychopathy* (pp. 533–554). New York: Guilford.

Ducro, C. & Pham, T. (2006). Evaluation of the SORAG and the Static-99 on Belgian sex offenders committed to a forensic facility. *Sexual Abuse: A Journal of Research and Treatment*, 18(1), 15–26.

Dvoskin, J. A. & Heilbrun, K. (2001). Risk assessment: Release decision-making toward resolving the great debate. *Journal of the American Academy of Psychiatry and the Law*, 29(1), 6–10.

Epperson, D. L., Kaul, J. D., Huot, S. J., Hesselton, D., Alexander, W., & Goldman, R. (1995). *Minnesota sex offender screening tool (MnSOST)*. St. Paul, MN: Minnesota Department of Corrections.

Epperson, D. L., Kaul, J. D., Huot, S. J., Hesselton, D., Alexander, W., & Goldman, R. (2000). *Minnesota sex offender screening tool revised (MnSOST-R)*. St, Paul, MN: Minnesota Department of Corrections.

Epperson, D. L., Kaul, J. D., Huot, S., Goldman, R., & Alexander, W. (2003). *Minnesota sex offender screening tool—Revised (MnSoST-R): Development, validation, and recommended risk level cut scores*. Technical Paper, St. Paul, MN: Minnesota Department of Corrections.

Ferguson, G. E., Eidelson, R. J., & Witt, P. H. (1998). New Jersey's sex offender risk assessment scale: Preliminary validity data. *Journal of Psychiatry & Law*, 26(3), 327–351.

Furby, L., Weinrott, M. R., & Blackshaw, L. (1989). Sex offender recidivism: A review. *Psychological Bulletin*, 105(1), 3–30.

Gottfredson, S. D. & Moriarty, L. J. (2006). Statistical risk assessment: Old problems and new applications. *Crime & Delinquency*, 52, 178–200.

Grisso, T. (2000). *Ethical issues in evaluations for sex offender re-offending*. Paper presented at the Paper presented at the Sex Offender Re-Offence Risk Prediction Training, Sinclair Seminars, Madison, WI.

Grisso, T. & Tomkins, A. J. (1996). Communicating violence risk assessments. American Psychologist, 51, 928–930.

Grove, W. M. & Meehl, P. E. (1996). Comparative efficiency of informal (subjective, impressionistic) and formal (mechanical, algorithmic) prediction procedures: The clinical-statistical controversy. *Psychology, Public Policy, and Law*, 2(2), 293–323.

Grubin, D. & Wingate, S. (1996). Sexual offence recidivism: Prediction versus understanding. *Criminal Behaviour and Mental Health*, 6(4), 349–359.

Hajek, A. & Hall, N. (2002). Induction and probability. In P. Machamer & M. Silerstein (Eds.), *The Blackwell Guide to the Philosophy of Science* (pp. 149–172). London: Blackwell.

Hanson, R. K. (1997). The development of a brief actuarial risk scale for sexual offense recidivism (User report 1997–04). *Ottawa: Department of the Solicitor General of Canada*.

Hanson, R. K. (1998). What do we know about sex offender risk assessment. *Psychology, Public Policy, and Law*, 4(1/2), 50–72.

Hanson, R. K. (2006). The Static-99 scoring and interpretation. Presented at the 8th annual Massachusetts District Attorneys Association conference on Sexually Dangerous Persons, Waltham, MA.

Hanson, R. K. & Bussiere, M. T. (1996). Predictors of sexual offender recidivism: A meta-analysis (User report 1996–04). *Ottawa: Department of the Solicitor General of Canada*.

Hanson, R. K. & Bussiere, M. T. (1998). Predicting relapse: A meta-analysis of sexual offender recidivism studies. *Journal of Consulting and Clinical Psychology*, 66(2), 348–362.

Hanson, R. K. & Thornton, D. (1999). Static 99: Improving actuarial risk assessments for sex offenders (User report 1999–02). *Ottawa: Department of the Solicitor General of Canada*.

Hanson, R. K. & Thornton, D. (2000). Improving risk assessment for sex offenders: a comparison of three actuarial scales. *Law and Human Behavior*, 24(1), 119–136.

Hanson, R. K. & Harris, A. J. (2000). *The sex offender need assessment rating (SONAR): A method for measuring change in risk levels (User report: 2000–1)*. Ottawa: Department of the Solicitor General of Canada.

Hanson, R. K. & Harris, A. J. R. (2001). A structured approach to evaluating change among sexual offenders. *Sexual Abuse: A Journal of Research and Treatment*, 13(2), 105–122.

Hanson, R. K. & Thornton, D. (2003). Notes on the devlopment of Static-2002 (User report 2003–01). *Ottawa: Department of the Solicitor General of Canada*.

Hanson, R. K. & Morton-Bourgon, K. E. (2005). The Characteristics of Persistent Sexual Offenders: A Meta-Analysis of Recidivism Studies. *Journal of Consulting and Clinical Psychology*, 73(6), 1154–1163.

Hare, R. D. (2003). *Hare psychopathy checklist-revised (PCL-R): 2nd Edition*. New York: Multi-Health Systems Inc.

Harris, A., Phenix, A., Hanson, R. K., & Thornton, D. (2003a). Static-99 coding rules revised-2003. Ottawa: Department of the Solicitor General of Canada.

Harris, G., Rice, M. E., & Quinsey, V. L. (1998). Appraisal and management of risk in sexual aggressors: Implications for criminal justice policy. *Psychology, Public Policy, and Law*, 4(1/2), 73–115.

Harris, G. T., Rice, M. E., Quinsey, V. L., Lalumiare, M. L., Boer, D., & Lang, C. (2003b). A Multisite Comparison of Actuarial Risk Instruments for Sex Offenders. *Psychological Assessment*, 15(3), 413–425.

Hart, S. D. (2003). Actuarial risk assessment: Commentary on Berlin et al. *Sexual Abuse: A Journal of Research and Treatment*, 15(4), 383–388.

Hart, S. D., Kropp, R., Laws, D. R., Klaver, J., Logan, C., & Watt, K. A. (2003). The risk for sexual violence protocol (RSVP): Structured professional guidelines for assessing risk of sexual violence. Simon Fraser University, Mental Health, Law and Policy Institute.

Hart, S. D., Michie, C., & Cooke, D. (2007). Precision of actuarial risk assessment instruments: Evaluating the "Margins of Error" of group versus individual predictions of violence. *British Journal of Psychiatry*, 190, s60–s65.

Heilbrun, K. (1992). The role of psychological testing in forensic assessment. *Law and Human Behavior*, 16, 257–272.

Hilton, N. Z., Carter, A. M., Harris, G. T., & Sharpe, A. J. B. (2008). Does using nonnumerical terms to describe risk aid violence risk communication? Clinician agreement and decision making. Journal of Interpersonal Violence, 23, 171–188.

Janus, E. S. & Meehl, P. E. (1997). Assessing the legal standard for predictions of dangerousness in sex offender commitment proceedings. *Psychology, Public Policy, & Law*, 3(1), 33–64.

Kansas v. Hendricks, 117 S.Ct. 2072 (1997).

Kropp, P. R. & Hart, S. D. (2000). The Spousal Assault Risk Assessment Guide (SARA): Reliability and validity in adult male offenders. *Law and Human Behaviour*, 24(1), 101–118.

Langton, C. M., Barbaree, H. E., Hansen, K. T., Harkins, L., & Peacock, E. J. (2007a). Reliability and validity of the Static-2002 among adult sexual offenders with reference to treatment status. *Criminal Justice and Behavior*, 34(5), 616–640.

Langton, C. M., Barbaree, H. E., Harkins, L., Seto, M. C., & Peacock, E. J. (2002). *Evaluating the predictive validity of seven risk assessment instruments for sexual offenders.* Paper presented at the Paper presented at the 21st Annual Research and Treatment Conference of the Association for the Treatment of Sexual Abusers, Montreal, Quebec, Canada.

Langton, C. M., Barbaree, H. E., Seto, M. C., Peacock, E. J., Harkins, L., & Hansen, K. T. (2007b). Actuarial assessment of risk for reoffense among adult sex offenders: Evaluating the predictive accuracy of the Static-2002 and five other instruments. *Criminal Justice and Behavior*, 34(1), 37–59.

Långström, N. (2004). Accuracy of actuarial procedures for assessment of sexual offender recidivism risk may vary across ethnicity. *Sexual Abuse: Journal of Research and Treatment*, 16(2), 107–120.

Litwack, T. R. (2001). Actuarial versus clinical assessments of dangerousness. *Psychology, Public Policy, and Law*, 7, 409–443.

Looman, J. (2006). Comparison of two risk assessment instruments for sexual offenders. *Sexual Abuse: A Journal of Research and Treatment*, 18(2), 193–206.

Matson, S. & Lieb, R. (1997). *Megan's Law: A review of state & federal legislation*: Washington State Institute for Public Policy.

McGrath, R. J. & Hoke, S. E. (2001). *Vermont assessment of sex offender risk manual (Research edition).* Middlebury, Vermont: Author.

McGrath, R. J., Hoke, S. E., Livingston, J. A., & Cumming, G. F. (2001). *The Vermont Assessment of sex offender risk (VASOR): An initial reliability and validity study.* Paper presented at the Paper presented at the 20th annual research and treatment conference of the association for the treatment of sexual abusers, San Antonio, TX.

Mendel, M. P. (1995). *The male survivor: The impact of sexual abuse.* Thousand Oaks, CA, US: Sage Publications, Inc.

Monahan, J. (1996). Violence prediction: The last 20 years and the next 20 years. *Criminal Justice and Behavior*, 23, 107–120.

Mossman, D. (1994). Assessing predictions of violence: Being accurate about accuracy. *Journal of Consulting and Clinical Psychology*, 62(4), 783–792.

Mossman, D. (2006). Another look at interpreting risk categories. *Sexual Abuse: A Journal of Research and Treatment*, 18, 41–63.

National Institute of Justice. (2000). *Full Report of the Prevalence, Incidences, Consequences of Violence Against Women.* Washington, DC.

Nunes, K. L., Firestone, P., Bradford, J. M., Greenberg, D., & Broom, I. (2002). A comparison of modified versions of the Static-99 and the Sex Offender Risk Appraisal Guide. *Sexual Abuse: A Journal of Research and Treatment*, 14(3), 253–269.

Olver, M. E., Wong, S. C. P., Nicholaichuck, T., & Gordon, A. (2007). The validity and reliability of the Violence Risk Scale – Sexual Offender Version: Assessing sex offender risk and evaluating therapeutic change. *Psychological Assessment*, 19(3), 318–329.

Packard, R. & Gordon, A. (1999, September). An investigation of actuarial risk scales: Concordance and factor analysis. Paper presented at the 18th Annual Research and Treatment Conference of the Association for the Treatment of Sexual Abusers, Lake Buena Vista, FL.

Prentky, R. A., Lee, A. F., & Knight, R. A. (1997). Risk factors associated with recidivism among extrafamilial child molesters. *Journal of Consulting and Clinical Psychology*, 65(1), 141–149.

Prentky, R. A., Barbaree, H., Janus, E., Schwartz, B. K., Kafka, M. P. (2006). Sexually violent predators in the courtroom: Science on trial. *Psychology, Public Policy, & Law*, 12, 357–393.

Quinsey, V. L., Harris, G. T., Rice, M. E., & Cormier, C. A. (1998). *Violent offenders appraising and managing risk.* Washington, DC: American Psychological Association.

Rice, M. E. & Harris, G. T. (1997). Cross-validation and extension of the Violence Risk Appraisal Guide for child molesters and rapists. *Law and Human Behavior*, 21(2), 231–241.

Roberts, C. F., Doren, D. M., & Thornton, D. (2002). Dimensions associated with assessments of sex offender recidivism risk. *Criminal Justice and Behavior*, 29(5), 569–589.

Sjostedt, G. & Langstrom, N. (2001). Actuarial assessment of sex offender recidivism risk: A cross-validation of the RRASOR and the Static-99 in Sweden. *Law and Human Behavior*, 25(6), 629–645.

Stadtland, C., Hollweg, M., Kleindienst, N., Dietl, J., Reich, U., & Nedopil, N. (2005). Risk assessment and prediction of violent and sexual recidivism in sex offenders: Long-term predictive validity of four risk assessment instruments. *Journal of Forensic Psychiatry & Psychology*, 16(1), 92–108.

Starnaman v. Penetanguishene Mental Health Centre (1995), 100 C.C.C. (3d) 190 (Ont. C.A.) Swets, J.A. (1988). Measuring the accuracy of diagnostic systems. Science, 240, 1285–1292.

Whitman, C. T. & Farmer, J. J. (2000). Attorney general guidelines for law enforcement for the implementation of sex offender registration and community notification laws. New Jersey: Office of the Attorney General.

Wong, S. C. P., Olver, M. E., Nicholaichuck, T., & Gordon, A. (2003). Violence Risk Scale–Sexual Offender Version (VRS-SO). Saskatoon, Saskatchewan, Canada: Regional Psychiatric Centre and University of Saskatchewan.

Chapter 7

Laboratory Measurement of Penile Response in the Assessment of Sexual Interests

J. Paul Fedoroff, Michael Kuban, and John M. Bradford

If the pathognomonic feature of all paraphilic sexual disorders is deviant sexual arousal, and if increased blood in the penis is associated with sexual arousal in men, then the objective measurement of changes in penile blood volume would appear to be an essential tool for clinicians and researchers in the field of pathologic sexual behaviors. Surprisingly, the merits and use of laboratory measurement of penile tumescence in the lab versus other methods of sexual preference measurement have proven to be somewhat complicated (Hanson, 2002; Johnson & Listiak, 1999; Konopasky & Konopsaky, 2000; Laws, 1989, 2003; Seto, 2001).

One reason for the confusion is the fact that measurement of changes in penile blood volume in response to external stimuli has gone by many names. These include "phallometry" (Freund & Watson, 1991); "penile tumescence testing" (PTT); and "penile plethysmography" (PPG).

While techniques vary concerning types of stimuli and methods of presenting them, instructions given, and ways of estimating changes in penile blood volume, all terms refer to the process of attempting to measure penile tumescence during presentation of sexual stimuli. For the purposes of this chapter, unless otherwise noted, the abbreviation "PPG" will be used. Several comprehensive reviews of PPG have been published (e.g., Barbaree, 1990; Barker & Howell, 1992; Fernandez & Marshall, 2003; Marshall & Fernandez, 2000a, 2000b; Murphy et al., 1984; Simon & Schouten, 1991).

HISTORICAL OVERVIEW

Kurt Freund (1957), a Czechoslovakian sexologist, pioneered phallometric testing in the 1950s, after being asked by government officials to help identify

Sections of this chapter are paraphrased from a grant application on which Susan Curry was a coauthor.

heterosexual men who were avoiding military service by claiming to be homosexual—an exclusionary condition at that time. Dissatisfied with other psychological or "projective" testing methods, Freund investigated differentiation of sexual orientation on the basis of physiological measures of penile responses to heterosexual and homosexual stimuli. He invented a technique in which he could reliably measure changes in penis volume by placing the penis in a sealed glass cylinder and monitoring the resulting air pressure changes (air displacement) within the cylinder as men viewed potentially erotic stimuli (nude male or female photographs). By correlating change in penis volume with the stimuli being presented, Freund (1963) showed that he could reliably assess sexual orientation. The success of this technique and stability of responses convinced Freund that sexual arousal patterns were physiologically determined and he subsequently (and successfully) fought to repeal laws criminalizing homosexuality in Czechoslovakia in 1961. This early success led Freund to extend this method's use in the 1960s toward measurement of sexual partner age preference on the basis of the hypothesis that offenders against children had pedophilic preferences, despite their understandable reluctance to admit having them (Freund, 1965, 1967, 1991).

Freund's work with "volumetric plethysmography" was soon followed by the development of circumferential plethysmography (Bancroft, Jones, & Pullan, 1966), in which a small tube filled with an electrical conductance liquid (mercury or indium/gallium) is placed around the penile shaft. Electrical resistance changes proportionally as the gauge is expanded allowing dynamic measurement of "circumferential" changes in penis size.

Soon after, the Barlow metal gauge was designed (Barlow, Becker, Leitenberg, & Agras, 1970). In this method, a metal "U" shaped device, calibrated to detect pressure changes, is placed over the penile shaft. Pressure changes on the device have been shown to correlate with change in penis size.

These three techniques have been used since the 1960s and continue to be used today, though now, by far the most widely used measurement is some variant of the circumferential method.

MEASUREMENT TECHNIQUES

Some debate has remained over the relative accuracy of volumetric versus circumferential measurements,

with initial impressions being that the volumetric method was more accurate, largely due to its ability to detect penile elongation that precedes circumferential enlargement during early stages of arousal. Kuban et al. (1999) examined the issue in detail, concluding that both volumetric and circumferential measurement apparati produced identical test outcomes provided there was at least a 10% (2.5 mm) increase in penis size. However, the volumetric apparatus was found to be more accurate in detecting changes in penis diameter less than 2.5 mm.

As noted earlier, circumferential measurements are now used much more widely. The reasons include the fact that volumetric testing is technically more difficult to conduct, and is considered by most to be a more invasive intervention due to the elaborate setup procedures. The Kurt Freund Phallometric lab in Toronto, Canada, annually assesses 250 to 300 new patients using the volumetric method, but is now one of the very few functioning labs in the world relying on volumetric testing.

In contrast, the comparative ease of use of circumferential strain gauges has led them to become the industry standard, circumferential test apparatus are commercially available, fairly inexpensive, and of equal reliability to volumetric measurements except at the lowest levels of penile tumescence.

Measurement, scoring, and interpretation of PPG data remains an issue since they were first reviewed. Howes (1995) reported results from a mailed questionnaire survey of 48 PPG labs. The study found considerable inconsistency across labs. In addition few labs had published (or even measured) standardization values such as sensitivity and specificity and there was noted inconsistency on basic parameters such as the minimum response requirements (ranging often from a low of 0% to 30% of erection).

Scoring methods also differed (Earls, Quinsey, Castonguay, 1987). Labs were found to vary in terms of the weight placed on "absolute" versus "relative" penile responses. In general, "absolute" response refers to simple measured change in penile circumference or volume. Since penile responsivity has a great deal of interindividual variance, most labs use "relative" measurements in which measured changes in penis circumference or volume in response to the test stimulus are compared with the changes in response to "neutral" or "normal" (nondeviant) stimuli. They also varied in terms of how the data were analyzed (e.g., area under response curves, use of z-scores, use of differential scores vs. quotient scores, diagnostic cutoff criteria). Labs also differed in terms of the interpretation of response values. In part this may be due to an inherent conflict between interpretation of results on the basis of group data and the interpretation of results based on individual data. For example, does an 80% response to child stimuli compared with adults represent a pathologic response pattern? Would equal responses to child and adult stimuli be of concern? What about two men, one of whom responds 50% to child stimuli and 100% to adult stimuli while the second man responds 20% to child stimuli but only 10% to adult stimuli? Which is more pedophilic? More important, which is more dangerous? As Launay (1999) commented about PPG testing, "No sooner is a review published to recommend its use, than another more critical publication urges caution…" (pp. 254).

Stimulus Sets

Laboratories vary widely in their stimulus sets, many having developed "idiosyncratic" assessment batteries (Howes 1995; Launay, 1999). Stimuli may involve visual slides/images (Freund, 1967), audiotapes (Abel, Becker, Murphy, & Flanagan, 1981), or movies/videotapes (Abel, Becker, Blanchard, & Djenderedjian, 1978). Opinions vary about the efficacy of each stimulus modality. Concerns have also been raised about the content of stimulus sets (Maletsky, 1995) to the extent that work is also now underway to develop stimuli based on multisensory virtual reality stimulus sets (Renaud et al., 2005).

Clearly, since different presentation modalities elicit different degrees of response and different levels of discriminative efficiency, the choice of modality of presentation is important. Movie depictions are reported to generate the greatest response both in men with paraphilic sexual interests and in men with nonparaphilic interests (Abel, Blanchard, & Barlow, 1981). Paradoxically, of possible stimulus modalities, while videotape stimuli are generally the most arousing, they also present the most specific information. For this reason, it has been hypothesized that they may not be most suitable for testing sadism or coercive sexual preferences, due to the potentially idiosyncratic nature arousal characteristics (e.g., body type of victim, or victim reaction). Of three violence tests conducted on hundreds of patients in Freund's laboratory in the early 1990s, only the audio version of one rape test produced sufficiently reliable documentation for publication (Seto & Kuban, 1996).

In spite of these findings, there are some validated PPG stimulus sets indicating that age and gender preferences are best assessed with pictures depicting males and females at different stages of development (Freund & Blanchard, 1989; Harris, Rice, Quinsey, Chaplin, & Earls, 1992). Notable validated sets include the Farrall stimuli, the Oak Ridges stimuli (Penetanguishine, Ontario), and the Freund audiovisual stimuli set. Attempts to standardize the use of the same stimuli across correctional services in Canada have been undertaken, as have attempts to standardize recording equipment and stimulus materials in a set of over a dozen sites in the United Kingdom. The final outcome of these larger studies involving identical stimulus sets is still pending. However, past attempts at large-scale multisite comparisons have been fraught with problems (Laws, Gulayets, & Frenzel, 1995).

Testing Sexual Arousal to Coercion

As noted earlier, "rape proneness" may be most accurately assessed using audio stimuli, with the most valid stimuli including graphic depictions of violent coercive sex (Lalumière & Harris, 1998; Rice, Chaplin, Harris, and Coutts, 1994). Lalumière et al. (2005) discuss problems in detecting sadism as opposed to rape proneness, arguing that the difficulty in clinically identifying sadism on PPG is the potentially idiosyncratic nature of sadistic fantasies.

The issue is further complicated by the differences between individuals who are aroused by consensual sadistic scenes and those who are aroused by nonconsensual sadistic activities since most studies to date have assessed primarily criminal men. Even within the criminal subsection of the population, rapists commit their offenses for a variety of reasons. Prentky and Knight (1991) attempted to taxonomize rapists into several mutually exclusive subtypes based on a variety of factors. Since then, the possible etiologies of rape have been further explored (Lalumière et al., 2005). If a "preferential rape pattern" exists within some males then it may be expected that such men will show greater relative phallometric responses to coercive nonconsenting interactions than to consenting sexual scenarios.

PPG studies with stimuli depicting consenting sex, rape, nonsexual violence, and neutral scenarios have varied widely over the past 30 years (e.g., Abel, Barlow, Blanchard, & Guild, 1977; Barbaree, Marshall, & Lanthier, 1979; Quinsey & Chaplin, 1982, 1984).

Lalumière et al. (2003) reviewed the earlier literature and reported on two large-scale meta-analyses involving published studies of PPG testing for sexual coerciveness in which the dependent variable was the "rape index," a ratio of responses to stimuli depicting rape and responses to stimuli depicting consensual sexual scenarios. The overall effect sizes were 0.71 (Hall, Schondrick, & Hirshman, 1993–9 studies) and 0.82 (Lalumière & Quinsey, 1994–16 studies). These results are generally considered to represent "moderate to large" effects (Cohen, 1992). The different effect sizes were related to individual study differences, such as whether rapists were compared with other sex offenders or to nonsex offenders (Hall et al., 1993), or to the particular stimuli set (Lalumière & Quinsey, 1994).

Not surprisingly, there have often been mixed and controversial results with regard to "rape testing." As reviewed by Lalumière et al. (2005), rapists as a group have been shown, relative to control subjects, to respond more to coercive stimuli than cwonsenting stimuli (Abel et al., 1977; Eccles, Marshall, & Barbaree, 1994; Freund, Scher, Racansky, Campbell, & Heasman, 1986; Quinsey & Chaplin, 1984; Quinsey, Chaplin, & Varney 1981; Rice et al., 1994).

However, other studies have found no difference (Baxter, Marshall, Barbaree, Davidson, & Malcolm, 1984; Murphy et al., 1984; Seto & Barbaree, 1993). These contradictory findings have brought into question the validity and utility of rape testing. In fact, following years of testing with video assessment stimuli for sadism and coerciveness, Freund discontinued development of a stimulus set that could distinguish between men with criminal sadism and those without. He concluded that too many "normals" respond highly to sexually coercive stimuli (personal communication, 1994).

Nevertheless, research on the identification of rape proneness via PPG testing has continued with some success. Current research indicates that the best discrimination between rapists and controls is obtained when the stimuli involve more extreme violence that emphasizes the victim's suffering (Harris, Rice, Chaplin, & Quinsey, 1999). Lalumière et al. (2003) concluded that since all studies reviewed in his study produced positive effect sizes—rapists always had a higher rape index than the comparison group—"it is incontestable that rapists differ from nonrapists in their responses to sexually coercive stimuli." This study also examined the most recent

PPG rape literature, and found three of the five "new" studies showed greater responding to rape scenarios, while one showed no difference, and a fifth showed greater responses to coercive interactions among the nonsex offending controls. On the basis of this literature review it was concluded that, "even though some studies show small differences, the general conclusion remains that rapists tend to be much more aroused to scenarios depicting coercive sex than do controls."

Questions also remain about the relationship between response to sadistic stimuli and actual (enacted) criminal activity. Two studies examined men who "self-reported" interest in rape (Malamuth & Check, 1983) or who said they had "sadistic" sexual fantasies but had not acted on their interests (Seto & Kuban, 1996). Both studies found these men responded more to coercive "stories" than to consensual "stories." In fact, the latter study found the sexually sadistic "admitters" to have greater responses to coercive stimuli than did rapists who had committed assaults but who denied sexually sadistic or coercive fantasies.

In a separate study, Lalumière et al. (2003), compared 24 sexual assaulters to 11 nonsexual offenders and 19 community volunteers. Using graphic sexual stimuli from the Rice et al. (1994) stimulus set, it was found that the two comparison groups scored similarly—in that they responded more to consenting sexual scenarios than rape scenarios.

However, men in the rapist group responded similarly to rape categories and consenting categories when the events were described from the female (victim) point of view, slightly more to rape scenarios than consensual scenarios. The Cohen's effect size was $d = 1.50$. Effect size is technically defined as a measure of the magnitude of a "treatment" that is independent of sample size. By usual criteria, 1.50 indicates a large effect size. Further, the test's sensitivity was determined to be 0.63, while the specificity was 0.84 and 0.91, based on the control group of "community men" and the known assaulters, respectively. Thus, 63% of rapists compared to 13% of nonrapists had a rape index larger than zero. Consistent with findings from the other sets of meta-analytic studies reviewed, these authors concluded that as a group, relative to controls, rapists, could be shown to respond more on PPG testing to forced, nonconsenting sexual behavior, particularly when the test stimuli are of a very graphic and violent nature, and are described from the woman's point of view.

Faking and Dissimulation

The intentional manipulation of testing, mentally or physically, certainly contributes to the acknowledged poor sensitivity of PPG in the assessment of sex offenders. This is important since the sensitivity (correct identification of true positives) of PPG testing has consistently been found to be much lower than its specificity (correct identification of true negatives). It is generally accepted that only 50% of child molesters who do not admit pedophilic interests may be correctly identified, while more than 95% of men with no known child victims are found on PPG testing to be nonpedophilic. One reason for such a low sensitivity is that penile tumescence is partially subject to voluntary control (Adams, Motsinger, McAnulty, & Moore, 1992; Freund, 1961; Freund; 1963; Freund, 1967, Lalumière & Earls; 1992; Mahoney & Strassberg, 1991 McAnulty & Adams, 1991; Quinsey & Chaplin, 1988). In fact, voluntary suppression could be why so many subjects display very low penile responses, (roughly one-third in most laboratories are found to be "low responders," also referred to in the field as "flat liners") (Kuban et al., 1997).

Other methods of manipulating PPG results include "stimulus avoidance" (looking away from the visual images), "fantasy manipulation" (thinking of arousing themes to increase penile response or thinking about sexually aversive themes to suppress penile response), "pumping" (contracting perineal musculature in an attempt to voluntarily produce penile erection (Freund, Watson, & Rienzo, 1988), or direct manual gauge manipulation (such as pulling on the circumferential gauge).

Management of PPG response (faking) manipulation by clinicians and researchers has taken a variety of forms. The earliest method was through the use of low-light cameras to consensually observe and ensure subjects to ensure that they were actually looking at the presented visual stimuli and that they were not manipulating the test apparatus. It should be noted that, standard testing excludes visual monitoring of the penis. Typically the subjects' genital region remains covered during the entire test. Subjects often comment that the lack of visual feedback about their erectile response is disconcerting. Moreover, modern strain gauges and highly sensitive data acquisition equipment (such as 16-bit sensors) make physical manipulation of the equipment readily detectable by the examiner. Visual monitoring of the subject by the PPG technician has become standard, and even when subjects are listening to audio narratives, observational cameras can show if headphone or other equipment manipulation occurs.

The use of more "potent" stimuli is another way to potentially decrease dissimulation, as videotapes with audio normally produce higher levels of arousal than audiotapes alone (Abel, Barlow, Blanchard, & Mavissakalian, 1975; Card & Farrall, 1990). According to this theory, the more potent the stimuli, the more penile response elicited, the less likely the incidence of low responses, and the better discrimination that can be observed (Freund & Blanchard, 1989; Harris et al., 1999). However, use of explicit sexual stimuli, particularly those depicting illegal themes, is limited by moral, legal, and ethical considerations.

In addition to obvious physical attempts at test manipulation, attempts have been made to detect dissimulation or manipulation by identification of unusual test outcomes. Freund et al. (1988) described several signs that he associated with "faking." The most obvious is evidence from the printed test curves that intentional perineal contractions were occurring during the test. These muscular contractions appear as small "spikes" during the section of the test in which the man is hoping to show arousal (usually the adult female category). These have been identified as attempts to voluntarily produce or enhance erections by men who do not find adult females sexually arousing. Of course, men with erectile dysfunction may also be tempted to use similar methods even if their primary arousal is toward adult females. This motivation would be particularly important in cases in which there are legal implications from the test results.

Other signs identified by Freund included results in which the highest response score is to visually neutral stimuli (such as landscapes). This has been interpreted to be the result of voluntary suppression to any of the sexual stimuli. It is hypothesized that subsequent relaxation of efforts to suppress erection during neutral scenes may then result in higher relative responses to the neutral stimuli. Cases in which the highest responses occur during presentation of neutral stimuli may be considered grounds for test invalidation (Freund et al., 1988; Lalumière & Harris, 1998). Again, while a "rebound effect" is one possible interpretation of this phenomenon, it does not exclude other explanations such as the possibility that neutral stimuli "unmask" fantasies. Evidence to support this alternative explanation comes from studies of women who were shown to demonstrate greater arousal on female vaginal plethysmography when given distracting tasks (Laan, 1994).

While more controversial, Freund also reported that "faking" might be suspected in cases where the highest responses (during PPG testing) are to an adult, and in which the second highest response is to stimuli depicting an adult of the opposite gender. Among control subjects, Freund and others, (see Lalumière et al., 2005) observed that in nonpedophilic men, pubescent age minors of the most preferred gender produced much higher penile responses on PPG than opposite gender stimuli. As a result, Freund concluded that a test profile in which the two highest responses were to adults (both male and female) sex should be considered evidence of response suppression to minors. Again, this interpretation is based on the now somewhat controversial assumption that true bisexuality never occurs in males.

Prior experience with PPG by men being tested also factors into PPG test validity. Subjects with prior experience in being assessed by PPG testing are believed to be better able to manipulate their responses (Freund et al., 1988; Golde, Strassberg, & Turner, 2000). A further uninvestigated question concerns whether the increased availability of pornographic materials (e.g., through the Internet) has had the effect of reducing the salience of the test stimuli used in most PPG labs.

Assessment of Pedophiles

Research on the assessment of pedophiles has undoubtedly been complicated by the fact that not all pedophiles molest children and not all child molesters are pedophiles. Early studies reporting accurate classification of offenders (Abel et al., 1977; Abel et al., 1978; Abel, Becker, & Skinner, 1980; Barbaree et al., 1979) failed to show the same degree of accuracy in replication studies (e.g., Avery-Clark & Laws, 1984; Baxter et al., 1984; Murphy et al., 1984) Some studies have been criticized on the basis of small, select samples. Others failed to replicate their findings in other studies, such as Quinsey et al. (1984), and Letourneau (2002), the focus was on particularly dangerous and violent offenders incarcerated in maximum security institutions. These data suggested that the validity of PPG testing in the assessment and treatment of sexual offenders required further empirical support and none

of these studies supported the application of PPG technology for the assessment of suspected offenders.

Mussack et al. (1987) attempted to determine the validity of the penile tumescence testing using a sample of 24 comparison subjects with no known paraphilic interests, recruited from the general population, and 34 heterosexual child molesters. The assessment procedure consisted of gathering interview and psychometric data, along with measures of sexual responses to visual and auditory stimuli using PPG. They conducted a discriminant function analysis on the sexual arousal measures using "group" as the dependant variable. The analysis correctly classified 73% of the subjects (p < .004) (67% of the comparison subjects and 77% of the child molesters). In a small cross validation sample, six out of six of the comparison subjects and seven out of eight of the child molesters were correctly classified.

In a later study, Laws et al. (2000) assessed the extent to which the use of multiple measures of pedophilic interest, including penile tumescence testing, improved on the diagnostic accuracy of any one measure alone. The authors found that PPG testing with slides yielded a sensitivity of 86.1%, and the use of PPG testing with audio resulted in a sensitivity of 81%. Overall classification accuracy was increased to 91.7% when PPG testing with both slides and audio stimulus sets were analyzed together with a card sort assessment procedure. Similarity in efficacy between audio and slide stimuli was replicated in a study by Looman and Marshall (2001), which found that both stimulus sets were equally effective in discriminating child molesters from a group of rapists.

Firestone and associates (2000) examined the ability of PPG to discriminate between 216 child molesters and a comparison group of 47 nonoffenders from the community. They found that child molesters (both homicidal and nonhomicidal) had significantly higher pedophile index scores than the comparison group (p < .05).

Blanchard et al. (2001) conducted a similar study using 82 male sex offenders against women, 172 offenders against unrelated children, and 70 offenders against their own biological children or stepchildren. Using PPG assessments, they obtained a specificity of 96% for offenders against adult women, with a calculated minimum sensitivity of 61% for positive diagnoses of pedophiles.

In another study, two groups, child molesters and normal control subjects, were compared using visual stimuli (Grossman, Cavanaugh, & Haywood, 1992). Although the pedophilic group was significantly discriminated from the control group, a significant interaction effect also showed that nonincestuous pedophiles responded more to child stimuli than either the control group or the incestuous fathers (both of which scored similarly). Furthermore, the nonincestuous pedophiles scored higher than the incestuous fathers on sexual interests toward adults, although they scored lower than the control group of men with no known paraphilias or criminal history. These results support the potential importance of PPG in the assessment of non incestuous child molesters. A similar effect was found by Letourneau (2002), in which PPG using audio stimuli resulted in significantly lower arousal to female child stimuli for men with female child victims than that of men with other victim types (boys or both boys and girls).

Regrettably, many studies involving PPG do not include sufficient data to calculate the sensitivity and specificity of the test. The results of several studies in which sensitivity and specificity data were presented are summarized in Table 7.1. Inspection of the studies in Table 7.1, reveal that the majority exclude cases in which the results are "faked" or insufficient to interpret. Arguably, this artificially inflates the reported sensitivity of the test.

FORENSIC ISSUES

Most labs conduct the majority of their PPG assessments on men accused or convicted of sex crimes. Therefore, any assessment of PPG testing should consider the potential forensic implications. For more on this topic see Simon and Schouten (1992).

The Association for the Treatment of Sexual Abusers (ATSA) discusses PPG testing in its "Practice Standards and Guidelines for Members of the Association for the Treatment of Sexual Abusers" (2004) (www.atsa.com). Concerning PPG testing, Section 22 of the document indicates that informed consent to undergo PPG testing must be obtained before proceeding and that the results should not

TABLE 7.1 Sensitivity and Specificity of PPG Tests for Pedophilia

Study	Groups (N)	Sensitivity (%)	Specificity (%)	Comments
Seto et al., 1999	Mixed incest and extrafamilial (64)	56.3	80	Other groups had lower sensitivity Excluded "technical problems," "faking," psychosis, and MR
Seto et al, 2000	Adolescent offenders against children (75) Young adult offenders against children(39) "Comparison" controls (39)	42	92	Control includes 23 rapists Rates higher for admitters Adolescent offenders with only female victims similar to control group Excluded "technical problems"
Blanchard et al., 2001	Rapists (82) Sex Offenders against children (172) Incest offenders (70)	61	96	Excluded "technical problems," "uncooperativeness," "Nonresponsiveness." "Invalid" profiles
Barsetti et al., 1998	Child molesters (39) Nonoffenders (18)	66.7	95	Excluded nonresponders
Chaplin et al., 1995	Child molesters (15) Unemployed men (15)	100	100	No exclusions Discrimination on the basis of violent stimuli
Freund & Watson, 1991	Sex Offenders against 2 + girls (27) Sex offenders against 2 + male minors (22) Sex Offenders against women (41) Paid Volunteers (50)	78.2 88.6	97 80.6	Exhibitionists excluded Psychosis, MR excluded Pedophiles were "nonadmitters" "Faking" or "low output" excluded

be used as the "sole criterion for estimating client risk…, making recommendations to release (or not release) clients to the community, or deciding that clients have completed a treatment program."

The question of whether PPG testing constitutes "degrading treatment" under Article 3 of the Convention of Human Rights, has been considered by the Court of the Council of Europe (1999) (http://hudoc.echr.coe.int). The case involved a prisoner with "sexual identity problems" who alleged that he was coerced into "submitting" to PPG testing which he found humiliating and degrading. Part of the prisoner's argument was that refusal to undergo PPG would have slowed acceptance into a sex offender treatment program. The Court did not find in favor of the prisoner, though it did comment that it would have been "more reasonable for the test to have been conducted by a male technician" (Gazan, 2002).

Concerns have also been raised about the use of stimulus materials that involve children and other sexually prohibited themes (see ATSA (2005) for discussion and comments). One of the most widely used stimulus sets used primarily in the United States and published by Farrall Instruments has been banned because it included nude pictures of children. Prohibition against the possession and dissemination of "child pornography" has impeded the standardization of PPG stimulus sets. Remarkably, studies investigating PPG with stimuli that do not include nudity have never been published.

Notwithstanding the issues raised in the preceding paragraphs, the primary forensic concerns about PPG, have involved its admissibility in court. In North Carolina, the Court of Appeals considered a lower court's decision to exclude the evidence of a doctor who had argued that an accused was "not a pedophile" on the basis of negative PPG results:

In view of the lack of general acceptance of the plethysmograph's reliability and utility and therefore, its reliability for forensic purposes in the scientific community in which it is employed, we hold that the trial court did not abuse its discretion in finding the defendant's plethysmograph testing data insufficiently reliable to provide a basis for the opinion testimony which defendant sought to elicit from (the doctor) (State of North Carolina vs. Robert Earl Spencer, 1995).

Since then many, but not all courts in the U.S. have rejected the admissibility of PPG evidence (see Smith, 1998 for review of cases).

CONCLUSION

Aside from substance abuse disorders, sleep disorders, and a handful of psychiatric disorders resulting from medical illnesses, sexual disorders are the only group of psychiatric disorders with verified physiologic markers: abnormalities on PPG testing. In spite of this, abnormalities on PPG testing are not part of the DSM of ICD diagnostic criteria for any of the paraphilias and many, if not most, treatment programs for sex offenders do not use PPG testing. Similarly, the trend in judicial decisions appears to be to exclude evidence based solely on PPG test results.

The reason is that in spite of a concerted research effort over the past half century, the sensitivity of PPG testing is insufficient and the specificity while certainly higher, is not known for certain. This state of affairs should come as no surprise since PPG testing has never been intended to determine guilt or innocence in criminal matters. Nor has the potential sensitivity and specificity of PPG testing ever been established in the way most other psychological or medical tests are standardized. What would happen if the validity of blood glucose testing were based on studies of men, some with diabetes and some without, at various stages of treatment, in which blood glucose levels were compared to the self-report of the men about whether they had diabetes? What if the same men also had varying motivations to attempt to trick or mislead the lab? The problem for validation of PPG testing is further compounded by the fact that the relationship between penile tumescence and sexual arousal is far from direct, even in healthy men on no medications.

Will PPG testing go the way of dexamethasone suppression testing for mood disorders? Probably. Future research needs to focus on physiologic changes associated with sexual arousal that occur before penile tumescence results. One important candidate is nitric oxide, a gaseous neurotransmitter involved in the cascade of physiologic events that culminate in penile tumescence. In addition, work needs to be done to establish standard stimulus sets with equivalent versions. This is important since the salience of stimulus sets decrease with repeat administration, making reliability testing problematic and decreasing the utility of PPG testing as a means to measure response to treatment. Further research on the effect of alcohol on PPG testing would also make sense since many sex offenders are intoxicated at the time of their crimes (Wormith, Bradford, Pawlak, Borzecki, & Zohar 1988). Further work on the refinement of stimulus sets, especially ones that do not involve illegal images, will likely be necessary if PPG testing is to become more widely employed (Renaud et al., 2005).

In the meantime, clinicians should be vigilant to guard against overinterpreting results. In its current form, PPG testing remains an investigational tool. Results of PPG testing in isolation will never be sufficient to prove the guilt or innocence of a suspect. As with any tool, the utility of PPG testing depends on the skill of the ones who use it. In combination with clinical judgment and other investigational procedures (e.g., psychological testing, eye-tracking, polygraphy, etc.), PPG may be invaluable.

References

Abel, G. G., Barlow, D. H., Blanchard, E. B., & Mavissakalian, M. (1975). Measurement of sexual arousal in male homosexuals: The effects of instructions and stimulus modality. *Archives of Sexual Behavior*, 4, 623–629.

Abel, G. G., Barlow, D., Blanchard, E., & Guild, D. (1977). The components of rapists' sexual arousal. *Archives of General Psychiatry*, 34, 895–903.

Abel, G. G., Becker, D. H., Blanchard, E. B., & Djenderedjian, D. A. (1978). Differentiating sexual aggressives with penile measures. *Criminal Justice and Behaviour*, 5, 315–332.

Abel, G. G., Becker, J. V., & Skinner, L. J. (1980). Aggressive behaviour and sex. *The Psychiatric Clinics of North America*, 3, 133–151.

Abel, G. G., Becker, J. V., Murphy, W. D., & Flanagan, B. (1981). Identifying dangerous child molesters. In R. Stuart (Ed.), *Violent behavior*. New York: Brunner/Mazel.

Abel, G. G., Blanchard, E. B., & Barlow, D. H. (1981). Measurement of sexual arousal in several paraphilias: the effects of stimulus modality, instructional set and stimulus content on the objective. *Behaviour Research and Therapy*, 19,25–33.

Adams, H. E., Motsinger, P., McAnulty, R. D., Moore, A. L. (1992). Voluntary control of penile tumescence among homosexual and heterosexual subjects. *Archives of Sexual Behavior*, 21(1), 17–31.

The Association for the Treatment of Sexual Abusers (ATSA). (2005). Practice Standards and Guidelines for Members of the Association for the Treatment of Sexual Abusers. (www.atsa.com).

Avery-Clark, C. & Laws, D. R. (1984). Differential erection response patterns of child abusers to stimuli describing sexual activities with children. *Behaviour Therapy*, 15, 71–83.

Bancroft, J. H., Jones, H. G., & Pullan, B. R. (1966). A simple transducer for measuring penile erection, with comments on its use in the treatment of sexual disorder. *Behaviour Research and Therapy*, 4, 239–241.

Barbaree, H. E., Marshall, W. L., & Lanthier, R. D. (1979). Deviant sexual arousal in rapists. *Behaviour Research and Therapy*, 17, 215–222.

Barbaree, H. E. (1990). Chapter 8. Stimulus control of sexual arousal. Its role in sexual assault. In W. L. Marshall, D. R. Laws & H. E. Barbaree (Ed.), *Handbook of sexual assault. Issues, theories, and treatment of the offender*. 233 Spring Street, New York, NY 10013, Plenum Press, New York: 115–142.

Barker, J. G. & R. J. Howell (1992). The plethysmograph: A review of recent literature. *The Bulletin of the American Academy of Psychiatry and the Law*, 20(1), 13–25.

Barlow, D. H., Becker, R., Leitenberg, H., & Agras, W. S. (1970). A mechanical strain gauge for recording penile circumference change. *Journal of Applied Behaviour Analysis*, 3, 73–76.

Barsetti, I., Earls, C. M., Lalumière, M. L., & Bèlanger, N. (1998). The differentiation of intrafamilial and extrafamilial heterosexual child molesters. *Journal of Interpersonal Violence*, 13(2), 275–286.

Baxter, D. J., Marshall, W. L., Barbaree, H. E., Davidson, P. R., & Malcolm, P. B. (1984). Deviant sexual behaviour: Differentiating sex offenders by criminal and personal history, psychometric measures, and sexual response. *Criminal Justice and Behavior*, 11, 477–501.

Blanchard, R., Klassen, P., Dickey, R., Kuban, M. E., & Blak, T. (2001). Sensitivity and specificity of the phallometric test for pedophilia in nonadmitting sex offenders. *Psychological Assessment*, 13(1), 118–126.

Card, R. D. & Farrall, B. S. (1990). Detecting faked penile responses to erotic stimuli: A comparison of stimuli conditions and response measures. *Annals of Sex Research*, 3, 381–396.

Chaplin, T. C., Rice, M. E., & Harris, G. T. (1995). Salient victim suffering and the sexual responses of child molesters. *Journal of Consulting and Clinical Psychology*, 63(2), 249–255.

Cohen, J. (1992). A power primer. *Psychological Bulletin*, 112, 155–159.

Court of the Council of Europe. (1999). Article 3: Convention of Human Rights. (http://hudoc.echr.coe.int).

Earls, C. M., Quinsey, V. L., & Castonguay, L. G. (1987). A comparison of three methods of scoring penile circumference changes. *Archives of Sexual Behavior*, 16(6), 493–500.

Eccles, T., Marshall, W. L., & Barbaree, H. E. (1994) Differentiating rapist and non-offenders using the rape index. *Behaviour Research and Therapy*, 32, 539–546.

Fernandez, Y. M. & Marshall, W. L. (2003). Victim empathy, social self-esteem, and psychopathy in rapists. *Sexual Abuse: A Journal of Research and Treatment*, 15(1), 11–26.

Firestone, P., Bradford, J. M., Greenberg, D. M., & Larose, M. R. (2000). Differentiation of homicidal child molesters, nonhomicidal child molesters, and nonoffenders by phallometry. *American Journal of Psychiatry*, 157(11), 1847–1850.

Freund, K. (1957). Diagnostika Homosexuality U muzu. *Cs. Psychiatrica*, 53, 382–393.

Freund, K. (1961). A laboratory differential diagnosis of homo- and heterosexuality—an experiment with faking. *Review of Medicine*, 7, 20–31.

Freund, K. (1963). A laboratory method for diagnosing predominance of homo- or hetero-erotic interest in the male. *Behaviour Research and Therapy*, 12, 355–359.

Freund K. (1965). A simple device for measuring the volume changes of the male genital. *Cs. Psychiatrica*, 61, 164–167.

Freund, K. (1967). Erotic preference in pedophilia. *Behaviour Research and Therapy*, 5, 339–348.

Freund, K. (1991). Reflections on the development of the phallometric method of assessing erotic preferences. *Annals of Sex Research*, 4, 221–228.

Freund, K., Scher, H., Racansky, I. G., Campbell, K., & Heasman, G. (1986). Males disposed to commit rape. *Archives of Sexual Behavior*, 15, 23–35.

Freund, K., Watson, R., & Rienzo, D. (1988). Signs of feigning in the phallometric test. *Behaviour research and therapy*, 26(2), 105–12.

Freund, K. & Blanchard, R. (1989). Phallometric diagnosis of pedophilia. *Journal of Consulting and Clinical Psychology*, 57, 100–105.

Freund, K. & Watson, R. J. (1991). Assessment of the sensitivity and specificity of a phallometric test: An update of phallometric diagnosis of pedophilia. *Psychological Assessment: A Journal of Consulting and Clinical Psychology*, 3(2), 254–260.

Gazan, F. (2002). Penile plethysmography before the European Court of Human Rights. *Sexual Abuse: A Journal of Research and Treatment*, 14(1), 89–93.

Golde, G. A., Strassberg, D. S., & Turner, C.M. (2000) Psychophysiological assessment of erectile response and its suppression as a function of stimulus media and previous experience with plethysmography. *Journal of Sex Research*, 37, 53–59.

Grossman, L. S., Cavanaugh, J. L., & Haywood, T. W. (1992). Deviant sexual responsiveness on penile plethysmography using visual stimuli: Alleged child molesters vs. normal control subjects. *The Journal of Nervous and Mental Disease*, 180(3), 207–208.

Hall, G. C. N., Shondrick, D. D., & Hirschman, R. (1993). The role of sexual arousal in sexually aggressive behaviour: A meta-analysis. *Journal of Consulting and Clinical Psychology*, 61, 1091–1095.

Hanson, E. K. (2002). Associate editor's introduction to E.J. Letourneau, A comparison of objective measures of sexual arousal and interest: Visual reaction time and penile plethysmography. *Sexual Abuse: A Journal of Research and Treatment*, 14(3), 205.

Harris, G. T., Rice, M. E., Quinsey, V. L., Chaplin, T. C., & Earls, C. (1992). Maximizing the discriminant ability of phallometric assessment data. *Psychological Assessment*, 4, 502–511.

Harris, G. T., Rice, M., Chaplin, T., & Quinsey, V. (1999). Dissimulation in Phallometric Testing of Rapists' Sexual Preferences. *Archives of Sexual Behavior*, 28(3), 223–232.

Howes, R. (1995). A survey of plethysmographic assessment in North America. *Sexual Abuse: A Journal of Research and Treatment*, 7, 9–24.

Johnson, S. A. & Listiak, A. (1999). Chapter 26: The measurement of sexual preference—a preliminary comparison of phallometry and the Abel Assessment. The Sex Offender. In B. K. Schwartz (Ed.), *Theoretical Advances, Treating Special Populations and Legal Developments*. 4490 U.S. Route 27, P.O.Box 585, Kingston, NJ 08258, Civic Research Institute. III, 26–1 - 26–20.

Konopasky, R. J. & Konopasky, A. W. B. (2000). Chapter 15. Remaking penile plethysmography. D. R. Laws, S. M. Hudson, & T. Ward (Ed.), *Remaking relapse prevention with sex offenders. A sourcebook*. 2455 Teller Road, Thousands Oaks, California 91320, Sage Publications, Inc., 257–284.

Kuban, M., Barbaree, H. E., & Blanchard, R. (1997). A comparison of volume and circumference phallometry: Response magnitude and method agreement. *Archives of Sexual Behavior*, 28, 345–357.

Kuban, M., Barbaree, H. E., & Blanchard, R. (1999). A comparison of volume and circumference phallometry: Response magnitude and method agreement. *Archives of Sexual Behavior*, 28(4), 345–359.

Laan, E. (1994). Determinants of Sexual Arousal in Women: Genital and subjective components of sexual response. Faculteit der Psychologie. Amsterdam, Universiteit van Amsterdam: pp. 189.

Lalumière, M. L. & Earls, C. M. (1992). Voluntary control of penile responses as a function of stimulus duration and instructions. *Behavioral Assessment*, 14, 121–132.

Lalumière, M. & Harris, G. (1998). Common questions regarding the use of phallometric testing with sexual offenders. *Sexual Abuse: A Journal of Research and Treatment*, 10, 227–237.

Lalumière, M. L. & Quinsey, V. L. (1994). The discriminability of rapists from nonoffenders using phallometric measures: A meta-analysis. *Criminal Justice and Behavior*, 21, 150–175.

Lalumière, M. L., Quinsey, V. L., Harris, G. T., Rice, M. R., & Trautrimas, C. (2003). Are rapists differentially aroused by coercive sex in phallometric assessments? *Annals of the New York Academy of Science*, 989, 211–224.

Lalumière, M. L., Harris, G. T., Quinsey, V. L., & Rice, M. E. (2005). *The causes of rape*. Washington, DC: American Psychological Association.

Launay, G. (1999). The phallometric assessment of sex offenders: An update. *Criminal Behaviour and Mental Health*, 9, 254–274.

Laws, D. R. (1989). *Direct monitoring by penile plethysmography. Relapse Prevention with Sex Offenders.* D. R. Laws. 72 Spring Street, New York, NY 10012, The Guildford Press: 105–114.

Laws, D. R. (2003). 5. Penile plethysmography. Will we ever get it right? Sexual Deviance. T. Ward, D. R. Laws, & S. M. Hudson (Ed.), *Issues and controversies.* 2455 Teller Road, Thousand Oaks, California 91320, Sage Publications, Inc., 82–102.

Laws, D. R., Gulayets, M. J., & Frenzel, R. R. (1995). Assessments of sex offenders using standardized slide stimuli and procedures: A multi-site study. *Sexual Abuse: A Journal of Research and Treatment*, 7, 45–66.

Laws, D. R., Hudson, S. M., & Ward, T. (2000). *Remaking relapse prevention with sex offenders. A sourcebook.* Thousands Oaks, CA: Sage Publications, Inc.

Letourneau, E. J. (2002). A comparison of objective measures of sexual arousal and interest: Visual reaction time and penile plethysmography. *Sexual Abuse: A Journal of Research and Treatment*, 14(3), 207–223.

Looman, J. & Marshall, W. (2001). Phallometric Assessments Designed to Detect Arousal to Children: The Responses of Rapists and Child Molesters. *Sexual Abuse: A Journal of Research and Treatment*, 13(1), 3–13.

Mahoney, J. M. & Strassberg, D. S. (1991). Voluntary control of male sexual arousal. *Archives of Sexual Behavior*, 20, 1–16.

Malamuth, N. M. & Check, J. V. (1983). Sexual arousal to rape depictions: Individual differences. *Journal of Abnormal Psychology*, 92, 55–67.

Maletsky, B. M. (1995). Editorial:Stimulus materials and the protection of victims. *Sexual Abuse: A Journal of Research and Treatment*, 7, 109–111.

Marshall, W. L. & Fernandez, Y. M. (2000a). Phallometric testing with sexual offenders: Limits to its value. *Clinical Psychological Review*, 20, 807–822.

Marshall, W. L. & Fernandez, Y. M. (2000b). Phallometry in forensic practice. *Journal of Forensic Psychological Practice*, 1, 77–87.

McAnulty, R. D. & Adams, H. E. (1991). Voluntary control of penile tumescence: Effects of an incentive and a signal detection task. *The Journal of Sex Research*, 28(4), 557–577.

Murphy, W. D., Krisak, J., Stalgaitis, S. J., & Anderson, K. (1984). The use of penile tumescence measures with incarcerated rapists: Further validity issues. *Archives of Sexual Behavior*, 13(6), 545–554.

Mussack, S. E., Bays, L., & Hindman, J. (1987) An investigation of the criterion validity of the penile plethysmograph as a tool for diagnosing sexual orientation in males. Paper presented at the Annual Conference of the A.B.T.S.A., May, Newport, Oregon.

Prentky, R. A. & Knight, R. A. (1991). Identifying critical dimensions for discriminating among rapists. *Journal of Clinical and Consulting Psychology*, 59, 643–661.

Quinsey, V. L., Chaplin, T. C., & Varney, G. (1981). A comparison of rapists' and non-sex offenders' sexual preferences for mutually consenting sex, rape, and physical abuse of women. *Behavioral Assessment*, 3, 127–135.

Quinsey, V. L. & Chaplin, T. C. (1982). Penile responses to nonsexual violence among rapists. *Criminal Justice and Behaviour*, 9, 312–324.

Quinsey, V. L. & Chaplin, T. C. (1984). Stimulus control of rapists' and non-sex offenders' sexual arousal. *Behavioural Assessment*, 6, 169–176.

Quinsey, V. L., Chaplin, T. C., & Upfold, D. (1984). Sexual arousal to nonsexual violence and sadomasochistic themes among rapists and non-sex-offenders. *Journal of Consulting and Clinical Psychology*, 52, 651–657.

Quinsey, V. L. & Chaplin, T. C. (1988). Penile responses of child molesters and normals to descriptions of encounters with children involving sex and violence. *Journal of Interpersonal Violence*, 3, 259–274.

Renaud, P., Proulx, J., Rouleau, J.-L., Bouchard, S., Madrigrano, G., Bradford, J., et al. (2005). The recording of observational behaviors in virtual immersion: A new clinical tool to address the problem of sexual preferences with paraphiliacs. *Annual Review of Cybertherapy and Telemedecine*, 3, 85–92.

Rice, M. E., Chaplin, T. C., Harris, G. T., & Coutts, J. (1994). Empathy for the victim and sexual arousal among rapists and nonrapists. *Journal of Interpersonal Violence*, 9, 435–449.

Seto, M. C. (2001). The value of phallometry in the assessment of male sex offenders. *Journal of Forensic Psychology Practice*, 1(2), 65–75.

Seto, M. C. & Barbaree, H. E. (1993). Victim blame and sexual arousal to rape cues in rapists and nonoffenders. *Annals of Sex Research*, 6, 167–183.

Seto, M. C. & Kuban, M. (1996). Criterion-related validity of a phallometric test for paraphilic rape and sadism. *Behaviour Research and Therapy*, 34, 175–183. Seto, M. C., Lalumière, M. L., & Kuban, M. (1999). The sexual preferences of incest offenders. *Journal of Abnormal Psychology*, 108(2), 267–272.

Seto, M. C., Lalumière, M. L., & Blanchard, R. (2000). The discriminative validity of a phallometric test for pedophilic interests among adolescent sex offenders against children. *Psychological Assessment*, 12(3), 319–327.

Simon, W. T. & Schouten, P. G. W. (1991). Plethysmography in the assessment and treatment of sexual deviance: An overview. *Archives of Sexual Behavior*, 20(1), 75–91.

Simon, W. T. & Schouten, P. G. (1992). Problems in Sexual Preference Testing in Child Sexual

Abuse Cases. *Journal of Interpersonal Violence, 7,* 503–516.

Smith, S. (1998). http://www.smith-lawfirm.com/Scientific_Evidence_Brief.html

State v. Spencer, 119 N.C. App. 662, 459 S.E. 2d 812 (1995).

Wormith, J. S., Bradford, J. M., Pawlak, A., Borzecki, M., & Zohar, A. (1988). The assessment of deviant sexual arousal as a function of intelligence, instructional set and alcohol ingestion. *Canadian journal of psychiatry. Revue canadienne de psychiatrie, 33*(9), 800–808.

Chapter 8

Visual Reaction Time: Development, Theory, Empirical Evidence, and Beyond

Gene G. Abel and Markus Wiegel

This chapter discusses the theoretical foundations for, development of, empirical evidence for, and the continued development of visual reaction time (VRT) as a measure of sexual interest. The evaluation of paraphilic sexual interests must adapt to scientific and technical advances, as well as to the cultural and societal attitudes, sociopolitical context, and the legal environment in which these advances occur. The thorough evaluation of individuals with possible paraphilias must include assessment of their sexual interest patterns, especially evaluation of any sexual interest in children. Some sexual abusers are highly motivated to conceal their sexual interest and, therefore, objective instruments that are difficult to fake are essential. In 1987, the assessment of possible sexual abusers was dominated by circumferential penile plethysmography (PPG) measures of adult males in the United States and circumferential and volumetric PPG measures of adult males in Canada. Neither standardized PPG stimuli, nor standard questionnaires, existed for evaluating the broad spectrum of

paraphilias. In addition, standardized systems for assessing adult females, adolescent males, and adolescent females were lacking. That year, The Behavioral Medicine Institute of Atlanta was formed to research VRT as a potential psychological test to assist clinicians in determining the sexual interests of individuals with potential paraphilias. The most critical objective of our research was to determine if a brief, valid screening instrument could be developed to identify those with sexual interests in children who were applying to organizations that work with youth, such as the Boy Scouts of America, Big Brothers and Big Sisters, the Catholic Church, the Civil Air Patrol, and so on.

Our scientific research had to adapt to a variety of nonscientific factors while developing this system. Since a number of clergy were being evaluated following accusations of sex offenses against children, their superiors (especially in the case of the Catholic Church) were reluctant to have their priests, who were to remain celibate, view nude images. The FBI and the State agencies began threatening arrests at those laboratories using slides of nude children to assess potential sexual abusers. Very importantly, those working with survivors of child sexual abuse were outraged by images of nude children being used in assessment and were concerned that the use of such images was a revictimization of the children depicted (beyond the original taking of the pictures). These and other factors culminated in the Governor of Nebraska demanding that the Farrell Instruments Company of Grand Island, Nebraska, who supplied most of the slides used in PPG laboratories in North America, terminate selling such depictions.

THEORETICAL FOUNDATIONS

While the criminal justice system is essentially concerned with determining whether an individual is guilty of a sex crime, for example, whether someone has sexually touched a child, the clinical evaluation of alleged child sexual abusers is concerned with whether the individual has sexual interest in children. Sexual behavior is influenced by a multitude of factors, both internal and external to the person. To understand these factors, there are a number of concepts that need to be defined and distinguished from one another. These include sexual desire, sexual arousal, sexual interest, and sexual attraction. Sexual desire can be conceptualized as a motivation to experience sexual sensations, sexual arousal, and potentially orgasm. Thus, sexual desire can be seen as one motivation to engage in sexual behavior. Singer and Toates (1987) conceptualize sexual motivation as following the rules of general incentive-based (as opposed to drive-based) models of motivation, but allowing for sexual desire to be determined by multiple factors, for example, hormones, satiation, and deprivation, as well as personality and social factors. Sexual arousal is probably the most complex to define. It has been conceptualized among the emotions, in that it involves preconscious processing of stimuli, cognitive appraisal of stimuli, autonomic arousal (genital as well as other peripheral autonomic arousal), and a subjective feeling state (Everaerd, 1988; Everaerd, Laan, & Spiering, 2000; Singer, 1984). Sexual arousal, like other emotional reactions, depends on appraisal of stimuli, which includes memory and attentional processes interacting with each other. As such, any stimuli is not intrinsically sexual, but must be appraised or interpreted as such, occurring at preconscious and conscious levels of awareness (Everaerd et al., 2000). It is this appraisal or interpretation of specific stimuli as sexual that is the essence of sexual interest. It is unknown whether sexual interests are already determined at birth; however, it is clear that we are born with a sensitivity for "sexual stimuli," (e.g., genital touch). This sensitivity strengthens during development, becoming prominent at puberty and continuing, although attenuated, through old age. A person's interactions with the environment, as well as internal rehearsal (fantasy), build up experience and potentiation of sexual stimuli (Everaerd et al., 2000). We prefer the term sexual interest to the terms sexual orientation and sexual preference, because orientation connotes more of a biological etiology, while preference connotes a more learned and even voluntary nature. Sexual interest refers to the result of biopsychosocial processes (hormonal, genetic, conditioned, and socially learned) that guide the appraisal of stimuli as "sexual stimuli."

The etiology of specific sexual interests may vary depending on the nature of the stimuli. For example, a shoe fetish or preference for sexual partners with a particular hair color are more determined by conditioning and learning, while sexual attraction to a specific gender (i.e., heterosexual vs. homosexual), especially in men, seems to be more biologically determined. A person's sexual interests determine what they find sexually attractive. Singer (1984) conceptualized three stages of sexual attraction: (1) increased visual attention to the stimulus, (2) movement toward the stimulus, and (3) resulting genital response.

Conceptually, PPG assesses the third of Singer's stages of attraction and is based on the assumption that sexual arousal, as measured by penile circumference or volume change, to a stimulus (e.g., image, film, or audiotaped scenario) is evidence of sexual attraction to the type of person or activity represented by the stimulus. In contrast, attentional measures of sexual interest are concerned with the first of Singer's three stages of attraction and are based on the assumption that the greater a person's attraction to a stimulus, the more attentional resources will be devoted to attending to that stimulus. Attentional measures of sexual interest can be divided into three categories: (1) direct measures of attending, for example, stimulus viewing time (Abel, Rouleau, Lawry, Barrett, & Camp, 1990; Abel, Lawry, Karlstrom, Osborn, & Gillespie, 1994; Abel, Huffman, Warberg, & Holland,

1998; Abel, Phipps, Hand, & Jordan, 1999; Quinsey, Ketsetzis, Earls, & Karamanoukian, 1996), (2) measures of stimulus interference (distraction) while performing another task, for example, choice reaction time (CRT; Wright & Adams, 1994, 1999), and (3) measures of preconscious processing of stimuli (rapid serial stimulus presentation and stimulus priming) (Kalmus, 2003; Spiering & Everaerd, 2007).

The measurement of stimulus viewing time, also called VRT, involves the respondent viewing images of different aged and gendered individuals presented via a slide projector or computer monitor. The images are advanced by the respondent via a laptop computer. Thus, respondents determine the length of time that each stimulus is presented (and presumably viewed) while the computer measures the amount of time that each stimulus is presented. Respondents are not informed about the measurement of VRT. It is assumed that the longer a person views an image, the greater his or her sexual interest in the type of individual represented in the image. In addition to viewing the images, respondents may be asked to rate their sexual attraction to each image for comparison with the VRT measure of sexual interest. On the Abel Assessment *for sexual interest*™ (AASI), after viewing a set of images once, respondents are asked to go through the set a second time to rate each image on a 7-point Likert scale (1 = very sexually disgusting to 7 = very sexually attractive). Acquiring the subjective ratings also helps to ensure that the respondent is processing the stimuli with a sexual mindset. Creating such a mindset through the instructional set before the VRT assessment and through the use of subjective ratings is particularly important when the stimuli include non-nude images of individuals.

Early Development and Validity of VRT

The AASI refers to a specific assessment instrument developed to evaluate sexual interest in children that utilizes information from both a detailed and standardized questionnaire and from a VRT measure. However, in the early stages of its development, the focus was on developing and validating a brief screen for sexual interest in children based on VRT. The ascent of the microcomputer, the availability of nude and non-nude slides from Farrell Instrument Company, an extensive pool of patients with paraphilias undergoing assessment or treatment, and staff privileges at a community hospital with an Institutional

Review Board, allowed us to investigate whether an individual's attention to visual stimuli depicting males and females of various ages suggested the individual's sexual interest. These initial studies did not stem from an extensive review of the scientific literature, but instead, from the researcher's simple observation that humans spend more time looking at individuals to whom they are more attracted. At first, this screening tool, named the Abel Screen, was developed using slides of nude individuals. However, as the political climate changed and Farrell Instruments ceased business, we explored the possibility of using non-nude stimuli. We developed our first set of non-nude stimuli depicting males and females from ages 8 to 10 and upwards, and depicting the major ethnicities in the United States (Caucasian and African-American), through a modeling agency.

An additional compound was that the cultural makeup of the United States was changing with an increasing number of Hispanic and Latino Americans, and we feared that the AASI may not be sensitive to this growing ethnic group. We, therefore, conducted a number of studies where new images of Latino adults and children were compared with the images of Caucasians already in use. To our surprise, Latino individuals were more responsive to images of Caucasians than they were to images of Latinos and we, therefore, did not alter our basic set of 160 images. By the mid 1990s, we were concerned that preschool-aged children were not depicted in our standard set of 160 images. Initially, we had included three categories of couples that could be used to determine adult sexual preference (two non-nude males hugging, two females hugging, a heterosexual couple hugging); all other slides depicted non-nude, single individual characters showing no sexual behavior). Believing that determining adult sexual preference in this manner, beyond an individual's awareness, was unethical, these three couple categories and a neutral category (depicting landscapes) were replaced by depictions of male and female children of preschool age, which completed our current set of stimuli.

The stimuli currently used in the VRT assessment of the AASI include 160 images, which depict a frontal view of the individual in a bathing suit without depictions of sexual activity or arousal. The images portray males and females of Caucasian and African-American ethnicity and include individuals who are preschool aged, grade school aged, adolescents, and adults. The stimulus set includes seven images of each category (e.g., seven images of Caucasian preschool girls, seven images of Caucasian grade school girls, etc.). In addition, the AASI includes images depicting six types of nonchild related paraphilic sexual behavior (exhibitionism, voyeurism, fetishism, frotteurism, sadomasochism targeting females, and sadomasochism targeting males).

On the basis of our work as well as others, there is ample evidence that VRT using images of non-nude individuals has construct validity, as well as discriminant validity for identifying individuals with a sexual interest in children. Early studies found that, as the erotic content of heterosexual images increases, so does VRT by both men and women (Brown, 1979; Brown, Amoroso, Ware, Pruesse, & Pilkey, 1973). Landolt et al. (1995) found viewing time to increase linearly with attractiveness ratings of images depicting only the head and shoulders of male and female adults. On the basis of samples of heterosexual men, VRT correlated significantly with ratings of image attractiveness, sexual arousal, and sexual stimulation (Lang, Searles, Lauerman, & Adesso, 1980; Quinsey, Rice, Harris, & Reid, 1993; Quinsey et al., 1996). On the basis of the results of four independent samples, Quinsey and colleagues (1996) also calculated the mean Pearson correlation (r) between image sexual attractiveness ratings and viewing time to be $r = 0.72$, range $= 0.54$ to 0.91. Additional support for the validity of VRT as a measure of sexual interest comes from convergent validity analyses between VRT and PPG assessments. On the basis of a sample of heterosexual, university-aged men ($N = 24$), the correlations between VRT and PPG ranged from $r = -0.05$ to $r = 0.84$, with a mean correlation of $r = 0.42 \pm 0.27$ (Quinsey et al., 1996).

The ability of VRT to discriminate between individuals with different sexual interest is of particular importance in regard to the practical application of VRT as a measure of sexual interest. Studies comparing individuals with opposite-sex and same-sex sexual orientation/preferences found that each group viewed stimuli depicting their preferred gender longer than stimuli depicting their nonpreferred gender (Abel et al., 1990; Wright & Adams, 1994, 1999). Using a CRT paradigm (another type of attentional assessment of sexual interest), Wright and Adams (1994) demonstrated that various groups (e.g., gay men, heterosexual men, lesbian women, and heterosexual women) had significantly longer reaction times to nude slides of their preferred gender. They

replicated these findings using slides of clothed individuals in addition to images of nudes (Wright & Adams, 1999). The pattern of results was the same for both images of nude and clothed individuals, but the effect was stronger for nude images. The CRT had an 87.5% accuracy in differentiating between individuals with same and opposite gender sexual orientation/preference using nude slides and a 75% accuracy using clothed slides.

Most importantly, VRT measures are sensitive to age preferences (Abel et al., 1990; Abel et al., 1998; Harris, Rice, Quinsey, & Chaplin, 1996; Quinsey et al., 1996). VRT has been shown to discriminate between male child sexual abusers and community men (Abel et al., 1994; Harris et al., 1996) and between male child sexual abusers and nonchild related sex offenders (Abel et al., 1998). Harris and colleagues (1996) examined VRT and PPG (penile circumference) discriminant validity between child sexual abusers and nonsexual abuser, community male adults. The sample included 26 child sexual abusers and 25 nonsexual abuser heterosexual men. The VRT stimuli included nude images of males and females, aged 5 to 8 years, pubescent aged (partial sexual development), and adult aged, with 10 slides in each category. The authors calculated a deviance index for VRT by subtracting the longest mean VRT for a child category from the longest mean VRT for an adult category. Child sexual abusers had a significantly smaller deviance index score ($M = 0.14 \pm 0.97$) than community volunteers ($M = 1.26 \pm 1.47$), indicating that relative to adult stimuli, child sexual abusers viewed child stimuli significantly longer, $p < .01$. The magnitude of this statistical difference (effect size) was large (Cohen's $d = 1.0$) and corresponded to 55.4% of the scores obtained by child sexual abusers and community volunteers not overlapping. Similarly, a deviance index was calculated for PPG by subtracting the greatest erectile response (in z-scores) to child stimuli from the greatest erectile response to adult stimuli (also in z-scores). Again, child sexual abusers ($M = -0.47 \pm 1.12$) differed significantly from the community volunteers ($M = 1.88 \pm 1.14$) on the PPG deviance index, $p < .001$. The effect size was also considered large (Cohen's $d = 2.1$) and corresponded to 81.1% of the scores for child sexual abusers not overlapping with those of community volunteers. It is unclear why the authors transformed penile tumescence into z-scores before calculating the deviance index, but used the raw mean visual reaction times for each category to calculate the VRT deviance index.

It is not only important to demonstrate significant differences in VRT to adult and child stimuli between child sexual abusers and nonchild sexual abusers, but of greater interest is the ability to correctly classify individuals with and without sexual interest in children based on VRT. Letourneau (2002) compared the ability to classify sex offenders on the basis of the VRT portion of the AASI and the results from PPG (penile circumference) assessments for 57 men incarcerated for sexual offenses in a maximum security military prison. The AASI was administered using the standardized procedures and stimuli. The AASI includes images of Caucasian and African-American males and females in preschool, grade school, adolescent, and adult age categories. Internal reliability (measured by Cronbach's alpha) is a measure of the degree of association of the images within a category. Typically, alphas above 0.80 are considered acceptable. The alphas for the VRT as assessed by the AASI were as follows: Caucasian preschool female α = 0.87, African-American preschool female α = 0.72, Caucasian grade school female α = 0.86, African-American grade school female α = 0.87, Caucasian adolescent female α = 0.85, African-American adolescent female α = 0.83, Caucasian adult female α = 0.80, African-American adult female α = 0.79, Caucasian preschool male α = 0.60, African-American preschool male α = 0.72, Caucasian grade school male α = 0.75, African-American grade school male α = 0.87, Caucasian adolescent male α = 0.90, African-American adolescent male α = 0.87, Caucasian adult male α = 0.90, African-American adult male α = 0.87.

The PPG assessments were conducted in accordance with the standards of The Association for the Treatment of Sexual Abusers (ATSA, 1997, pp. 44–52) and utilized commercially available ATSA audiotapes. The ATSA audiotapes consist of 16 three-minute vignettes that describe a male engaging in masturbation or sexual activity with another individual in four categories: (1) Adult female consenting, (2) adult male consenting, (3) minor female (compliant and coercive), and (4) minor male (compliant and coercive). The tapes do not explicitly mention the age of the target person, but instead the examiner instructs the respondent to think of a child "just the age he likes." The internal consistency of tumescence response (PPG) for each of the stimulus

categories for the ATSA tapes was as follows: Adult female consenting α = 0.85, adult male consenting α = 0.91, minor female α = 0.82, and minor male α = 0.91.

To assess the validity of the AASI and PPG, each participant was assigned to one of four classifications based on the characteristics of the person against whom they offended: abusers of girls (n = 34), abusers of boys (n = 10), abusers of adolescent females (n = 9), and abusers of adult females (n = 8). Three participants were included in more than one classification because two participants abused individuals in two different categories and one participant abused individuals in three categories. Letourneau (2002) calculated the correlations between PPG (penile tumescence change score from baseline) and the AASI (VRT raw scores, in milliseconds). The PPG change scores and AASI VRTs were significantly correlated for female child stimuli (r = 0.28, p < .05), male child stimuli (r = 0.61, p < .01), and the adult female rape stimuli (r = 0.38, p < .01), but not for the female adolescent stimuli (r = 0.18, p = ns). In addition, Letourneau (2002) compared the offender classification on the basis of victim characteristics with the predicted classification based on the results of the PPG assessment and the VRT portion of the AASI. *Kappa* is a measure of agreement that takes into account agreement due to chance. The *kappa* coefficients comparing classification based on victim and classification based on VRT were nonsignificant for abusers of girls (*kappa* = 0.19), abusers of adolescent females (*kappa* = 0.01), and abusers of adult females (*kappa* = −0.08). In contrast, there was a significant degree of agreement between the two means of classification for abusers of boys (*kappa* = 0.65, p < .001), indicating a degree of agreement above and beyond that expected by chance. Similarly, the coefficients of agreement between classification based on PPG and classification based on the victim's age and gender were significant for abusers of boys (*kappa* = 0.61, p < .001), but nonsignificant or in the wrong direction for abusers of girls (*kappa* = −0.37, p < .01), abusers of adolescent females (*kappa* = 0.19), and abusers of adult females (*kappa* = 0.21). The extremely low degree of agreement between classification based on VRT and based on choice of victim was due to the finding that, based on VRT, all but one of the participants were classified as having sexual interest in adolescent females. This is not altogether surprising since men without sexual interest in children (i.e., normative controls) tend to look at the adolescent images as long or longer than adult images (Feierman, 1990; Freund, McKnight, Langevin, & Cibiri, 1972). It is also interesting that the *kappa* coefficient for abusers of girls based on PPG compared to victim choice was significant, but in the opposite direction. One would have expected that PPG should be positively correlated with victim choice.

The methods and findings from this study raise some important and interesting issues regarding the two objective measures of sexual interest. Letourneau (2002) converted the raw tumescence data into change from baseline scores and considered a 10% or more mean increase above baseline for a stimulus category as evidence of sexual arousal to that category. Some PPG evaluation centers consider a response of less than 10% to all the stimulus categories as signifying nonresponders. How to operationally define sufficient erectile response is to some degree dependent on the type of stimuli used. Erotic films tend to elicit the greatest erectile response in studies of non-sex offender men, with images and audiotapes typically eliciting a weaker response. As a result, for stimuli predicted to elicit strong erectile responses, a change score of 10% or less might indicate a lack of arousal, and for stimuli predicted to elicit a weaker response, a change score of 10% or greater might be considered a substantial response. Harris and colleagues (1992) found that while nonchild sexual abusers evidenced their greatest erectile tumescence to appropriate adult stimuli, they obtained greater tumescence to the deviant stimuli than did the sex offenders, based on a comparison of raw penile circumference change scores (in millimeters). This is one of the reasons why the use of z-scores and deviation indexes, rather than responses to individual stimulus categories has been recommended for obtaining the maximum discriminant validity of PPG (Harris, Rice, Quinsey, Chaplin, & Earls, 1992).

To determine whether a respondent had sexual interest in a particular stimulus category on the basis of VRT, Letourneau (2002) employed the "method of thirds" (Abel, 1997), which involves the interpretation of z-score converted visual reaction times relative to the categories with the highest and lowest z-scores. The method of thirds states that any child stimulus z-score that exceeds one-third the difference between the highest adult/adolescent VRT z-score and the lowest VRT z-score among all categories is

indicative of possible sexual interest in that child category. This method has been criticized because it attempts to interpret ordinal scores (i.e., ranks, which should not be used to compare the magnitude of responses) as if they were scale scores (i.e., with an absolute zero point and defined distances between points) (Fischer & Smith, 1999, p. 196). The use of empirically derived logistic regression models that include the raw visual reaction times (in milliseconds) or ratios of the raw VRT, rather than z-scores, is one of the ways this criticism has been addressed by *Abel Screening, Inc.* (Abel, Jordan, Hand, Holland, & Phipps, 2001; Abel, Wiegel, & Jordan, 2004). These regression models also integrate the AASI questionnaire data with the VRT data to assess pedophilic sexual interests. Thus, the discriminant validity of the AASI as reported in Letourneau (2002) does not reflect the methods used by the AASI as it is currently marketed, but instead describes the convergent and discriminant validity of only VRT using the AASI images.

Abel and colleagues (1998) administered a measure of VRT to a sample of 157 admitted sexual abusers, 56.7% of whom had admitted to having sexual contact with children and/or adolescents. The slide categories included male and female grade school, adolescent, and adult individuals, with seven slides per category. All images were of individuals in bathing suits, standing in front of a blue background. The internal consistency for the stimulus categories ranged from $\alpha = 0.84$ for adolescent female stimuli to $\alpha = 0.90$ for child female stimuli ($\alpha > 0.80$ are considered acceptable). On the basis of regression analyses, the measure of VRT resulted in the highest overall percentage correctly categorized (child sexual abuser vs. nonchild sex offender) for child sexual abusers of male adolescents (91.2% correctly classified). The rate of true-positives (i.e., correctly categorized as child sexual abusers) was 60%, with 6.5% incorrectly classified as child sexual abusers. Similarly, the percentage of the sample correctly classified for child sexual abusers of boys was also high at 90.6%. However, the rate of true-positives (sensitivity) was only 38% for abusers of boys, but because the rate of false-positives was very low, with only 4.4% false-positives, the overall percentage correctly classified remained high. For child sexual abusers of female children and female adolescents, the percentages correctly classified were 65.6% and 76.7%, respectively. The rate of true-positives was adequate (female child 67.4% and female adolescent 60%); however, based on VRT, a fairly high percentage of non–child related sex offenders were incorrectly classified as child sexual abusers of girls (35.2%) and as child sexual abusers of female adolescents (20.8%). The higher rate of false-positives in the female adolescent category is not that surprising because nonsex offender, heterosexual men show sexual interest in and arousal to adolescent female stimuli (Feierman, 1990; Freund, McKnight, Langevin, & Cibiri, 1972). Of greater concern is the unacceptably high rate of classifying non–child related sex offenders as child sexual abusers of female children. Demonstrating a low rate of false-positives is critical for any measure used in the assessment of child sexual abusers because the consequences of being falsely categorized as a child sexual abuser are very serious. One of the limitations of this study and what may have contributed to the higher rates of false-positives was that the comparison group was composed of admitted sexual abusers who were accused of non–child related sexual offenses (e.g., exhibitionism, voyeurism, etc.) rather than nonsexual abusing men. Abel and colleagues (1998) also administered PPG assessments to 56 of the participants and found comparable results between VRT and PPG.

In contrast to Abel and colleagues (1998), who found good discriminant validity for the female child stimuli, Letourneau (2002) found poor agreement between the classification based on VRT and the criterion classification based on choice of victim. The difference in findings may be due to the different comparison groups used in the two studies. Letourneau (2002) used all sex offenders who were not in the category of interest as the comparison group. Therefore, her results are reflective of the ability of VRT to discriminate between child sexual abusers of female children and child sexual abusers of male children, female adolescents, and female adults. In contrast, Abel et al. (1998) used a sample of nonchild related sex offenders as the comparison group. Thus, the findings by Abel et al. (1998) are reflective of VRT's ability to discriminate between sex offenders against children and offenders against adults.

Johnson and Listiak (1999) conducted a further study comparing the AASI and PPG (penile circumference) procedures based on a sample of 24 incarcerated male sex offenders. They used similar procedures as Letourneau (2002), but evaluated two commercially available PPG stimulus sets that utilize videotaped images of non-nude models. Johnson and Listiak (1999), like Letourneau (2002), used the rule of thirds as the criteria for determining significant response based on the VRT portion of the AASI. Johnson and Listiak (1999) defined an erectile circumference change of 5 mm or greater as indicating a significant response on the PPG assessments. The authors reported that, based on the VRT portion of the AASI, 94% of the child molester category were correctly identified on the basis of the age and gender of the abuse victim for which they were convicted. The two sets of PPG stimuli each categorized 62% correctly in terms of age and gender of their victim. Caution in interpreting these results is warranted because of the small sample size, nonuse of z-scores or deviation indices for the PPG data, and the particular criteria used to determine significant response on the AASI and PPG assessments.

When taken together, the reviewed studies indicate that VRT shows acceptable levels of being able to discriminate between child sexual abusers and non–child related abusers. The accuracy of VRT alone is similar to that of PPG, but avoids problems of so called "flat-liners" (a failure to show erection responses to any category of stimulus) and is less intrusive.

FROM SCREEN TO ASSESSMENT INSTRUMENT: THE ADDITION OF QUESTIONNAIRES

In the early 1990s when we presented the initial "Abel Screen" at the annual conference of the ATSA, the largest organization of individuals working with sexual abusers, we were startled to find minimal interest in developing a screening methodology (Abel et al., 1990). This lack of interest probably emanated from ATSA members focusing predominantly on evaluating potential sexual abusers (including child sexual abusers), but within the clinical setting of evaluating and treating such individuals, not screening large numbers for potential risk in working with children. The Catholic Church scandal relating to child sexual abuse by Catholic priests had not broken to the media and most therapists working in the area focused on sexual abusers after they had committed sex crimes and were not focused on identifying predilections for sex with children among individuals who had not been accused of child molestation. A further problem was that funding for our initial research studies came from profits from private psychiatric care and, as the financial costs for our research mounted and the lack of interest in screening continued, we temporarily refocused our research efforts to adapting the Abel Screen so that it could be used by clinicians evaluating and working with alleged sexual abusers.

At the time, there were no commercially available systematic questionnaires that evaluated the broad range of paraphilias, the cognitive distortions held by sexual abusers (especially child sexual abusers), and those being examined were attempting to give "socially desirable" responses. On the basis of clinical experience since the late 1960s, a detailed questionnaire for adult males was added to the VRT assessment to create the Abel assessment for sexual interest (AASI). Including a standardized and detailed self-report questionnaire in any assessment of suspected sexual abusers is important because individuals may be more forthcoming on a questionnaire completed in private, as compared to a face-to-face clinical interview. In addition, such a questionnaire allows for the efficient assessment of a wide range of problematic sexual behaviors, which is important since many individuals engaging in one paraphilia tend to also be involved with other paraphilic behaviors (Abel, Becker, Cunningham-Rathner, Mittelman, & Rouleau, 1988).

The questionnaire is divided into four sections. Section I contains items that inquire about the respondent's demographics, social relationships as a teenager, past sexual abuse and sexual coercive behavior of the respondent, child sexual abuse related cognitive distortions, their sexual attraction, sexual fantasies, and masturbation activity. Section II contains five items that assess the respondent's subjective appraisal of his social skills and of the role of alcohol and pornography in his sexual behavior. Section III gathers information about the following 21 sexual behaviors: exhibitionism, public masturbation, fetishism, frotteurism, voyeurism, zoophilia, telephone scatologia (obscene phone calls and letters), necrophilia, sexual masochism, coprophilia, adult–child sexual contact (the respondent as the perpetrator), coercive sexual behavior (rape), sexual sadism, transvestic fetishism, professional sexual misconduct, sex with prostitutes, sexual affairs, sex with strangers, use of pornography, calling telephone sex lines, and gender identity dysphoria (transsexualism). Section IV includes items that ask respondents to rate each of the 21 sexual behaviors described in Section III regarding

how sexually arousing each is and amount of sexual fantasy to each type of behavior, as well as legal history (i.e., convictions, arrests, or accusations). Section IV also includes 20 items that assess social desirability, the individual's willingness to admit to minor violations of common social mores.

Including a questionnaire that assessed a variety of paraphilic and problematic sexual behaviors in a standard manner, including age of onset, number of times engaged in the behavior, number of victims, and the relationship between the respondent and the victim, has resulted in the systematic collection of data on a large sample of alleged sexual abusers presenting for evaluation. Analyses of this continually growing database resulted in the Abel and Harlow Stop Child Molestation Prevention Study (Abel & Harlow, 2001, 2002), which summarized the findings based on a sample of 3952 admitted male sexual abusers of children. Currently, the database contains information on almost 50,000 individuals evaluated throughout North America using the AASI who admitted to a variety of paraphilic and sexually problematic sexual behaviors (see Table 8.1). The results indicate that individuals seeking evaluation are more likely to have been involved in child sexual abuse relative to any other paraphilia.

In 1995, the research and development arm for VRT, called *Abel Screening, Inc.*, was established as a separate entity from the Behavioral Medicine Institute of Atlanta. After 8 years of preliminary research, the company sold its first product for objectively measuring a variety of sexual interests, using VRT and gathering information on a number of sexually problematic behaviors, cognitive distortions, and social desirability. Having a separate research company that operated as a free-standing company rather than as a research center in a clinical setting has resulted in two advantages. First, it allowed the availability of specific staff who were able to exclusively focus on providing technical assistance and customer service to clinicians who had purchased and were using the AASI in their practice. Second, it allowed for ongoing research regarding how to best improve the AASI, which was funded by the revenue generated through sales of the evaluation technology. Over the years, funneling all the profits back into research and development has led to a number of advances in using the AASI in the evaluation of potential sexual abusers. These include developing a standardized assessment system for adult women, as well as male

TABLE 8.1 Problematic Sexual Behaviors Assessed by the AASI and their Associated Prevalence in Sexual Abusers Presenting for Evaluation

Problematic Sexual Behavior	Males (N = 47,265)		Females (N = 1,684)	
	Count	Percent (%)	Count	Percent (%)
Exhibitionism	4762	10.1	105	6.2
Public masturbation	3904	8.3	44	2.6
Fetishism	4069	8.6	56	3.3
Frotteurism	2966	6.3	28	1.7
Voyeurism	6525	13.8	43	2.6
Sex with animals	2706	5.7	82	4.9
Obscene phone calls/letters	2670	5.6	88	5.2
Sex with dead bodies	92	0.2	1	0.1
Sexual masochism	815	1.7	63	3.7
Sex involving urine/excrement	649	1.4	17	1.0
Child sexual abuse	13901	29.4	268	15.9
Rape	1354	2.9	17	1.0
Sexual sadism	971	2.1	28	1.7
Transvestism	2036	4.3	17	1.0
Professional sexual misconduct	738	1.6	32	1.9
Use of prostitutes	12,285	26.0	45	2.7
Sexual affairs	17,038	36.0	496	29.5
Affairs with strangers	12,806	27.1	305	18.1
Phone sex	2,448	5.2	25	1.5
Use of pornography	12,519	26.5	166	9.9
Transsexualism	882	1.9	49	2.9

and female adolescents; the development of probability values for comparison of a client's pattern of responses to those of known child sexual abusers; and the development of an assessment system specifically designed for the evaluation of individuals with intellectual disabilities.

THE AASI AND THE COURTS

Since 1993, the *Daubert* standard (*Daubert vs. Merrell Dow Pharmaceuticals*) is used in many state and federal cases as the criteria for evaluating whether expert testimony is admissible in a particular court case. The *Daubert* standard is a two-pronged approach that states that the science on which the testimony is based must be reliable and valid, and that the testimony must be relevant to the issues of the case. Thus, expert testimony in a case can be excluded on the basis of lack of scientific merit or lack of relevance. The *Daubert*

standard establishes some guidelines in evaluating scientific merit. These include (1) whether the underlying theory or technique is empirically testable and has been tested, (2) whether the theory or technique has been subjected to peer review, (3) whether the theory or technique has a known or potential error rate and associated safeguards and standards controlling its operation, and (4) whether the theory or technique is generally accepted in the scientific community.

The results of *Daubert* motions for the AASI have been mixed. The AASI has passed the *Daubert* standard in some federal and state court cases, and has been excluded in others. In *U.S. versus Robinson*, 2000, the court decided that AASI met all four of the suggested guidelines to judge scientific merit and that the testimony and the AASI results were relevant to the case. However, in *U.S. versus White Horse*, 2001, and *U.S. versus Birdsbill*, 2003, the AASI was judged not to pass the *Daubert* standard. This was due in part to the lack of evidence that the AASI, and in particular VRT, were valid among Native American test-takers, since among some Native American cultures it is impolite to make prolonged eye contact, which could affect the validity of the VRT. The latter case, excluded expert testimony based on the AASI, both for lack of relevance and lack of scientific merit, citing the *Ready versus Commonwealth of Massachusetts* ruling. In *Ready versus Commonwealth of Massachusetts*, 2002, the AASI was found not to meet the *Daubert* standard for scientific validity because the original research study that developed the "rule of thirds" used to score the VRT, was never published. However, the "rule of thirds" was also used by Letourneau (2002), which was published in a peer review journal. In addition, the court found that because the defendant had abused boys aged 6 to 12, and that this age range is not represented in the AASI VRT images, that the test was neither valid nor relevant for this defendant. Furthermore, the court felt that the method used to remove outliers in the VRT data had not been adequately tested by researchers who were not connected with Dr. Abel. Lastly, the court found that the defendant's AASI results were not relevant to the issues of the case which pertained to sexually dangerous persons (SDP), future dangerousness, and risk to reoffend. Interestingly, in Ohio the AASI is a standard part of the state's sexual predator evaluation, and the results are routinely accepted as one aspect of the evidence used to judge as to whether a person qualifies as a sexual predator. Since *Ready versus Commonwealth of Massachusetts*, the AASI has been admitted as evidence in at least one Massachusetts case, *Commonwealth of Massachusetts versus Lyons aka Swimm*, 2002. In addition, testimony regarding the AASI results were admissible in several federal cases, for example, *U.S. versus Graves*, 2005 and *U.S. versus Stoterau*, 2008.

EVALUATING FEMALE SEXUAL ABUSERS

While the vast majority of sexual abusers appear to be males, there have been increasing reports by both male and female abuse survivors that their abuser was female, and more attention is being paid to the clinical assessment and treatment of female sexual abusers (Grayston & De Luca, 1999). Finkelhor and Russell (1984) reviewed 17 studies regarding the prevalence of women who sexually abuse children. After reviewing possible sources of bias, they concluded that, by best estimates, 14% to 27% of cases involving male survivors and 0% to 10% of cases involving female survivors could be attributed to female perpetrators. Laumann et al. (1994), in a nationally representative survey, found that 3% of the total sample had been sexually touched as a child by an adolescent female and 1% by an adult female. The survey also asked respondents whether they had ever forced someone to do something sexual that the other person did not want to do. Only 0.1% of the female respondents reported forcing sexual contact with a female and 1.5% reported having forced a male into sexual contact, as compared to 2.8% and 0.2% of male respondents, respectively.

In contrast to the clinical and empirical work done with male sexual abuses, sexual interest in or attraction to children is rarely examined and has not been well studied in female child sexual abusers. Even when sexual attraction to children by women is acknowledged, it is frequently discounted. For example, Mathews et al. (1989) reported that 11 of 16 women in their study acknowledged either arousal to or sexual fantasies about the children they sexually abused; however, according to the authors, the majority of these women reported that sexual arousal was not a main motivating factor. Similarly, based on interviews with 67 incarcerated female child sexual abusers, Davin (1999) concluded that, even though over 25% of the women who sexually abused children without a cooffender (*n* = 30) experienced orgasms while offending, sexual gratification was not a motivating factor in the offenses. While there are a number of social, cultural, and political factors that make it more difficult to acknowledge that women, and mothers in particular, are sexually attracted to children, another factor contributing to the dearth of empirical work focusing on sexual attraction and sexual interest in female child sexual abusers stems from the lack of empirically validated and reliable objective measures of female genital sexual arousal.

As mentioned, the PPG (circumferential or volumetric) is a common method of measuring genital sexual arousal in men. Vaginal photoplethysmography is the corresponding method of measuring female genital arousal (Janssen, 2002; Laan, Everaerd, & Evers, 1995; Sintchak & Geer, 1975). The vaginal pulse amplitude (VPA) signal is a measure of the moment-to-moment blood flow to the genitals (Janssen, 2002; Laan et al., 1995). Measures of genital sexual arousal are based on the assumption that sexual arousal in response to a specific stimulus is indicative of sexual interest in the type of person or activity depicted in the stimulus. This assumption is probably valid in men; that is, male sexual arousal is category specific. However, recent research findings suggest that genital sexual arousal in women may not be category specific. Chivers and colleagues (2004) measured genital sexual arousal in heterosexual and gay/lesbian men and women, as well as male-to-female transsexuals in response to male–male, female–female, and male–female sexual stimuli. The results indicated that heterosexual and gay men evidenced their greatest erectile tumescence to stimuli depicting their preferred gender. In contrast, VPA did not differ significantly between the three types of stimuli in heterosexual women. Additionally, heterosexual and lesbian women evidenced significantly lower correlations between self-reported sexual preference and genital arousal. To rule out that these findings were due to differences in the method of measuring genital sexual arousal (i.e., PPG vs. vaginal photoplethysmography), Chivers and colleagues (2004) included a group of male-to-female transsexuals, since these individuals were biologic males but with female genitalia and, thus, their genital arousal would be measured using photoplethysmography. The results indicated that male-to-female transsexuals showed a similar category specific pattern of arousal, as did the heterosexual and gay men. The authors concluded that women have a "nonspecific pattern of sexual arousal that is quite different from men's category specific pattern" (p. 741). On the basis of these findings, one would predict that using photoplethysmography to assess genital sexual arousal in adult female child sexual abusers would result in sexual arousal responses to most stimulus categories, and thus be insufficiently specific to discriminate a woman's sexual interest pattern.

To date, only one published study has utilized vaginal photoplethysmography in the assessment of a female sexual abuser. Cooper et al. (1990) presented a case report of a 20-year-old female pedophile with multiple comorbid paraphilias. The results of the physiologic assessment using VPA revealed high physiologic sexual arousal to all categories of stimuli presented (e.g., adults as well as children, and males as well as females). The authors concluded that the woman's responses indicated "polymorphous eroticism, with sadistic, masochistic, and pedophilic elements" (p. 336). Alternatively, the VPA data could be interpreted as supporting the findings by Chivers and colleagues (2004) that female vaginal response is not category specific.

The validity of using vaginal photoplethysmography for female sexual abuser evaluations is ultimately an empirical question that requires well controlled studies. However, if female genital arousal lacks category specificity as suggested by Chivers and colleagues (2004), then VPA would not be well suited for assessing female sexual interest patterns. A method of measuring sexual interest that is not dependent on vaginal sexual arousal, yet still not easily dissimulated or misrepresented, is needed for female sexual abuser evaluations. Attentional measures of sexual interest provide that alternative.

VRT measures of sexual interest have also been shown to have some validity in women. Brown (1979) showed slides of varying erotic content to male and female college students. The slides ranged from images of dressed couples to explicit images of group sex, and also included images of same sex sexual activity. The female participants viewed all but the male same sex images for less time than their male counterparts and evidenced greater variability in their VRT. However, there was an overall trend for VRT of the female participants to increase with increased erotic explicitness of the images. Quinsey and colleagues (1996) measured VRT and subjective ratings of attractiveness of images depicting nude adult, pubescent, and child males and females in a sample of heterosexual male and female college students. The results indicated that female participants evidenced their longest VRT to adult images of their preferred gender, with decreasing VRTs as age of the depicted male decreased, and they viewed nonpreferred gender images of all age groups for a similar amount of time. While male participants had longer VRTs than female participants for adult images of their preferred gender, this difference was not statistically significant. However, male participants viewed pubescent images of their preferred gender significantly longer than female participants. The average correlation between VRT and image attractiveness ratings was significantly higher among male participants (Pearson $r = 0.80$) than among female participants (Pearson $r = 0.60$).

The earlier studies are evidence that, in women, VRT is a valid measure of sexual interest when using images of nude individuals or images with sexual content. There is also some evidence for the validity of attentional measures of sexual interest when using non-nude images of individuals. Using images showing just the head and shoulders of individuals that had previously been rated as unattractive, moderately attractive, and attractive, female college students evidenced a linear relationship between z-transformed VRT and image attractiveness rating, with more attractive images viewed for longer time periods (Landolt et al., 1995). Additionally, Wright and Adams (1994) assessed a measure related to VRT, and found that CRT discriminated opposite sex from same-sex sexual orientation in both men and women. Attentional measures of sexual interest, including VRT, require further validation and study in samples of female sexual abusers, specifically female child sexual abusers.

Amassing an adequate sample of admitted adult female child sexual abusers to validate VRT takes a lot longer because of their lower prevalence. However, to date, we have collected a sample of 81 adult women who admit to having sexually abused at least one child, and the results look promising. On the basis of an overall sample of 411 women who were evaluated for problematic sexual behaviors, the internal reliability (Cronbach's alpha) of the visual reaction times for the different age and gender categories were all above $\alpha = 0.85$. The adolescent male category had the least internal reliability with an $\alpha = 0.85$, while the 14 images in the preschool boys category (seven Caucasian and seven African-American boys) had the greatest degree of internal reliability with an $\alpha = 0.93$, and the remaining categories having Cronbach's alphas around $\alpha = 0.90$ (see Table 8.2).

The sample of 411 adult female sexual abusers included 81 women who admitted to sexually abusing at least one child (younger than 14 years), 94 women who admitted to sexually abusing at least one adolescent (age 14 to 17), and 236 women who were evaluated for non–child related problematic sexual behaviors (e.g., exhibitionism, sadomasochism, multiple sexual affairs, etc.). These three groups of sexual abusers were compared on VRT to child and adult stimuli by using the natural log transformed VRT. When examining objective measures of sexual interest, whether PPG or VRT, it is clinically most useful to analyze the relative sexual interest in inappropriate stimuli to the sexual interest in appropriate sexual stimuli by either using a sexual deviance difference score (e.g., child minus adult) or a sexual deviance ratio (child divided by adult). As a result, the three

TABLE 8.2 Cronbach's Alphas for VRT Categories in Adult Female Sexual Abuser Sample (N = 411)

VRT Category	Cronbach's Alpha	No. of Images
Preschool males	0.925	14
Grade school males	0.914	14
Adolescent males	0.851	14
Adult males	0.902	14
Preschool females	0.896	14
Grade school females	0.908	14
Adolescent females	0.877	14
Adult females	0.913	14

groups were compared on the ratio of child VRT to adult VRT. A between-groups analysis of variance (ANOVA) indicated that the three groups significantly differed on the child/adult VRT ratio, $F(2,408) = 22.38, p > .001$. Bonferroni-adjusted follow-up tests revealed that the adult female sexual abusers of children evidenced significantly greater child/adult VRT ratios (i.e., greater relative sexual interest in children) than the nonchild related sexual abusers and the sexual abusers of adolescents. However, adult female child sexual abusers of adolescents did not differ significantly from either of the other two groups. To get a better understanding of these differences, the three groups were compared on their natural log transformed VRTs to adult males, adult females, child males, and child females. The between-groups ANOVA indicated significant differences on the VRT to adult females, $F(2,408) = 5.34, p > .01$, as well as, on the VRT to child females, $F(2,408) = 15.74, p > .001$, and child males, $F(2,408) = 19.16, p > .001$. Bonferroni-adjusted follow-up t-tests found that none of the groups differed on their natural log transformed VRT to adult males. However, adult female sexual abusers of children evidenced significantly longer VRTs to adult females, female children and male children. Again the group of admitted sexual abusers of adolescents evidenced VRTs in between those of the child sexual abusers and the nonchild related sexual abusers, which did not differ significantly from either of the other two groups.

These data, while preliminary, indicate two important findings. First, VRT seems to be a promising measure for evaluating the sexual interest of adult women who have sexually abused children (younger than 14 years) since these women had significantly higher child/adult VRT ratios from non–child related sexual abusers. Second, sexual interest in children by female child sexual abusers may play a more important role in the factors influencing sexually abusive behavior by adult women towards children than has previously been reported in the scientific literature. Certainly, further rigorous empirical studies of female sexual abusers are needed to confidently draw these conclusions.

THE ADDITION OF PROBABILITY VALUES

Our next scientific advancement occurred with the development of probability values. Probability values are calculated using logistic regression equations that are developed on the basis of samples of known groups of child sexual abusers and nonchild related sexual abusers or nonsexual abusers (i.e., community volunteers without a history of sexual behavior with minors). The logistic regression models include information from both VRT and the questionnaire. The integration of different types of information results in several advantages. First, it makes it more difficult to "fake good," since respondents would not only need to keep track of the relative VRTs to 160 images, but also would need to know how to specifically answer questionnaire items, many of which are not apparent as being related to sexual interest in children. Second, the use of more information results in a higher accuracy of classification. In one preliminary study, including questionnaire data in addition to VRT data in logistic regression modeling, on average, increased the area under the receiver operator characteristic (ROC) curve from 0.778 to 0.843 (Abel et al., 1999). ROC curves plot the true-positive rate (sensitivity) against the false-positive rate (one minus the specificity). The area under the ROC curve is a measure of the instrument's ability to differentiate between the two groups. Last, the integration of VRT and questionnaire data by the AASI allows for the construction of empirically derived regression equation models for different types of child sexual abusers and an associated probability value for each respondent. Thus, a probability value represents a method for integrating self-reported information with objective measures of sexual interest and using the resulting score to help answer the question, "What is the likelihood that this person has sexually touched a child in the past?"

The development of probability values began with a sample of admitted child sexual abusers and a comparison group of nonchild related sexual abusers (e.g., exhibitionists, voyeurs, etc.). These admitter probability values were of minimal clinical utility from an assessment standpoint, since they only substantiated the self-reported sexual behavior of the individual. However, developing the first probability values on the basis of a sample of admitted child sexual abusers allowed us to test the construct validity of the probability value. Much more clinically relevant is a probability value developed to discriminate between child sexual abusers who appear to have sexually abused a child but deny their alleged offenses and those who have not sexually touched a child. We empirically derived one regression model for differentiating between nonchild related sexual abusers and admitted child sexual abusers of girls, and a second model for differentiating between non–child related sexual abusers and admitted child sexual abusers of boys (Abel et al., 2001). On the basis of those two admitter logistic regression models, the first denier-dissimulator model was derived for differentiating between non–child related sexual abusers and suspected child sexual abusers who deny committing their offenses, but were thought to have sexually touched a child. Information was gathered from those individuals who had been accused of child sexual abuse and denied culpability, but whose interview or explanation of the allegations appeared preposterous, they had been found guilty of child sexual abuse, or at least two different families had accused them of child sexual abuse. These individuals were called *denier-dissimulators*, because their clinician, based upon the sum total of information, concluded that they had indeed committed child sexual abuse, but were attempting to deny the same. This group was different than individuals who denied culpability but no determination could be made regarding whether they had indeed been involved in child sexual abuse; these latter individuals were simply labeled as deniers, and excluded from the denier-dissimulator group.

The three logistic regression models were based on a sample of 747 men undergoing sex offender evaluation for a variety of offenses. Forty-one percent (n = 308) were being evaluated for nonchild related sexual offenses or problematic sexual behaviors (e.g., exhibitionism, voyeurism, or excessive affairs), 30.79% of the sample (n = 230) admitted to sexually abusing girls (below age 14), 6.16% of the sample

($n = 46$) admitted to sexually abusing boys (below age 14), 4.15% of the sample ($n = 31$) admitted to abusing both boys and girls, and 17.4% were denier-dissimulator child sexual abusers ($n = 130$). Incest child sexual abusers were excluded from the samples used to develop the models for admitted child sexual abusers of girls and admitted child sexual abusers of boys, thus none of the admitted child sexual abusers had offended exclusively against family members. However, genders, ages, or relationship type (incest or nonfamilial) of the children abused were not known for the denier-dissimulator child sexual abusers. Thus, individuals in the denier-dissimulator sample probably included both extrafamilial and incest child sexual abusers, as well as abusers of adolescents and/or children. Half the total sample was randomly assigned to a model building sample, while the other half was assigned to a holdout sample.

The first logistic regression equation was based on men who admitted sexually abusing girls below 14 years of age (Abel et al., 2001). The model included the following predictors: VRT for images depicting grade school girls (coefficient = 0.29), cognitive distortion score (coefficient = 1.34), self-reported attraction to grade school girls (coefficient = 0.31), self-reported attraction to adult males (coefficient = −0.20), number of times married (coefficient = 0.39), and the response to the item "I feel that I am someone children look up to" (coefficient = −0.68). The second logistic regression equation was developed using men who admitted sexually abusing boys under the age of 14 years (Abel et al., 2001). In this model, VRT of grade school boys (coefficient = 0.53), cognitive distortion score (coefficient = 1.30), being the survivor of child abuse (coefficient = 2.43), and a measure of hobbies and interests (coefficient = 0.31) were included as predictors for classifying sex offenders.

The last regression model was developed for the denier-dissimulator group (Abel et al., 2001). Predictors for this first denier-dissimulator model included a measure of hobbies and interests (coefficient = 0.27), the higher of the predicted values from the previous two models (coefficient = 3.97), a behavior denier scale score (coefficient = −0.14), and a variable representing the combination (interaction term) of the behavior denier scale and the higher of the predicted value from the previous two models (coefficient = −1.22).

The holdout sample was used to determine the specificity and sensitivity of each of the models. The use of higher or lower cut points with each logistic regression model results in different sensitivity and specificity values. A cut point for the logistic regression score of 0.48 applied to the child sexual abuser of girls model resulted in a sensitivity of 74% and a specificity of 73%. Using a higher cut point of 0.88 increased the specificity to 99%, indicating that 99% of nonchild sexual abusers were correctly classified as nonchild sexual abusers in the holdout sample. The higher specificity unfortunately comes at a cost of the sensitivity, which was reduced to 25%, on the basis of a cut point of 0.88. Similarly, for the child sexual abuser of boys model, a cut point of 0.21 had a sensitivity of 86% and specificity of 86%. Obtaining a specificity of 99% required a cut point of 0.83, which resulted in a sensitivity of 28%, indicating that only 28% of sexual abusers of boys would be correctly identified. A cut point of 0.32 with the denier-dissimulator model resulted in a sensitivity of 75% and a specificity of 76%, while a cut point of 0.83 resulted in a specificity of 99%, indicating that 99% of nonchild sexual abusers would correctly be classified as nonchild sexual abusers; however a cut point of 0.83 results in a sensitivity of 22%, meaning that only 22% of denier-dissimulators would be classified as such. The first two models, for child sexual abusers who admit sexually touching children, are important primarily as demonstrating criterion validity for the AASI, while the model for denier-dissimulator child sexual abusers has practical applications for identifying nonadmitting child sexual abusers.

The first set of three logistic regression models demonstrated that the AASI probability values could discriminate between child sexual abusers and sex offenders being evaluated for non–child related offenses; however, it was unclear how well the AASI discriminates between child sexual abusers and non-sex offender controls (community volunteers).

A further study was subsequently designed to develop a logistic regression equation based on a sample of 2356 men suspected of sexually abusing minors and 170 nonsex offender men recruited from the community (Abel et al., 2004). All of the suspected child sexual abusers denied having sexually abused minors or having sexual interests in children and they met the criteria for being denier-dissimulator child sexual abusers. This second denier-dissimulator model was developed in such a way that it would be free of race bias and respondent age bias. The resulting maximum likelihood logistic regression equation included nine predictor variables. The overall model likelihood ratio *chi-square* was significant, χ^2 (9, N = 2526) = 236.61, $p<$ .0001. The model was found to have an acceptable goodness of fit. The nine model predictor variables included the ratio of child stimuli VRT to frotteurism stimuli VRT (coefficient = 3.04); VRT for frotteurism (coefficient = 0.43); marital status (coefficient = 1.49); cognitive distortion score (coefficient = 0.86); hobbies and interest score (coefficient = 0.78); respondent having been sexually abused as a child (coefficient = 0.98); and the responses to the single items, "I talk to children on their level" (coefficient = 0.36), "I enjoy being around children" (coefficient = 0.23), and "I would rather spend my time with children" (coefficient = 0.23). The area under the ROC curve for this denier-dissimulator learning model was 0.83. Rather than using half of the sample as a holdout sample, a ten-fold cross-validation method was used to determine the sensitivity and specificity of the model. The mean area under the ROC curves based on the ten-fold cross-validation was 0.81, indicating good cross validation. Using a cut point of 0.3 for the model, the sensitivity was 87%, with a specificity of 45%. A predicted value cut point of 0.6 resulted in a sensitivity of 61% and specificity of 86%. Thus, on the basis of a child sexual abuser prevalence of 50% (i.e., 50% of the population of men referred for sex offender evaluation are child sexual abusers), a person whose model score was 0.3 would have a 22.4% probability of being a denier-dissimulator child sexual abuser, whereas an individual whose model score was 0.6 would have a 81.3% probability of being a denier-dissimulator child sexual abuser.

The use of a probability score dramatically increases the clinical applicability of the AASI results because it avoids having to choose one cut point and making an either/or determination. The newer AASI denier-dissimulator probability value can then be integrated into a client's overall assessment results, adding another tool to help clinicians discriminate those who have actually sexually touched a child in the past from those who have not (an important issue to the average evaluator). As described earlier, every test and measure has false-positives, and must be interpreted in the context of all of the information gathered during an assessment from a variety of sources. Unfortunately, some clinicians have taken the denier-dissimulator scores into the courtroom, where it was inappropriately being used to argue guilt or innocence of a charge of child sexual abuse. This of course, is not a valid use of the denier-dissimulator probability values, since they can only indicate the likelihood that a person has sexually touched a child in the past, but not whether the individual has sexually touched any one particular child. Guilt or innocence of an alleged child sexual abuser is always an issue for the judge or jury to determine, never by a clinician or a psychological test.

THOSE WITH A LEARNING DISABILITY AND THOSE WHO ARE ILLITERATE

Individuals with intellectual disabilities or who are illiterate represent a major challenge for testing and evaluation. These underserved populations are often prone to carry out inappropriate sexual behaviors, often because of a lack of understanding of cultural norms. In addition, only limited evaluative instruments have been available for them (Blasingame, 2005).

In collaboration with Gerry D. Blasingame, who is an expert in the field of assessing and treating individuals with intellectual disabilities, the Abel–Blasingame Assessment System *for individuals with intellectual disabilities*™ (ABID) was developed. Blasingame was especially experienced with the language and the common problems experienced by individuals with intellectual disabilities, as well as the unique challenges inherent in their evaluation. In developing an assessment system for this population, it was important that the assessment went beyond identifying the self-reported inappropriate sexual behaviors, and also assessed education and training, living arrangements, sexual education and experience, cognitive beliefs about sexual behavior, alcohol and substance abuse, and very importantly, the respondent's own history of being sexually abused. Additionally, the assessment system needed to be flexible enough to be comprehensible to individuals with a wide range of intellectual disabilities and functional levels, not only by using easy language but also by giving the evaluator the opportunity to get direct feedback about the client's understanding of the items and provide clarification when needed.

The ABID is intended to assist in the assessment of individuals with intellectual disabilities who are being evaluated for problematic sexual behaviors. The ABID represents a system of evaluation tools or components that include the following:

- Demographic information and presenting problem
- Psychosexual history (self-report)

- Assessment of the client's history of being sexually abused (self-report)
- Objective assessment of sexual interest (visual reaction time)
- Items inquiring in detail about 16 problematic sexual behaviors (self-report)
- Sexual fantasy ratings (self-report)
- Cognitive–Distortion Scale (related to sexually abusing children)
- Social Desirability Scale
- Substance use history (self-report)
- Assessment of the client's ability to distinguish between different ages and genders (using images)
- Assessment of conduct disorder/antisocial behaviors

The ABID is administered on a laptop computer and includes three parts: (1) an evaluator section, (2) a self-report questionnaire (which is read aloud to the client), and (3) an objective assessment of sexual interest that is measured beyond the client's awareness (VRT assessment).

The ABID's development took over 2 years and, based on the field testing, it seems to be an effective tool for evaluating individuals with individuals whose full scale IQ (FSIQ) is as low as 60. The ABID may also be appropriate for individuals with FSIQ lower than 60, but further research and clinical experience using this new assessment are needed. Since the evaluator reads the questions to the client, the client does not need to be able to read or write. The ABID can be used with both adults and adolescents. No lower age limit has been set because in individuals with intellectual disabilities, chronological age is not always a good indicator of functioning ability. For example, many adults with mild intellectual disabilities function cognitively at the developmental levels of early adolescence (Blasingame, 2005). The comprehension level for the ABID is measured at approximately the second or third grade reading level.

COMPLETING A SCREEN FOR THOSE WHO WOULD BE WORKING WITH CHILDREN

The recent scandal associated with the Catholic Church has continued to dominate the media for the past 5 years, emphasizing the importance of having a screening system for determining individuals who are at risk of sexually abusing children. Almost two decades after beginning to work on a brief screen for sexual interest in children, we have now come full circle and are proceeding with developing such a screen, called "The Diana Screen®." However, at this point we can build on our database of denier-dissimulator child sexual abusers and community volunteers (those not referred because of some type of sexual problem) as well as the benefit of years of experience researching and using VRT. The screening system was field tested for 3 years. The screen is based on the assumption that anyone attempting to gain access to children out of sexual interest in children or a desire to sexually touch children will be highly motivated to hide such sexual interest from potential employers, as well as conceal it during any sort of testing. As a result, The Diana Screen®, similar to the denier-dissimulator probability value on the AASI, uses logistic regression models to integrate information from approximately 100 specific self-report items and results from a VRT assessment. The screen itself takes only about 60 minutes to complete and is easy to administer.

Due to the complexity of and variability in employment laws across the United States, we decided to test the efficacy of The Diana Screen® exclusively in situations involving churches (where most aspects of employment law do not apply) and only in situations in which the individual has already been incorporated into the church system (postulates, permanent deaconates, and deacons). The successful outcome of this 3-year test indicates that the screen could expand into use by secular organizations. However, The Diana Screen® is not designed to function as a stand-alone assessment, but as a screen to determine which individuals may need further assessment before an organization makes any final decision regarding their hiring.

CONCLUSION

We have tried to accomplish two objectives in this chapter. First, we have outlined the development of these assessment systems within the climate of the scientific, political, legal, and cultural attitudinal environments at the time. We have tried to show how scientific developments, especially dealing with sex research, must adapt, modify, and change as a result of a multitude of factors, beyond pure science. As our culture adapts, these factors will change themselves further, requiring the developers of assessment systems to remain responsive. Second, we have shown the scientific support that now exists for the development of the various VRT-related instruments that currently assess not only adult males but also adult females, adolescent males and females; probability values that help the clinician predict the likelihood that a patient has actually molested a child; assessment of the intellectually disabled patient; and now, full circle, we are clarifying the development of a screening instrument to evaluate the risk that individuals might pose to children in their workplace. We have focused on the AASI since it is broadly used throughout the United States and we obviously have been intimately aware of the problems in developing such a system, given the current climate in the United States.

Given our own experience, it is almost impossible to predict what scientific advancements will occur in this area. We have already noticed presentations dealing with CRT (Wright & Adams, 1994, 1999) and rapid serial stimulus presentation and stimulus priming (Kalmus, 2003; Spiering & Everaerd, 2007). It is highly probable that scientific focus on all these areas will be productive in the assessment of paraphiliacs.

References

Abel, G. G. (1997). *Memorandum November 12, 1997*. Atlanta, GA: Abel Screening Inc.

Abel, G. G., Becker, J. V., Cunningham-Rathner, J., Mittelman, M. S., & Rouleau, J. L. (1988). Multiple paraphilic diagnoses among sex offenders. *Bulletin of the American Academy of Psychiatry and the Law*, 16(2), 153–168.

Abel, G. G., Rouleau, J., Lawry, S. S., Barrett, D. H., & Camp, N. L. (1990). *A non-invasive physiologic measure of adult sexual preference*. Paper presented at the Sixteenth Annual Meeting of the International Academy of Sex Research. Sigtuna, Sweden.

Abel, G. G., Lawry, S. S., Karlstrom, E. M., Osborn, C. A., & Gillespie, C. F. (1994). Screening tests for pedophilia. *Criminal Justice and Behavior*, 21(1), 115–131.

Abel, G. G., Huffman, J., Warberg, B., & Holland, C. L. (1998). Visual reaction time and plethysmography as measures of sexual interest in child molesters. *Sexual Abuse: A Journal of Research and Treatment*, 10(2), 81–94.

Abel, G. G., Phipps, A. M., Hand, C. G., & Jordan, A. D. (1999). *The reliability and validity of visual reaction time as a measure of sexual interest in children*. Paper presented at the 18th Annual Conference of the Association for the Treatment of Sexual Abusers. Lake Buena Vista, FL.

Abel, G. G., Jordan, A. D., Hand, C. G., Holland, L. A., & Phipps, A. (2001). Classification models of child molesters utilizing the Abel Assessment for Sexual Interest. *Child Abuse & Neglect*, 25, 703–718.

Abel, G. G. & Harlow, N. (2001). *The stop child molestation book*. Philadelphia, PA: Xlibris Corporation.

Abel, G. G. & Harlow, N. (2002). *The Abel and Harlow stop child molestation prevention study. Revised text edition*. Retrieved November 1, 2005, from the Child Molestation Research and Prevention Institute website: http://www.childmolestationprevention.org/pages/study.pdf

Abel, G. G., Wiegel, M., & Jordan, A. D. (2004). *Classification model of male denier-dissimulator child molesters utilizing the Abel assessment for sexual interest*. Unpublished manuscript, Atlanta, GA.

Association for the Treatment of Sexual Abusers. (1997). *Ethical standards and principles for the management of sexual abusers* (pp. 44–52). Beaverton, WA: ATSA.

Blasingame, G. (2005). *Developmentally disabled persons with sexual behavior problems, 2nd Edition*. Oklahoma City, OK USA: Wood & Barnes Publishing.

Brown, M. (1979). Viewing time of pornography. *The Journal of Psychology*, 102, 83–95.

Brown, M., Amoroso, D. M., Ware, E. E., Pruesse, M., & Pilkey, D. W. (1973). Factors affecting viewing time of pornography. *Journal of Social Psychology*, 90, 125–135.

Chivers, M. L., Rieger, G., Latty, E., & Bailey, J. M. (2004). A sex difference in the specificity of sexual arousal. *Psychological Science*, 15(11), 736–744.

Commonwealth of Massachusetts versus Aron Lyons aka Roy Swimm, Docket: PLCV2002–00396 (Super. MA June, 2002).

Cooper, A. J., Swaminath, S., Baxter, D., & Poulin, C. (1990). A female sex offender with multiple paraphilias: A psychologic, physiologic (laboratory sexual arousal) and endocrine study. *Canadian Journal of Psychiatry*, 35, 334–337.

Davin, P. A. (1999). Secrets revealed: A study of female sex offenders. In E. Bear (Ed.), *Female sexual abusers: Three views* (pp. 9–134.). Brandon, VT: Safer Society Press.

Everaerd, W. (1988). Commentary on sex research: Sex as an emotion. *Journal of Psychology and Human Sexuality*, 1, 3–15.

Everaerd, W., Laan, E. T. M., & Spiering, M. (2000). Male sexuality. In L. T. Szuchman & F. Muscarella (Eds.). *The Psychological Science of Human Sexuality* (pp. 60–100). New York: Wiley.

Feierman, J. R. (Ed.). (1990). *Pedophilia: biosocial dimensions*. New York: Springer-Verlag.

Finkelhor, D. & Russell, D. (1984). Women as perpetrators: Review of the evidence. In D. Finkelhor (Ed.). *Child sexual abuse: New theory and research* (pp. 171–187.). New York: Free Press.

Fischer, L. & Smith, G. (1999). Statistical adequacy of the Abel Assessment for Interest in Paraphilias. *Sexual Abuse: A Journal of Research and Treatment,* 11(3), 195–205.

Freund, K., McKnight, C. K., Langevin, R., & Cibiri, S. (1972). The female child as surrogate object. *Archives of Sexual Behavior,* 2, 119–133.

Grayston, A. D. & De Luca, R. V. (1999). Female perpetrators of child sexual abuse: A review of the clinical and emperical literature. *Aggression and Violent Behavior,* 4(1), 93–106.

Harris, G. T., Rice, M. E., Quinsey, V. L., Chaplin, T. C., & Earls, C. M. (1992). Maximizing the discriminant validity of phallometric assessment data. *Psychological Assessment,* 4(4), 502–511.

Harris, G. T., Rice, M. E., Quinsey, V. L., & Chaplin, T. C. (1996). Viewing time as a measure of sexual interest among child molesters and normal heterosexual men. *Behaviour Research and Therapy,* 34(4), 389–394.

Janssen, E. (2002). Psychophysiological measurement of sexual arousal. In M. W. Wiederman & B. E. Whitley Jr. (Eds.). *Handbook for conducting research on human sexuality* (pp. 139–171). Mahwah, NJ: Lawrence Erlbaum Associates.

Johnson, S. A. & Listiak, A. (1999). The measurement of sexual preference—A preliminary comparison of phallometry and the Abel Assessment. In B. K. Schwartz & H. R. Cellini (Eds.). *The sex offender* (Vol. 3, pp. 26.21–26.20). Kingston, NJ: Civic Research Institute.

Kalmus, E. (2003). *Developing a computer-based assessment using rapid serial visual presentation and attentional phenomena: a new means of measuring sexual interest?* Unpublished doctoral thesis, University of Birmingham, UK Birmingham, UK.

Laan, E., Everaerd, W., & Evers, A. (1995). Assessment of female sexual arousal: Response specificity and construct validity. *Psychophysiology,* 32, 476–485.

Landolt, M. A., Lalumiere, M. L., & Quinsey, V. L. (1995). Sex differences in intra-sex variations in human mating tactics: An evolutionary approach. *Ethology & Sociobiology,* 16(1), 3–23.

Lang, A. R., Searles, J., Lauerman, R., & Adesso, V. (1980). Expectancy, alcohol, and sex guilt as determinants of interest in and reaction to sexual stimuli. *Journal of Abnormal Psychology,* 89(5), 644–653.

Laumann, E. O., Gagnon, J. H., Michael, R. T., & Michaels, S. (1994). *The social organization of sexuality: sexual practices in the United States.* Chicago: The University of Chicago Press.

Letourneau, E. J. (2002). A comparison of objective measures of sexual arousal and interest: Visual reaction time and penile plethysmography. *Sexual Abuse: A Journal of Research and Treatment,* 14(3), 207–223.

Mathews, R., Matthews, J. K., & Speltz, K. (1989). *Female sexual offenders: An exploratory study.* Brandon, VT: Safer Society Press.

Quinsey, V. L., Rice, M. E., Harris, G. T., & Reid, K. T. (1993). The phylogenetic and ontogenetic development of sexual age preferences in males: Conceptual and measurement issues. In H. E. Barbaree, W. L. Marshall, & S. M. Hudson (Eds.). *The Juvenile Sex Offender* (pp. 143–163.). New York: Guilford Press.

Quinsey, V. L., Ketsetzis, M., Earls, C., & Karamanoukian, A. (1996). Viewing time as a measure of sexual interest. *Ethology & Sociobiology,* 17(5), 341–354.

Ready versus Commonwealth of Massachusetts, 2002 Mass. Super. LEXIS 557, May 17, 2002, Decided, Affirmed by Ready, 2005 Mass. App. LEXIS 261 (Mass. App. Ct., Mar. 24, 2005) (MA 2002).

Singer, B. (1984). Conceptualizing sexual arousal and attraction. *Journal of Sex Research,* 20, 230–240.

Singer, B. & Toates, F. M. (1987). Sexual Motivation. *Journal of Sex Research,* 23, 481–501.

Sintchak, G. & Geer, J. H. (1975). A vaginal plethysmograph system. *Psychophysiology,* 12, 113–115.

Spiering, M. & Everaerd, W. (2007). The sexual unconscious. In E. Janssen (Ed.), *The Psychophysiology of Sex* (pp. 166–184). Bloomington, IN Indiana University Press.

United States versus Jeremy Shane Birdsbill, 243 F. Supp. 2d 1128; 2003 U.S. Dist. LEXIS 12614 (D. MT 2003).

United States versus Anthony Graves, 2005 D.C. Super. LEXIS 14 (Super. D.C. 2005).

United States versus Lamont Robinson, 94 F. Supp. 2d 751; 2000 U.S. Dist. LEXIS 7923; 54 Fed. R. Evid. Serv. (Callaghan) 412 (W.D. LA 2000).

United States versus Joseph Stoterau, 524 F.3d 988; 2008 U.S. App. LEXIS 9247 (C. D. CA 2008).

United States versus Guy Randy White Horse, 2001 DSD 38; 177 F. Supp. 2d 973; 2001 U.S. Dist. LEXIS 19564 (W.D. SD 2001).

Wright, L. W. & Adams, H. E. (1994). Assessment of sexual preference using a choice reaction time task. *Journal of Psychopathology & Behavioral Assessment,* 16(3), 221–231.

Wright, L. W. & Adams, H. E. (1999). The effects of stimuli that vary in erotic content on cognitive processes. *Journal of Sex Research,* 36(2), 145–151.

Chapter 9

Mental Illness and Sex Offending

Fred S. Berlin, Fabian M. Saleh,
and H. Martin Malin

The terms "sex offending" and "mental illness" are sometimes inextricably linked, often in improper ways. For example, the legal term "Mentally Disordered Sex Offender," or some variant, known in the popular parlance as a "sexual predator," is now widely used to justify civil commitment for some sex offenders who have completed their sentences in penal institutions.

The basis for the civil commitment of sex offenders is that some offenders are deemed at high risk to reoffend if released into the community because many have not had adequate treatment while incarcerated. Some of these civilly committed offenders have identifiable paraphilic disorders or other Axis I diagnoses (such as impulse control disorders) that could predispose them to commit sex offenses.

Others do not carry Axis I diagnoses and are civilly committed because it is believed that their underlying personality structure (Axis II traits or disorders) places them at risk to offend again. Additionally, other sex offenders who have a variety of other diagnoses that are deemed dangerous to society are civilly committed.

The utility, as well as aspects of the legality, of civil commitment as a modality for managing sex offenders and reducing recidivism continues to be a topic of considerable debate. (For a general discussion of the civil commitment of sex offenders in see Falk, 1999; for a cross-cultural discussion comparing civil commitment practices in the United States and Rumania, see Loue, 2002).

Strictly speaking, personality disorders are considered to be mental disorders, coded on Axis II, (American Psychiatric Association, 2000). However, in practice many use the term "mental disorder" to refer only to Axis I conditions, as opposed to personality disorders or mental retardation. This chapter will largely focus on sex offending by patients with an Axis I diagnosis who do not have an Axis II personality disorder, but will also include some discussion of patients who engage in sex offending behaviors related to an Axis III medical condition.

There is general agreement among treatment professionals that sex offense recidivism can be reduced with appropriate psychological and psychopharmacological treatments, at least for some kinds of offenders. Although it is not always possible to accurately predict in advance the precise recidivism risk for any specific individual it is often possible to reduce whatever risk may have been present by means of proper treatment, monitoring and supervision (Berlin, Galbreath, Geary, & McGlone, 2003).

SEX OFFENSES IN THE CONTEXT OF MAJOR MENTAL ILLNESS

It is sometimes overlooked that some sex offenders commit their acts in the context of an Axis I major mental illness, rather than in the context of an Axis I paraphilic disorder or an Axis II personality disorder (which can sometimes be more refractory to treatment). That is not necessarily to say that the major mental illness itself directly "causes" the sex offense, but just as postpartum depression can sometimes predispose to irrational and even illegal acts, major mental illness can sometimes also predispose to sexual misconduct. Treatments and social interventions over time have sometimes been organized on the assumption that the targeted class of individuals are "socially-sick" (Sutherland, 1950).

The flip side of the coin is that sex offenders come in many varieties. Many sex offenders have co-occurring conditions, whether or not directly related to their instant sexual offenses. There is the risk that these disorders could go untreated in conventional cognitive-behavioral, or relapse prevention sex offender treatment programs which are designed specifically to identify cyclical patterns of behavior resulting in reoffense. Co-occurring conditions (e.g., depression or alcoholism) left untreated may increase the chances of sex offense recidivism. We will discuss this aspect of mental illness in sex offenders later in this chapter.

Among the commonly seen Axis I major mental disorders are those which significantly disrupt cognitive processes such as schizophrenia (Glaser, 1985; Henderson & Kalichman, 1990) or bipolar disorder, and other conditions such as traumatic brain injury (DelBello et al., 1999). Such cognitive disruptions can be of significant importance in the commission of sex offenses and ex offenses committed in the context of a major mental illness have been well documented. Less common Axis I diagnoses, some still a source of controversy, may also contribute to sex offending. One example includes sex offenses committed by individuals while sleeping ("sexsomnias") a phenomenon that has been reported in the literature on parasomnias (Ebrahim, 2006; Fenwick, 1996; Rosenfeld & Elhajjar, 1998; Schenck & Mahowald, 1992).

Berlin (1986) has documented the case of one bipolar rapist whose delusional system and command hallucinations while in a manic phase had resulted in a series of rapes. That case can serve as an instructive example of patients who commit sex offenses as the result of nonparaphilic major mental illnesses.

The patient, who had no prior history of any criminal activity, began to experience altered states of consciousness as a young man during what he had termed a "nervous breakdown." In between episodes of increasingly severe mania, he led a normal, if sometimes confused life. He considered himself to be a moral person who participated actively in his church, and had committed no prior crimes.

In the grips of his illness, however, he had delusions of being "special," and he had come to believe that he was a "biblical hero," a role he believed other people intuitively understood even if they did not react to him differently. He had spent time under the night sky convinced that he had had special God-given powers and that he could move meteorites via his mental abilities.

As his illness had progressed, he began to hear clear voices of a darker sort telling him that he was somebody else. The voices, which by now he had believed were perhaps Satanic, told him to shave off his moustache and beard, which he did. The voices insisted that he become "the other me." He described racing thoughts, increasing in intensity, "like sirens going off in your head." The voices insisted that he was their agent and told him "you're going to do this for me." He struggled to make sense out of the voices, at one time concluding that he was part of a struggle between the forces of God and Satan, and at other times believing that he was being controlled by the Russians.

During a 4-week period in which he raped several women, he had come to believe that the women were actually seeking him out, or for some reason were being sent to him. He believed that he had to find victims. He reported "It was like I was in a picture show, and I was going through the movements but it wasn't me. There was something telling me what to do and doing it in me."

He described himself as a "lion" and his victims as "lambs." He said "When I was a lion I was being a part of the lamb. I could smell the lamb's flesh and want it's blood…like a ritual…the sexual contact was part of the battle or the conquest," between the forces of good and evil. During a prior manic episode, while in the military in Turkey, he had been seen running about the canteen totally naked.

Treatment Considerations

Clearly, conventional sex offender treatment regimens will not be much help with patients who offend in the context of a nonparaphilic Axis I major mental illness. In such cases, directly addressing the Axis I disorder is the treatment of choice. Subsequent counseling, however, either individually or in groups can also be helpful.

Sex offenses in the context of Axis I disorders appear to occur most frequently in those cases in which there is an altered state of mind with respect to the perception of reality. Sex offenses have been reported in the context of substance abuse, mania, depression, delusional states, hallucinations, obsessions, and compulsions.

Treatment depends on the primary diagnosis. For mood disorders, antidepressants and mood stabilizers are the pharmacotherapy of choice. Most individuals with mood disorders will also benefit from psychotherapy.

For psychotic disorders such as schizophrenia or drug-induced psychoses, antipsychotics can be the cornerstone of initial treatment. Many individuals with psychotic disorders will benefit from psychotherapy once their hallucinations or delusions have been medically controlled. Patients with substance-induced psychoses will also need substance abuse treatment, and possibly, management during drug withdrawal.

A good social support system can also be useful in the treatment of individuals with these Axis I disorders. Individual and group psychotherapy, designed to break through patients' denial about suffering from a significantly impairing major mental illness, while emphasizing the importance of continuing to take medications even if they do not feel that they need them at the moment, can also be important. Helping

them build close family, community, and peer-support systems, and working through the emotional trauma of realizing that they are not "OK," not "normal," and not like "other people" can be crucial as well.

When such patients can be taught how to treat their illnesses by means of both psychotherapy and medication, they, or their families, may then be able to recognize the signs of impending abnormal psychotic episodes. That can enable them to seek out additional treatment, perhaps even brief hospitalizations, should they be slipping toward a period in which they could become a danger to themselves or others.

SEX OFFENSES IN THE CONTEXT OF A PARAPHILIC MENTAL DISORDER

Paraphilias are Axis I mental disorders that are qualitatively quite different from the other Axis I mental illnesses that we have discussed earlier. The major difference is that sex offenses arising from the paraphilias are motivated behaviors linked to sex hormones. In that sense, to some extent, they may be conceptualized as disorders of appetite.

Paraphilias are sexual disorders characterized by uncommon or unusual erotic appetites involving a wide range of behaviors with animate or inanimate "partners." Approximately 50 paraphilias have been described in the literature.

The term, "paraphilia," (from the Greek *para* [beside] *philos* [love]) is an English translation of a word first used by the physician Wilhelm Stekel around 1925 to describe what he saw as "sexual aberrations." Stekel had not wanted to resort to the already pejorative term "perversion" that had been in use among the Freudians of his day—terminology that nevertheless continued to be used in psychiatric circles until the 1950s.

The fourth revision of the *Diagnostic and Statistical Manual of Mental Disorders* (DSM-IV-TR) specifies that a paraphilia must include "recurrent, intense sexual urges, fantasies or behaviors that involve unusual objects, activities or situations." Paraphilias can also cause "clinically significant distress or impairment in social, occupational or other important areas of functioning (Association, 2000)." Thus, paraphilic behavior may be the manifestation of a mental disorder both because (1) cravings for the preferred "partner" are highly unusual (e.g., corpses or shoes) and because (2) the presence of those cravings can lead to impaired sexual functioning with a socially defined suitable partner. Paraphilias are often associated with volitional impairment (e.g., in exhibitionism, impairment of the ability to consistenly resist cravings to expose). They can also be associated with cognitive impairment (e.g., in pedophilia, impairment in the ability to objectively appreciate the immature developmental level of a young child). Although there are exceptions, paraphilias primarily afflict men (Berlin & Malin, 1991).

The intrusive thoughts, fantasies, and behaviors that are so often sexually exciting to a person with a paraphilia may either be not sexually arousing at all or be repugnant to most individuals. Although the "average individual" might be capable of exposing publicly, he is not driven by recurrent, intense sexual urges to do so. Similarly, while most people would find just the idea of having sex with a corpse repugnant, the paraphilic necrophile experiences recurrent cravings to do just that (Rosman & Resnick, 1989).

Like the term "perversion" before it, the term "paraphilia" is becoming increasingly more pejorative. While pedophilia has a precise psychiatric definition, even mental health professionals can confuse the terms "paraphile" or "paraphiliac" with the term "pedophile." It is not uncommon for mental health professionals, as well as the lay public and others, such as lawyers and journalists, to conflate the terms "pedophile," "child molester," "paraphiliac," "sex offender," and "sexual predator."

The phenomenology of paraphilic arousal dictates that a satisfactory sexual response cycle, ending in orgasm, may either invariably, or at least sometimes, be dependent upon fantasizing about, or acting on, paraphilic imagery. Borrowing from legal vocabulary, paraphilic imagery in masturbatory fantasies is more or less a "condition precedent" to making a diagnosis of a paraphilia.

Failure to appreciate this phenomenological (mental state) aspect of paraphilias can lead to significant diagnostic errors. It can also lead to treatment errors as well (Saleh, Malin, Berlin, & Thomas, 2007).

Much of the misunderstanding stems from a lack of appreciation that phenomenology is paramount in the diagnosis of the paraphilias. While behaviors emphasized by DSM-IV-TR are the "symptoms" of the psychiatric affliction that will typically bring a person with a paraphilia to the attention of clinicians or civil authorities, the internal phenomenological experience is the defining factor of a paraphilic

disorder. Paraphilic behavior has traditionally been considered by the criminal justice system to be entirely volitional, and will usually elicit little sympathy during a judicial sentencing proceeding. That is the case even though, paradoxically, the justification for civilly committing some persons with paraphilias for treatment at the conclusion of a prison term has been based, in no small part, upon the concept of volitional impairment.

It is certainly possible to describe a behavior—for example, genital exposure—and to prescribe social consequences for it, without resorting to phenomenology. But to qualify as a paraphilia, the phenomenology underlying the behavior must have some erotosexual valence for the individual experiencing it (Saleh, Malin, Berlin, & Thomas, 2007).

For example, there are many instances in which a person could choose to expose his genitals—some as commonplace as a physical examination. Others, like "mooning," are not strictly legal but are socially tolerated to some degree. Yet others, such as masturbating in public, are considered to be sexually offensive and are illegal.

Civil authorities will generally deal differently with different manifestations of genital exposure. However, they may not appreciate the phenomenological difference between paraphilic and nonparaphilic exposing. Unfortunately, when a clinician fails to make such a distinction, treatment errors can occur.

If the paraphilic behavior is not illegal, such as enacting a shoe fetish, it is often viewed as nuisance behavior. Nevertheless, the individual in question may face significant social ostracism, including dissolution of a marriage, loss of employment, and loss of other community support, should his condition come to light. In addition, many members of the general public, as well as some professionals, may unjustifiably fear an inevitable escalation of relatively harmless paraphilic behaviors to more serious ones.

If the behavior is illegal, a person with a paraphilia can often expect to experience the full weight of the criminal justice system (Berlin, 1994). On the other hand, depending upon the severity of the illegal behaviors, some patients may be ordered into treatment by the Court with criminal justice oversight. Sometimes even the nature of the treatment itself is not so subtly influenced by civil authorities. Paraphilic patients who commit more serious offenses can expect to be incarcerated, often without the benefit of treatment, or in some cases executed.

Treatment Considerations

Conventionally the treatment of paraphilic patients includes some form of behaviorally based group treatment (e.g., cognitive behavioral therapy or relapse prevention therapy), sometimes combined with medication intended to suppress sexual appetite. Some treatment models do not make use of testosterone-lowering medications, but instead rely entirely on behavior-based interventions. However, failure to provide informed consent to a patient about the possible benefits of sex drive–lowering medications should not be considered a form of "best practice." No current treatment models rely solely upon pharmacological interventions. Treatment methods intended to "recondition" erotic arousal patterns, though previously in wide use, have not proved themselves to be generally effective.

The treatment of sexually disordered (paraphilic) sexual offenders can be a challenging task. The main consideration should be community safety. The goal is to reduce sexual recidivism by increasing the person's ability to exert better behavioral control.

Most psychologically based therapies are designed both to support patients who are typically undergoing significant emotional distress and to confront patterns of denial that may impede the patient's ability to adopt more appropriate behavioral patterns. Therapies designed to challenge and change patients' distorted thoughts, belief patterns, and behaviors fall into several broad categories. These include cognitive behavioral therapy (to confront "thinking errors" that can lead to abusive behaviors), relapse prevention (to identify triggers and to intervene early in the cycle that can lead to abusive behaviors), and behavioral therapy (to condition or decondition fantasies, urges, and behaviors).

Psychodynamic and psychoanalytic treatment modalities have produced disappointing results with paraphilic patients. Therefore, they have largely been abandoned in favor of therapies that have been able to demonstrate concrete, prosocial behavioral change.

Behavioral therapy, an outgrowth of social learning theory, primarily concerns itself with "deviant" acts without respect to what the underlying cause of that behavior might be. With dangerous paraphilic patients the rationale for behavioral therapy is that, although a patient might thoroughly understand the antecedents of his behavior, such understanding by itself will not necessarily facilitate change.

Among the techniques of behavioral therapy are desensitization, aversion therapy, biofeedback, masturbatory satiation, and covert sensitization. Each involves a somewhat different method.

Covert sensitization, for example, pairs paraphilic sexual fantasies with mental images of their potential negative consequences (e.g., jail, social ostracism). The hope is that this will give the patient sufficient incentive to use other techniques (e.g., "thought blocking") to block the paraphilic fantasy, and to not permit himself/herself to be aroused by it. Covert sensitization is a form of aversion therapy in which imagining what will happen if the paraphilia comes to light is aversive, in and of, itself. Other tools, such as olfactory conditioning, might be used adjunctively to help make it easier to "give up" the paraphilic fantasy.

Masturbatory satiation is a two-part process that begins with instructing a patient to masturbate to orgasm (if possible) only in response to appropriate sexual fantasies. Following orgasm, the patient is instructed to continue masturbating, switching to his paraphilic fantasy.

Since the patient is typically in the refractory phase of his sexual cycle following orgasm, reaching orgasm again will likely be difficult, if not impossible. Masturbation during the refractory period is usually not pleasant and may even be painful. Orgasm is assumed to be a powerful reinforcer of fantasies (possibly a false assumption) so that the expectation is that the nonparaphilic fantasies will be enhanced, whereas the paraphilic fantasies will be extinguished. However, is it really the case that sexual interest is only present because of the reinforcing aspects of arousal and orgasm? When a heterosexual man masturbates while looking at a centerfold picture of a woman, does his doing so reinforce his interest in women, or is that simply indicative of the fact that he has had such an interest in the first place? Certainly, he would not be expected to lose that interest, were he to simply refrain from masturbating.

Virtually all of the methods that have been used to try to "recondition" a person's erotic make-up have been based on Pavlov's model of classical conditioning. Indeed, Pavlov did demonstrate that certain conditioned physiological responses (e.g., salivation to the sound of a bell) could be "deconditioned." However, some physiological responses are, in effect, "stamped in," via a "learning" process known as imprinting. Such physiological responses, even if learned, cannot ordinarily be unlearned. That may be true as well with respect to one's sexual make-up. How many heterosexual men could be successfully "deconditioned" so as to lose their interest in women (assuming that such an interest was even learned in the first place)?

In the past, efforts to "recondition" homosexuality were a clear failure. The same would appear to be true of methods intended to "recondition" paraphilic conditions such as pedophilia. Instead, other methods may often be more helpful.

Cognitive Behavior Therapy and Relapse Prevention

Cognitive therapy posits that distorted cognitions help to maintain paraphilic behaviors. Cognitive therapy attempts to change thinking errors and beliefs, and to disrupt unacceptable thought processes, through techniques such as cognitive restructuring and thought stopping. Thought stopping is a technique intended to interrupt paraphilic thoughts and to encourage their replacement with appropriate thoughts.

Relapse prevention is premised on the assumption that without treatment, paraphilic sex offending behaviors will almost certainly recur after a period of absence, much like "falling off the wagon" for an alcoholic who was previously able to stop drinking. According to that theoretical model, relapses will likely occur unless they are actively prevented from doing so. That can be accomplished by teaching a patient about the cyclical nature of relapses, and the antecedents to them. The goal of relapse prevention is to make the patient aware of this cycle and to provide tools for containing paraphilic thoughts and behaviors early in the cycle at a time during which they are presumably easier to control.

In addition to the therapies mentioned earlier, victim empathy, assertiveness training, and social skills training are often integrated into treatment programs for paraphilic patients. However, not all patients with a paraphilic disorder lack either victim empathy or social skills. Beyond that, teaching either assertiveness or better social skills to a patient with pedophilia could backfire, should that enable him to more assertively approach a child in a skillful fashion. All of the psychological therapies can be provided in either an individual or a group setting, although group treatment is generally preferred because it provides an environment in which patients can be both supported in their struggles as well as challenged by their peers. It is believed that peer confrontation and support, with adjunctive professional guidance from trained therapists, carry additional weight and may not be so actively opposed by some, since the "authority figure" is not the therapist but a peer group member.

BIOLOGICAL TREATMENTS

Biologically based sex drive–lowering treatments are a powerful intervention many paraphilic patients. They should be offered to those patients whose cravings are so strong that they experience difficulties in successfully resisting them. They should also be offered to persons who have no acceptable form of sexual release (e.g., those whose erotic attractions are directed exclusively toward children, especially in cases in which masturbation serves only to whet sexual appetite). Many patients will need to be maintained on "sexual appetite suppressants" indefinitely, while in other instances, especially as the individual grows older, it may be appropriate to consider whether the patient can be safely weaned off.

In the past, the only effective biological treatment methods available to physicians had been orchiectomy (surgical castration, which is removal of the testes), and in rare instances, stereotaxic hypothalamotomy (brain surgery). It is clear, from past studies, that orchiectomy can dramatically decrease sex offender recidivism. Orchiectomy has become somewhat more widespread in recent years as offenders have sometimes requested it, possibly in some cases at least, hoping that a judge may lessen a sentence.

However, the use of orchiectomy alone, particularly in nonparaphilic patients, may not ensure that an individual will not recidivate sexually. Surreptitious testosterone replacement in orchiectomized patients is often a simple matter of ordering it over the Internet, from a country where supplies of exogenous testosterone may be obtained without a prescription. Testosterone replacement therapy may even be obtained legally in this country from physicians who may be misled concerning all of the facts involved with an orchiectomized patient. Although some testosterone is normally manufactured in the adrenal glands, that amount is ordinarily insufficient to support much intensity of sexual drive.

Finally, it should be pointed out that on rare occasions it has been possible for an orchiectomized patient with no detectable free testosterone in his blood to commit a sexual offense. While studies have shown that orchiectomy substantially decreases a sex offender's risk for sexual recidivism, with rates ranging between 50% to 60% for nonorchiectomized and 1% to 3% for orchiectomized sex offenders, the recidivism rate is still not zero.

Orchiectomy is not the only intervention for reducing testosterone. Equally efficacious results can be obtained using testosterone-lowering medications including progesterone derivatives, such as Depo-Provera, and gonadotropin releasing hormone analogues, such as leuprolide (Depo-Lupron). Depo-Lupron would appear to be a more powerful agent with fewer side effects. Some clinicians have suggested that serotonergic agents, many of which have the side effects of both lowering libido and of being anti-obsessional, may also be helpful in treating paraphilias. However, evidence about the efficacy of testosterone-lowering medications as a means of suppressing sexual drive is far more compelling.

Serotonergic agents may play a role in managing some patients, however, including those who may be suffering from depression or other conditions co-occuring with their paraphilia. Furthermore, it is important to keep in mind that the obsessional ruminations that are so often part of a paraphilic disorder are eroticized obsessions and as such may be responsive to treatment with serotonergic agents.

LIAISONING WITH THE CRIMINAL JUSTICE SYSTEM

Many treatment models also include a variety of monitoring strategies by law enforcement, particularly parole and probation officials. These may include random drug-screening when appropriate, electronic surveillance, polygraphs, and periodic unannounced searches of premises and equipment, such as computers for contraband, including pornography or evidence of inappropriate "chat room" participation. From a psychological perspective, however, it is undemonstrated that limiting exposure to, or possession of, adult pornography, is, in itself, a therapeutically useful intervention (Linz, Malamuth, & Beckett 2002).

In some instances, it has become increasingly more difficult to define boundaries between legal interventions as an aid to therapy, as opposed to mandated therapy as a component of legal proscription.

Nowhere, perhaps, have the boundaries between traditional values of psychiatric intervention, as opposed to community-driven social control strategies, become more blurred than in the treatment of certain paraphilic sexual offenders. For example, in those states that civilly commit individuals for treatment rather than releasing them to the community at the conclusion of their criminal sentences, is the desire to treat or to further confine? If the intent is to treat, then why have so many incarcerated offenders not been offered treatment while still serving their sentences?

For these reasons, the concept of stand-alone "treatment" as applied to paraphilic sex offenders seems to be declining, even among individuals trained as psychiatric professionals, in favor of the more inclusive sociological term "offender management." Individuals, who were traditionally considered to be "patients," are now more likely to be labeled "clients," or "perpetrators," even by mental health professionals. (For a general discussion of the ramification of some of these linguistic changes, see Slavney & McHugh, 1987.) In our judgment, conditions such as pedophilia are legitimate psychiatric disorders, and afflicted patients in treatment are deserving of the status of "patient." In general, we do not believe that treatment that supports a "we versus they" attitude has been shown to be helpful. For those patients who are on either parole or probation, however, we do support a close working relationship between therapists and parole/probation agents.

COMORBID PSYCHIATRIC ILLNESS AMONG NONPARAPHILIC AND PARAPHILIC SEX OFFENDERS

Comorbid psychiatric illness is prevalent among sex offenders in psychiatric treatment, including among those who do not have a paraphilia. Such comorbidity, if untreated, might reasonably be expected to negatively impact subsequent treatment success, and to increase recidivism rates. However, there has been little research to date concerning this aspect of sex offender treatment.

The available research focuses largely upon discerning the prevalence of specific comorbid psychiatric conditions such as depression or alcoholism in sex offenders, particularly in prison settings. In many instances, treating these comorbid conditions has not, as yet, been integrated into mainstream models of sex offender treatment. To the contrary, practitioners sometimes "select out" seriously psychotic patients or provide adjunctive treatment for severely depressed patients. The literature concerning these patients is sometimes difficult to interpret, for a variety of reasons.

Research into the area of psychiatric comorbidity has been limited, and methodological problems, such as small size and sample heterogeneity, have confounded studies. One problem in research designed to assess for comorbidity is that much of it has been carried out with large heterogeneous populations of "sex offenders," "child molesters," or "sexual predators," without providing any sort of diagnostic clarity. To date, there have been no large-scale studies on the Axis I and Axis II base rates within clinically relevant subgroups of nonparaphilic sexual offenders.

McElroy and his colleagues (1999) looked for comorbidity in a small heterogeneous group (n = 36) of convicted sex offenders in a residential treatment center. Of the sample, 97% met criteria for a nonparaphilic Axis I diagnosis, and 94% qualified for an Axis II diagnosis. In a smaller subset of paraphilic sex offenders (n = 21), they found a high rate of comorbidity with mood, anxiety, and eating disorders.

In a larger heterogeneous sample Dunseith evaluated 113 consecutive male patients convicted of sexual offenses (Dunseith et al., 2004). Patients had been referred from prison, jail, or probation to a residential treatment facility. There, they had undergone structured interviews designed to assess for Axis I and II disorders, including sexual disorders. Of the total sample, 84 (74%) had a paraphilia.

That study compared offenders with and without paraphilias. The overall sample displayed a high incidence of lifetime Axis I and II disorders, including substance use disorder (85%), mood disorder (58%), bipolar disorder (35%), and depressive disorder (24%). In addition, 38% had an impulse control disorder, 23% an anxiety disorder, 9% an eating disorder, and 56% a personality disorder. In this study, the presence of a paraphilia correlated positively with mood disorder, major depression, bipolar I disorder, anxiety disorder, impulse control disorder, and avoidant personality disorder. It did not correlate with either antisocial personality disorder or with narcissistic personality disorder.

When considering comorbidity, it is helpful to recall the nosology delineated in the Diagnostic and Statistical Manual of Mental Disorders of the American Psychiatric Association, (Association, 2000). Not all comorbid psychiatric conditions are limited to Axis I. As some of the studies cited here have shown, Axis II personality disorders can also be present in sex offenders. While impaired intellectual functioning is typically not considered a "mental illness," mental retardation is defined as an Axis II mental disorder. Lindsay and colleagues (2004) looked at a group of 184 men who were either mentally retarded or learning disabled. They found a subgroup of 106 who had committed a sexual offense. The 78 others had committed a nonsexual offense. Of those intellectually compromised men who had committed a sexual offense, one-third had at least one comorbid nonparaphilic Axis I disorder.

COMORBID PSYCHIATRIC ILLNESS AMONG PARAPHILIC SEX OFFENDERS

Raymond et al. (1999) examined the rate of comorbid Axis I and Axis II disorders in a small, homogeneous (n = 42) sample of men with a diagnosis of pedophilia from several outpatient, and one inpatient, residential treatment programs. They found that 93% of men with pedophilia met the diagnostic criteria for an additional Axis I diagnosis over their lifetime, with 55% exhibiting symptoms that met criteria for five or more comorbid psychiatric disorders. Mood and anxiety disorders were the most common diagnoses in this sample. They also determined that 33% of the sample met criteria for one or more of the paraphilias in addition to pedophilia. Sixty-seven percent had only pedophilia. Over half of the sample (60%) met criteria for an Axis II disorder as well. However, of note, only a small percentage met the criteria for either narcissistic personality disorder or antisocial personality disorder.

In another study of a dichotomous sample (n = 120) of outpatients with paraphilic (PA) or paraphilic-related disorders (PRD) such as "sexual addiction" Kafka and his colleagues found that the PA patients experienced significantly higher rates of inpatient hospitalizations for either substance abuse or other psychiatric illnessess (Kafka & Hennen, 2002). When the overall study sample was further subdivided into those who had been criminally charged with a sexual offense, and those who had not, the sex offender group (n = 66) had a significantly higher rate of inpatient psychiatric hospitalization. A smaller study (n = 60) found high rates of both mood and anxiety disorders, as well as a high prevalence of both attention-deficit/hyperactivity disorder (ADHD) and dysthymia, among paraphilic patients (Kafka & Prentky, 1998). Not all of those paraphilic patients were sexual offenders.

THE RELATIONSHIP BETWEEN AXIS III (MEDICAL DISORDERS) AND THE PARAPHILIAS

Axis III pathology can also be a contributor to sex offending behavior in some instances. A few documented cases of traumatic brain injuries and diffuse central nervous system lesions (e.g., multiple sclerosis) have been linked to changes in sexual drive and associated behaviors.

Burns and Swerdlow (2003) reported the case of a patient with an orbitofrontal tumor who presented de novo with pedophilic behaviors. His pedophilic interests and behaviors had ceased after his tumor had been removed. Huws et al. (1991) reported on a patient with multiple sclerosis who had developed a foot fetish and hypersexuality in the context of that illness. An MRI revealed lesions in both his temporal and frontal lobes.

In a 5-year retrospective study Simpson et al. (1999) reviewed the case files of 445 patients who had sustained a traumatic brain injury (TBI). Of those patients, 29 (6.5%) engaged in sex offending behaviors following their TBI (Miller, Cummings, McIntyre, Ebers, & Grode, 1986). Similarly, Miller reported on patients presenting with aberrant sexual behaviors after suffering from a TBI (...). In one such case, a 39-year-old man began to engage in public masturbation following rapture of an anterior communicating arterial aneurysm. Another male patient had become hypersexual following surgical resection of a frontal meningioma, as had a woman who had suffered a right-sided stroke.

Temporal lobe pathology, including epilepsy, is sometimes associated with paraphilia-like behavior (e.g., fetishism, and exhibitionism). In one study, a patient with temporal lobe epilepsy presented with cross-dressing and fetishistic behaviors. Symptoms decreased following temporal lobectomy (Mitchell, Falconer, & Hill, 1954).

Mendez and colleagues (2000) reported two cases of men with both frontotemporal dementia and bilateral hippocampal sclerosis who had developed late-onset homosexual pedophilia. Positron emission tomography (PET) scan using the ligand 18-fluorodeoxyglucose subsequently confirmed hypometabolic activity in the right temporal lobe.

These cases manifesting Axis III pathology offer tantalizing clues to the underlying biology. Similarly, the few, small-scale studies of otherwise healthy patients who have exhibited sexual misconduct in the context of an episode of major mental illness reminds us of how much more there is to be learned. In spite of the significant implications for treatment, and a better understanding of etiology, risk assessment and patient management, there have been very few studies to shed light on some of these areas.

CONCLUSION

Treatment of sex offenders is an evolving process, and recently, thoughtful critiques have begun to emerge about treatment practices that have assumed the level of "Standards of Care" over the past two decades. Vivian-Byrne (2004), for example, has "strongly challenged" the core tenets of behavioral "treatment" for sexual offenders as initially conceptualized by McGuire and Priestly (1985). Instead, he invites us to examine "our assumptions about psychological treatment in therapy in general." However, we should not "throw out the baby with the bathwater." In the 1960s Szasz (1960) suggested that conditions such as schizophrenia should, perhaps, not be thought of as mental disorders, speaking instead, about "the myth" of mental illness. He was wrong. Schizophrenia is a serious mental disorder and so are many of the paraphilias. In addition, though not curable, many can be successfully treated.

There is some consensus that state-of-the-art treatment can be effective in reducing sexual recidivism. Clearly, that is the case with respect to sex-drive-lowering interventions. Group therapy has also produced promising results. Berlin and colleagues (1991) published a study that included more than 400 men with pedophilia, (only some of whom had had sex-drive-lowering treatments). Most had been in group therapy, and that study documented low rates of sexual recidivism. Other investigators (e.g., Hanson et al., 2002; Maletzky & Steinhauser, 2002; Saleh & Berlin 2003) have also documented good outcomes. At the same time, results assessing the efficacy of essentially psychological treatments must be interpreted cautiously, in part, because of the low base-rate of sexual offending in the population at large. That is so, despite seemingly high numbers of sex offenses reported by criminal justice agencies and the large numbers of incarcerated sex offenders who make up about 20% to 25% of the more than 2 million males incarcerated in the United States. However, the fact that sexual offenses of varying degrees of severity may be quite prevalent does not constitute evidence that those who have entered into treatment are continuing to reoffend.

Studies in prison populations have consistently demonstrated that a significant number of sex offenders have major mental health problems. Beyond that, according to Human Rights Watch, one in six prisoners—between 200,000 and 300,000 men and women in U.S. prisons—suffer from serious mental disorders, including such illnesses as schizophrenia, bipolar disorder, and major depression. An estimated 70,000 are psychotic on any given day (Abramsky, 2003; Lamb & Weinberger, 1998; Pinta, 2000). These figures do not appear to include the specifically sexual mental disorders (i.e., the paraphilias). Many of those individuals have been additionally confined via the process of civil commitment.

Additional studies on large, properly diagnosed and assessed samples are needed to further clarify the relationships between major mental illness, the paraphilias, and sex offending behaviors, and to design future treatment regimens that will continue to be increasingly more effective.

References

Abramsky, S. & Fellner, F. (2003). Ill Equipped: U.S. Prisons and Offenders with Mental Illness. New York: Human Rights Watch.

American Psychiatric Association. (2000). *Diagnostic and Statistical Manual of Mental Disorders, 4th Edition, Text Revision*. Washington, DC: American Psychiatric Association.

Berlin, F. (1986). Interviews with five rapists. *American Journal of Forensic Psychiatry*, 41, 11–41.

Berlin, F. (1994). Jeffrey Dahmer: Was he ill? Was he impaired? Insanity revisited. *American Journal of Forensic Psychiatry*, 15, 1–25.

Berlin, F. S. & Malin, H. M. (1991). Media distortion of the public's perception of recidivism and psychiatric rehabilitation. *The American Journal of Psychiatry*, 148(11), 1572–1576.

Berlin, F. S., Hunt W. P., Malin, H. M., Dyer, A., Lehne, G. K., & Dean, S. (1991) A five-year plus follow-up survey of criminal recidivism within a treated cohort of 406 pedophiles, 611 exhibi-tionists, and 109 sexual aggressives: Issues and Outcome. *American Journal of Forensic Psychiatry*, 12, 5–28.

Berlin, F. S., Galbreath, N. W., Geary, B., & McGlone, G. (2003). The use of actuarials at civil commitment hearings to predict the likelihood of future sexual violence. *Sex Abuse*, 15(4), 377–382.

Burns, J. M. & Swerdlow, R. H. (2003). Right orbitofrontal tumor with pedophilia symptom and constructional apraxia sign. *Archives of Neurology*, 60(3), 437–440.

DelBello, M. P., Soutullo, C. A., Zimmerman, M. E., Sax, K. W., Williams, J. R., McElroy, S. L., et al. (1999). Traumatic brain injury in individuals convicted of sexual offenses with and without bipolar disorder. *Psychiatry Research*, 89(3), 281–286.

Dunseith Jr, N., Nelson, E. B., Brusman-Lovins, L., Holcomb, J., Beckman, D., Welge, J., et al. (2004). Psychiatric and legal features of 113 men convicted of sexual offenses. *Journal of Clinical Psychiatry*, 65(3), 293–300.

Ebrahim, I. O. (2006). Somnambulistic sexual behaviour (sexsomnia). *Journal of Clinical Forensic Medicine* 13(4) 219–224.

Falk, A. (1999). Notes and comments: Sex offenders, mental illness and criminal responsibility: The constitutional boundaries of civil commitment after Kansas v. Hendricks. *American Journal of Law and Medicine*, 25, 117.

Fenwick, P. (1996). Sleep and sexual offending. *Medicine, Science, and the Law*, 36(2), 122–134.

Glaser, W. F. (1985). Admissions to a prison psychiatric unit. *The Australian and New Zealand Journal of Psychiatry*, 19(1), 45–52.

Hanson, R. K., Gordon, A., Harris, A., Marques, J., Murphy, W., Quinsey, V., et al. (2002). First report of the collaborative outcome data project on the effectiveness of psychological treatment for sex offenders. *Sex Abuse*, 14(2), 169–194.

Henderson, M. C. & Kalichman, S. C. (1990). Sexually deviant behavior and schizotypy: A theoretical perspective with supportive data. *The Psychiatric Quarterly*, 61(4), 273–284.

Huws, R., Shubsachs, A. P., & Taylor, P. J. (1991). Hypersexuality, Fetishsim and Multiple Sclerosis. *British Journal of Psychiatry*, 158: 280–281.

Kafka, M. P. & Prentky, R. A. (1998). Attention-deficit/hyperactivity disorder in males with paraphilias and paraphilia-related disorders: A comorbidity study. *The Journal of Clinical Psychiatry*, 59(7), 388–396; Quiz 397.

Kafka, M. P. & Hennen, J. (2002). A DSM-IV Axis I comorbidity study of males (n = 120) with paraphilias and paraphilia-related disorders. *Sex Abuse*, 14(4), 349–366.

Lamb, H. R. & Weinberger, L. E. (1998): Persons with severe mental illness in jails and prisons: A review. *Psychiatric Services*, 49, 483–492.

Lindsay, W. R., Smith, A. H., Law, J., Quinn, K., Anderson, A., Smith, A., et al. (2004) Sexual and nonsexual offenders with intellectual and learning disabilities: A comparison of referral patterns and outcomes. *Journal of Interpersonal Violence*, 19(8) 875–90.

Linz, D., Malamuth, N., & Beckett, K. (2002). Civil liberties and research on the effects of pornography In P. Tetlock & P Suedfelds (Eds.), *psychology and social policy* (pp 149–164). New York, NY: Hemisphere.

Loue, A. (2002). The involuntary civil commitment of mentally ill persons in the United States and Romania. *Journal of Legal Medicine*, 23, 211–250.

Maletzky, B. M. & Steinhauser, C. (2002). A 25-year follow-up of cognitive/behavioral therapy with 7,275 sexual offenders. *Behavior Modification*, 26(2), 123–147.

McElroy S. L., Soutello, C. A., Taylor Jr, P., Nelson, E. B., Beckman, D. A., Brusman, L. A., et al. (1999). Psychiatric features of 38 men convicted of sexual offenses. *Journal of Clinical Psychiatry*, 60(6):412–20: quiz 421–2.

McGuire, J. & Priestly, P. (1985). Offending behavior: Skills and strategems for going straight. London: Batsford.

Mendez, M. F., Chow, T., Ringman, J., Twitchell, G., & Hinkin, C. H. (2000). Pedophilia and temporal lobe disturbances. *The Journal of Neuropsychiatry and Clinical Neurosciences*, 12(1), 71–76.

Miller, B. L., Cummings, J. L., McIntyre, H., Ebers, G., & Grode, M. (1986). Hypersexuality or altered sexual preference following brain injury. *Journal of Neurology, Neurosurgery, and Psychiatry*, 49(8), 867–873.

Mitchell, W., Falconer, M. A., & Hill, D. (1954). Epilepsy with fetishism relieved by temporal lobectomy. *Lancet*, 267(6839), 626–630.

Pinta, E. R. (2000). Prison mental disorder rates – what do they mean? *Correctional Mental Health Report*, 1:81, 91–92.

Raymond, N. C., Coleman, E., Ohlerking, F., Christenson, G. A., & Miner, M. (1999). Psychiatric comorbidity in pedophilic sex offenders. *The American Journal of Psychiatry*, 156(5), 786–788.

Rosenfeld, D. S. & Elhajjar, A. J. (1998). Sleepsex: A variant of sleepwalking. *Archives of Sexual Behavior*, 27(3), 269–278.

Rosman, J. & Resnick, P. (1989). Sexual attraction to corpses: A psychiatric review of necrophilia. *The Bulletin of the American Academy of Psychiatry and the Law*, 17, 153–163.

Saleh, F., Malin, H., Berlin, F., & Thomas, K. (2007) Paraphilias and Paraphilia-Like Disorders In Gabbard, G. (Ed.), *Gabbard's Treatments of Psychiatric Disorders, Fourth Edition*. Washington, CD: American Psychiatric Press, Inc

Saleh, F. M. & Berlin, F. S. (2003) Sex hormones, neurotransmitters, and psychopharmacological treatments in men with paraphilic disorders. *Journal of Child Sexual Abuse*, 13(3–4), 233–253.

Schenck, C. H. & Mahowald, M. W. (1992). Sleepwalking and indecent exposure. *Medicine, Science, and the Law*, 32(1), 86–87.

Simpson, G., Blaszczynski, A., & Hodgkinson, A. (1999). Sex offending as a psychosocial sequela of traumatic brain injury. *The Journal of Head Trauma Rehabilitation*, 14(6), 567–580.

Slavney, P. R. & McHugh, P. R. (1987). *Psychiatric polarities: Methodology and practice*. Baltimore: The Johns Hopkins University Press.

Sutherland, E. H. (1950). The diffusion of sexual psychopath laws. *American Journal of Sociology*, 56, 142–148.

Szasz, T. (1960). The myth of mental illness. *American Psychologist*, 15, 113–118.

Vivian-Byrne, S. (2004). Changing people's minds. *Journal of Sexual Aggression*, 10(2), 181–192.

Chapter 10

The Assessment of Psychopathy and Response Styles in Sex Offenders

Michael J. Vitacco and Richard Rogers

Studies have demonstrated a robust relationship between high scores on the Psychopathy Checklist-Revised (PCL-R) (Hare, 2003) and violent recidivism (Salekin, Rogers, & Sewell, 1996). However, these predictions are complex and multidetermined. As described by Hart (1998, p. 133), "psychopathy is a necessary but not sufficient factor in the assessment of violence risk." In some cases of sexual violence, "the violence may be related more to disturbances of normal attachment processes rather than the pathological lack of attachment associated with psychopathy" (Hemphill & Hart, 2003). In summary, psychopathy plays a critical role in sexual violence for a minority of sex offenders. Objectives for assessing psychopathy among sex offenders are threefold in evaluating (a) the risk of recidivism, (b) institutional adjustment, and (c) treatment needs and outcome.

OVERVIEW OF PSYCHOPATHY

Psychopathy is defined by a "constellation of affective, interpersonal, and behavioral characteristics, including egocentricity; impulsivity; irresponsibility; shallow emotions; lack of empathy, guilt, or remorse; lying; manipulativeness; and the persistent violation of social norms and expectations" (Hare, 1996, p.25) and is the longest standing recognized personality syndrome. The diagnosis of psychopathy originated in the eighteenth century (Pinel, 1801) with the first systematic criteria authored by Cleckley (1941). Hare (1985, 2003), based on the work by Cleckley, developed the Psychopathy Checklist (PCL and PCL-R), a semistructured interview that is widely considered the gold standard in psychopathy measurement (Rogers, 2001a).

As a group, psychopaths are characterized by moderate levels of violence (Salekin et al., 1996) with longstanding problems evidenced from adolescence to adulthood (Gretton, Hare, & Catchpole, 2004; Vitacco, Neumann, & Jackson, 2005). However, many psychopaths have virtually no history of violent behavior. In the next section, we discuss how psychopathy relates to sex offending.

THE APPLICATION OF PSYCHOPATHY TO SEX OFFENDERS

Subtyping Sex Offenders

The classic study by Abel et al. (1986) categorized sex offenders by their primary motivation into three groups: psychotic, antisocial, and paraphilic. Of special interest to this chapter, nearly one-third (29%) were motivated predominantly by their antisocial personalities. Extrapolating from Abel et al. we surmise that facets of their psychopathy motivate a substantial minority of sex offenders.

Theoretically, psychopathy is likely to be particularly relevant to a subset of sex offenders who are "generalists." Generalists engage in a broad range of criminal activities and have poor work histories and unstable relationships. Psychopathy is least likely to be relevant for sex offenders who specialize in child offenses (see Miller, Geddings, Levenston, & Patrick, 1994) but are otherwise unremarkable with respect to criminal lifestyles.

Several formulations have been proposed to understand the motivation of dynamics for psychopathic rapists. Meloy (2002) posited multiple determinants including callousness, lack of bonding, sense of entitlement, and sensation seeking. From a very different perspective, Prentky and Knight (1991) conceptualized the psychopathic rapist as guided by impulsivity in many areas of criminal behavior, including sexual offenses. Psychopathic sex offenders are viewed as both predatory and impulsive. Offering a third perspective, Brown and Forth (1997) found psychopathic rapists to be opportunistic in their offending and predominantly angry.

Psychopathic rapists can also be described by their offense behavior. For example, Langevin (2003) found sex offenders who used violence to control victims, were substantially higher on psychopathy when compared to general sex offenders. Psychopathic sex offenders

often demonstrate a pattern of escalation beginning with noncontact sex offenses culminating in contact offenses (MacPherson, 2003). Moreover, Porter et al. (2002) posited that the psychopathic offending behavior is motivated by thrill seeking rather than paraphilias. Combining across investigators, the prototypical cases of psychopathic sex offender are typified by control, opportunism, and thrill seeking. Recognizing the heterogeneity of psychopathy, other sexual psychopaths are likely to exhibit very different patterns.

Psychopathy and Recidivism in Sex Offenders

In general, most offenders, but specifically sex offenders, including recidivists, are *not* psychopaths. Hare (2003) provides a useful summary of sex offenders and recidivism.[1] On average, sexual recidivists scored substantially lower than the threshold (PCL-R> 30) for psychopathy: (a) 21.4 (Langevin et al., 2001), (b) 23.4 (Hanson & Harris, 2000), (c) 21.5 (Dempster, 1998), 23.2 (Simourd & Malcolm, 1998), and (d) 21.7 (Firestone, Bradford, & McCoy, 1999). The unweighted average is 22.0, far short of the *minimum* level for the classification of psychopathy. As expected, nonrecidivating sex offenders substantially lower PCL-R scores than recidivists. For the four studies cited previously, nonrecidivists had average PCL-R scores of 15.7, 16.7, 13.3, and 16.3. With an unweighted average of 15.5 and reported SDs from 5.9 to 8.7, very few of these sex offenders likely qualified as psychopaths.

Walters (2003) conducted the most recent meta-analysis of the PCL-R factor scores and sexual recidivism. With five studies, the effect sizes were quite modest for both Factor 1 (weighted $M r = 0.05$) and Factor 2 (weighted $M r = 0.08$). These correlations account for less than 10% of the variance. Overall, these studies suggest that PCL-R factor scores are generally not helpful in identifying sexual recidivism but that PCL-R total scores may be moderately helpful in differentiating groups.

Can the PCL-R be used to predict the risk of sexual violence in an *individual* case? Forensic practitioners are likely to be divided on this issue. It is instructive to examine closely the conclusions of two prominent investigators who are closely associated with Hare. Hemphill and Hart (2003, p. 96) offered the following conclusions.

It is important to note that there is no good scientific evidence (contrary to some claims; e.g., Harris, Rice, & Quinsey, 1993) that diagnoses or traits of psychopathy, including scores on the PCL-R, can be used either on their own or in combination with other variables to estimate the absolute likelihood of future violence for a given individual with any reasonable degree of scientific or professional certainty. This is particularly important given the practice of some professionals to use diagnoses of psychopathy or antisocial personality disorder to support the conclusion that an individual is "more likely than not" (i.e., more than 50% likely) to commit acts of future violence or sexual violence. In some jurisdictions, such a conclusion is used to justify indeterminate civil commitment of a sexual predator (e.g., Janus, 2000) or even capital punishment (Cunningham & Reidy, 1998, 1999). Such a practice is simply unfounded and unethical at the present time.

Hemphill and Hart (2003) appear concerned about the overall accuracies of risk assessments and the substantial danger of false-positives. Their conclusions apply to both the PCL-R alone and attempts to combine the PCL-R scores with other actuarial measures, specifically the Violence Risk Appraisal Guide (VRAG) and the Sex Offender Risk Appraisal Guide (SORAG) (see also Quinsey, Rice, & Harris, 1995).

Character pathology rather than psychopathy per se may contribute to sexual recidivism. In a meta-analysis of 87 studies of sex offender recidivism, Hanson and Bussiére (1998) found antisocial personality disorder ($r = 0.14$), total number of prior offenses ($r = 0.13$), and sexual interest in children ($r = 0.33$) predicted sexual offense recidivism. This meta-analysis offers a competing hypothesis to psychopathy.

In summary, sex offenders often have multiple motivations for their deviant behavior. In a subset of sex offenders, psychopathic traits appear to play an important contributory role. At present, we do not know which psychopathic traits or facets are most responsible for predicting continued sex offending.

ASSESSING PSYCHOPATHY IN SEX OFFENDERS

This section provides a selective review that focuses on the three primary measures of psychopathy in adult populations. These measures are comprised of the PCL-R (Hare, 2003), Psychopathy Personality Inventory (PPI; Lilienfeld & Andrews, 1996), and the Self-Report of Psychopathy-2nd Edition (SRP-II; Hare, 1991). In addition, we summarize research on two popular multiscale inventories, specifically the Minnesota Multiphasic Personality Inventory-Second Edition (MMPI-2; Butcher, Dahlstrom, Graham, Tellegen, & Kaemmer, 1989) and the Personality Assessment Inventory (PAI; Morey, 1996).

The Psychopathy Checklist-Revised

The PCL-R is a 20-item semistructured interview measuring four inter-related facets (i.e., affective, interpersonal, lifestyle, and antisocial behavior) of psychopathy. In addition to the PCL-R, two other versions include the PCL: Screening Version (PCL:SV; Hart, Cox, & Hare, 1995) and the PCL-Youth Version (PCL-YV; Forth, Kosson, & Hare, 2003). The PCL-R is the most frequent measure used to assess psychopathy. Strengths of the PCL-R include extensive data on its reliability, validity, and generalizability. Regarding its reliability, Rogers (2001a) reviewed 21 investigations of the PCL-R. Overall, the studies found excellent inter-rater reliability for the total scores ranging from 0.77 to 0.98. PCL-R factor scores were substantially lower (0.55 to 0.86) but still good. In examining PCL-R criteria, the results for inter-rater reliability are decidedly mixed with two studies in the 0.3 range and three studies in the 0.5 range. Relatively little data are available on test–retest reliability; for PCL-R total scores, three studies range from moderate (0.63 for a 2-year interval) to excellent (0.80 and 0.94 for 1-month intervals).

The PCL-R has generally demonstrated similar factor structures and item response theory (IRT) analyses across gender and racial cultural groups (e.g., Cooke & Michie, 1999; Cooke, Kosson, & Michie, 2001; Jackson, Rogers, Neumann, & Lambert, 2002; Kosson, Smith, & Newman, 1990). The critical question is whether gender and racial cultural groups are similar in their expression of psychopathy and attendant risks. Clearly, women and Europeans have much lower rates than North American men with less associated violence in those classified as psychopaths (Cooke, 1998; Salekin et al., 1996). Racial differences require more research; Rogers (2001a) found variable results mostly limited to African Americans and European Americans. On this point, Hare (2003) cited unpublished research finding differences in Factor 2 scores.

Clinicians must be aware of potential limitations when drawing conclusions from PCL-R data. Some psychologists simply neglect the standard error of measurement (S_{EM}) for the PCL-R in their offender evaluations. The official test standards require that S_{EM} be considered (see American Psychological Association 1999). The S_{EM} for the total PCL-R score is approximately 3 (Hare, 2003) or 3.25 (Hare, 1991). Hart (1998), a close associate of Hare and the coauthor of PCL:SV, recommended that predictions of violent recidivism take into account 1 S_{EM}. Based on this recommendation, only offenders with PCL-R total scores >33 would be considered psychopathic and potentially at higher risk than nonpsychopaths. As observed by Rogers and Shuman (2005), even this recommendation leads to a false positive rate of approximately 16%.

The PCL-R should be only used in forensic consultations when its semistructured interview is compared with corroborative records. Use of the PCL-R interview alone is unacceptable (Hare, 2003). Use of the records alone is vulnerable to insufficient or biased information. The recommended format is helpful in addressing the minimization and denial often used by sex offenders attempting to portray themselves as less sexually deviant (see Wasyliw, Grossman, & Haywood, 1994; Marshall, 1994). The effects of defensiveness on PCL-R scores of sex offenders have not been adequately evaluated. The only study to formally address defensiveness found that delinquents were able to lower their scores significantly ($M = 5.03$ points) on the PCL:YV with minimal coaching (Rogers et al., 2002).

The Psychopathic Personality Inventory

The Psychopathic Personality Inventory (PPI) is a relatively recent multiscale instrument consisting of 187 items designed to measure psychopathy. The primary focus of the PPI is the measurement of psychopathic personality traits (Lilienfeld & Andrews, 1996). The PPI consists of eight psychopathy scales: Machiavellian Egocentricity (ME), Social Potency (SP), Coldheartedness (CH), Carefree Nonplanfulness (CN), Fearlessness (FE), Blame Externalization (BE), Impulsive Nonconformity (IN), and Stress Immunity (SP). These scales were intended to assess two broad

psychopathic facets (a) social dominance and level-headedness and (b) aggression and unconventional attitudes (Benning, Patrick, Hicks, Blonigen, & Krueger, 2003).

The PPI concurrent validity with the PCL-R yielded disappointing results. Of its eight scales, only the ME evidences a moderate relationship (0.56), with three modest correlations (i.e., SP = 0.37, CH = 0.37, and IN = 0.31) and four nonsignificant ones (Poythress, Edens, & Lilienfeld, 1998). These results indicate that the PPI cannot be used to measure psychopathy, as measured by the PCL-R.

Construct validity, investigated by Sandoval et al. (2000) with 100 inmates yielded mixed results. Most promising was the significant correlations between several scales of the PPI (i.e., total [0.60], ME [0.64], FE [0.37], BE [0.63], and IN [0.51]) and the Aggression Questionnaire. Focusing on correctional populations, Edens et al. (2001) found the total score of the PPI to modestly predict institutional infractions (rs from 0.26 to 0.37). Despite small to moderate correlations with the PCL-R, the only study documenting inter-rater reliability was in the initial sample of 1,104 undergraduates. The lack of reliability studies severely constrains the applicability of the PPI with sex offenders.

A potential strength of the PPI is the presence of validity scales measuring both fake-good and fake-bad indices. Two validity indices, Unlikely Virtues and Deviant Responding, measure defensiveness and malingering, respectively. However, studies analyzing the validity scales on the PPI have consisted of analogue studies and have lacked clinical comparisons (Baldwin & Roys, 1998; Edens, Buffington, Tomicic, & Riley, 2001).

Pending further investigations, the PPI is not currently recommended for clinical use in evaluating sex offenders. Its limitations include (a) lack of concurrent data with the PCL-R and (b) absence of research on sex offenders. Its potential usefulness for evaluating defensiveness among sex offenders should be explored.

The Self-Report of Psychopathy-2nd Edition (SRP-II)

The SRP-II (Hare, 1991) is a 60-item self-report scale of psychopathy. It is administered in a paper and pencil format with a very low reading level (3.70). The SRP-II was designed to parallel the original factor structure of the PCL-R (Zagon & Jackson, 1994). Efforts to apply the SRP-II to correctional samples have proved unsuccessful. While initial results produced moderate correlations with the PCL-R total and factor scores, subsequent studies have found only modest to low moderate relationships and limited information addressing reliability (Hare, 2003). In applying the SRP-II to mentally disordered offenders, Vitacco (2003) found low internal consistencies and poor convergence with the PCL-R. The SRP-II is currently undergoing substantial revisions (Paulhus, Hemphill, & Hare, in press) which may improve its reliability and validity. Presently, it should not be employed as either a measure or a screen for psychopathy.

Multiscale Inventories

Clinicians are often tempted to use multiscale inventories in forensic assessments because they conveniently evaluate different aspects of psychopathology and impairment. The two commonly used multiscale inventories are the MMPI-2 (Butcher et al., 1989) and the PAI (Morey, 1991). When using measures designed to address a spectrum of clinical correlates, the key issue is bandwidth fidelity (Widiger & Frances, 1987); as the breadth of a measure increases, its accuracy for specific clinical construct decreases.

The MMPI-2 is a 567-item multiscale inventory that is widely employed to assess patterns of psychopathology, clinical correlates, and response styles. One clinical scale, Psychopathic Deviance (Pd), may be mistakenly used as a measure of psychopathy. Despite its name, the Pd scale was *not* developed or validated to assess psychopathy as it is currently conceptualized. Instead, the Pd scale was intended as a measure of chronic but relatively minor delinquency. Not surprisingly, the MMPI-2 Pd scale has a low correlation $(r = 0.26)$ with the PCL-R total score (Hare, 2003).

The PAI is a 344-item multiscale inventory designed to assess for psychopathology, treatment needs, and response styles. Its advantages over the MMPI-2 include its easy reading level (fourth grade), use of multiple gradations, and the homogeneity of its scales and subscales (i.e., high alphas and low inter-item correlations). Extensive research (Morey, 1996, 2003) provides strong evidence of its reliability and validity.

The PAI has an Antisocial Features (ANT) scale that was designed to measure two core elements of psychopathy (Egocentricity and Stimulus Seeking) and evidence of social deviance (Antisocial Behaviors). Conceptually, these subscales correspond roughly to Hare's two-factor model of psychopathy. Edens et al. (2000) examined the usefulness of the ANT scale in evaluating sex offenders. They found that only the Antisocial Behaviors subscale was significantly correlated with the PCL:SV $(r = 0.54)$ and PCL-R $(r = 0.40)$ total score. Contrary to expectations, two psychopathically based scales were not significantly related to psychopathic personality measured by the PCL-R.

In summary, multiscale inventories are not recommended for the assessment of psychopathic sex offenders or other forensic populations. However, many practitioners will use these measures to assess to evaluate psychopathology and response styles. Importantly, validity scales of the MMPI-2 and PAI offer no information about the denial or minimization of sexual deviance. In particular, "normal" validity indicators do not suggest that sex offenders are forthcoming about their sexual practices. Likewise, "defensive" validity indicators do not suggest sex offenders are hiding information about their sexual practices.

PSYCHOPATHY AND SEXUAL PREDATOR LAWS

In the United States the treatment and indefinite containment of sex offenders has had two distinct movements. Beginning in the 1930s, many states passed laws focused on sexual psychopaths. The purpose of this legislation was to offer treatment to sex offenders. Although they were labeled "psychopaths," this term should not be confused with modern conceptualizations of psychopathy.

The second movement began with the Washington statute (Washington Revised Code 7 1.09.020(1)) and emphasized indefinite containment in locked hospitals rather than treatment. The Supreme Court in *Kansas versus Hendricks* (1997) upheld the right of states to civilly commit convicted sex offenders deemed likely to reoffend. In clarifying volitional impairment, the Supreme Court ruled in *Kansas versus Crane* (2001) that the inability to control sexual behavior need not be absolute. Since these landmark decisions, 17 states have developed statutes authorizing the civil commitment of sex offenders (Doren, 2002; Schopp & Slain, 2000).

These sexual violent predator (SVP) laws vary by jurisdiction but typically include three prongs, (a) the presence of a mental condition (e.g., a mental disorder or mental abnormality) and (b) a concomitant loss of volitional abilities, which leads to (c) a substantial likelihood of engaging in a sexual offense. Despite the SVP designation, states vary whether the sexual offense must be violent. Rogers and Shuman (2005) discuss two major concerns regarding SVP laws: the unknown error rate associated with specific SVP commitments and the absence of research congruent with the SVP standards.

SVP statutes have largely discarded psychopathy, although it may still play a role in these commitment proceedings. Levenson (2003) concluded that psychopathy was a strong determinant of which sex offenders were committed under Florida's sexual predator law. Analogue research by Guy and Edens (2003) suggested that any designation as "high-risk psychopath" may increase the perceived risk of sexual recidivism offenses, irrespective of the actual risk.

The assessment of psychopathy, via the PCL-R or other measures, does *not* take into account the requirements of SVP statutes for three reasons. First, these measures do not evaluate the broad range of clinical conditions as set forth in the SVP criteria. Second, the loss of volitional impairment resulting from psychopathy remains unknown. Third, the individualized risk of sexual recidivism posed by a particular SVP candidate is largely speculative. Beyond these pivotal issues, a low psychopathy score does not rule out recidvism (Edens, 2001; Porter, Fairweather, Hughes, Angela, & Birt, 2000). If psychopathy is assessed as part of SVP evaluations, forensic clinicians have a professional responsibility to clarify its marginal role in these determinations.

Rogers (2001b) observed that comprehensive risk assessments must include both *risk* (e.g., variables that increased the likelihood of recidivism) and *protective* (e.g., variables that reduced the likelihood of recidivism) factors. Unfortunately, research on sex offenders has virtually ignored protective factors. As a result, risk assessments of sexual recidivism are skewed by their unbalanced design.

Psychopathy can play a useful role in determining *general* risk of recidivism. Clinicians must be alert to practitioners who improperly attempt to extrapolate from this general risk to sex offender recidivism. In the evaluation of sex offenders, we present the following clinical recommendations:

1. Clinicians should only consider psychopathy as a peripheral issue in SVP determinations. They have an ethical responsibility to ensure that their assessment results are not misused or misinterpreted by others.

2. Beyond SVP determinations, psychopathy should be evaluated selectively. It may be very helpful in decisions regarding institutional placement and in development of specific treatment intervention aimed at the most malleable traits.

3. Psychologists involved in program development must consider the complex interplay of paraphilias, psychopathology, and facets of psychopathy. The offenders' readiness for change should also be incorporated into any intervention.

4. The measurement of psychopathy is not precise, as documented by the S_{EM}. Training and supervision are required for both PCL-R and PCL:SV; otherwise, problems with imprecision are magnified.

PSYCHOPATHY AND ITS ROLE IN THE MANAGEMENT AND TREATMENT OF SEX OFFENDERS

Recent research by Hill et al. (2004) demonstrated that patients in a maximum-security forensic hospital with Axis I disorders and comorbid psychopathy committed more institutional infractions including verbal abuse, verbal threats, and fighting (see also Caperton, Edens, & Johnson, 2004; Edens, Buffington-Vollum, Colwell, Johnson, & Johnson, 2002; Hildebrand, Ruiter, & Nijman, 2004; Walters, 2003). In applying these result to sex offenders, Buffington-Vollum et al. (2002) discovered modest biserial correlations between psychopathy ratings and nonaggressive ($r = 0.37$), verbally aggressive ($r = 0.40$), and physically aggressive institutional infractions ($r = 0.23$). Institutional programs that deliberately ignore these data may put staff and other offenders at undue risk.

Psychopathic sex offenders are problematic to treat in generic programs that do not take into account their psychopathy (Gacono, Nieberding, Owen, Rubel, & Bodholdt, 1997). Historically, psychopaths have been faulted for not responding to intervention programs that are not designed to treat their psychopathy. Rather than criticizing the naiveté of the interventions, psychopaths are often labeled untreatable. However, two recent reviews underscore the potential treatability of psychopaths. Using 44 independent samples, Salekin (2002) discovered many examples of psychopaths improving with treatment. Most notably, improvements occurred through implementation of a variety of psychotherapeutic interventions. Independent of treatment modality, Salekin (2002) found that successful programs included intensive individual therapy lasting at least 1-year and augmented with group interventions. In fact, those studies suggesting the intractability of psychopaths lack sound methodology and do not implement specific treatment for psychopathy (D'Silva, Duggan, & McCarthy, 2004).

Seto and Barbaree (1999) offered the same cognitive-behavioral interventions to both psychopaths and nonpsychopaths. Without modifying their interventions to address psychopathy, their findings were predictable. In particular, the explicit nature of some cognitive-behavioral programs makes them easily vulnerable to manipulation. Many psychopaths were able to graduate from the program without any real improvement. Not surprisingly, their recidivism rate did not substantially decrease.

Care must be taken not to blame treatment oversights on sex offenders. Scholars (Lösel & Schmucker, 2005) have provided programmatic guidelines including using cognitive-behavioral techniques that encourage patient accountability and focus on maladaptive behaviors. On the basis of their recommendations we provide the following guidelines for developing treatment programs for psychopathic sex offenders.

- Treatment should target cognitive distortions (Beck, Freeman, & Davis, 2004) that are frequently employed to minimize responsibility.
- Treatment should target the affective deficits that impair the psychopaths' ability to experience the emotions of others, including their victims.
- Treatment must be long-term with specific components aimed at improving psychopathic personality traits.
- Treatment should also target issues related general recidivism, perhaps within the paradigm of the transtheoretical model of change (Prochaska, DeClemente, & Norcross, 2003).

PSYCHOPATHY AND RESPONSE STYLES

Some evidence exists suggesting that individuals high on psychopathy are more likely than other offenders to engage in significant distortions and fake psychopathology (see Gacono, Meloy, Sheppard, & Speth, 1995). Unfortunately, many clinicians simply assume that the presence of psychopathy indicates response distortion. Engaging in this type of *ad hominem fallacy* (Rogers & Vitacco, 2002) compromises the clinician's ability to conduct an objective and thorough evaluation. In addition, forensic clinicians may be vulnerable to countertransference. Therefore, we recommend that clinicians be aware of their own emotional responses and rely only on empirically validated methods when assessing psychopathy and response styles.

Kropp and Rogers (1993) found that most psychopaths are no more effective at malingering (i.e., "faking bad") or engaging in defensiveness (i.e., "faking good"). To illustrate this, Poythress et al. (2001) discovered low correlations between malingering on standardized tests and scores on the PPI in a sample of prison inmates. Likewise, Kropp (1994) found that psychopaths were not more likely to malinger than nonpsychopaths; however, he also found a trend indicating successful feigners were more likely to be from the psychopathic group. In explaining Kropp's findings on psychopathy, Rogers and Cruise (2000) suggested that "the capacity to deceive is well represented in certain variants of this classification" (p. 271). In other words, specific symptoms of psychopathy may be associated with malingering, but the classification as a whole is not.

To assist clinicians in assessments of malingering with psychopathic offenders, Rogers and Cruise (2000) provided two overarching recommendations. First, clinicians should differentiate between general deceptions, designed to enhance self-image or to deny criminal activity, and specific malingering. Second, clinicians should not discount genuine Axis I symptoms in psychopaths; psychopathy and psychopathology are not mutually exclusive. Clinicians following these recommendations can (1) conduct comprehensive evaluations of risk and mental health, (2) tease out symptoms of criminal thinking and behavior from malingering, and (3) avoid unethical practice by prematurely discontinuing the evaluation of comorbid Axis I disorders.

Overview of Response Styles and Sex Offenders

Sex offenders often engage in gross misrepresentations of their offending behavior. Specific strategies include outright denial of sexual deviation or minimization of the offending behavior on their victims

(Happel & Auffrey, 1995; Lanyon, 2001). Kennedy and Grubin (1992) performed a cluster analysis of 102 sex offenders engaged in denial and four primary groups emerged. The largest group completely denied committing a sex offense. Other groups included (a) those who admitted the offense but denied any harm to the victim, (b) offenders who admitted the offense but blamed others, and (c) those who offered excuses for their offending (e.g., diminished mental state). Although rarely utilized by sex offenders, malingering of extreme psychopathology may be employed to excuse the offense or mitigate sentencing.

Owing to the prevalence of defensiveness and denial among sex offenders, Sewell and Salekin (1997) recommended that response styles should be evaluated in conjunction with physiological indices, such as deviant arousal. Offenders who deny sexual deviance may also minimize other personality difficulties (Haywood, Grossman, & Hardy, 1993). Therefore, assessments of defensiveness should include both general as well as specific indicators. This section of the chapter focuses on assessing response distortion in sex offenders. It includes the following:

- Definitions of response styles frequently observed in sex offenders
- Explanatory models for understanding dissimulation in sex offenders
- General measures and instruments employed in evaluating defensiveness in sex offenders
- Information on specific psychophysiological measures used in sex offender evaluations

Definition of Response Styles Utilized by Sex Offenders

Sex offenders will frequently engage in distortions to minimize or externalize responsibility for their criminal behavior. Three response styles that may be encountered when evaluating sex offenders: defensiveness, hybrid responding, and malingering.

- *Defensiveness* is defined by purposeful denial or severely minimizing symptoms to achieve an external goal. Both outright denial and minimization of sexual deviance are frequently encountered in sex offender evaluations and treatment (Tierney & McCabe, 2001). For instance, an offender may deny having a sexual attraction to children or minimize the impact of their behavior on their victims.

- *Hybrid Responding* (Rogers & Vitacco, 2002) refers to employing a variety of response styles. For instance, a sex offender may exaggerate their own histories of sexual and physical abuse, be forthright about their depression, but completely deny their offending behavior. Hybrid responding is common among sex offenders and complicates their evaluation and treatment.

- *Malingering* (American Psychiatric Association, 1999) refers to the deliberate production of false symptoms or exaggeration of symptoms to obtain an external goal. Although rare, sex offenders may fabricate psychotic symptoms in attempting to deny responsibility for their illegal behavior. Clinicians are urged to consult the text by Rogers (2008) for comprehensive chapters on assessing malingering.

EXPLANATORY MODELS OF RESPONSE STYLES IN SEX OFFENDERS

Rogers and Dickey (1991) described three explanatory models that seek to understand the motivations of sex offenders when they attempt to deny and discount sexually deviant behavior. These models are criminological, pathogenic, and adaptational models. Sewell and Salekin (1997) proposed a fourth motivation, specifically the socioevaluative model. Understanding these underlying motivations may assist in treating sex offender distortions.

The Criminological Model

The criminological model posits that antisocial persons engage in a broad range of deceptions. The denial and defensiveness of sex offenders is simply a subset of these deceptions. For some clinicians, the criminological model has intrinsic appeal that is possibly exacerbated by feelings of countertransference. Despite its intrinsic appeal, we believe this model only explains a small minority of distortions found in sex offenders. One danger of the criminological model is a fostering of cynicism (Vitacco & Rogers, 2005), which can hinder clinical assessment and subsequent interventions.

The Pathogenic Model

Rogers and Dickey (1991) proposed that a small number of sex offenders may engage in denial and minimization to protect themselves from the enormity of their actions. For instance, a male intrafamilial child molester may find it difficult to acknowledge or cope with the psychological damage he caused his young daughters. As such, denial becomes a defense mechanism to protect the offender against his unforgivable and reprehensible actions. It may also explain why some sex offenders continue to hold adamantly onto cognitive distortions, even after their convictions (Sewell & Salekin, 1997).

The pathogenic model may serve to protect sex offenders from devastatingly negative self-images. Ward and colleagues (Ward, Hudson, Marshall, & Siegert, 1995; Ward, Louden, Hudson, & Marshall, 1995) explained how denial wards off negative self-evaluative thoughts and thereby contributes to further offending. It may also have some utility in explaining the pervasive denial found in some pedophiles.

The Adaptational Model

The adaptational model assumes that the sex offender is caught in a highly adversarial set of circumstances and is seeking a favorable outcome. In pretrial evaluations, a full admission of sexual deviance may lead to further criminal sanctions. A complete denial of sex deviance may lead to negative characterizations (e.g., callous and remorseless) with no access to treatment. Some sex offenders struggle with what to admit and what to deny in an attempt to secure the least negative outcome. After conviction, pedophiles are particularly vulnerable to prison abuse. They face another set of challenges in their denials or admission of sexual deviance. Those sex offenders, forthcoming in treatment of the extensiveness of their deviant thinking and practices, may find their self-disclosures are subsequently used against them in SVP commitments.

The Socioevaluative Model

Sewell and Salekin (1997) proposed the socioevaluative model and described its application to sex offenders. Closely aligned to the adaptational model, the socioevaluative model posits that "dissimulation is a learned response to any evaluative stimulus" (Sewell & Salekin, 1997, p. 332). This model goes beyond the adaptational model by not requiring an adverse situation, only the presence of the offender's judgment. Once detected, sex offenders are routinely scrutinized for any additional evidence of maladaptive behavior. Aligned with this model, Marshall (1994) found sex offenders used less denial when they believe they would not be rejected for their admissions. This finding has treatment implications in explaining how sex offenders may respond to perceived rejection by clinicians.

ASSESSING DEFENSIVENESS AND DENIED SEXUAL DEVIATIONS

This section reviews measures and instruments used to assess sex offenders' response styles. We focus predominantly on defensiveness, given its prevalence among sex offenders.

General Tests of Defensiveness

The MMPI-2 is the one widely used to assess general defensiveness. The MMPI-2 contains 12 indices of underreporting. These indices include standard validity scales (i.e., Lie [L] and Correction [K] scales), their derivatives (i.e., $L - K$, $F - K$, and $L + K$) and several specialized scales of defensiveness. Baer and Miller (2002) conducted an extensive review of underreporting and defensiveness on the MMPI-2. Two specialized scales were more effective than the standard validity indices: the Wiggins Social Desirability Scale ($d = 1.56$) and the Positive Malingering ($d = 1.36$). Archer et al. (2004) found the Superlative (S) scale to add incremental validity in assessing underreporting among psychiatric inpatients. Importantly, the MMPI-2 scales evaluate general defensiveness as specific denials of sexual deviance.

- The PAI (Morey, 1993) contains two scales designed to assess general defensiveness, the Positive Impression Management (PIM) scale and the *Defensiveness* Index (DEF). Peebles and More (1998) found good classification rates for each scale. However, PIM requires a lower cut score (see also Cashel, Rogers, Sewell, & Martin-Cannici, 1995). Like the MMPI, the PAI is only designed to evaluate general defensiveness.
- The Paulhus Deception Scale (PDS; Paulhus, 1998) consists of two scales measuring defensiveness. First, Impression Management (IM) assesses attempts to conform to social norms. Second, Self-Deceptive Enhancement Scale (SDE) attempts to

measure unconscious biases leading to positive self portrayals. Its usefulness with correctional (Richards & Pai, 2003) and clinical (Salekin, 2000) populations requires further testing.

Sex Offender Specific Tests of Defensiveness

- Multiphasic Sex Inventory-II (MSI-II, Nichols & Molinder, 2000) contains 12 validity scales that measure aspects of response distortion.) demonstrated that the MSI-II possess some effectiveness at assessing denial in sex offenders. While the original MSI was designed to assess offenders who "acknowledge culpability" (Nichols and Molinder, 1984) the MSI-II is not hindered by such limitations (Molinder, personal communication, October 2004). However, the MSI-II is hindered by a lack of studies demonstrating its accuracy.
- The Penile Plethysmograph (PPG) records differential penile responses of "normal" and deviant sexual stimuli. PPG stimuli can be presented either audibly or visually. Different assessment laboratories may use PPG different stimuli and equipment thereby constraining the generalization of research findings. Among the strongest evidence, Laws et al. (2000) found a 91.7% correct classification rate for child molesters when the PPG was combined with a card-sorting self-report technique assessing sexual interests. Clearly, the PPG can play an important role monitoring deviance in sex offenders undergoing treatment.
- Polygraph Testing is often used in sex offender treatment programs to assess forthrightness of sex offenders in making full and complete disclosures of their sexual deviances. Blasingame (1998) found that disclosures were increased during interview before the polygraph. Thus the polygraph may motivate more self-disclosures, despite weaknesses in its reliability and validity (see also Ahlmeyer, Heil, McKee, & English, 2000). Use of the polygraph in treatment may assist in controlling deviant behaviors (Grubin, Madsen, Parsons, Sosnowski, & Warberg 2004). Without the polygraph, Hindman and Peters (2001) concluded, adults minimize their participation in juvenile and adult offense and exaggerate their history of childhood victimization. The polygraph should be used in treatment but not court evaluations, given problems with its validity and admissibility (Iacono & Lykken, 1997; Saxe & Ben-Shakhar, 1999).

Final Caution on Measuring Defensiveness

Research on defensiveness has consistently indicated that assessment methods are imprecise and less accurate than malingering (Baer & Miller, 2002; Nicholson et al., 1997). To address its imprecision, Nicholson et al. (1997) recommended multiple sources be used for any determination of defensiveness. In a sex offender evaluation, these sources could include standardized tests with validity scales, psychophysiological measures, and structured interviews with the alleged perpetrator.

CONCLUSION

Psychopathy and response styles are important albeit distinct clinical constructs that are critical to the evaluation and treatment of offender populations. Among sex offenders in particular, antisocial and psychopathic motivations can play an important role in a minority of cases. In contrast, issues of denial and defensiveness are very common among sex offenders irrespective of their motivations or type of paraphilias. The motivations of paraphilias and the separate motivations for deception must be considered in any comprehensive assessment of sex offenders.

In closing, forensic clinicians should be aware that many practitioners are guided by intuitively appealing ideas that are not supported by the empirical literature. Given its far-reaching implications, the assessment and treatment of sex offenders requires both specialized knowledge and methods. Clinicians should insure their instruments and methodologies have been properly validated on sex offenders and apply them appropriately.

Notes

1. We did not consider the Canadian studies at the Oak Ridge Division where many insane acquittees were forced to participate in extremely coercive interventions that included elements of involuntary treatment, deprivation, and restraint.

References

Abel, G. G., Rouleau, J. L., & Cunningham-Rathner, J. (1986). Sexually aggressive behavior. In W.J. Curran, A.L. McGarry, & S.A. Shah (Eds.), *Forensic psychiatry and psychology: Perspectives and standards for interdisciplinary practice* (pp. 289–313). Philadelphia: F.A. Davis.

Ahlmeyer, S., Heil, P., McKee, B., & English, K. (2000). The impact on polygraphy on admissions of victims and offenses in adult sexual offenders. *Sexual Abuse: Journal of Research and Treatment*, 12, 123–138.

American Psychological Association (1999). Standards for educational and psychological testing. Washington DC: author.

Archer, R. P., Handel, R. W., & Couvadelli, B. (2004). An evaluation of the incremental validity of the MMPI-2 Superlative (S) Scale in an inpatient psychiatric sample. *Assessment*, 11, 102–108.

Baer, R. A. & Miller, J. (2002). Underreporting of psychopathology on the MMPI-2: A meta-analytic review. *Psychological Assessment*, 14, 16–26.

Baldwin, K. & Roys, D. T. (1998). Factors associated with denial in a sample of alleged adult sexual offenders. *Sexual Abuse: Journal of Research and Treatment*, 10, 211–226.

Beck, A., Freeman, A., & Davis, D. (2004). *Cognitive therapy of personality disorders* (2nd ed.). New York, NY: Guilford Press.

Benning, S. D., Patrick, C. J., Hicks, B. M., Blonigen, D. M., & Krueger, R. F. (2003). Factor structure of the psychopathic personality inventory: Validity and implications for clinical research. *Psychological Assessment*, 15, 340–350.

Blasingame, G. D. (1998). Suggested clinical uses of polygraphy in community-based sexual offender treatment programs. *Sexual Abuse: Journal of Research and Treatment*, 10, 37–45.

Brown, S. L. & Forth, A. E. (1997). Psychopathy and sexual assault: Static risk factors, emotional precursors, and rapist subtypes. *Journal of Consulting and Clinical Psychology*, 65, 848–857.

Buffington-Vollum, J., Edens, J. F., & Johnson, J. (2002). Psychopathy as a predictor of institutional misbehavior among sex offenders: A prospective replication. *Criminal Justice and Behavior*, 29, 497–511.

Butcher, J., Dahlstrom, G., Graham, J., Tellegen, A., & Kaemmer, B. (1989). *MMPI-2 manual for administration and scoring*. Minneapolis, MN: University of Minnesota Press.

Caperton, J. D., Edens, J. F., & Johnson, J. K. (2004). Predicting sex offender institutional adjustment and treatment compliance using the Personality Assessment Inventory. *Psychological Assessment*, 16, 187–191.

Cashel, M., Rogers, R., Sewell, K., & Martin-Cannici, C. (1995). The Personality Assessment Inventory (PAI) and the detection of defensiveness. *Assessment*. 2, 333–342.

Cleckley, H. (1941). The *mask of sanity*. St. Louis, MO. Mosby Books.

Cooke, D. J. (1998). Cross-cultural aspects of psychopathy. In T. Millon and E. Simonsen (Eds). *Psychopathy: antisocial, criminal, and violent behavior* (pp. 260–276). New York: The Guilford Press.

Cooke, D. J. & Michie, C. (1999). Psychopathy across cultures: North America and Scotland compared. *Journal of Abnormal Psychology*, 108, 58–68.

Cooke, D. J., Kosson, D. S., & Michie, C. (2001). Psychopathy and ethnicity: Structural, item, and test generalizability of the Psychopathy Checklist-Revised (PCL-R) in Caucasian and African American participants. *Psychological Assessment*, 13, 531–542.

Cunningham, M. & Reidy, T. (1998). Integrating base rate data in violence risk assessments at capital sentencing. *Behavioral Sciences & the Law*, 16, 71–95.

Cunningham, M. & Reidy, T. (1999). Don't confuse me with the facts: Common errors in violence risk assessment at capital sentencing. *Criminal Justice and Behavior*, 26, 20–43.

Dempster, R. J. (1998). *Prediction of sexually violent recidivism: A comparison of risk assessment instruments*. Unpublished master's thesis, Simon Frasier University.

Doren, D. M. (2002). *Evaluating sex offenders: A manual for civil commitment and beyond*. Thousand Oaks, CA: Sage Publications.

D'Silva, K., Duggan, C., & McCarthy, L. (2004). Does treatment really make psychopaths worse? A review of the evidence. *Journal of Personality Disorders*, 18, 163–177.

Edens, J. (2001). Misuses of the Hare Psychopathy Checklist-Revised in court: Two case examples. *Journal of Interpersonal Violence*, 16, 1082–1093.

Edens, J. F., Hart, S. D., Johnson, D. W., Johnson, J. K., & Oliver, M. E. (2000). Use of the Personality Assessment Inventory to assess psychopathy in offender populations. *Psychological Assessment*, 12, 132–139.

Edens, J. F., Buffington, J. K., Tomicic, T. L., & Riley, B. D. (2001). Effects of positive impression management on the Psychopathic Personality Inventory. *Law and Human Behavior*, 25, 235–256.

Edens, J. F., Poythress, N. G., & Watkins, M. M. (2001). Further validation of the Psychopathic Personality Inventory among offenders: Personality and behavioral correlates. *Journal of Personality Disorders*, 15, 403–415.

Edens, J. F., Buffington-Vollum, J., Colwell, K. W., Johnson, D. W., & Johnson, J. K. (2002). Psychopathy and institutional misbehavior among incarcerated sex offenders: A comparison of the Psychopathy Checklist-Revised and the Personality Assessment Inventory. *International Journal of Forensic Mental Health*, 1, 49–58.

Firestone, P., Bradford, J. M., & McCoy, M. Prediction of recidivism in incest offenders. *Journal of Interpersonal Violence*, 14, 511–531.

Forth, A. E., Kosson, D. S., & Hare, R. D. (2003). The *psychopathy checklist: youth version manual*. Toronto: Multi-Health Systems.

Gacono (Ed). *The clinical and forensic assessment of psychopathy: A practitioner's guide* (pp. 269–284). Manwah, NJ: Lawrence Erlbaum Associates.

Gacono, C. B., Meloy, J. R., Sheppard, K., & Speth, E. (1995). A clinical investigation of malingering and psychopathy in hospitalized insanity acquittees. *Bulletin of the American Academy of Psychiatry and the Law*, 23, 387–397.

Gacono, C. B., Nieberding, R. J., Owen, A., Rubel, J., & Bodholdt, R. (1997). Treating conduct disorder, antisocial, and psychopathic personalities. José Ashford and Bruce Sales (Eds). *Treating adult and juvenile offenders with special needs* (pp. 99–129). Washington DC: American Psychological Association.

Gretton, H. M., Hare, R. D., & Catchpole, R. (2004). Psychopathy and offending from adolescence to adulthood: A 10-year follow-up. *Journal of Consulting and Clinical Psychology*, 72, 636–645.

Grubin, D., Madsen, L., Parsons, S., Sosnowski, D., & Warberg, B. (2004). A prospective study on the impact of polygraphy on high-risk sexual behaviors in adult sex offenders. *Sexual Abuse: Journal of Research and Treatment*, 16, 209–222.

Guy, L. S. & Edens, J. F. (2003). Juror decision-making in a mock sexually violent predator trial: Gender differences in the impact of divergent types of expert testimony. *Behavioral Sciences and the Law*, 21, 215–237.

Hanson, K. R. & Bussiére. M. T. (1998). Predicting relapse: A meta-analysis of sexual offender recidivism studies. *Journal of Consulting and Clinical Psychology*, 66, 348–362.

Hanson, K. R. & Harris, J. R. (2000). Where should be intervene? Dynamic predictors of sexual assault recidivism. *Criminal Justice and Behavior*, 27, 6–35.

Happel, R. & Auffrey, J. (1995). Sex offender assessment: Interpreting the dance of denial. *American Journal of Forensic Psychology*, 13, 5–22.

Hare, R. D. (1985). *The Hare psychopathy checklist*. Toronto: Multi-Health Systems.

Hare, R. D. (1991). *Self-report of psychopathy, 2nd Edition*. Toronto, ON: Multi-Health Systems.

Hare, R. D. (1996). Psychopathy: A clinical construct whose time has come. *Criminal Justice and Behavior*, 23, 25–54.

Hare, R. D. (2003). *The Hare psychopathy checklist-revised, 2nd Edition*. Toronto, ON: Multi-Health Systems.

Harris, G. T., Rice, M. E., & Quinsey, V. L. (1993). Violent recidivism of mentally disordered offenders: The development of a statistical prediction instrument. *Criminal Justice and Behavior*, 20, 315–335.

Hart, S. (1998). The role of psychopathy in assessing risk for violence: Conceptual and methodological issues. *Legal and Criminological Psychology*, 3, 121–137.

Hart, S., Cox, D., & Hare, R. D. (1995). *Manual for the psychopathy checklist:screening version (PCL:SV)*. Toronto: Multi-Health Systems.

Haywood, T., Grossman, L. S., & Hardy, D. W. (1993). Denial and social desirability in clinical examinations of alleged sex offenders. *Journal of Nervous and Mental Disease*, 181, 183–188.

Hemphill, J. F. & Hart, S. D. (2003). Forensic and clinical issues in the assessment of psychopathy. In A. M. Goldstein (ed.), *Handbook of psychology: forensic psychology, Volume 11* (pp. 87–107). New York: John Wiley and Sons.

Hildebrand, M., Ruiter, C., & Nijman, H. (2004). PCL-R psychopathy predicts disruptive behavior among male offenders in a Dutch forensic psychiatric hospital. *Journal of Interpersonal Violence*, 19, 13–29.

Hill, C. D., Neumann, C. S., & Rogers, R. (2004). Confirmatory factor analysis of the Psychopathy Checklist: Screening Version with axis I disorders. *Psychological Assessment*, 16, 90–95.

Hindman, J. & Peters, J. (2001). Polygraph testing leads to better understanding of adult and juvenile sex offenders. *Federal Probation*, 65, 17–34.

Iacono, W. G. & Lykken, D. T. (1997). The validity of the lie detector: Two surveys of scientific opinion. *Journal of Applied Psychology*, 82, 426–433.

Jackson, R., Rogers, R., Neumann, C. S., & Lambert, P. (2002). Psychopathy in Women: An investigation of its underlying dimensions. *Criminal Justice and Behavior*, 29, 692–704.

Janus, E. (2001). Sex offender commitments and the "inability to control"—Developing legal standards and a behavioral vocabulary for an elusive concept. In, A. Schlank (Ed.), *Sexual predator* (pp. 11–30). Kingston, NJ: Civic Research Institute.

Kansas v. Hendricks, 521 U.S. 346 (1997).

Kansas v. Crane, 534 U.S. 407 (2002).

Kennedy, F. & Grubin, D. (1992). Patterns of denial in sex offenders. *Psychological Medicine*, 22, 191–196.

Kosson, D. S., Smith, S. S., & Newman, J. P. (1990). Evaluating the construct validity of psychopathy in black and white male inmates: Three preliminary studies. *Journal of Abnormal Psychology*, 9, 250–259.

Kropp, R. (1994). The relationship between psychopathy and malingering of mental illness. *Dissertation Abstracts International*, 54, 5594.

Langevin, R. (2003). A study of the psychosexual characteristics of sex killers: Can we identify them before it is too late? *International Journal of Offender Therapy and Comparative Criminology*, 47, 366–382.

Langevin, R., Curnoe, S., Federoff, P., Bennett, R., Peever, C., et al. (2004). Lifetime sex offender recidivism: A 25-Year Follow-Up Study *Canadian Journal of Criminology and Criminal Justice*, 46, 531–552.

Lanyon, R. I. (2001). Dimensions of self-serving misrepresentation in forensic assessment. *Journal of Personality Assessment*, 76, 169–179.

Laws, D. R., Hanson, K., Osborn, C. A., & Greenbaum, P. E. (2000). Classification of child molesters by plethysmographic assessment of sexual arousal and a self-report measure of sexual preference. *Journal of Interpersonal Violence*, 15, 1297–1312.

Levenson, J. S. (2003). Factors predicting recommendation for civil commitment of sexually violent predators under Florida's Jimmy Ryce Act. *Dissertation Abstracts International*, 64, 1079.

Lilienfeld, S. O. & Andrews, B. P. (1996). Development and preliminary validation of a self-report measure of psychopathic personality traits in noncriminal populations. *Journal of Personality Assessment*, 66, 488–524.

Lösel, F. & Schmucker, M. (2005). The effectiveness of treatment for sexual offenders: A comprehensive meta-analysis. *Journal of Experimental Criminology*, 1(1), 117–146. Lorenz, A. R. & Newman, J. P. (2002). Deficient response modulation and emotional processing in low-anxious Caucasian psychopathic offenders: Results from a lexical decision task. *Emotion*, 2, 91–104.

MacPherson, G. (2003). Predicting escalation in sexually violent recidivism: Use of the SVR-20 and PCL:SV to predict outcome with non-contact recidivists and contact recidivists. *Journal of Forensic Psychiatry and Psychology*, 14, 615–627.

Marshall, W. L. (1994). Treatment effects on denial and minimization in incarcerated sex offenders. *Behaviour Research and Therapy*, 32, 559–564.

Meloy, J. R. (2002). The polymorphously perverse psychopath: Understanding a strong empirical relationship. *Bulletin of the Menninger Clinic*, 66, 273–289.

Miller, M. W., Geddings, V. J., Levenston, G. K., & Patrick, C. J. (1994). *The Personality characteristics of psychopathic and nonpsychopathic sex offenders*. Paper presented at the American Psychology and Law Society Biannual Conference, Santa Fe.

Morey, L. C. (1991). *The personality assessment inventory manual*. Odessa, FL: Psychological Assessment Resources.

Morey, L. C. (1996). *An interpretive guide to the personality assessment inventory*. Odessa FL: Psychological Assessment Resources.

Morey, L. C. (2003). *Essentials of PAI assessment*. Hoboken, New Jersey: John Wiley & Sons.

Nichols, H. R. & Molinder, I. Multiphasic Sex Inventory, Technical Manual. Nichols & Molinder Assessments, Tacoma, WA.

Nicholson, R. A., Mouton, G. J., Bagby, M., Buis, T., Peterson, S., & Buigas, R. (1997). Utility of MMPI-2 indicators of response distortion: Receiver operating characteristic analysis. *Psychological Assessment*, 9, 471–479.

Paulhus, D. L. (1998). Paulhus Deception Scales (PDS): *The balanced inventory of desirable responding-7*. North Tonawanda, NY: Multi-Health Systems.

Paulhus, D. L., Hemphill, J. F., & Hare, R.D. (in press). *Scoring manual for the Hare self-report psychopathy scale-III*. Toronto: Multi-Health Systems.

Peebles, J. & Moore, R. (1998). Detecting socially desirable responding with the personality assessment inventory: The positive impression management scale and the defensiveness index. *Journal of Clinical Psychology*, 54, 621–628.

Pinel, P. (1801). *Traite Medico-Philosophique Sur l'Alientation Mentale*. Paris: Caille et Ravier.

Poythress, N. G., Edens, J., & Watkins, M. M. (2001). The relationship between psychopathic personality features and malingering symptoms of major mental illness. *Law and Human Behavior*, 25, 567–582.

Poythress, N., Edens, J., & Lilienfeld, S. (1998). Criterion-related validity of the Psychopathic Personality Inventory in a prison sample. *Psychological Assessment*, 10, 426–430.

Prentky, R. A. & Knight, R. A. (1991). Identifying critical dimensions for discriminating among rapists. *Journal of Consulting and Clinical Psychology*, 59, 643–661.

Porter, S., Fairweather, D., Hughes, H., Birt, Angela, & Boer, D. P. (2000). Profiles of psychopathy in incarcerated sex offenders. *Criminal Justice and Behavior*, 27, 216–233.

Porter, S., Campbell, M., Woodworth, M., & Birt, A. (2002). A new psychological conceptualization of the sexual psychopath. In, S. Shohov (Ed). *Advances in psychological research*. New York, NY: Nova Science Publishers.

Prochaska, J., DiClemente, C., & Norcross, J. (1992). In search of how people change: Applications to addictive behaviors. *American Psychologist*, 47, 1102–1114.

Quinsey, V. L., Rice, M. E., & Harris, G. T. (1995). Actuarial prediction of sexual recidivism. *Journal of Interpersonal Violence*, 10, 85–105.

Richards, H. & Pai, S. M. (2003). Deception in prison assessment of substance abuse. *Journal of Substance Abuse Treatment*, 24, 121–128.

Rogers, R. (2001a). *Handbook of diagnostic and structured interviewing*. New York, NY: The Guilford Press.

Rogers, R. (2001b). The uncritical acceptance of risk assessment in forensic practice. *Law and Human Behavior*, 24, 595–605.

Rogers, R. (2008). *Clinical assessment of malingering and deception (3rd ed.)*. New York, NY: Guilford Press.

Rogers, R. & Dickey, R. (1991). Denial and minimization among sex offenders: A review of competing models of deception. *Annals of Sex Research*, 4, 49–63.

Rogers, R. & Cruise K. (2000). Malingering and deception among psychopaths. In C. Rogers, R. & Shuman, D.W. (2005). *Fundamentals of forensic practice: Mental health and criminal law*. New York, NY: Springer.

Rogers, R. & Vitacco, M. J. (2002). Forensic assessment of malingering and related response styles. In B. Van Dorsten (Ed.). *Forensic psychology: From classroom to courtroom* (pp. 83–104). New York, NY: Kluwer Academic Press.

Rogers, R., Vitacco, M. J., Jackson, R. L., Martin, M., Collins, M., & Sewell, K. W. (2002). Faking psychopathy? An examination of response styles with antisocial youth. *Journal of Personality Assessment*, 78, 31–46.

Salekin, R. T. (2000). Test review: The Paulhus Deception Scales. *American Psychology-Law Society News*, 20, 8–11.

Salekin, R. T. (2002). Psychopathy and therapeutic pessimism: Clinical lore or clinical reality? *Clinical Psychology Review*, 22, 79–112.

Salekin, R. T., Rogers, R., & Sewell, K. W. (1996). A review and meta-analysis of the Psychopathy Checklist and Psychopathy Checklist-Revised: Predictive validity of dangerousness. *Clinical Psychology: Science and Practice*, 3, 203–215.

Sandoval, A. R., Hancock, D., Poythress, N., Edens, J. F., & Lilienfeld, S. (2000). Construct validity of the Psychopathic Personality Inventory in a correctional sample. *Journal of Personality Assessment*, 74, 262–281.

Saxe, L. & Ben-Shakhar, G. (1999). Admissibility of polygraph tests: The application of scientific standards post- Daubert. *Psychology, Public Policy, and Law*, 5, 203–223.

Schopp, R. F. & Slain, A. J. (2000). Psychopathy, criminal responsibility, and civil commitment as a sexual predator. *Behavioral Sciences and the Law*, 18, 247–274.

Seto, M. C. & Barbaree, H. E. (1999). Psychopathy, treatment behavior, and sex offender recidivism. *Journal of Interpersonal Violence*, 14, 1235–1248.

Sewell, K. W. & Salekin, R. T. (1997). Understanding and detecting dissimulation in sex offenders. In R. Rogers (Ed). *Clinical assessment of malingering and deception, 2nd edition* (pp. 328–350). New York, NY: The Guilford Press.

Simourd, D. & Malcolm, P. (1998). Reliability and validity of the Level of Service Inventory—Revised among federally incarcerated sex offenders. *Journal of Interpersonal Violence*, 13, 261–274.

Tierney, D. W. & McCabe, M. P. (2001). An evaluation of self-report measures of cognitive distortions and empathy among Australian sex offenders. *Archives of Sexual Behavior*, 30, 495–519.

Vitacco, M. J. (2002). Construct validity of psychopathy in mentally disordered offenders: A multi-trait multi-method approach. *Dissertation Abstracts International*, 64, 2945.

Vitacco, M. J., Neumann, C. S., & Jackson, R. (2005). Development of a four-factor model of psychopathy: Associations with ethnicity, gender, violence, and intelligence. *Journal of Consulting and Clinical Psychology*, 73, 466–476.

Vitacco, M. J. & Rogers, R. (2005). Assessment of Malingering in Correctional Settings. In C. Scott (Ed.). *Clinical handbook of correctional psychiatry* (pp 133–150). Arlington, VA: American Psychiatric Publishing Press.

Walters, G. D. (2003). Predicting institutional adjustment and recidivism with the Psychopathy Checklist factor scores: A meta-analysis. *Law and Human Behavior*, 27, 541–558.

Ward, T. U., Hudson, S., Marshall, W. L., & Siegert, R. (1995). Attachment style and intimacy deficits in sexual offenders. *Sexual Abuse: Journal of Research and Treatment*, 7, 317–335.

Ward, T. U., Louden, K., Hudson, S., & Marshall, W. L. (1995). A descriptive model of the offense chain for child molesters. *Journal of Interpersonal Violence*, 10, 452–472.

Wasyliw, O. E., Grossman, L. S., & Haywood, T. W. (1994). Denial of hostility and psychopathology in the evaluation of child molestation. *Journal of Personality Assessment*, 63, 185–190.

Widiger, T. A. & Frances, A. (1987). Interviews and inventories for the measurement of personality disorders. *Clinical Psychology Review*, 7, 49–75.

Zagon, I. K. & Jackson, H. J. (1994). Construct validity of a psychopathy measure. *Personality and Individual Differences*, 17, 125–135.

Chapter 11

The Role of Personality Disorder in Sexual Offending

Roy J. O'Shaughnessy

Persons who commit sexual offenses are a heterogeneous group of individuals who may demonstrate various underlying psychiatric illnesses or personality disturbances described in other chapters of this book. Sexual assaults are complicated behaviors that result from the interaction of various factors, including sexual thoughts and interests, social and cultural values, psychological needs and desires as well as possible underlying psychiatric illness or disturbances in personality. While many individuals commit sexual assault simply because they do not conform their conduct to the requirements of law and social values, many offenders also demonstrate significant psychopathology that may or may not be related to their sexual offending behavior. In many individuals there is a complex relationship between their underlying personality traits and/or personality disorders and psychiatric illnesses such as paraphilia. The focus of this chapter will be to demonstrate the role of personality traits and disorders in sexual offending behavior.

DEFINING PERSONALITY DISORDER

Personality disorder is defined by the DSM-IV (American Psychiatric Association, 2000) as an "enduring pattern of inner experience and behavior that deviates markedly from the expectations of the individual's culture, is pervasive and inflexible, has an onset in adolescence or early adulthood, is stable over time, and leads to distress or impairment." DSM defines "personality traits" as

> enduring patterns of perceiving, relating to, and thinking about the environment and oneself that are exhibited in a wide range of social and personal contexts. Only when personality traits are inflexible and maladaptive and cause significant functional impairment or subjective distress do they constitute Personality Disorders (American Psychiatric Association, 2000).

The decision in DSM-III (American Psychiatric Press) to code personality disorders on a separate axis from other psychiatric illness led to greater research interest in personality disorders, which resulted in substantive changes in the research literature for DSM-IV. Further research is now influencing the formulation of personality disorders for DSM-V (Livesley, 2003).

Categorical Models of Assessment

The initial DSM-III concept of personality disorder was challenged by subsequent research that illustrates a number of deficits in the early diagnostic model. In particular, research data led to questions regarding the reliability and validity of the different DSM-III personality disorders (Livesley, 1991). The categorical diagnostic approach used in DSM-III was not supported by data that suggested a dimensional view of personality was more accurate (Schroeder, Wormworth, & Livesley, 1992; Zimmerman, & Coryell, 1990).

Comprehensive review by Zimmerman (1994) outlined the research pertaining to the reliability and stability of DSM-III-R personality disorder diagnoses. While studies suggested that joint interviews using standardized interview formats showed good to excellent inter-rater reliability, other research demonstrated that clinicians not using standardized instruments only achieved poor to fair inter-rater reliability. Studies examining self-report measures of personality and those examining informant descriptions of personality showed marked differences in the descriptions of usual personality functioning. Information available was insufficient to justify which perception, self-report, or informant, would be more accurate. Zimmerman also noted marked variability between the DSM-III-R disorders and instruments available at that time to measure Personality Disorder. Further, different Personality instruments lacked concordance with each other and with DSM criteria and coverage of the disorders. Concern was also noted regarding state versus trait bias in individuals' responses to various self-report personality measures and inventories. Despite concerns about the lack of empirical support for the DSM-III-R approach to Personality Disorder, few changes were made in DSM-IV.

Further criticisms of the DSM-III-R model was noted pertaining to the diagnosis of Antisocial Personality Disorder (APD) (Duggan, 1993, Widiger & Corbitt, 1994). Specifically, DSM-III-R chose to focus primarily on antisocial behavior as opposed to

underlying personality traits such as described previously by Cleckley (1976). Paradoxically, the focus on actual behaviors led to improved inter-rater reliability in the diagnosis of APD compared to other DSM Personality Disorders. As a consequence of focusing only on behavior, the APD description was somewhat bereft of the richness in personality traits one would hope to achieve in order to adequately understand and describe the complexity of APD.

DSM-IV TR acknowledged some of the criticisms of earlier research (American Psychiatric Association, 2000). In the preamble, DSM-IV TR noted that the clustering of Personality Disorders into different groupings had not been consistently validated and individuals frequently presented with "co-occurring Personality Disorders from different clusters." It was acknowledged that the diagnosis of Personality Disorder often required multiple interviews focusing on the person's enduring pattern of traits over the course of time. The complication of diagnosing a Personality Disorder when the individual does not perceive their traits to be problematic was also identified It was recognized that features of Personality Disorder usually can be seen in adolescence but caution was voiced in making such a diagnosis given that many such traits do not persist into adult life. DSM-IV also documented the difficulties in external validity in which many of the traits of Personality Disorder are in fact found in other Axis I mental disorders and are not exclusive to Personality Disorders. , Accordingly, DSM-IV advised caution in diagnosing Personality Disorders during episodes of Mood or Anxiety Disorders.

DSM-IV TR also recognized the research demonstrating that dimensional models of Personality Disorders seem to be more appropriate than categorical models, and suggested that the DSM-IV Personality Disorder clusters "may also be viewed as dimensions representing spectra of personality dysfunction on a continuum with Axis I mental disorders." DSM-IV proposed that the integration and utility of dimensional models need further investigation.

Livesley (2001) has done an extensive review of the literature on personality disorders and offers cogent criticisms of the DSM-IV diagnostic process. Multivariate studies of individuals do not offer empirical support for the categories defined by DSM-IV. Further, psychometric properties and in particular inter-rater reliability is relatively poor, unless individuals apply structured interviews that are rarely used in clinical settings. He also noted the lack of validity of most personality disorder categories. Internal validity, or the extent to which the diagnostic criteria identify a homogenous group, is relatively poor. DSM-IV personality disorders are diagnosed by affirming a certain number of diagnostic criteria within a list of traits. Two individuals who meet the minimum threshold to diagnose a "Personality Disorder" may in fact demonstrate very different traits of personality. The external validity, or the extent to which a diagnosis of one personality disorder differs from other diagnoses, is also very questionable. There is a substantial overlap between the traits in certain personality disorders and other Axis I disorders. Likewise, there is substantial overlap in traits between different personality disorders. Further, individuals meeting the minimum threshold of traits to diagnose a personality disorder are not substantially different from those individuals who fail to meet the threshold by one or two criteria. These issues have critical import in forensic settings where a diagnostic category such as personality disorder may play a substantial role in social and legal proceedings.

Dimensional Models of Assessment

Dimensional models of personality argue that personality traits are on a continuous distribution depending on the extent of the presence or absence of certain traits. Much of the research is derived from "normal" populations as opposed to clinical populations in attempts to understand personality generally. Dimensional models of normal personality are derived from multivariate analysis of personality traits that are grouped to form clusters or factors. Different researchers have placed varying emphasis on the factors that have emerged from multivariate analyses.

The three factor approach (Eysenck, 1987) identified a number of specific traits that Eysenk organized into three higher order factors: extraversion, neuroticism, and psychoticism. These three higher order factors then interacted in a manner to define personality and behavior. The five factor approach (Costa & McCrae, 1992; Widiger, 2000) identified five higher order factors including neuroticism, extraversion, openness to experience, agreeableness, and conscientiousness. Each of these specific factors was in turn subdivided into six facets. While clearly multivariate analysis affirmed the traits and the specific

factors, there has never been a model that allows these factors to be adequately assessed in clinical populations or to be clinically useful.

Multivariate studies have also been conducted on clinical populations to evolve a dimensional model of Personality Disorder. Item analysis of DSM-IV items (Livesley, Jang, & Vernon, 1998; Mulder & Joyce, 1997) identified a four factor model of Personality Disorder. These included asthenia or emotional disregulation, antisocial or dissocial factor, asocial or inhibited factor, and an anakastic or compulsivity factor.

Another method of examining dimensional models has been the use of prototype descriptions of personality. Prototypes based on the five factor model (Widiger & Lyna, 1998) have been tested in clinical samples. Prototypes generated by clinicians showed good agreement with profiles generated by self-report and showed convergent validity with a semistructured interview. Patients with Borderline Personality Disorder according to DSM-IV criteria were compared with other patients with Personality Disorder and a general control group (Pukrop, Herpertz, Sass, & Steinmeyer, 1998). Patients with Borderline Personality Disorder showed specific profiles compared to other groups and gave support to the view that a dimensional approach had sufficient sensitivity and specificity.

Dimensional models remain very difficult to implement. Livesley (2003) argues for alternative categories, for example, the establishment of prototypes that would have more favor within clinical settings. Prototypes would be those disorders in which clinicians would have high agreement on specific features. Patients would then be graded as to their fit within the prototype. Recent methodology utilizing Q sort (Schedler & Westn, 2004; Westn & Schedler, 2003) offers a potential methodology for prototype classification that seems more congruent with views of what is clinically important. Clinicians were asked to rate 200 descriptive statements into eight categories on the basis of their degree of fit. This resulted in seven clusters of "prototypes" including dysphoria, schizoid, antisocial, obsessional, paranoid, histrionic, and narcissistic. They argued that this methodology was clinically relevant because it is built on clinicians' strengths of observations and the richness of psychological experiences that would not otherwise be captured by structured interviews or self-report instruments. Although using very different methodology, a similar outcome can be seen in the use of the Psychopathy Check List-Revised (Hare, 1991). Hare took the initial traits described by Cleckley and operationalized them in an instrument that has proven to demonstrate good inter-rater reliability and validity. The discussion of "psychopathy" is addressed in a separate chapter and only noted here as a potential methodology to more accurately describe underlying personality traits and/or disorder on a continuum of traits that has empirically validated support.

PREVALENCE OF PERSONALITY DISORDER

Prevalence studies of personality disorders have been limited and constrained by the same methodological issues related to diagnostic issues. Studies have varied substantially in estimates of frequency of specific disorders (Mattin & Zimmerman, 2001). Of note is that APD, the most common personality disorder associated with criminal behavior, is the most frequently studied personality disorder. Prevalence rates of APD vary from 2.5% to 3.5% of the population. Most patients with Personality Disorder also had Axis I disorder (Maier, Minges, Lichtermann, & Heun, 1995). Swanson et al. (1994) found individuals meeting the criteria of APD were three times more likely to also be diagnosed with an Axis I disorder although the majority of these were substance abuse disorders. Nonetheless, 25% of patients with APD had an Axis I diagnosis of a mood disorder.

Despite the limitations in diagnostic validity and reliability regarding personality disorders, forensic clinicians are often required to assess personality disorders and proffer opinions in a variety of legal proceedings. Sexual Violent Predator legislation has now been enacted in a number of states and Dangerous Offender legislation is in effect in Canada. Individuals may be declared a Sexual Violent Predator (SVP) if they meet the criteria of having a psychiatric illness or a personality disorder that renders them more likely to engage in sexual offending behavior in the future (Tucker & Brakel, 2003). Individuals may be declared a dangerous offender (DO) if they demonstrate a pattern of persistently aggressive behavior risking death, injury or severe psychological damage to others through failing to restrain his or her behavior in the future.

Further, many risk instruments used in predicting whether an individual will reoffend rely heavily on diagnoses of APD or other personality disorders.

In SVP, DO or other sentencing hearings, the prosecution may be required to prove that an accused or convicted person meets the criteria for personality disorder as a threshold test to be declared likely to reoffend with a resultant different penalty than might be imposed if the person fails to meet the criteria. Considerations of dangerousness are often reflected in longer jail sentences that may be at the upper level of what is appropriate for the offense. Testimony in sentencing or SVP hearings often involves debate over whether a person meets the minimum criteria for APD or any other personality disorder. The controversies over diagnosis, reliability, and validity are not simply academic exercises but rather carry meaningful and possibly severe consequences for affected individuals. It is incumbent upon the forensic clinician involved in such processes to be fully familiar with the limitations in the diagnosis of personality disorder, especially when using a categorical approach such as DSM-IV. In keeping with ethical standards (AAPL Ethics Code) the forensic clinician has a duty to explain the current limitations in diagnosis.

PERSONALITY DISORDER IN SEXUAL OFFENDING

A number of studies of sexual offenders have pointed to personality disorder or at least personality traits as being predictive for sexual recidivism by sexual offenders. While much of the research has focused on the use of the PCL-R as a measurement of psychopathy (Serin, Milloux, & Malcolm 2001; Seto & Barbaree, 1999), other personality traits and disorders have also been identified as predictive for sexual reoffending (Craig, Brown, & Stringer, 2003).

Hanson (2004) has updated a meta-analysis that involved a total of 31,000 sexual offenders in various recidivism and follow-up studies. The strongest predictor was sexual deviancy although it was recognized that not all sexual offenders in fact had enduring patterns of sexually deviant fantasy or behavior. The other factors predictive for future reoffending tended to be personality traits including antisocial orientation, intimacy deficits, and sexual attitudes. In many of the studies any personality disorder was grouped with the APD categories. Specific subtraits included difficulties in self-regulation such as lifestyle instability and impulsivity, unstable employment, substance abuse, and hostility. Intimacy deficits and conflicts in intimate relationships also predicted for reoffending. In review of the data, it appears that the definitions of personality disorder were more broadly applied and not necessarily conformed to DSM-IV categories. What perhaps is more relevant, especially for clinical psychiatry, is the identification of specific traits that have been identified as predictive for reoffending as these will understandably be the focus of clinical attention for both treatment purposes and risk assessment.

Studies using various personality inventories have demonstrated marked heterogeneity and variability among sexual offenders. Earlier studies failed to differentiate between sexual offenders and nonsexual offenders (Ridenour, 1997). Studies comparing sexual offenders with nonsexual violent offenders demonstrated that sexual offenders tended to be more introverted than violent offenders (Gudjensson & Sigurdson, 2000). In a large study comparing over 7,000 nonsexual offenders incarcerated in the Colorado Department of Corrections with almost 700 sexual offenders, sexual offenders were found to have much more varied personality traits and psychopathology than nonsexual offenders (Ahlmeyer, Kleinsasser, Stoner, & Retzlaff, 2003). Sexual offenders had higher incidence of schizoid, avoidant, depressive dependent, self-defeating, and schizotypal traits while most nonsexual offenders had more classical symptoms compatible with APD. Multivariate analysis demonstrated that traits consistent with dependent, narcissistic, antisocial, and schizotypal scales were the most differentiating between the groups. Sexual offenders also had more affective symptoms with significant overlap between mood disorders, anxiety, and post-traumatic stress disorders. The authors concluded that while sexual offenders and other offenders had high rates of psychopathology, the sexual offenders were more broadly pathological with increased evidence of social inadequacy, dependency, and affective disturbances. Comparisons between child molesters and rapists showed increased rate of psychopathology in child molesters.

Recent efforts to subdivide sexual offenders into more homogenous groups have helped further our knowledge about specific subtypes of offenders. Assessments of individuals with and without deviant

sexual fantasies (Curnoe & Langevin, 2002) compared sexual offenders with reported deviant fantasy with those who did not demonstrate symptoms of deviant fantasy. Those offenders who acknowledged deviant fantasy showed significantly elevated MMPI scales Sc, Pd, Mf, and Pa. Individuals with deviant fantasies also scored higher on social and emotional alienation and had higher history of family discord with evidence of increased general neuroticism. The authors raised the question as to whether individuals with deviant fantasy retreated into the deviant fantasies to escape the reality of their limited social and family involvement.

Issues of psychopathy in sexual offenders are described elsewhere in this text. What is evident from the general literature is the high rate of nonsexual offending behavior committed by sexual offenders. In studies examining antisocial attitudes, however, sexual offenders tended to endorse fewer antisocial or criminal attitudes than did nonsexual offenders (Mills, Anderson, & Kroner, 2004). Within the sexual offender group, child molesters endorsed fewer antisocial attitudes than rapists although these differences disappeared when controlled for age. Incarcerated sexual offenders with antisocial attitudes have higher rates of general and major infractions than sexual offenders who score lower on antisocial orientation (Caperton, Edens, & Johnson, 2004). An interesting study out of Finland comparing antisocial attitudes and testosterone levels amongst sexual offenders demonstrated a positive correlation between APD and the mean saliva testosterone levels (Aromaki, Lindman, & Eriksson, 2002).

Studies comparing child molesters with controls and/or other sexual offenders consistently demonstrate that child molesters show higher rates of psychopathology than the offenders who assault teenagers or adults (Cohen, Gans, & McGeoch, 2002; Kalichman, 1991). Likewise, elderly sexual offenders were differentiated from nonsexual offenders by increased rates of schizoid, obsessive–compulsive, and avoidant traits and relatively fewer antisocial traits (Fazel, Hope, O'Donnell, & Jacoby, 2002).

In examining the antisocial dimension in sexual offenders, one would assume that those who murdered and/or exhibited sexual sadistic behaviors would likely be higher on measurements of antisocial behavior or psychopathy. In a study of 20 sexually sadistic serial murderers, Warren et al. (1996) in fact found that 65% had no prior arrest history, unlike the pattern of other sexual offenders who have a high rate of nonsexual offenses. The authors argue that sexually sadistic serial murderers form a distinct subgroup that does not fit comfortably within our continuums. In contrast, Langevin (2003) studied 33 sex killers compared to 80 sexually aggressive, 23 sadists, and 611 general sexual offenders and found sexual killers showed higher rates of antisocial orientation and behavior as well as showing higher rates of paraphilic behaviors. The most common associated diagnosis was APD but he that found only 15.2% of the group met the criteria of "psychopathy." He also noted high rates of neuropsychiatric impairment and academic underachievement and possible learning disorders. Berger et al. (1999) studied 70 sexual offenders including 19 diagnosed with sadistic personality disorder. There is a high overlap between the diagnosis of sadistic personality disorder, APD, and borderline personality disorder. A factor analysis revealed four major factors that did not support a separate diagnosis of sadistic personality disorder as a discreet category but rather as an important subdimension of an APD category. Our understanding of sexually sadistic killers is curtailed by the limited numbers available for study that likely in turn lead to sample biasing.

Increasing interest has been given to identification and treatment of adolescent sexual offenders (O'Shaughnessy, 2002). Adolescent sexual offenders are clearly a heterogeneous group who are difficult to differentiate from other nonsexual offending delinquent youth. Attempts at developing typologies and path analysis have demonstrated that adolescent sexual offenders who assault prepubescent victims had increased deficits in psychosocial functioning compared to offenders choosing teen or peer-related victims (Hunter, Figuerdo, Malamuth, & Becker, 2003). The data also indicated high rates of significant depression and anxiety. Attempts at subclassifying adolescent sexual offenders into those who are primarily antisocial versus those who demonstrate deviant sexual arousal have been entertained (Becker & Murphy, 1998; Seto & Barbaree, 1997). Butler et al. (2002) did affirm that adolescent sexual offenders who only committed sexual offenses had fewer conduct disorder symptoms before the offense than those who also engaged in other antisocial behaviors. Studies generally support the model that adolescent sexual offenders in particular had difficulties in intimacy and social competence and that sexual

misbehavior in this group may be more suggestive of compensatory behavior than the true beginnings of paraphilia or APD (Hunter & Figuerdo, 2000).

PERSONALITY TRAITS IN SEXUAL OFFENDING

Attempts at differentiating sexual offenders have not been successful in clearly identifying a particular subgroup but rather have been instrumental in identifying specific traits that seem to be more relevant to certain types of offending. Traits including impulsivity and compulsivity as well as traits related to impairment in empathy and impairment in social intimacy, and relationship seem to be most frequently identified in the literature as being relevant in the assessment, and in particular, treatment of sexual offenders.

Impulsivity

Various studies, however, have held different definitions of impulsivity as a personality trait. Moeller et al. (2001) argue for three descriptive dimensions of impulsivity including (1) "decreased sensitivity to negative consequences of behavior," (2) "rapid unplanned reactions to stimuli before complete processing of information," and (3) "lack of regard for long-term consequences." Impulsivity is seen more as a predisposition or part of a general pattern as opposed to a single act. They argued for treatment of impulsivity as a trait disturbance through pharmacological interventions affecting serotonin regulation. Swann et al. (2002) identified two subdimensions of impulsivity related to psychiatric illness. Reward delay impulsivity was defined as the inability to wait for a larger reward. Rapid response impulsivity was defined as behavior occurring without adequate reflection or assessment of context. Rapid response type of impulsivity was clearly associated with lifetime Axis I or Axis II diagnoses but reward delay impulsivity was not clearly associated with psychiatric impairment. Impulsivity has in turn been associated with deficits in serotonin functioning in individuals with borderline personality disorder (Coccaro, 2001) and APD (Dolan, 2001). What is noted, however, is that a dimensional relationship between serotonin function and impulsivity seems to be applicable and raises the question as to whether serotonin agents may benefit in offenders with higher impulsivity scores.

Disorders of impulsivity have been implicated in a wide variety of psychiatric disorders including conduct disorders, personality disorders, substance abuse disorders, bipolar disorders, and various disorders of impulse control (Coccaro, 2001).

The trait of "impulsivity" must be clearly differentiated from the behavior of failure to control a sexual impulse. Different definitions of "impulsivity" have been used in the literature. Prentky and Knight (1986) identified three measures including a general lifestyle of impulsive behavior, the capacity to anticipate consequences for one's behavior, and a third dimension they described as a sense of transiency with unstable employment and aimlessness. They noted that many rapists in fact planned their activities quite carefully whereas other sexual offenders who appeared more aggressive or angry engaged in unplanned or more spontaneous sexual assaults. They postulated that the planned sexual assault was more consistent with individuals whose assault arose from underlying fantasies that had been rehearsed. They anticipated that sexual offenders with higher impulsivity often reacted out of anger and attacked victims of opportunity. The lifestyle of impulsivity domain manifested in individuals with high frequency of antisocial behavior in adolescence and adulthood and closely correlated with antisocial personality traits. Such individuals were clearly involved in serious sexual offenses. The final subtrait, transiency, was uncorrelated with the other measures and more closely associated with child molesters who had significant social and interpersonal defects characterized as schizoid-like and seclusive.

Cohen et al. (2002) questioned whether pedophiles displayed an impulsive aggressive disorder because of failure to control sexual impulses. They used standardized measurements of impulsivity as well as positron emission tomography (PET) scans in a small group of child molesters and controls. There were no differences on executive functioning although some of the scales supported an increase in impulsive personality traits in pedophiles. Overall, however, the data was more suggestive of broad interpersonal deficits amongst child molesters.

Compulsion

Sexual offending behavior has been postulated as being related to the underlying compulsive behavior (Bradford, 2001). Bancroft and Vukadinovic (2004) critically reviewed the concepts of sexual compulsivity

and impulsivity and studied a small sample of self-defined "sex addicts." This study revealed increased rates of sexual interest while individuals were in states of depression or anxiety and that out of control sexual behavior seemed to be the product of multiple factors thought to be more related to mood than compulsivity. Raymond et al. (2002) investigated compulsive sexual behavior defined as excessive sexual behavior or thoughts that lead to subjective distress or social or occupational dysfunction. In his small sample, 88% met the criteria for an Axis I disorder with predominant Mood and Anxiety Disorders. The group demonstrated more traits of impulsivity than compulsivity although it is evident that mood and anxiety disorders seemed to be more relevant to their behavior. Small case studies using serotonin uptake inhibiting antidepressants have demonstrated improvement in sexual functioning in individuals with "compulsive behaviors" (Aboush, 1999). The role of impulsivity and/or compulsivity in sexual offensive behaviors appears to be important in some offenders. Larger scale studies are required before any meaningful conclusion can be drawn about the overall significance of these traits to general sexual offending. While lifestyle impulsivity certainly is clearly associated with antisocial behaviors in individuals who commit both sexual and other nonsexual offenses, there is no clear association between impulsivity traits and sexual offending behavior.

Empathy

The role of empathy or lack of empathy in sexual misbehavior is quite complicated. Hanson (2004) in his meta-analysis did not find the lack of empathy to be significantly related to reoffending. By the same token, clinicians would be hard-pressed to accept that a sexual offender who clearly lacks any empathic awareness or concern regarding his victims would be anything less than a significant risk to reoffend. The apparent failure of correlation with lack of empathy and subsequent offending may be more related to difficulties in measuring empathy. Further, sexual offenders who have normal empathy in other zones are very effective at rationalizing their conduct to believe their behavior is not harmful to their victims.

Goliffe and Farrington (2003) completed a review and meta-analysis of research studies on empathy in general offending and sexual offending. Twenty-one studies measuring cognitive empathy and 14 measuring affective empathy were reviewed. Low scores on cognitive empathy were strongly related to general offending while affective empathy scores were only weakly related to offending. This relationship, however, was much stronger for violent offenders and tended to disappear after controlling for intelligence and socioeconomic status. They concluded that better measures of empathy were required.

Fernandez and Marshall (1999) developed a Child Molester Empathy Measure (CMEM) that designed questions to assess empathy towards the child injured in a car accident versus molested by an unknown assailant versus molested by the offender himself. In the study of 61 child molesters, the CMEM suggested relative deficit in empathy towards the offender's own victims but intact empathy to the other victims. In a follow-up study (Marshall, Hamilton, & Fernandez, 2001) child molesters showed greater cognitive distortions and empathy deficits towards their own victims compared to a sample of nonsexual offenders and nonoffending controls. There was a close association between the apparent lack of empathy and scores on a cognitive distortions scale. In contrast, Curwen (2003) examined reliability and validity of three scales including empathic concern, perspective taking, and personal distress subscales of the Interpersonal Reactivity Index. The results were counterintuitive and the authors advised caution in interpretation because of the likelihood of socially desirable responding contaminating the results. Hanson (2003) offered a model to think through the problems of perceived empathy deficits in sexual offenders. In noting the lack of empirical foundation to any relationship between measures of victim empathy and reoffending, he concluded that we needed to have a different understanding of empathy deficits in a particular individual consistent with the heterogeneity of offenders and their different types of deficits. Specifically, he noted that some offenders simply are indifferent to the pain they may be causing the victims while others simply fail to appreciate that they have caused harm or are too ashamed to admit it. He argued that treatment should focus specifically on those deficits of empathy in the particular individual.

Interpersonal Relations

Core to any deficit in personality functioning or personality disorder are deficits in interpersonal relationships. A number of studies have demonstrated impaired abilities to form and maintain adult attachments (Araji & Finklehore, 1985[1995 is correct]; Marshall & Barbaree, 1990; Marshall, 1996). Marshall (2000) viewed the impaired development of interpersonal relationships as a critical factor in the genesis of sexual offending. Marshall borrowed heavily from attachment theory to suggest that children who form insecure attachments to their parents develop impaired self-esteem and self-image as well as difficulties in social skills and building and maintaining relationships. Their need for attention led them to be vulnerable to other forms of abuse including sexual abuse. As the child matured, the sexual fantasy became contaminated with the previous sexual abuse experiences. As they experienced difficulties in attaining and maintaining stable interpersonal relationships due to their self-esteem and relationship deficits, they would turn more to sexual fantasies as a retreat. This in turn led to increased sexual preoccupation and an increased vulnerability or risk for sexual offending behavior, especially if accompanied by disinhibition. This model emphasized the confluence of multiple, different factors leading to impairment in personality functioning and interpersonal skills in addition to development of deviant sexual fantasies.

A number of studies have documented the subjective reports of increased rates of sexual abuse in the background of sexual offenders (Ryan, Miyoshi, Krugman, & Fryer, 1996; Wolfe & McGee, 1994; Worling, 1995). For the same reason, it is clear that the vast majority of individuals who have been sexually abused as children do not become sexual offenders but rather display evidence of personality disorder, substance abuse difficulties, or anxiety and mood disorders (Kendall-Tackett, Williams, & Finkelhor, 1993). Observations by Marshall on the interaction between impaired parent–child relationships and sexual abuse, however, have been in part supported by subsequent research. Craissati et al. (2002) studied sexual offenders with a measurement of parent bonding and demonstrated a significant increased rate of affectionless control style of parental bonding with sexual offenders even without any history of sexual abuse. Stirpe et al. (2003) reviewed the combined childhood victimization experiences with family of origin characterized in a Canadian forensic hospital and noted significant increase in reported sexual abuse by child molesters compared to other types of offenders. Child molesters also reported increased rates of physical discipline at home. Lambie et al.

(2002) looked at the problem by examining resiliency in those child sexual abuse survivors who did not go on to become offenders compared to a group who were offenders. Consistent with the theory by Marshall, was the observation that the nonoffender group was less likely to have fantasized and/or masturbated about the sexual abuse and had greater family and social supports and better relationship with peers. Lee et al. (2002) researched an Australian group and found similar support with data that demonstrated childhood emotional abuse and family dysfunction as well as childhood sexual abuse were developmental risk factors for sexual offending behavior, especially in child molesters. The linkage between childhood adverse experiences and personality dysfunction has long been established. Adding the dimension of child abuse or other exposure to inappropriate sexual activity seems to have increasing support as a significant risk factor for the subsequent development of deviant sexual arousal and/or sexual offending behaviors.

CONCLUSION

The two decades since the development of DSM-III have seen a substantial growth in research on personality traits and personality disorder that has challenged our assumptions and diagnostic classifications and has increased our awareness and understanding of the complexity of personality formation and pathology. The previous debates on how much a personality trait is nature versus nurture have been, in part, answered by genetic studies demonstrating significant genetic component to core personality traits (Jang & Vernon, 2001). It is also clear, however, that adverse childhood events lead to increased rates of psychiatric disorder and personality dysfunction including antisocial behaviors of all types. Research continues to identify underlying neuro-developmental and neural pathways and transmitters that play substantive roles in the manifestation of personality traits and behaviors. Over the next decade it is likely that we will move further away from viewing personality disorder in a categorical model and will increasingly recognize the value of dimensional models emphasizing specific identification of core traits and facets that in turn may be more closely related to target behaviors and treatment goals. The ability to identify specific traits related to target antisocial behaviors has specific value in forensic psychiatry, especially in the areas of risk assessment and in planning and implementing treatment and management programs for violent persons including sexual offenders. There is promise that richer clinical information regarding personality traits and functioning will substantially improve our current risk assessment process that relies far too heavily on static historical factors. As we become more adept at identifying potentially changeable factors that are empirically related to likelihood of reoffending, we will in turn be better prepared and able to monitor these traits and/or measure the impact of treatment and rehabilitation.

Increasing knowledge regarding genesis of personality traits related to subsequent antisocial behavior and sexual offending also carries great potential for the implementation of early treatment and prevention programs for youth at risk. When one looks at many of the empirically proven risk factors for sexual abuse, one is struck that there are substantial shared factors that are associated with the genesis of juvenile delinquency and general antisocial functioning as well as substance abuse. It is probable that multiple risk factors are required and that no single risk factor is sufficient to explain the genesis of sexual offending behavior. In his important paper on prediction of sexual recidivism, Hanson noted that although a number and different variety of factors are associated with sexual offending, the "breeding ground" remained an adverse family environment associated with neglect, abuse, and lack of nurturance and guidance. This family environment then leads to significant disturbance in personality formation and interpersonal relationships characterized by insecure attachments, social rejection, loneliness, and impaired social functioning. He considered that sexuality developed in such an atmosphere of deficit of intimacy would likely show similar deficits and even be associated with rage or anger. This background coupled with attitudes that permit antisocial behavior, limit empathic awareness, or lead to indifferent attitudes about the suffering of others would then result in sexual offending behavior. This model is consistent with current models of personality formation and description in which various traits along a continuum coalesce to form specific patterns of behavior.

References

Aboush, A. & Clayton, A. (1999). Compulsive voyeurism and exhibitionism: A cliical response to paroxetine. *Archives of Sexual Behavior*, 28(1), 23–30.

Ahlmeyer, S., Kleinsasser, D., Stoner, J., & Retzlaff, T. (2003). Psychopathology of incarcerated sex offenders. *Journal of Personality Disorders*, 17(4), 306–318.

American Academy of Psychiatry and the Law. *Ethics guidelines for the practice of forensic psychiatry*, Bloomfield Ct: American Academy of Psychiatry and the Law *(revised* May 2005).

American Psychiatric Association. (2000). *Diagnostic and statistical manual of mental disorders, 4th Edition*, text revision. Washington, D.C.: American Psychiatric Association.

American Psychiatric Association. (1980). *Diagnostic and statistical manual of mental disorders, 3rd Edition*. Washington, D.C.: American Psychiatric Association.

Araji, S. & Finkelhor, D. (1985). Explanations of pedophilia: Reviews of empirical research. *Bulletin of the American Academy of Psychiatry and Law*, 13(1), 17–38.

Aromaki, A. S., Lindman, R. E., & Eriksson, C. G. (2002). Testosterone, sexuality, and antisocial personality in rapists and child molesters: A pilot study. *Psychiatry Research*, 110(3), 239–247.

Bancroft, J. & Vukadinovic, Z. (2004). Sexual addiction, sexual compulsivity, sexual impulsivity, or what? Toward a theoretical model. *Journal of Sex Research*, 41(3), 225–234.

Becker, J. & Murphy, W. D. (1998). What we know and do not know about assessing and treating sex offenders. *Psychology, Public Policy, and Law*, (4), 116–137.

Berger, P., Berner, W., Bolterauer, J., & Berger, G. (1999). Sadistic personality disorder in sex offenders: Relationship to antisocial Personality Disorder and sexual sadism. *Journal of Personality Disorder*, 13(2), 175–186.

Bradford, J. (2001). The neurobiology, neuropharmacology, and pharmacological treatment of paraphilias and compulsive sexual behaviour. *Canadian Journal of Psychiatry*, 46(1), 26–34.

Butler, S. M. & Seto, M. C. (2002). Distinguishing two types of adolescent sex offenders. *Journal of the American Academy of Child and Adolescent Psychiatry*, 41(1), 83–90.

Caperton, J. D., Edens, J. F., & Johnson, J. K. (2004). Predicting sex offender institutional adjustment and treatment compliance using the Personality Assessment Inventory. *Psychological Assessment*, 16(2), 187–191.

Cleckley, H. (1976). *The mask of sanity, 5th Edition*. Mosby, MO: St. Louis.

Coccaro, E. F. (2001). Biological and treatment correlates. In W. Livesley (Ed.), *Handbook of Personality Disorders: theory, research, and treatment*. New York, NY: The Guildford Press.

Cohen, L. J., Gans, S. W., McGeoch, P. G. (2002). Impulsive personality traits in male pedophiles versus healthy controls: Is pedophilia an impulsive/aggressive disorder? *Comprehensive Psychiatry*, 43(2), 127–134.

Costa, P. T. & McCrae, R. R. (1992). Revised NEO personality inventory and the NEO 5-factor inventory. *Psychological Assessment Resources*. Florida, FL: Odessa.

Craig, L. A., Browne, K. D., & Stringer, I. (2003). Treatment and sexual offence recidivism. *Trauma, Violence, and Abuse*, 4(1), 70–89.

Craissati, J., McClurg, G., & Browne, K. (2002). Characteristics of perpetrators of child sexual abuse who have been sexually victimized as children. *Sex Abuse*, 14(3), 225–239.

Curnoe, S. & Langevin, R. (2002). Personality and deviant sexual fantasies: An examination of the MMPI's of sex offenders. *Journal of Clinical Psychology*, 58(7), 803–815.

Curwen, T. (2003). The importance of offence characteristics, victimization history, hostility, and social desirability in assessing empathy of male adolescent sex offenders. *Sex Abuse*, 15(4), 347–364.

Dolan, M. (2001). Relationship between 5H-T function and impulsivity and aggression in male offenders with Personality Disorders. *British Journal of Psychiatry*, (178), 352–359.

Duggan, C. (1993). Personality Disorder. *Current Opinion in Psychiatry*, 6, 764–768.

Eysenck, H. J. (1987). The definition of Personality Disorders and the criteria appropriate to their definition. *Journal of Personality Disorders*, 1, 211–219.

Fazel, S., Hope, T., O'Donnell, I., & Jacoby, R. (2002). Psychiatric, demographic, and personality characteristics of elderly sex offenders. *Psychological Medicine*, 32, 219–226.

Fernandez, Y. M. & Marshall, W. L. (1999). The child molester empathy measure: Description and examination of its reliability and validity. *Sex Abuse*, 11(1), 17–31.

Gudjensson, G. & Sigurdson, J. (2000). Differences and similarities between violent offenders and sex offenders. *Child Abuse and Neglect*, 24(3), 363–372.

Hanson, K. (2003). Sexual offender empathy deficits, a conceptual model. *Journal of Sexual Aggression*, 9(9), 13–23.

Hanson, K. & Morton-Bourgon, K. (2004). Predictors of sexual recidivism: An updated meta-analysis. Published by Public Safety and Emergency Preparedness Canada, Public Works and Government Services Canada.

Hare, R. D. (1991). The Hare Psychopathy Check List, Revised. Toronto, Ontario, *Multi-Health Systems*.

Hunter, J. A. & Figuerdo, A. J. (2000). The influence of personality and history of sexual victimization and the prediction of juvenile perpetrated child molestation. *Behaviour Modification*, 24(2), 241–263.

Hunter, J. A., Figuerdo, A. J., Malamuth, N. M., & Becker, J. V. (2003). Juvenile sex offenders: Towards a development of a typology. *Sexual Abuse: A Journal of Research and Treatment*, 15(1), 27–48.

Jang, K. & Vernon, P. A. (2001). Genetics. In W. J. Livesley (Ed.), *Handbook of Personality Disorders*, *theory, research, and treatment.* New York, NY: The Guildford Press.

Joliffe, D. & Farrington, D. (2004). Empathy and offending: A systematic review and meta-analysis. *Aggression and Violent Behaviour,* 9(5), 441–476 Elsevior Limited.

Kalichman, S. (1991). Psychopathology and personality characteristics of criminal sexual offenders as a function of victim age. *Archives of Sexual Behaviour,* 20(2), 187–197.

Kendall-Tackett, K. A., Williams, L. M., & Finkelhor, D. (1993). Impact of sexual abuse on children: A review and synthesis of recent empirical studies. *Psychological Bulletin,* (113), 164–180.

Lambie, I., Seymour, F., Lee, A., & Adams, P. (2002). Resiliency in the victim-offender cycle in male sexual abuse. *Sex Abuse,* 14(1), 31–48.

Langevin, R. (2003). A study of the psychosexual characteristics of sex killers: Can we identify them before it is too late? *International Journal of Offender Therapy and Comparative Criminology,* 47(4), 366–382.

Lee, J. K., Jackson, H. J., Pattison, P., & Ward, T. (2002). Developmental risk factors for sexual offending. *Child Abuse and Neglect,* 26(1), 73–92.

Livesley, W. J. (2001). Conceptual and taxonomic issues. In W. J. Livesley (Ed.), *Handbook of Personality Disorders. Theory, research, and treatment.* New York, NY: The Guildford Press.

Livesley, W. J. (2003). Diagnostic dilemmas in classifying Personality Disorder. In K. Phillips, M. First, & H. Pinkus (Eds.), *Advancing DSM Dilemmas in Psychiatric Diagnosis.* Washington, WA: American Psychiatric Association.

Livesley, W. J., Jackson, D. N., & Schroeder, M. L. (1991). Dimensions of personality pathology. *Canadian Journal of Psychiatry,* 36, 557–562.

Livesley, W. J., Jang, K. L., & Vernon, P. A. (1998). The phenotypic and genetic architecture of traits delineating Personality Disorder. *Archives of General Psychiatry,* 55, 941–948.

Maier, W., Minges, J., Lichtermann, D., & Heun, R. (1995). Personality Disorders and personality variations in relatives of patients with Bipolar Affective Disorder. *Journal of Affective Disorders,* 53, 173–181.

Marshall, W. L. (1996). Assessment, treatment, and theorizing about sexual offenders. *Criminal Justice and Behaviour,* (23), 162–199.

Marshall, W. L. & Barbaree, H. E. (1990). An integrated theory of the etiology of sexual offending. In W. L. Marshall, D. R. Laws, & H. E. Barbaree (Ed.), *Handbook of Sexual Assault: Issues, theories, and treatment of offenders* (pp. 257–275). New York, NY: Plenum.

Marshall, W. L. & Marshall, L. E. (2000). The origins of sexual offending. *Trauma, violence, and abuse. A Review Journal,* (1), 250–263.

Marshall, W. L., Hamilton, K., & Fernandez, Y. (2001). Empathy deficits and cognitive distortions in child molesters. *Sex Abuse,* 13(2), 123–130.

Mattin, J. & Zimmerman, M. (2001). Epidemiology. In W. J Livesley (Ed.), *Handbook of Personality Disorders, theory research, and treatment.* New York, NY: The Guildford Press.

Mills, J. F., Anderson, D., & Kroner, D. J. (2004). The antisocial attitudes and associates of sex offenders. *Criminal Behaviour and Mental Health,* 14(2), 134–145.

Moeller, F. G., Barratt, E. S., Dougherty, D. M., Schmitz, J. M., Swann, A. C. (2001). Psychiatric aspects of impulsivity. *American Journal of Psychiatry,* (158) 1783–1793.

Mulder, R. T. & Joyce, P. R. (1997). Temperament and the structure of Personality Disorder symptoms. *Psychological Medicine,* 27: 99–106.

O'Shaughnessy, R. (2002). Violent adolescent sexual offenders. In *Child and adolescent psychiatric clinics of North America* (pp. 749–766). Philadelphia, PA: W.B. Saunders Company.

Pukrop, R., Herpertz, S., Sass, H., Steinmeyer, E. M. (1998). Special feature: Personality and Personality Disorders: A facet theoretical analysis of the similarity relationship. *Journal of Personality Disorders,* 12, 226–246.

Prentky, R. A. & Knight, R. A. (1986). Impulsivity and the lifestyle and criminal behaviour of sex offenders. *Criminal Justice and Behaviour,* 13(2), 141–164.

Raymond, N. C., Coleman, E., & Miner, M. H. (2003). Psychiatric comorbidity and compulsive/impulsive traits in compulsive sexual behaviour. *Comprehensive Psychiatry,* 44(5), 370–380.

Raymond, N. C., Grant, J. E., Kim, S. W., & Coleman, E. (2002). Treatment of compulsive sexual behaviour with neltrexone and serotonin re-uptake inhibitors: Two case studies. *International Clinical Psychopharmacology,* 17(4), 201–205.

Ridenour, T. A., Miller, A. R., Joy, K. L., & Dean, R. S. (1997). Profile analysis of the personality characteristics of child molesters using the MMPI-2. *Journal of Clinical Psychology,* 53(6), 575–586.

Ryan, G., Miyoshi, T. J., Krugman, R. D., & Fryer, G. E. (1996). Trends in a national sample of sexually abusive youth. *Journal American Academy of Child and Adolescent Psychiatry,* 35, 17–25.

Schedler, J. & Weston, D. (2004). Dimensions of personality pathology: An alternative to the five factor model. *American Journal of Psychiatry,* 161, 1743–1754.

Schroeder, M. L., Wormworth, J. A., & Livesley, W. J. (1992). Dimensions of Personality Disorder and their relationship to the big five dimensions of personality. *Psychological Assessment,* (4), 47–53.

Serin, R. C., Milloux, D. L., & Malcolm, P. B., (2001). Psychopathy, deviant sexual arousal, and recidivism among sexual offenders. *Journal of Interpersonal Violence,* 16, 234–246.

Seto, M. C. & Barbaree, H. E. (1999). Psychopathy, treatment behaviour, and sex offender recidivism. *Journal of Interpersonal Violence*, 14, 1235–1248.

Stirpe, T. S. & Stermac, L. E. (2003). An exploration of childhood victimization and family of origin characteristics of sexual offenders against children. *International Journal of Offender Therapy and Comparative Criminology*, 47(5), 542–55.

Swann, A. C., Bjork, J. M., Moeller, F. G., & Dougherty, D. M. (2002). Two models of impulsivity: Relationship to personality traits and psychopathology. *Biological Psychiatry*, 51(12), 988–994.

Swanson, M. C., Bland, R. C., & Newman, S. C. (1994). Antisocial Personality Disorder. *Acta Psychiatrica Scandinavica*, 376 (Supplement) 63–70.

Tucker, D. E. & Brakel, S. J. (2003). Sexually violent predator laws. In R. Rosner (Ed.), *Principles and practice of forensic psychiatry*. London: Arnold Press.

Warren, J. I., Hazelwood, R. R., & Dietz, T. (1996). The sexually sadistic serial killer. *Journal of Forensic Sciences*, 41(6), 970–974.

Weston, D. & Schedler, J. (2003). Personality diagnoses in adolescents: DSM-IV Axis II diagnosis and an empirically-derived alternative. *American Journal of Psychiatry*, 160(5), 52–66.

Widiger, T. (2000). Personality disorder in the 21st Century. *Journal of Personality Disorders*, 14, 3–16.

Widiger, T. & Corbitt, E. (1994). Norman versus abnormal personality from the perspective of the DSM. In S. Strack & M. Lorr (Eds.), *Differentiating normal and abnormal personality*. New York, NY: Springer Press.

Widiger, T. & Lyna, M. (1998). Psychopathy and the five factor model of personality. In T. Millon, E. Simonsen, M. Birket-Smith, & R.D. Davis (Eds.), *Psychopathy: Antisocial, criminal, and violent behaviour* (pp. 171–187). New York, NY: Guildford Press.

Wolfe, D. A. & McGee, R. (1994). Dimensions of child maltreatment and their relationship to adolescent adjustment. *Developmental Psychopathology*, (6), 165–181.

Worling, J. R. (1995). Sexual abuse histories of adolescent male sex offenders: Differences on the basis of age and gender of their victims. *Journal Abnormal Psychology*, (104) 610–613.

Zimmerman, M. (1994). Diagnosing Personality Disorders. A review of issues and research methods. *Archives of General Psychiatry*, 51, 225–244.

Zimmerman, M. & Coryell, W. (1990). Diagnosing Personality Disorders in the community. *Archives of General Psychiatry*, 47, 527–531.

Part IV

Treatment

Chapter 12

Psychological Treatment
of Sexual Offenders

*William Marshall, Liam E. Marshall,
Geris A. Serran, and Matt D. O'Brien*

Early psychological approaches to the treatment of sexual offenders represented a variety of theoretical views (Barbaree & Marshall, 1998). However, very few of these reports provided convincing evidence of their efficacy. At that time there was little awareness of the possibility that women could offend sexually. This view persisted until very recently, so the focus of this chapter will be restricted to male sexual offenders and more specifically to adult males who offend sexually.

It was only with the advent of behavior therapy approaches in the late 1950s that a devoted concern for empirically evaluating treatment emerged (Laws & Marshall, 2003). These early behavioral programs focused on little more than the modification of sexual interests, it being accepted at the time that sexual offending resulted from acquired (through classical conditioning) deviant sexual preferences (McGuire, Carlisle, & Young, 1965). Indeed, Bond and Evans (1967) declared that it was enough to simply reduce sexual interest in deviant acts to effectively treat sexual offenders. They further claimed that once deviant sexual interests were reduced "normal outlets for the control of sexual arousal will develop" (p. 1162). Quite soon after this declaration, clinicians working with sexual offenders began to realize that the assumption that normal interests would simply emerge, was naive. Marshall (1971) was the first to point to the fallibility of this notion. He argued that if the goal was to have child molesters, for example, develop normative sexual interests, then it would be wise to have, as part of treatment, training in the skills, confidence, and attitudes necessary to function effectively in adult sexual relations. Subsequently numerous other clinicians made similar claims and, as a consequence, the 1970s saw an expansion of behaviorally-based programs to include modifications of distorted cognitions, enhancements of the capacity for empathy, and (albeit rather limited) social skills training (for a history of these early developments, see Marshall & Laws, 2003).

Leading the way in the 1970s was Gene Abel, an American psychiatrist who was instrumental in convincing various funding agencies to support research directed at furthering the understanding of sexual offenders and in developing treatment programs for these men. Descriptions of the psychological treatment approach by Abel (Abel, Blanchard, & Becker, 1978), had the effect of encouraging those providing psychological treatment of sexual offenders to include a broad range of targets in their programs. Over the subsequent years these approaches, soon called "*cognitive behavioral programs*," continuously expanded the range of treatment targets.

In the early 1980s, Janice Marques (1982) introduced the field of sexual offender treatment to the relapse prevention approach of Alan Marlatt (1982) that he used with substance abusers. On the basis of its intuitive appeal, rather than sound evidence, the relapse prevention (RP) approach was rapidly adopted by almost all cognitive behavioral programs in North America. The focus of RP was primarily on strategies for maintaining offense-free behavior after discharge from treatment. Clients were taught skills to escape from, or avoid, risky situations. The emphasis was on developing a set of avoidance plans to minimize risk.

The views underlying the RP, and the strategies associated with such an approach, was detailed in a book edited by Richard Laws (1989). Later the RP approach was criticized in a series of papers by Ward and his colleagues (Ward & Hudson, 1996; Ward, Hudson, & Marshall, 1994; Ward, Hudson, & Siegert, 1995) culminating in another edited book (Laws, Hudson, & Ward, 2000) in which a broad range of authors took issue with almost every facet of the RP approach. In that book, Marshall and Anderson (2000) demonstrated that there was no convincing evidence that the RP model enhanced the effectiveness of cognitive behavioral treatment. More importantly, the evaluation by Marques et al. (2005) of her own rather restricted RP program, failed to demonstrate any benefits within a random controlled trial. This ought to have ended the romance among sexual offender treatment providers with the RP model but, unfortunately, evidence does not always drive therapeutic endeavors, and RP lives on as the framework around which most current psychological programs operate (see survey by McGrath, Cumming, & Burchard, 2003).

As a result of changes in etiological theories of sexual offending (see Ward, 2006 for a review of such theories and their changing face over the past 30 years), as well as research indicating a broad range of dysfunctional attributes of these clients, and clinical innovations that introduced more effective procedures for changing behavior, current treatment approaches target a quite comprehensive range of issues with quite sophisticated procedures. Included in treatment are procedures aimed at: changing distorted cognitions; enhancing empathy; increasing self-esteem; equipping offenders with better coping skills; providing them with knowledge about healthy sexual functioning and about the features and benefits of enhanced intimacy; and reducing deviant sexual interests while increasing sexual arousal to adult consenting sex (see Marshall, Anderson, & Fernandez, 1999 for a detailed description of these current treatment targets). Some of these comprehensive programs appear to be more effective than others.

CONTENTIOUS ISSUES

Several issues have emerged in recent years that have generated disagreement and discussion. As is often the case in science, some of these debates, while not yet resolved, have served to increase awareness of the complexities of psychological treatment with this difficult population and have led to the development of gradually divergent treatment approaches. We will consider some of these issues here.

As mentioned earlier, despite the evidence suggesting that RP approaches may not be effective, many programs remain steadfastly wedded to this model. Among other things, this model emphasizes the need to (a) help each client develop a detailed analysis of his pattern of offending; (b) assist each offender in identifying a broad range of what are called "*high risk situations*" which are derived from his "patterns of offending"; and (c) work with each client to develop strategies for avoiding his high risks or escaping from unanticipated risks. The offense analysis is primarily concerned with identifying the offender's specific thoughts, feelings, and behaviors that occur within his typical offense chain. From this the client is assisted in recognizing the kinds of situations or events that put him at risk to reoffend and then he is given help in generating an extensive list of avoidance plans.

Critics of the RP approach have, among other things, suggested that this is a far too sophisticated process for most of the clients seen in sexual offender treatment programs (Ward & Hudson, 1996). Perhaps more importantly it has been suggested that the emphasis on avoidance goals is misplaced. Mann and her colleagues (Mann, 1998; Mann, Webster, Schofield, & Marshall, 2004) have demonstrated that having approach goals rather than avoidance goals as the primary targets of sexual offender treatment is most effective. Basic psychological research had already demonstrated that avoidance strategies are not only difficult to maintain, they are associated with repeated disappointments resulting in gloomy prospects regarding the future (Austin & Vancouver, 1996; Wegner, 1994). Approach strategies, on the other hand are easier to maintain and typically generate optimism about the future (Emmons, 1999).

This recent emphasis on approach goals is consistent with another recently introduced concept. Ward, in a series of papers (Ward & Gannon, in press; Ward & Marshall, 2004; Ward & Stewart, 2003; Ward, Vess, Collie, & Gannon, 2006) has provided evidence that humans characteristically seek what has been called a "good life" which is described as being made up of the pursuit of a list of needs covering various areas of life functioning (e.g., knowledge, mastery, autonomy, inner peace, relatedness, happiness, sexual satisfaction). Ward suggests that sexual offenders commit their offenses in the vain hope of achieving some or all of these goals; that is, he proposes that sexual offenders are seeking to meet, by their offending, the same needs that all other people seek to meet. From this Ward concludes that treatment should aim at assisting each sexual offender in identifying a unique set of positive (i.e., approach) goals that will meet his needs. Therapists can then plan treatment around providing each offender with the knowledge, skills, self-confidence and attitudes necessary to meet his needs in prosocial ways. It is Ward's belief that such an approach will eliminate the need to stamp out deviance. He argues that "a focus on the promotion of specific goods or goals in the treatment of sexual offenders (i.e., developing a good life) is likely to automatically eliminate...risk factors" (Ward et al., 2006, section in parentheses added). This approach to treatment is consistent with claims made by Marshall some time earlier (1989, 1996) and detailed in the latest book by him and his colleagues (Marshall, Marshall, Serran, & Fernandez, 2006).

Ward has consistently set his Good Lives Model approach to treatment in opposition to the so-called "Risk/Needs Model". This latter model is most clearly spelled out by Canadian researcher Don Andrews and his colleagues (Andrews & Bonta, 2001; Gendreau & Andrews, 1990). The Risk/Needs Model derives from a series of comprehensive meta-analyses of what works in the rehabilitation programs for all types of offenders, and involves three principles: (1) the *Risk Principle* which states that treatment intensity should be adjusted according to each offender's risk level (high, moderate, or low); (2) the *Need Principle* which states that treatment should address primarily (or perhaps even only) those potentially modifiable factors that have been shown to predict risk (i.e., the so-called dynamic risk factors); and (3) the *Responsivity Principle* that points to the importance of adjusting the treatment approach to the unique features (e.g., motivation, learning style, culture, and day-to-day fluctuations) of each individual.

Ward believes that the Good Lives approach, through enhancing the client's skills necessary to attain his good life, would eliminate the issues relevant to the need principle. In fact, all of the features identified so far in research on dynamic risk factors, and therefore appropriate treatment targets within the Risk/Needs model, can be seen as targets for treatment consistent with the goals of the Good Lives Model. The basic disagreement between the two models is that Ward's approach emphasizes generating approach goals whereas the Risk/Needs Model has been seen by many as more consistent with treatment based on the Relapse Prevention Model. Recent research by Mann and Webster (2002) has offered support for Ward's views. They found that many sexual offenders who refuse treatment said they would willingly enter a program if it focused on giving them a better life (i.e., a program that enhances their chances of attaining a "good life"), rather than simply addressing their offending.

This shift in focus suggested by Ward also fits well with recent research indicating a significant role for therapeutic processes in the treatment of sexual offenders, but so also does the Risk/Needs Model with its emphasis on responsivity. Unless the therapist has the skill to readily adapt to the idiosyncrasies of each client (i.e., enact the responsivity principle), and motivate the client to build a better life (i.e., the good life), his/her effectiveness will be reduced.

Several researchers have recently examined the influence of process features in the treatment of sexual offenders. Beech and his colleagues (Beech & Fordham, 1997; Beech & Hamilton-Giachritsis, 2005) demonstrated that it was only those treatment groups that functioned cohesively and encouraged expressiveness (including emotional expressions) that generated the sought-after treatment changes. Cognitive behavioral treatment groups that did not have these features, failed to produce benefits. Pfäfflin et al. (2005) also found that emotional expressiveness was crucial to the attainment of beneficial treatment changes with sexual offenders. An examination of the influence of the therapist's behaviors in two studies (Marshall, Serran, Fernandez, Mulloy, Mann, & Thornton, 2002; Marshall, Serran, Moulden, Mulloy, Mann, & Thornton, 2003) revealed that therapists who were empathic, warm, rewarding, and somewhat directive, produced maximal benefits in their sexual offender clients. In addition, Marshall et al. found that an aggressive confrontational approach essentially eliminated any positive changes that might otherwise have occurred. Drapeau (2005) found that sexual offenders reported that while they found some of the procedures employed during treatment to be helpful, they believed it was the way the group therapist responded that was critical to them deriving benefits from the program. Essentially these offenders identified as crucial, the same therapist features that Marshall et al. (2002, 2003) had demonstrated to be effective.

Clearly the behavior of therapists plays a vital role in successful treatment programs for sexual offenders. Indeed, in the study by Marshall et al. (2002) the influence of the crucial therapist features was quite dramatic, accounting for as much as 60% of the variance in beneficial changes. This is dramatically more than is typically found in psychotherapy with other problem behaviors (usually approximately 20 to 25%) (Martin, Graske, & Davis, 2000). No doubt this is because sexual offenders are typically reluctant clients, at least in the early stages of treatment. Sexual offender therapists, therefore, need to have good motivational skills which characteristically include the display of warmth, empathy, and rewardingness. The introduction to the field of motivational interviewing approach by Miller and Rollnick (1991) and by Mann and her colleagues (Mann, 1996; Mann, Ginsberg, & Weekes, 2002; Mann & Rollnick, 1996) provided specific guidelines for engaging sexual offenders.

An additional contentious issue concerns the debate about the value, or otherwise, of providing therapists with detailed treatment manuals. When treatment is provided in several locations by the same service, it is usually considered necessary to ensure that all treatment providers deliver the same program. Similarly, agencies providing funding to evaluate treatment consistently demand that treatment integrity be guaranteed, again requiring detailed treatment manuals. Such manuals have become so widespread that some programs describe their treatment as "psychoeducational" (Green, 1995), where treatment involves a rather heavy emphasis on the imparting of knowledge and where all clients get precisely the same program. In treatment evaluation, those who advocate the use of the Random Controlled Trial design, likewise insist on the use of a highly detailed treatment manual.

This "one size fits all" approach has been critically evaluated by Laws and Ward (2006) and found to be seriously wanting. In fact, this manualized approach defies the responsivity principle of the Risk/Needs Model as well as the recent research findings showing the important influence of the therapist. The flexibility needed to follow the responsivity principle is eliminated by the requirement that the therapist rigidly follow the detailed manual, and as a result the influence of the therapist's style of delivery is diminished. In addition this "one size fits all" approach contradicts the idea that pretreatment assessments or case formulations (Drake & Ward, 2003) should guide differential foci in treatment on individually-determined needs. A more flexible approach, as demanded by both the Risk/Needs Model and the Good Lives Model, fits better with current knowledge about sexual offenders and their needs, than does the overly manualized approach.

The combination of the responsivity principle from the Risk/Needs Model, Ward's Good Lives Model, motivational interviewing, and the importance of therapeutic processes, has moved psychological treatments for sexual offenders to a new, and hopefully more effective, plane. This new approach has been outlined in two recent publications (Marshall et al., 2006; Marshall, Ward, Mann, Moulden, Fernandez, Serran, & Marshall, 2005). These two publications provide details of this more positive approach which downplays the need to focus on the offender's past offensive behaviors and shifts the emphasis to the future and to the development of a more fulfilling life. The following section briefly describes this recent approach.

AN INTEGRATED POSITIVELY-ORIENTED TREATMENT PROGRAM

First it is important to note that to be fully effective, a psychological treatment program must include the use of medications where necessary. Not only do many sexual offenders have comorbid disorders (Marshall, in press a) that require both medications and an adjustment to the treatment approach (i.e., the responsivity principle), some have such a strong sexual drive, or are so sexually preoccupied, that medications are required to either reduce libido or to reduce the compulsivity associated with sexual expression. The various antiandrogens or hormonal treatments can usefully serve to reduce sex drive intensity, while the selective serotonin reuptake inhibitors (SSRIs) can reduce compulsivity (Bradford, 2000; Greenberg & Bradford, 1997). However, it is necessary to develop guidelines for deciding when these medications are required. Bradford (2000) has described his algorithm for deciding when to use medications, and with whom to use these drugs, and we (Marshall & Hillen, 2002) have developed a guide to assist in similar decisions within a prison setting. Over the past 20 years fewer than 10% of our clients have been placed on antiandrogens or an SSRI.

Table 12.1 describes the offense-specific treatment targets and the offense-related problematic issues. All sexual offenders participate in psychological treatment that addresses the offense-specific targets while those who have problems with one or another of the offense-related issues are placed in one or another specialist-led programs.

Since there are numerous books that outline in detail the approaches to each of the offense-related problems (e.g., Brown, 2005; Carich & Calder, 2003; Marshall et al., 1999; Marshall et al., 2006), we will provide only a brief description of the procedures involved in targeting the issues. The reader should note that these procedures are implemented in a maximally effective way when the therapist displays empathy and warmth, is rewarding, and provides some degree of directiveness (see studies by Marshall et al., 2002, 2003, for the research bases for this claim).

TABLE 12.1 Treatment Targets

Offense-specific	Offense-related
Self-esteem.	Substance use/abuse.
Life history.	Anger management.
Acceptance of responsibility.	Cognitive skills
Offense pathways.	(Reasoning and
Coping/mood management.	rehabilitation).
Social and relationship	Other psychological
skills.	problems.
Sexual interests.	
Self-management plans.	

A motivational approach that is future-oriented and that encourages the client to be optimistic about his future, is also essential.

Self-Esteem

This is targeted first to enhance the client's belief that he has the strengths necessary to change. Also low self-esteem is predictive of relapse among sexual offenders (Thornton, Beech, & Marshall, 2004). We refer to our clients as men who have committed a sexual offense and we insist they use the same descriptor rather than referring to themselves as rapists or child molesters or exhibitionists. This serves to distinguish the client from his offensive behavior and reduces feelings of shame which have been shown to stand in the way of change (Tangney & Dearing, 2002). We also encourage clients to increase the range and frequency of their social activities and we assist them in identifying the small pleasures they enjoy; both these procedures have been shown to increase self-esteem (Marshall & Christie, 1982; Marshall, Christie, Lanthier, & Cruchley, 1982). In addition, we elicit from each client a list of at least 4 to 6 positive statements about himself and have him rehearse these statements several times each day. We have shown the combination of all these procedures to be effective in enhancing overall levels of self-confidence in sexual offenders (Marshall, Champagne, Sturgeon, & Bryce, 1997). An increase in self-esteem in sexual offenders is significantly correlated with improvements in empathy, intimacy, and loneliness (Marshall, Champagne, Brown, & Miller, 1997) and with reductions in deviant sexual arousal (Marshall, 1997).

Autobiography

Concurrent with enhancing self-esteem, clients are instructed to begin the process of generating an account of their life history. This autobiography is to encompass childhood, adolescence, and adult experiences focusing on issues such as relationships (including sexual relations), health, education, work, and leisure. From this the therapist helps the client identify events or problematic ways of living that can create a state where sexual offending seems attractive.

Acceptance Of Responsibility

This is a process that continues throughout treatment and involves firm but supportive challenges of antisocial or offense-supportive views or attitudes. However since denial bears no relationship to long-term recidivism (Hanson & Bussière, 1998; Hanson & Morton-Bourgon, 2004), clients should not be vigorously pressed to agree with every detail of the official statement of the offense. The goal is not so much rehashing the past but rather encouraging clients to take responsibility for all aspects of their life, most particularly their future.

Pathways To Offending

Therapists should begin quite early in treatment to help each client develop a set of pathways that describe the steps involved in their offending. Two sets of factors are relevant have: (1) Background factors that describe the disruptive events in their life (e.g., problems in adult relationships, loss of job, financial difficulties, psychological and emotional disorders) that might make them vulnerable to temptations to offend; and (2) the typical steps they take to offend when they are in their vulnerable state. Ward and Sorbello (2003) have outlined an empirically derived model describing several pathways that generates sexual offending, and the accuracy of this model has been independently confirmed (Bickley & Beech, 2002; Yates, Kingston, & Hall, 2003). The main point of Ward's model is that each offender may follow different pathways on different occasions; that is, sexual offenders do not seem to maintain a specific modus operandi nor is their need to offend constant nor always driven by the same background factors. This is important to keep in mind when identifying future potential risks; clients must be encouraged to develop a generic disposition toward risk rather than generate a limited list of specific risk factors derived solely from past experiences.

Victim Harm/Empathy

Research suggests that sexual offenders are not deficient in general empathy but rather they appear to suspend empathy toward their victims (Polaschek, 2003). Accordingly sexual offenders' lack of empathy for their victims can be best construed as yet another of their distorted cognitions that serves to allow them to continue to offend. Many sexual offenders, particularly child molesters, claim to have information indicating that their victim has not suffered any consequences of the abuse. In our view there are two

reasons why it is pointless to challenge clients on this issue. First, the therapist has no way of demonstrating that the victim did suffer damaging consequents however much he/she may believe that to be true; and second, it seems irrelevant to discuss possible harm in the past when what we are attempting to do is alert the offender to the very real possibility of harm should he offend again in the future. Consequently the best approach is to attempt to instill in the offender the idea that he can never be sure what the consequences to a future victim may be but he can be confident based on the evidence that the chances of harm are high. This is best achieved by having the group of offenders generate a list of all possible consequences to sexual abuse and the kind of features (often seemingly benign) that increase the negative consequences.

Nevertheless it may be useful to sensitize the client to the possibility that he has harmed his past victims. To do this, most programs have offenders write hypothetical letters from and to one of their victims. These letters should contain the specification of negative consequences and an indication of responsibility by the offender. These procedures have been shown to effectively enhance victim empathy (Marshall, O'Sullivan, & Fernandez, 1996).

Relationship Skills

The assumption underlying numerous theories of sexual offending is that these men lack the skills, confidence, and the attitudes necessary to meet their needs prosocially so they turn instead to deviant behaviors in a vain attempt to satisfy these vaguely understand needs (Marshall & Marshall, 2000; Smallbone, 2006; Ward, Hudson, & McCormack, 1997). If these theories are correct, and there is considerable evidence indicating a lack of intimacy and poor attachment in sexual offenders (Bumby & Hansen, 1997; Marshall, 1993; Ward, Hudson, & Marshall, 1996), then obviously increasing the capacity of these men to function effectively in intimate relationships should be an essential feature of sexual offender treatment.

In fact training in general social skills has long been part of such treatment programs (Abel, Blanchard, & Becker, 1978; Barlow, 1974; Marshall, 1971). Recently treatment has focused more specifically on training relationship skills with sexual offenders with most programs simply adopting procedures that have been developed within the more general field of marital and relationship counselling (Jacobson & Margolin, 1979). Assisting sexual offenders to develop skills related to communication, reciprocity, empathy, sexuality, and shared leisure activities is an essential feature of sexual offender treatment programs as are procedures to help them learn how to deal with being alone or with feelings of jealousy. Comprehensive approaches such as these have been shown to markedly increase the capacity for intimacy among sexual offenders as well as reduce their experience of loneliness (Marshall, Bryce, Hudson, Ward, & Moth, 1996).

Coping and Mood Management

Clients are provided a description of both functional and dysfunctional coping styles (see Parker & Endler, 1996) and assisted in identifying their typical style. They are taught how to employ good problem-solving skills and are given the opportunity to role-play possible responses to situations from their past with which they previously did not effectively cope. Where necessary, training in specific coping skills is introduced. It is quite common, for example, for rapists to respond to problems with anger while child molesters are frequently unassertive (Segal & Marshall, 1985), and both groups tend to turn to sex to deal with distressing experiences (Cortoni & Marshall, 2001).

In addition, sexual offenders have problems regulating their emotions (Ward & Hudson, 2000) and these difficulties have been identified as dynamic risk factors for sexual offending (Hanson & Harris, 2000). Emotional dysregulation has been shown to be related to various problems (Lewis & Haviland-Jones, 2000) many of which characterize sexual offenders. On the basis of a combination of therapeutic approaches that encourage emotional expression and the development of emotional regulation (e.g., Greenberg & Pavio, 1997; Kennedy-Moore & Watson, 1999) we have developed a component of our program that specifically addresses these issues (Marshall et al., 2006). We have evaluated these two components of our program (i.e., coping and mood management) and found that, indeed, they do produce the sought-after results (Serran, Firestone, Marshall, & Moulden, in press).

Sexual Interests

Behavioral procedures for reducing deviant sexual interests and enhancing interests in appropriate sexual activities include: foul odor aversion, ammonia aversion, covert sensitization, orgasmic reconditioning, and satiation therapy. These procedures have been described in detail elsewhere (Laws & Marshal, 1991; Marshall, Marshall, & O'Brien, in press), but, although they are in common use in sexual offender treatment programs (see McGrath et al., 2003), the evidence supporting their efficacy is generally rather weak. Satiation therapy (Marshall, 1979; Marshall & Lippens, 1977) has the strongest empirical support although there are well-controlled single case studies demonstrating the effectiveness of some of the other procedures. As noted earlier in this chapter, medications (e.g., antiandrogens, hormonal agents, and the SSRIs) can also be helpful in altering problematic sexual interests and their expression.

SELF-MANAGEMENT PLANS

Earlier we pointed to recent changes in the focus and emphases in sexual offender treatment. These changes are nowhere more evident than in this final stage of treatment where the introduction of the Good Lives Model and the focus on approach goals, has substantially altered this final element in treatment. It is still considered essential to identify some risk factors but the emphasis is on developing future goals, and the skills necessary to strive toward these goals, rather than on traditional relapse prevention plans. Child molesters, for example, must avoid being alone with children, and rapists must avoid situations within which they previously offended (e.g., the hitchhiker rapists must avoid driving alone where possible). Since the offenses of exhibitionists are not so situationally-bound (they often seize opportunities to expose in a wide variety of circumstances), risky situations are more difficult to identify, but it is possible to identify some circumstances to avoid.

The Good Lives Model identifies nine areas of functioning (see Table 12.2) that have been shown in the general psychological research literature to be functionally related to the achievement of a fulfilled life (Deci & Ryan, 2000; Emmons, 1999; Schmuck & Sheldon, 2001). Every target of sexual offender treatment is, in essence, providing these clients with the skills, self-confidence, and attitudes necessary to embark on the pursuit of each client's, individually-designed, good life. In the final stage of treatment, the therapist helps the client organize his future

TABLE 12.2 Focus of the Good Lives Model

A. *Human needs are* propensities in various areas of functioning that determine the necessary conditions for well-being and fulfillment.

B. *Areas of functioning* that are typically pursued in people who are moving toward fulfillment are as follows:

1. General healthy/optimal functioning.
2. Knowledge.
3. Mastery.
4. Autonomy.
5. Inner peace.
6. Relatedness.
7. Spirituality.
8. Happiness.
9. Creativity.

goals, identify each step in the plans necessary to move toward these goals, and pursue any future skills training (e.g., upgrade his education) that is required to achieve his goals.

In addition, the therapist works with the client to develop a support group, the members of which will assist him in reintegrating back into society. Each member of the support group should have an identified set of responsibilities commensurate with the support person's capacities. Some will be professionals (e.g., probation or parole supervisor, treatment provider) while others will be family or friends. Wilson and his colleagues (Wilson & Picheca, in press; Wilson, Stewart, Stirpe, Barrett, & Cripps, 2000) have developed what they call "Circles of Support and Accountability" for sexual offenders released from prison at the end of their sentence where there would otherwise be no supervision. They have shown this to be effective in reducing recidivism in these high risk offenders, and the program has been adopted by others.

CONCLUSION

Evaluating the long-term effectiveness of sexual offender treatment is beset with difficulties (Barbaree, 1997) and few programs have the resources or endurance to conduct a satisfactory evaluation. Some maintain that psychological treatment with sexual offenders has not yet been satisfactorily demonstrated to be effective (Rice & Harris, 2003), but these authors seem to set standards for what they would regard as satisfactory evaluations at a level beyond what most programs can implement. For example, they claim that the only basis for inferring treatment effectiveness rests on conducting a Random Controlled Trial (RCT). This design requires that volunteers for treatment be randomly allocated to treatment or no-treatment, and then released to the community for several years to determine how many reoffend. The practical, ethical, and design problems with this approach have been spelled out quite clearly both in the general clinical literature (Persons & Silberschatz, 1998; Seligman, 1995, 1996) and in the offender literature (Hollin, in press; Marshall, 2006, in press b), so we will not elaborate those discussions here.

The view taken by the committee appointed by the *Association for the Treatment of Sexual Abusers* (Hanson, Gordon, Harris, Marques, Murphy, Quinsey, & Seto, 2002) was that evaluations relying on official recidivism data and having a reasonably satisfactory comparison group, could enter a meta-analysis designed to determine the effects of treatment with sexual offenders. From a worldwide search 43 such studies were located, which, when combined, demonstrated an overall effect for treatment on both sexual and general recidivism. A further examination showed cognitive behavioral programs produced the most benefits and a subsequent, larger meta-analysis by Lösel and Schmucker (2005) demonstrated even greater effects for such programs. We (briefly reported in Marshall et al., 2006) recently evaluated our program operated in a Canadian federal prison. The actuarially calculated risk level of sexual offenders in this evaluation was 16.8% for sexual offenses and 40% for general nonsexual offending. Of our 534 treated sexual offenders released into the community for an average of 5.4 years, only 3.2% reoffended sexually and only 13.6% committed a subsequent nonsexual offense. Similar findings for the effectiveness of other sexual offender programs operated within Canadian federal prisons have been described (Barbaree, Langton, & Peacock, 2004; Looman, Abracen, & Nicholaichuk, 2000; Nicholaichuk, Gordon, Gu, & Wong, 2000).

There is, therefore, evidence that at the very least encourages optimism about the value of psychological treatment with sexual offenders. On the basis of accepting that sexual offender treatment has been shown to be effective, Marshall and McGuire (2003) demonstrated that the effect sizes of sexual offender treatment was comparable to the effect sizes produced by medical treatments for some common disorders and comparable to the treatment of various other psychological problems. Finally, when sexual offender treatment is effective, it not only saves future possible victims from suffering, it is also financially cost-effective (Marshall, 1992; Prentky & Burgess, 1990).

References

Abel, G. G., Blanchard, E. B., & Becker, J. V. (1978). An integrated treatment program for rapists. In I. R. Rada (Ed.), *Clinical aspects of the rapist* 9 (pp. 161–124). New York: Grupe & Stratton.

Andrews, D. A. & Bonta, J. (2001). *The psychology of criminal conduct, 3rd Edition.* Cincinnati, OH: Anderson.

Austin, J. T. & Vancouver, J. B. (1996). Goal constructs in psychology: Structure, process, and content. *Psychological Bulletin, 120,* 338–375.

Barbaree, H. E. (1997). Evaluating *treatment* efficacy with *sexual* offenders: The insessitivity of recidivism studies to treatment effects. *Sexual Abuse: A Journal of Research and Treatment, 9,* 111–128.

Barbaree, H. E., Langton, C., & Peacock, E. (2004, October). *The evaluation of sex offender treatment efficacy using samples stratified by levels of actuarial risk.* Paper presented at the 23rd Annual Research and Treatment Conference of the Association for the Treatment of Sexual Abusers. Albuquerque, NM.

Barbaree, H. E. & Marshall, W. L. (1998). Treatment of the sexual offender. In R. M. Wettstein (Eds.), *Treatment of offenders with mental disorders* (pp. 265–328). New York, NY: Guilford Press.

Barlow, D. H. (1974). The treatment of sexual deviation: Towards a comprehensive behavioral approach. In K. S. Calhoun, H. E. Adams, & K. M. Mitchell (Eds.), *Innovative treatment methods in psychopathology.* New York, NY: John Wiley & Sons.

Beech, A. R. & Fordham, A. S. (1997). Therapeutic climate of sexual offender treatment programs. *Sexual Abuse: A Journal of Research and Treatment, 9,* 219–237.

Beech, A. R. & Hamilton-Giachritsis, C. E. (2005). Relationship between therapeutic climate and treatment outcome in group-based sexual offender treatment programs. *Sexual Abuse: A Journal of Research and Treatment, 17,* 127–140.

Bickley, J. A. & Beech, A. R. (2002). An empirical investigation of the Ward and Hudson Self-regulation model of the sexual offence process with child abusers. *Journal of Interpersonal Violence, 17,* 371–393.

Bond, I. K. & Evans, D. R. (1967). Avoidance therapy: Its use in two cases of underwear fetishism. *Canadian Medical Association Journal, 96,* 1160–1162.

Bradford, J. M. W. (2000). The treatment of sexual deviation using a pharmacological approach. *Journal of Sex Research, 3,* 248–257.

Brown, S. (2005). *Treating sex offenders: An introduction to sex offender treatment programmes.* Cullumpton, UK: Willan Publishing.

Bumby, K. M. & Hansen, D. J. (1997). Intimacy deficits, fear of intimacy, and loneliness among sex offenders. *Criminal Justice and Behavior, 24,* 315–331.

Carich, M. S. & Calder, M. C. (2003). *Contemporary treatment of adult male sex offenders.* Lyme Regis, UK: Russell House Publishing.

Cortoni, F. A. & Marshall, W. L. (2001). Sex as a coping strategy and its relationship to juvenile sexual history and intimacy in sexual offenders. *Sexual Abuse: A Journal of Research and Treatment, 13,* 27–43.

Deci, E. L. & Ryan, R. M. (2000). The "what" and "why" of goal pursuits: Human needs and the self-determination of behavior. *Psychological Inquiry, 11,* 227–268.

Drake, C. R. & Ward, T. (2003). Treatment models for *sex* offenders: A move toward a formulation-based approach. In T. Ward, D. R. Laws, & S. M. Hudson (Eds.), *Sexual deviance: Issues and controversies* (pp. 226–243). Thousand Oaks, CA: Sage Publications.

Drapeau, M. (2005). Research on the processes involved in treating sexual offenders. *Sexual Abuse: A Journal of Research and Treatment, 17,* 117–125.

Emmons, R. A. (1999). *The psychology of ultimate concerns.* New York, NY: Guilford Press.

Gendreau. P. & Andrews, D. A. (1990). Tertiary prevention: What the meta-analyses of the offender treatment literature tell us about what works. *Canadian Journal of Criminology, 32,* 173–184.

Green, R. (1995). Psycho-educational modules. In B. K. Schwartz & H. R. Cellini (Eds.), *The sex offender: Corrections, treatment and legal practice* (pp. 13.1–13.10). Kingston, NJ: Civic Research Institute.

Greenberg, D. M. & Bradford, J. M. W. (1997). Treatment of the paraphilic disorders: A review of the role of the selective serotonin reuptake inhibitors. *Sexual Abuse: A Journal of Research and Treatment, 9,* 349–360.

Greenburg, L. S. & Pavio, S. (1997). *Working with emotions in psychotherapy.* New York, NY: Guilford Press.

Hanson, R. K. & Bussière, M. T. (1998). Predicting relapse: A meta-analysis of sexual offender recidivism studies. *Journal of Consulting and Clinical Psychology, 66,* 348–362.

Hanson, R. K., Gordon, A., Harris, A. J. R., Marques, J. K., Murphy, W. D., Quinsey, V. L., & Seto, M. C. (2002). First report of the Collaborative Outcome Data Project on the effectiveness of psychological treatment of sex offenders. *Sexual Abuse: A Journal of Research and Treatment, 14,* 169–195.

Hanson, R. K. & Harris, A. J. R. (2000). Where should we intervene? Dynamic predictors of sex offender recidivism. *Criminal Justice and Behavior, 27,* 6–35.

Hanson, R. K. & Morton-Bourgon, K. (2004). *Predictors of sexual recidivism: An updated meta-analysis.*

(Cat. No. P53–1/2004–2E-PDF) Ottawa: Public Works and Government Services Canada.

Hollin, C. R. Offending behaviour programmes and contention: Evidence-based practice, manuals, and programme evaluation. In C. R. Hollin & E. J. Palmer (Eds.), *Offending behaviour programmes: Development, application, and controversies.* Chichester, UK: John Wiley & Sons (in press).

Jacobson, N. S. & Margolin, G. (1979). *Marital therapy: Strategies based on social learning and behavior exchange principles.* New York, NY: Brunner/Mazel.

Kennedy-Moore, E. & Watson, J. C. (1999). *Expressing emotion: Myths, realities, and therapeutic strategies.* New York, NY: Guilford Press.

Laws, D. R. (Ed.). (1989). *Relapse prevention with sex offenders.* New York, NY: Guilford Press.

Laws, D. R., Hudson, S. M., & Ward, T. (Eds.). (2000). *Remaking relapse prevention with sex offenders.* Thousand Oaks, CA: Sage Publications.

Laws, D. R. & Marshall, W. L. (1991). Masturbatory reconditioning with sexual deviates: An evaluative review. *Advances in Behaviour Research and Therapy, 13,* 13–25.

Laws, D. R. & Marshall, W. L. (2003). A brief history of behavioral and cognitive-behavioral approaches to sexual offender treatment: Part 1. Early developments. *Sexual Abuse: A Journal of Research and Treatment, 15,* 75–92.

Laws, D. R. & Ward, T. (2006). When one size doesn't fit all: The reformulation of relapse prevention. In W. L. Marshall, T. M. Fernand, L. E. Marshall, & G. A. Serran (Eds.), *Sexual offender treatment: Controversial issues* (pp.241–254). Chishester, UK: John Wiley & Sons.

Lewis, M. & Haviland-Jones, J. (Eds.). (2000). *Handbook of emotions.* New York, NY: Guilford.

Looman, J., Abracen, J., & Nicholaichuk, T. P. (2000). Recidivism among treated sexual offenders and matched controls: Data from the Regional Treatment Centre (Ontario). *Journal of Interpersonal Violence, 15,* 279–290.

Lösel, F. & Schmucker, M. (2005). The effectiveness of treatment for sexual offenders: A comprehensive meta-analysis. *Journal of Experimental Criminology, 1,* 1–29.

Mann, R. E., (Ed.). (1996). *Motivational interviewing with sex offenders: A practice manual* NOTA, P.O. 508, Hull, UK.

Mann, R. E. (1998, October). Relapse prevention? Is that the bit where they told me all the things I couldn't do anymore? Paper presented at the 17th Annual Research and Treatment Conference of the Association for the Treatment of Sexual Abusers, Vancouver.

Mann, R. E. (2000). Managing resistance and rebellion in relapse prevention intervention. In D. R. Laws, S. M. Hudson & T. Ward (Eds.), *Remaking relapse prevention with sex offenders* (pp. 187–200). Thousand Oaks, CA: Sage Publications.

Mann, R. E., Ginsberg, J. I. D., & Weekes, J. R. (2002). Motivational interviewing with offenders. In M. McMurran (Ed.), *Motivating offenders to change: A guide to enhancing engagement in therapy* (pp. 87–102). Chichester, UK: John Wiley & Sons.

Mann, R. E. & Rollnick, S. (1996). Motivational interviewing with a sex offender who believed he was innocent. *Behavioral and Cognitive Psychotherapy, 24,* 127–134.

Mann, R. E. & Webster, S. (2002, October). Understanding resistance and denial. Paper presented at the 21st Annual Research and Treatment Conference of the Association for the Treatment of Sexual Abusers, Montreal.

Mann, R. E., Webster, S. D., Schofield, C., & Marshall, W. L. (2004). Approach versus avoidance goals in relapse prevention with sexual offenders. *Sexual Abuse: A Journal of Research and Treatment, 16,* 65–75.

Marlatt, G. A. (1982). Relapse prevention: A self-control program for the treatment of addictive behaviors. In R. B. Stuart (Ed.), *Adherence, compliance, and generalization in behavioral medicine* (pp. 329–378). New York, NY: Brunner/Mazel.

Marques, J. K. (1982, March). Relapse prevention: A self-control model for the treatment of sex offenders. Paper presented at the 7th Annual Forensic Mental Health Conference, Asilmoar, CA.

Marques, J. K., Weideranders, M., Day, D. M, Nelson, C., & van Ommeren, A. (2005). Effects of a relapse prevention program on sexual recidivism: Final results from California's Sex Offender Treatment and Evaluation Project (SOTEP). *Sexual Abuse: A Journal of Research and Treatment, 17,* 79–107.

Marshall, W. L. (1971). A combined treatment method for certain sexual deviations. *Behaviour Research and Therapy, 9,* 292–294.

Marshall, W. L. (1979). Satiation therapy: A procedure for reducing deviant sexual arousal. *Journal of Applied Behavior Analysis, 12,* 10–22.

Marshall, W. L. (1992). The social value of treatment for sexual offenders. *The Canadian Journal of Human Sexuality, 1*(3), 109–114.

Marshall, W. L. (1989). Intimacy, loneliness and sexual offenders. *Behaviour Research and Therapy. 27,* 491–503.

Marshall, W. L. (1993). The role of attachment, intimacy, and loneliness in the etiology and maintenance of sexual offending. *Sexual and Marital Therapy, 8,* 109–121.

Marshall, W. L. (1996). Assessment, treatment, and theorizing about sex offenders: Developments during the past 20 years and future directions. *Criminal Justice and Behavior, 23,* 162–199.

Marshall, W. L. (1997). The relationship between self-esteem and deviant sexual arousal in nonfamilial child molesters. *Behavior Modification, 21,* 86–96.

Marshall, W. L. (2006). Appraising treatment outcome with sexual offenders. In W. L. Marshall, Y. M. Fernandez, L. E. Marshall & G. A. Serran (Eds.),

Sexual offender treatment: Controversial issues (pp. 255–273). Chichester, UK: John Wiley & Sons.

Marshall, W. L. Diagnostic issues, multiple paraphilias, and comorbid disorders in sexual offenders: Their incidence and treatment. *Aggression and Violent Behavior: A Review Journal* (in press a).

Marshall, W. L. The random controlled trial: An optimal or problematic approach to the evaluation of the effectiveness of sexual offender treatment. *NOTA News* (in press b).

Marshall, W. L. & Anderson, D. (2000). Do relapse prevention components enhance treatment effectiveness? In D. R. Laws, S. M. Hudson & T. Ward (Eds.), *Remaking relapse prevention with sex offenders: A sourcebook* (pp. 39–55). Newbury Park, CA: Sage Publication.

Marshall, W. L., Anderson, D., & Fernandez, Y. M. (1999). *Cognitive behavioural treatment of sexual offenders.* Chichester, UK: John Wiley & Sons.

Marshall, W. L., Bryce, P., Hudson, S. M., Ward, T., & Moth, B. (1996). The enhancement of intimacy and reduction of loneliness among child molesters. *Legal and Criminological Psychology, 1,* 95–102.

Marshall, W. L., Champagne, F., Brown, C., & Miller, S. (1997). Empathy, intimacy, loneliness, and self-esteem in nonfamilial child molesters. *Journal of Child Sexual Abuse, 6,* 87–97.

Marshall, W. L., Champagne, F., Sturgeon, C., & Bryce, P. (1997). Increasing the self-esteem of child molesters. *Sexual Abuse: A Journal of Research and Treatment, 9,* 321–333.

Marshall, W. L. & Christie, M. M. (1982). The enhancement of social self-esteem. *Canadian Counsellor, 16,* 82–89.

Marshall, W. L., Christie, M. M., Lanthier, R. D., & Cruchley, J. (1982). The nature of the reinforcer in the enhancement of social self-esteem. *Canadian Counsellor, 16,* 90–96.

Marshall, W. L., & Hillen, J. (2002). Guidelines for medical and behavioral interventions for the reduction of deviant or excessive sexual expression in sexual offenders. Ontario, Bath: Bath Institution. Unpublished manuscript.

Marshall, W. L. & Laws, D. R. (2003). A brief history of behavioral and cognitive behavioral approaches to sexual offender treatment: Part 2. The modern era. *Sexual Abuse: A Journal of Research and Treatment, 15,* 93–120.

Marshall, W. L. & Lippens, K. (1977). The clinical value of boredom: A procedure for reducing inappropriate sexual interests. *Journal of Nervous and Mental Diseases, 165,* 283–287.

Marshall, W. L. & Marshall, L. E. (2000). The origins of sexual offending. *Trauma, Violence, & Abuse: A Review Journal, 1,* 250–263.

Marshall, W. L., Marshall, L. E., & O'Brien, M. D. Behavioral modification procedures. In A. R. Beech, L. A. Craig & K. D. Browne (Eds.), *Assessment and treatment of sexual offenders: A handbook.* Chichester, UK: John Wiley & Sons (in press).

Marshall, W. L., Marshall, L. E., Serran, G. A., & Fernandez, Y. M. (2006). *Treating sexual offenders: An integrated approach.* New York, NY: Routledge.

Marshall, W. L. & McGuire, J. (2003). Effect sizes in treatment of sexual offenders. *International Journal of Offender Therapy and Comparative Criminology, 46,* 653–663.

Marshall, W. L., O'Sullivan, C., & Fernandez, Y. M. (1996). The enhancement of victim empathy among incarcerated child molesters. *Legal and Criminological Psychology, 1,* 95–102.

Marshall, W. L., Serran, G. A., Fernandez, Y. M., Mulloy, R., Mann, R. E., & Thornton, D. (2003). Therapist characteristics in the treatment of sexual offenders: Tentative data on their relationship with indices of behaviour change. *Journal of Sexual Aggression, 9,* 25–30.

Marshall, W. L., Serran, G. A., Moulden, H., Mulloy, R., Fernandez, Y. M., Mann, R. E., & Thornton, D. (2002). Therapist features in sexual offender treatment: Their reliable identification and influence on behaviour change. *Clinical Psychology and Psychotherapy, 9,* 395–405.

Marshall, W. L., Ward, T., Mann, R. E., Moulden, H., Fernandez, Y. M., Serran, G. A., & Marshall, L. E. (2005). Working positively with sexual offenders: Maximizing the effectiveness of treatment. *Journal of Interpersonal Violence, 20,* 1–19.

Martin, D. J., Graske, J. P., & Davis, M. K. (2000). Relation of the therapeutic alliance with outcome and other variables: A meta-analytic review. *Journal of Consulting and Clinical Psychology, 68,* 438–450.

McGrath, R. J., Cumming, G. F., & Burchard, B. L. (2003). *Current practices and trends in sexual abuser management: Safer Society 2002 nationwide survey.* Brandon, VT: Safer Society Press.

McGuire, R. J., Carlisle, J. M., & Young, B. G. (1965). Sexual deviations as conditioned behavior: A hypothesis. *Behaviour Research and Therapy, 2,* 185–190.

Miller, W. R. & Rollnick, S. (Eds.). (1991). *Motivational interviewing: Preparing people to change addictive behavior.* New York, NY: Guilford Press.

Nicholaichuk, T., Gordon, A., Gu, D., & Wong, S. (2000). Outcome of an institutional sexual offender treatment program: A comparison between treated and matched untreated offenders. *Sexual Abuse: A Journal of Research and Treatment, 12,* 139–153.

Parker, J. D. A. & Endler, N. S. (1996). Coping and defense: A historical overview. In M. Zeidner & N. S. Endler (Eds.), *Handbook of coping: Theory, research, applications* (pp. 3–23). New York, NY: John Wiley & Sons.

Persons, J. B. & Silberschatz, G. (1998). Are results of randomized controlled trials useful to psychotherapists? *Journal of Consulting and Clinical Psychology, 66,* 126–135.

Pfäfflin, F., Böhmer, M., Cornehl, S., & Mergenthaler, E. (2005). What happens in therapy with sexual offenders? A model of process research. *Sexual Abuse; A Journal of Research and Treatment, 17,* 141–151.

Polaschek, D. L. L. (2003). Empathy and victim empathy. In T. Ward, D. R. Laws & S. M. Hudson (Eds.), *Sexual deviance: Issues and controversies* (pp. 172–189). Thousand Oaks, CA: Sage Publications.

Prentky, R. A. & Burgess, A. W. (1990). Rehabilitation of child molesters: A cost-benefit analysis. *American Journal of Orthopsychiatry.* 60, 80–117.

Rice, M. E. & Harris, G. T. (2003). The size and sign of treatment effects in sex offender therapy. *Annals of the New York Academy of Sciences,* 989, 428–440.

Schmuck, P. & Sheldon, K. M. (Eds.). (2001). *Life goals and well-being.* Toronto: Hogrefe & Huber.

Segal, Z. V. & Marshall, W. L. (1985). Self-report and behavioral assertion in two groups of sexual offenders. *Journal of Behavior Therapy and Experimental Psychiatry,* 16, 223–229.

Seligman, M. E. P. (1995). The effectiveness of psychotherapy: The Consumer Reports study. *American Psychologist,* 50, 965–974.

Seligman, M. E. P. (1996b). Science as an ally of practice. *American Psychologist,* 51, 1072–1079.

Serran, G. A., Firestone, P., Marshall, W. L., & Moulden, H. Changes in coping following treatment for child molesters. *Journal of Interpersonal Violence* (in press).

Smallbone, S. W. (2006). An attachment-theoretical revision of Marshall and Barbaree's integrated theory of the etiology of sexual offending. In W. L. Marshall, Y. M. Fernandez, L. E. Marshall & G. A. Serran (Eds.), *Sexual offender treatment: Controversial issues* (pp. 93–107). Chichester, UK: John Wiley & Sons.

Tangney, J. P. & Dearing, R. L. (2002). *Shame and guilt.* New York, NY: Guilford Press.

Thornton, D., Beech, A. R., & Marshall, W. L. (2004). Pre-treatment self-esteem and posttreatment sexual recidivism. *International Journal of Offender Therapy and Comparative Criminology,* 48, 587–599.

Ward, T. & Gannon, T. A. Rehabilitation, etiology, and self-regulation: The Comprehensive Good Lives Model of treatment for sexual offenders. *Aggression and Violent Behaviors: A Review Journal* (in press).

Ward, T. & Hudson, S. M. (1996). Relapse prevention: A critical analysis. *Sexual Abuse: A Journal of Research and Treatment,* 8, 177–200.

Ward, T. & Hudson, S. M. (2000). A self-regulation model of relapse prevention. In D. R. Laws, S. M. Hudson & T. Ward (Eds.), *Remaking relapse prevention with sex offenders: A sourcebook* (pp. 79–101). Thousand Oaks, CA: Sage Publications.

Ward, T., Hudson, S. M., & Marshall, W. L. (1994). The abstinence violation effect in child molesters. *Behaviour Research and Therapy,* 32, 431–437.

Ward, T., Hudson, S. M., & Marshall, W. L. (1996). Attachment style in sex offenders: A preliminary study. *Journal of Sex Research,* 33, 17–26.

Ward, T., Hudson, S. M., & McCormack, J. (1997). Attachment style, intimacy deficits, and sexual offending. In B. K. Schwartz & J. R. Cellini (Eds.), *The sex offender: New insights, treatment innovations, and legal developments* (Vol. II, pp. 2.1–2.14). Kingston, NJ: Civic Research Institute.

Ward, T., Hudson, S. M., & Siegert, R. J. (1995). A critical comment on Pithers' relapse prevention model. *Sexual Abuse: A Journal of Research and Treatment,* 7, 167–175.

Ward, T. & Marshall, W. L. (2004). Good lives, aetiology and the rehabilitation of sex offenders: A bridging theory. *Journal of Sexual Aggression,* 10, 153–169.

Ward, T. & Sorbello, L. (2003). Explaining child sexual abuse: Integration and elaboration. In T. Ward, D. R. Laws, & S. M. Hudson (Eds.), *Sexual deviance: Issues and controversies* (pp. 3–20). Thousand Oaks, CA: Sage Publications.

Ward, T. & Stewart, C. A. (2003). Good lives and the rehabilitation of sexual offenders. In T. Ward, D. R. Laws, & S. M. Hudson (Eds.), *Sexual deviance: Issues and controversies* (pp. 12–44) Thousand Oaks, CA: Sage Publications.

Ward, T., Vess, J., Collie, R. M., & Gannon, T. A. (2006). Risk management or goods promotion: The relationship between approach and avoidance goals in the treatment for sex offenders. *Aggression and Violent Behavior: A Review Journal,* 11, 378–393.

Wegner, D. M. (1994). Ironic processes of mental control. *Psychological Bulletin,* 101, 34–52.

Wilson, R. J. & Picheca, J. E. Circles of support and accountability: Engaging the community in sexual offender risk management. In B. K. Schwartz (Ed.), *The sex offender: Theoretical advances, treating special populations and legal developments* (Vol. V). Kingston, NJ: Civic Research Institute (in press).

Wilson, R. J., Stewart, L., Stirpe, T. S., Barrett, M., & Cripps, J. E. (2000). Community-based sex offender management: Combining parole supervision and treatment to reduce recidivism. *Canadian Journal of Criminology,* 42, 177–188.

Yates, P. M., Kingston, D., & Hall, K. (2003, October). Pathways to offending: Validity of Ward and Hudson's (1998) Self-regulation Model and relationship to static and dynamic risk among treated sexual offenders. Paper presented at the 22nd Annual Research and Treatment Conference of the Association for the Treatment of Sexual Abusers, St. Louis.

Chapter 13

Orchiectomy

Richard B. Krueger, Michael H. Wechsler, and Meg S. Kaplan

This chapter aims to review the rationale and data supporting bilateral orchiectomy as a possible treatment modality for sex offenders. Although the idea of orchiectomy, or surgical castration, evokes strongly negative emotional responses in many individuals, several reviews of biological treatments for sex offenders examining recidivism data from European studies have concluded that castration had very significant positive effects on recidivism (Bradford, 1985; Freund, 1980; Meyer & Cole, 1997). A recent meta-analysis by Lösel and Schmucker (2005) reviewed 69 studies and found that surgical castration and hormonal medication showed larger effects on sexual recidivism than psychosocial intervention. Finally, a recent review of pharmacotherapy in the treatment of sex offenders suggested that it might not be surprising if a "comeback" for surgical castration would occur (Rösler & Witztum, 2000) because of its efficacy and the low rates of recidivism reported by outcome studies.

Orchiectomy was selected as the title for this chapter because it more properly reflects the nature of the therapeutic procedure that will be discussed in depth. Orchiectomy (Hensyl, 1990, p. 1096) comes from the Greek, *orchis*, or testis, and *ektome*, or excision, and is referred to, alternatively, as orchidectomy, orchectomy, or testectomy, and consists of the removal of one or both testes.

The term "castration" comes from the Latin stem *castrare* meaning to castrate, prune, expurgate, deprive of vigor (Simpson & Weiner, 1989, p. 959) and has a broader meaning which includes mutilation, which undoubtedly has contributed to its negative associations. Castration for control, domination, punishment, mutilation, social advancement, and political reasons has been practiced since antiquity and has been the subject of several recent reviews (Ayalon, 1999; Marmon, 1995; Ringrose, 2003; Scholz, 2001; Taylor, 2000; Tougher, 2002; Tsai, 1996; Winslade, Stone, Smith-Bell, & Webb, 1998). Although castration is a term which is referred to in much of the literature cited in this article, unless otherwise indicated, it should be understood that insofar as can be determined bilateral orchiectomy was performed, and not a more extensive procedure.

Some of the literature also refers to "medical castration" by which is meant the use of hormonal or gonadotropin-releasing hormone agonist (GNRH) therapy to reduce testosterone to castrate levels. Finally, some of the literature on the treatment of prostate cancer refers to androgen deprivation therapy, which has the aim of reducing testosterone to castrate levels, and which can be accomplished by surgical or medical castration.

HISTORY

Europe

The first therapeutic castration based on a psychiatric indication was performed in 1892 by August Forel in Zurich for an "imbecilic" man who was on the verge of autocastration because of neurologic pains in his testes (Sturup, 1972). Denmark pioneered legalizing this treatment in 1929, followed by Germany (1933), Norway (1934), Finland (1935), Estonia (1937), Iceland (1938), Latvia (1938), and Sweden (1944) (Bradford, 1985; Heim & Hursch, 1979; Le Marie, 1956). Heim and Hursch (1979) reported that Switzerland, the Netherlands, and Greenland practiced this treatment without any legal mandate, sometimes quite extensively. For instance, Heim (1981) reported that the procedure was widely used in Switzerland and that in the Zurich region alone more than 10,000 patients had been castrated for various psychiatric reasons since 1910. Heim and Hursch (1979) reported that in Germany between 1934 and 1944 at least 2800 sex offenders were subjected to compulsory castration and that subsequently in West Germany, between 1955 and 1977, 800 sex offenders were castrated. They also reported 1100 cases of castration in Denmark since 1929. This procedure was also used in the Netherlands (Sturup, 1968a).

Castration has not been used in most countries for the treatment of sex offenders for several decades (Gijs & Gooren, 1996), although Germany was reported (Wille & Beier, 1989) to have been conducting five castrations annually since 1980 and the Czechoslovakian republic was reported, in a paper presented at a conference in 1995, to have conducted 84 such procedures since 1976 (Gijs & Gooren, 1996).

United States

In the late 1800s castration for criminals in the United States was more a subject of discussion in the penal literature than a practice, but many cases were reported (Gugliotta, 1998). Dr. Sharp in 1899 in Indiana began experiments on convicts (Le Marie, 1956). Although described as castration, his procedure, in fact, involved only vasectomy to prevent the loss of secretions from the testes and thus preserve the loss of the "elixir of life" to promote well-being and health. More than 450 vasectomies were performed on incarcerated men, both with and without explicit legal sanction (Gugliotta, 1998).

Elsewhere in the United States castration was practiced in California from 1937 to 1948. A study reporting on the outcome of 40 castrated males was recently published (Weinberger et al., 2005), but other reports suggest that that total number of inmates subjected to this procedure was in the neighborhood of 400 (Linsky, 1989).

More recently in 1996, in the United States, California became the first of nine states passing contemporary legislation authorizing the use of either medical or surgical castration for certain sex offenders (Scott & Holmberg, 2003). Of these nine states, four permit the use of medical castration only (Georgia, Montana, Oregon, and Wisconsin); four allow either medical castration or voluntary surgical castration (California, Florida, Iowa, and Louisiana); and only one (Texas) provides voluntary surgical castration as the only treatment option (Scott & Holmberg, 2003). While medical or surgical castration is described as mandatory in five of these states (Scott & Holmberg, 2003), issues of informed consent are often not addressed by these statutes. Moreover, we have been able to locate only one published description from one of these states, Oregon, on the use of these statutes (Maletzky, Tolan, & McFarlan, 2006). This group reported on a 5-year follow-up of men referred under Oregon House Bill 2500 enacted in 1999, for evaluation as to whether medical treatment with medroxyprogesterone acetate (MPA) was indicated to reduce their risk. Two hundred seventy-five men were evaluated, and sexual recidivism was established. Of these, 79 men were advised to receive

MPA and did, in fact, received it; none of this group recidivated sexually. One hundred forty-one were not referred for MPA treatment and 14% recidivated sexually; 55 were advised to have MPA treatment, but for a variety of reasons did not receive it, and 18% of this group recidivated sexually. This study lends support to the efficacy of antiandrogen treatment in reducing sexual recidivism. The lack of other published reports or information from the other eight states suggests that these laws are not being utilized.

RECENT CASES OF SEX OFFENDERS UNDERGOING ORCHIECTOMY

Aside from sporadic case reports of orchiectomy in the medical literature (Alexander, 1993; Joseph, 1993; Silcock, 1993) (of a British pedophile) or news media (CBS News, 2004) (of a pedophile in Texas) the authors know of only six recent cases , three of these were performed in canada, two on sex offenders (Bradford, 2006, personal communication) and another for the treatment of autoerotic asphyxia (Fedoroff, 2006, personal communication), three were performed in texas on individuals offered surgical castration under the recent Texas statute (Winslade, 2008, personal communication) Thus, the use and study of this procedure have fallen off extensively.

Ethical Issues and Use of Castration for Other Conditions

Castration has also quite continuously been the topic of many ethical debates and reviews (Alexander, 1993; Bingley, 1993; Bund, 1997; Cook, 1993; Eastman, 1993; Finch, 1993; Freund, 1980; Gaensbauer, 1973; Gandhi, Purandare, & Lock, 1993; Heim & Hursch, 1979; Hicks, 1993; Icenogle, 1994; Joseph, 1993; Klerman, 1975; Silcock, 1993; Tancredi & Weisstub, 1986; Taylor, 1993). In the United States, opponents of castration legislation cite First Amendment concerns involving the protection of a person's freedom of speech (including sexual expression); violation of the Eighth Amendment's ban on cruel and unusual punishment; and violation of the Fourteenth Amendment's guarantee of due process and equal protection (subjecting prisoners to castration without adequate process of protection) (Scott & Holmberg, 2003).

However, although the use of castration is controversial for sex offenders, it has achieved the status of an accepted surgical treatment for a variety of medical conditions. The Nobel Prize in physiology or medicine was awarded to Charles Huggins in 1966 for his investigations during the 1940s into the role of sex hormones on prostate cancer and for his use of bilateral orchiectomy to treat patients with metastatic prostate cancer. (Corbin & Thompson, 2003; Huggins & Hodges, 2002). Although hormonal therapy and GNRH agonists have largely supplanted the use of castration for prostate cancer, it is still a common urological procedure. Unilateral orchiectomy constitutes standard of care treatment for testicular cancer.

Furthermore, voluntary castration for a variety of motivations, including a feeling of control over one's sexual urges and appetite, a sense of calmness, and cosmetic reasons, has been described with 23 of 234 respondents to an Internet survey in 2002, indicating that they had actually undergone castration for some of these reasons (Wassersug, 2004). A treatise on the psychological and other advantages of castration was published recently (Cheney, 2004).

ANIMAL AND PRIMATE STUDIES

Rat and Canine Studies

Research studies in rats demonstrate that castration results in a loss of sex drive and an abolishment of mating behavior, and that this can be restored by testosterone (Davidson, Stefanick, & Sachan, 1978). Beach (1976) provided a review and rationale for cross-species comparison of sexual behavior and described a sequential reduction in ejaculation, intromission, and mounting in males of a variety of species following castration. He also summarized experiments on rats and dogs suggesting that previous sexual experience was not related to the variation in the effects of castration on animals (Beach 1970).

Primate Studies

The effects of castration in primates have been reviewed by Dixson (1998, pp. 392–397). Chemical or physical castration has been studied in six species, with quite attenuated sexual functioning being uniformly demonstrated. For example, castration of sexually experienced adult male rhesus monkeys results in a decline in sexual behavior, reversible with testosterone (Dixson, 1998, pp. 392–393). In the first 2 to

4 weeks frequencies of ejaculation and intromission are reduced; mounting behavior declines more gradually. However, there is marked individual variability with 5 out of 10 male rhesus monkeys studied by Phoenix (Phoenix, 1980; Phoenix, Slob, & Goy, 1973) still capable of intromission and three with ejaculatory responses, 1 year after the operation. Loy (1971) observed a castrated male rhesus monkey still capable of mounts, intromissions, and an ejaculatory pause characteristic of intact males 7 years after operation.

Taken together, these data suggest that orchiectomy can markedly reduce sexual behavior in rodents and primates, but that its effects can be readily reversed by exogenous testosterone and there is much individual variation, with some animals having sexual functioning extinguished and others continuing with it.

HUMAN STUDIES OF CASTRATION FOR MEDICAL CONDITIONS

Case Studies by Kinsey

Kinsey et al. (1953, pp. 731–745) reviewed a large amount of mostly anecdotal evidence on the effects of castration, including some of the European castration literature, and noted that there was large variability in the effects of the procedure. They described one male from their own studies who was married and normally sexually active 30 years after castration. They also noted that at 50 years of age, 7% of males were impotent and sexually unresponsive, whether castrated or not, and concluded that although castration was generally associated with reduced sexual functioning, castrated males were still capable of being aroused by tactile or psychological stimuli, and that the data did not justify an opinion that the public may be protected from socially dangerous types of sex offenders by castration laws.

TESTICULAR CANCER STUDIES

Treatment of testicular cancer provides some information on the psychological effects of castration. For patients with early stage testicular cancer, radical unilateral orchiectomy is virtually always the primary therapeutic intervention (Jones & Vasey, 2003). Van Basten et al. (1999) reported on 21 patients who

had undergone unilateral orchiectomy for testicular cancer, studying sex hormone levels and performing visual erotic stimulation (VES) tests and cavernosal artery duplex ultrasonography. They found that after a diagnosis of testicular cancer, sexual dysfunction was considerable, but within 1 year after treatment there was some improvement, and the results of the VES test suggested that sexual dysfunction was more psychological than organically based. Jonker-Pool et al. (2001) performed a meta-analysis of 36 studies of individuals treated for testicular cancer. Four of these studies reported on groups treated with unilateral orchiectomy followed by surveillance, with 25% of subjects reporting a loss of desire, 24% orgasmic dysfunction, 16% ejaculation dysfunction, and 11% a decrease in sexual activity. Unilateral orchiectomy has no effect on the endocrine system. The clinical experience of one of the authors (Wechsler, 2006, personal communication) is that patients recover quite well psychologically over time.

PROSTATE CANCER STUDIES

Studies of individuals treated with prostate cancer provide data that is more relevant because castration is bilateral. The classic form of androgen deprivation is surgical castration by bilateral orchiectomy, which is the most immediate method of reducing circulating testosterone by >90% within 24 hours (Maatman, Gupta, & Montie, 1985; Miyamoto, Messing, & Chang, 2004). Another summary indicates that surgical castration, estrogens and LHRH agonists equally decrease plasma testosterone to between 5% and 10% of its original value (Baltogiannis, Giannakopoulos, Charalabopoulos, & Sofikitis, 2004). However, the adrenal glands still produce testosterone, estimated at 5% to 10% of the total amount (Sanford et al., 1977; Santen, 2003; Young & Landsberg, 2001).

Side effects of this procedure are loss of libido and potency, hot flashes, osteoporosis, loss of muscle mass, fatigue, weight gain and anemia, and psychological symptoms associated with definitive castration (Miyamoto et al., 2004; Schroder, 1997).

Patient Preference of Medical over Surgical Treatment for Prostate Cancer

While orchiectomy is a relatively simple procedure with minor risks (Loblaw et al., 2004), it has fallen out of favor because of its psychological impact and the existence of viable medical alternatives (Mcleod, 2003; Sharifi, Gulley, & Dahut, 2005). Despite this, some authors have suggested that it is underused (Hellerstedt & Pienta, 2003; Miyamoto et al., 2004). Potosky et al. (2001) used questionnaires to assess quality of life issues, and compared men who had received surgical castration with men who had received medical castration with LHRH agonists. Men who chose LHRH agonist therapy reported greater problems with their overall sexual functioning than orchiectomy patients, despite both groups having a similar pretreatment level of functioning. The group receiving medical castration perceived themselves as less likely to be free of cancer. The authors suggested that these differences might have been partially related to regular injections that served as a constant reminder to the presence of disease. They also suggested that preference for injections over surgery might have been because of fear of permanent mutilation, the ability to discontinue injections, and/or the loss of a masculine self-image. Another study suggested that patients preferred this approach for reasons of convenience and cost (Chadwick, Gillatt, & Gingell, 1991).

It is clear, however, that when patients are given the choice of medical or surgical castration, most choose medical approaches first (Cassileth et al., 1989).

Studies of the Effects of Castration on Sexual Functioning in Patients Treated for Prostate Cancer

Greenstein et al. (1995) reported on a study of 16 men who had undergone physical (10, with posttreatment maintenance with flutamide) or hormonal (6, treated with diethylstilbestrol) castration. The mean interval from castration was 21 months. All patients had penile plethysmography while provided with erotic visual stimulation. Four of these patients achieved functional erections; all four of these had been physically castrated. All patients reported good erections and strong libido before castration with libido being markedly decreased after castration. In all patients the onset of erectile dysfunction was noticed a few weeks after castration. No patient reported spontaneous erections following castration and none had attempted intercourse.

Rousseau et al. (1988) administered a questionnaire and reported on biological and sexuality changes

in prostate cancer patients receiving flutamide with either surgical or medical castration with an LHRH agonist. Serum concentrations of testosterone were decreased to approximately 5% of pretreatment values with no difference in levels being found between those receiving orchiectomy and those with medical castration. The only difference was that there was a 2 to 3 week delay before castrate levels of serum androgens were achieved with LHRH agonists. In fact, a "flare" reaction is usually observed with the onset of GNRH agonist therapy for prostatic cancer, with a surge of testosterone during the first week or so after a depot injection, and some urologists will block this with a 1-week course of bicalutamide or a similar agent. Chabner et al. (2006) in Goodman & Gilman's Textbook the *Pharmacological Basis of Therapeutics* suggest a 2 to 4 week administration of androgen receptor blocking (ARB) agents (p. 1388) for this purpose. Other authorities using GNRH agonists for the control of sexual behavior have suggested that ARB agents may be used, or that, as an alternative to using ARB agents, patients or their caregivers may be advised of the risk of hypersexuality and appropriate protective measures could be taken (Krueger & Kaplan, 2001). A major reduction in their interest for sexual intercourse was noticed by 70% of subjects; however, 20% of patients reported continuing sexual activity and interest, although the time from initiation of treatment to the assessment of current functioning was not specified.

Cost–Benefit Analyses

Several cost-benefit studies have been performed on the use of different types of antiandrogen therapies for the treatment of prostate cancer (Hellerstedt & Pienta, 2003). A recent study evaluated the cost-effectiveness of six androgen suppression strategies to treat advanced prostate cancer. (Bayoumi, Brown, & Garber, 2000). Most provided similar outcomes in both survival and quality of life estimates. The annual cost of monotherapy with a GNRH agonist was $4995 in 2000; the cost has now fallen to approximately $3000. Orchiectomy had a one-time cost of $3360, which now in New York City is an outpatient procedure costing between $1500 and $2000. Cost concerns of medical castration led to the suggestion of surgical castration as an alternative (Oefelein & Resnick, 2003).

Degree of Androgen Suppression in Prostate Cancer

Androgen deprivation therapy in the treatment of prostate cancer has the aim of achieving serum testosterone levels as low as possible so as to minimize androgenic stimulation of prostate cancer cells. Serum testosterone concentrations that correspond to castration levels have been set at less than 50 ng/dL (1.7 nmol/L), given variability of values in various reference laboratories (Bubley et al., 1999; Sharifi, Gulley, & Dahut, 2005). Most men, however, achieve levels below 20 ng/dL (0.7 nmol/L) after orchiectomy and it has been suggested that castration levels be redefined to use this as a threshold (Sharifi, Gulley, & Dahut, 2005). Two studies suggested that for individuals treated with GNRH agonists who did not achieve castrate values of less than 20 ng/dL surgical castration should be considered (Oefelein, Feng, Scolieri, Ricchiutti, & Resnick, 2000; Oefelein & Resnick, 2003), although it is generally held that surgical and medical castration result in equivalent suppression of testosterone.

BIOLOGICAL AND BEHAVIORAL EFFECTS IN CASTRATED SEX OFFENDERS

In Czechoslovakia Zverina et al. (1991) examined 84 castrated "sexual delinquents" 1 to 15 years after castration. Eighteen percent of subjects were capable of occasional sexual intercourse, and 21% lived in a stable heterosexual relationship. One-half had occasional erections in the morning. More than a third masturbated occasionally. One quarter of the subjects had objections to the results of the castration, most frequently because sex was lacking in their life. The authors did not observe serious physical or mental consequences of castration in the examined men.

In Denmark Sturup (1968, 1968) reported on 900 cases, and found that "asexualization" was present in 97% of castrated individuals, with 90% of individuals being satisfied with the operation. Castration was seldom followed by obesity, but there was a gynecoid distribution of fat. Hot flashes and sweating were common; beard and body hair were diminished but not head hair. Some individuals reported an increase in head hair. It was noted that diminished vitality, energy, and initiative was not definitely seen, and several of the men were noted to have increased energy and to have built new careers. Although it was noted that serious psychological consequences were not observed, at least 5, or 1.8%, of the men committed suicide.

In Germany Heim (1981) authored one of the most detailed studies of the effects of castration on sex offenders released from prison. He studied 39 men who had consented to castration while imprisoned in West Germany. The mean age of the subjects at castration was 42.5 years, and the median time since release from prison was 4.3 years. Sexual desire and sexual arousability were perceived by the subjects as having been considerably impaired by castration, and the frequency of coitus, masturbation, and sexual thoughts were perceived as strongly reduced after castration. However, 11 of 35 castrates stated they were still able to engage in sexual intercourse, and rapists proved to be more sexually active after castration than homosexual or pedophiliacs. The results of this study led him to conclude that there was a strong effect on sexual behavior only if castration were performed on males between 46 and 59 years of age and that the sexual manifestations of castration varied considerably between individuals.

In Norway Heim and Hursch (1979) and Bremer (1958) reported on a group of 244 Norwegian castrates, 102 of which were sex offenders. A questionnaire interview with the castrate and/or information from those in contact with him and an analysis of documentary sources was conducted. In 66% of 157 persons for whom the effect of castration on sexual function could be judged, all sexual interest, reactivity, and activity had disappeared. Of 103 cases, 72% reported the effect immediately or just after the operation and 28% reported that it took a few months to a year for their sexual urges to disappear. However, 34% of the total group reported that their sexual interest and reactivity persisted for more than a year. Problems were reported in 18% of subjects after an observation period of 6 to 15 years, with weight gain, development of an aged appearance, climacteric symptoms, weakness, and deterioration in general health. There was an operative mortality of 2%, which nowadays would be considered extremely high and surgically unacceptable.

In Switzerland Heim and Hursch (1979) described details of a study by Cornu (1973), consisting of 127 sex offenders from Switzerland who were evaluated by psychiatrists and who had lived as castrates for at least 5 years after release from prison, with a comparison group of 50 who had refused to have their testes removed. Follow-up was 5 to 35 years. Criminal records and files from the court, police, and psychiatric hospitals were examined and 68 castrates were interviewed and medically examined. Cornu estimated the recidivism rate as being 4.13% after castration, in comparison with 52% in group of men who had had castration recommended to them, but refused, 10 years earlier. Of the 68 castrates, 63% said their libido and potency had been extinguished quickly after castration; 26% said there was a gradual decline; and 10% said they were able to have sexual intercourse 8 to 20 years after they were castrated. On medical examination, 51% were extremely overweight; gynecomastia was present in 10%; hair on the body was reduced in 63%. Thirty four percent of the castrates were adjudged to have a "castrate face," apparently because their skin had become softer, more pliable, and slacker. Sixty subjects had X-rays of their vertebral column and 82% of these had osteoporosis diagnosed. Forty-three percent mentioned bone pains, mainly in the vertebral column.

Of the 68 castrates 28% indicated that they had not experienced any psychological disorders; 40% had the opinion that castration had favorably influenced their moods, specifying that they felt calmer, happier, and more active than before the operation. Thirty two percent said that they felt miserable, with some indicating that they felt depressed, irritable, isolated, or maimed. Twenty two percent thought their capacity for work had deteriorated after castration; 16% thought that it had improved; and 61% thought there had been no change. Three men committed suicide. Seventy one percent said they were content with the operation because their abnormal sex drive had vanished, confinement was prevented, their state of health had improved, or marriage was possible for the first time; 16% were ambivalent; and 13% felt effeminate and mutilated.

RECIDIVISM STUDIES

A review of the recidivism literature is summarized in the accompanying table (Table 13.1). By today's standards for conducting prospective clinical trials, most of these studies suffer from significant methodological difficulties. The subject groups are heterogeneous, not well described, and not exclusively sex offenders. Some individuals appeared to have had schizophrenia or mental retardation as primary diagnoses. Assignment was not random and treatment was not blinded. Length of time at follow-up was not clear and outcome measures, whether rearrest or reconviction, were often not specified. There also are not for the most part good comparison or control groups. However, at the time these trials and studies were conducted, the methodology was current and acceptable. Furthermore, standards applicable to clinical trials are not necessarily appropriate for forensic populations. There are severe limitations on the conduct of research studies on such populations. Randomized and treatment blinded designs in situations where an outcome variable would involve victimization of an adult or child face substantial ethical challenge from institutional reviews boards. And many recidivism studies today use survival analysis techniques, which do not require control groups. It is clear that these studies are one of the most important sources of information concerning the effects of androgen deprivation therapy on sexually aggressive behavior. They do provide the equivalent of a series of retrospective analyses of open clinical trials conducted over very long periods of time (in many instances greater in duration of follow-up by a factor of at least three, compared with contemporary clinical studies (Bradford, 2006, personal communication), with assessments of the effects of this treatment on the most critical behavioral variable, commission of another sexual offense.

Czechoslovakia produced 2 studies (Taus & Susicka, 1973; Zverina, Zimanova, & Bartova, 1991) with small numbers, 5 and 84. Few details are available, but there were only 3 offenders relapsed out of these two groups for a very low recidivism rate.

Denmark yielded several studies (Hansen, 1991; Hansen & Lykke-Olesen, 1997; Le Marie, 1956; Ortmann, 1980; Sand, Dickmeiss, & Schwalbe-Hansen, 1964; Sturup, 1968, 1972; Weinberger et al., 2005), many with poorly defined or no control groups. All report a low recidivism rate with the largest by Sand who reported on 900 patients castrated from 6 to 30 years earlier and found a relapse rate of 1.1%, compared with relapse rates in comparison groups of 9.7%, 16.8%, or 50% depending on the study and group.

Germany has produced a number of detailed studies (Heim, 1981; Heim & Hursch, 1979; Langelüddeke, 1963, 1968; Wille & Beier, 1989) that again support

TABLE 13.1 Summary of Surgical Castration Studies and the Effects of Castration on Recidivism for Sexual Crimes

Nation/Study	Number of Subjects	Diagnoses	Precastration Crime Rate	Follow-up Period (Years)	Post Castration Recidivism (No. and/or %)	Recidivism of Noncastrates	Notes
Czechoslovakia (Taus & Susicka 1973)	5	"Sexually dangerous deviations"	Unknown	5	0	No comparison group	Article in Czechoslovakian; English summary only consulted.
Czechoslovakia (Zverina et al. 1991)	84	"Sexual offenders"	"100%" reoffense rate	1–15	3 offenders; 3.6%	No comparison group	Article in Czechoslovakian; English summary only consulted.
Denmark (Le Marie, 1956)	139 castrated out of 3,185	96 guilty of sexual offenses	Unknown	10	Of 91, two relapsed	16.8% recidivism rate for whole sample	Discussed in Bradford, 1985 and Ortman, 1981.
Denmark (Ortman, 1980)	738 castrated sex offenders	Half indecent offenses against children	Unknown	22– 52 years	1.4%–2.4%	9.7% or 16.8% or 50% depending on comparison group	Patients were castrated during 30-year period 1929–1959; this larger group included LeMarie's 1956 group. Time at follow-up and comparison groups not given.
Denmark (Sand et al., 1964)	900	42%, two or more convictions; 44% mental defectives; 25% psychopaths 13% sexually abnormal	Unknown	6 to more than 30 years	10 (1.1%) were real sexual recidivists; another 10 were borderline cases	No comparison	Report also cited by Sturup, 1968. This group encompasses the groups reported by Le Marie and Ortman. Ortman (1980) reports relapse rate of 9.7% in follow-up study of noncastrated offenders in Denmark. Report cited in Sturup (1968). 90% of subjects satisfied with their operation.
Denmark (Sturup, 1968)	38 (18 of these castrated) 11 non castrates	Rapists	Unknown	13–24 yrs 3 months–13yrs	0 of 11 castrated 1 of 5 not castrated No recidivism	1 of 5 not castrated recidivated; information on others not available	Group consists of all rapists received at Herstedvester Detention Center from 1935 to 1964; this group appears to be different from other groups studied in Denmark. "Forced castration" was never performed.

Study (reference)	Sample	Offender type	Offender history	Follow-up	Recidivism	Comparison group	Results / Notes
Denmark (Hansen, 1991; Hansen, & Lykke-Olesen, 1997)	43 (21 castrated, 22 not)	No information	Unknown	More than 15 years	10% (after 2 subjects took exogenous testosterone)	36%, 8 of 22 not castrated; sexual reoffense	Cited in Weinberger et al., 2005; Hansen, 1991; Hansen, & Lykke-Olesen, 1997.
Germany (Langelüddeke, 1963; 1968)	1,036 castrated released into the community; 1,618 (same group, reported in Sturup)	84% two or more convictions	Unknown	6 weeks–20 years 20/30	2.3% 46 2.8%	685 noncastrated released into the community; 39.1% reoffended	Langelüddeke, 1963, also reported by Heim & Hursch, 1979 and Sturup, 1972; 65% of 58 castrated males reported immediate decrease of libido; 17% gradual; 18% could have intercourse 20 years after castration. Primary reference and cited in Sturup, 1972.
Germany (Heim 1981)	39 released offenders from group reported by Langelüddeke	31% rapists; 51% pedophiliacs; 3% sexual murders; 15% homosexuals	15% first offenders 85% 2 or more sexual crimes	4 months–13 years; median time since release from prison 4.3 years	No reported recidivism	No comparison group	64% had additional "Protective measures" imposed because they were exceptionally dangerous. Frequency of coital behavior, rate of masturbation, frequency of sexual thoughts strongly reduced after castration. 31% of castrates were still able to engage in sexual intercourse.
Germany (Wille & Beier, 1989)	104 (25% of all orchidectomized sex offenders between 1970 and 1980)	70% pedophiles; 25% aggressive sex offenders; 3% exhibitionists; 2% homosexual	Unknown	11 years	3% "maximum"	46% noncastrated applicants (permission not granted or application canceled by applicant)	75% reported decreased sexual interest, libido, erection, and ejaculation within 6 months; 10% remained sexually active for years at diminished level; 15% reported sexual outlets over longer period of time. 70% "satisfied"; 20% "ambivalent"; 10% not satisfied.

(continued)

TABLE 13.1 Continued

Nation/Study	Number of Subjects	Diagnoses	Precastration Crime Rate	Follow-up Period (Years)	PostCastration Recidivism (No. and/or %)	Recidivism of Noncastrates	Notes
The Netherlands (Fischer van Rossum)	237	Unknown	Unknown	Unknown	3 1.3%	Unknown	Cited in Sturup, 1960 and in Meyer& Cole, 1997. Primary reference unavailable.
Norway (Bremer 1959, Part 1 and 2)	244 studied 102 males 28 females	13 rapists; 79 pedophiles; 10 others of females; 13 promiscuity; 14 for behavioral disturbances	58% Unknown	1–10 years	2.9%	No comparison group	Concluded indications for castration were too broad; that it did not work for females; and that it showed promise for sex offenders.
Sweden (Kinmark, 1949)	66	Unknown	Unknown	Unknown	0 0	Unknown	Cited in Sturup, 1968 and Meyer & Cole, 1997. Primary reference unavailable.
Sweden (Lidberg 1968)	241	"About half were first-time sex offenders"	Unknown	Unknown	2	Unknown	Also cited in Sturup, 1972.
Switzerland (Hackfield, Wolff, Colle)	83	Unknown	Unknown	Unknown	6 7.2%	No comparison group	Cited in Sturup, 1972. Primary reference unavailable.
Switzerland (Cornu, 1973)	127	77% 2 or more convictions	Unknown	5–35 years	7% or 4%	N = 50 (52%)	Cited in Heim & Hursch, 1979. Younger castrates appeared to have higher risk of recidivating than older. Primary reference unavailable.
United States, (Weinberger et al. 2005)	60	27.5% based on 40 of 60 subjects; 1 or more arrests or convictions	Unknown	2 months–13 years	0%	No comparison group	Reports follow-up 44 convicted sex offenders who underwent surgical castration in San Diego County, California, between 1937 and 1948.

castration's positive effect on recidivism. The largest, by Langeluddeke, reporting on patients in the community who had been castrated from 6 weeks to 20 years earlier reported a recidivism rate of 2.3% compared with a rate of 39.1% in 685 patients who were not castrated and released into the community. It should be noted that many of those castrated were under the Nazi regimen and were castrated involuntarily; this included individuals who were homosexuals.

A study is reported to have been done in the Netherlands (Meyer & Cole, 1997; Sturup, 1968) but details of this are not available beyond aggregate data.

Bremer (1958) reported on a group of 244 individuals castrated in Norway, 28 of whom were women, concluding that the indications, which, in addition to sex offenses, included schizophrenia and epilepsy, were too broad but that the procedure offered effective medical therapy to a subgroup of sex offenders.

Information is available from Sweden (Bremer, 1958; Lidberg, 1968; Meyer & Cole, 1997; Sturup, 1968), Switzerland (Cornu, 1973; Heim & Hursch, 1979; Sturup, 1972), and the Netherlands (Meyer & Cole, 1997; Sturup, 1968) which also suggest a dramatic effect on recidivism.

Finally, in California Weinberger et al. (2005) reported on the follow-up of 40 sex offenders castrated in San Diego County during the period 1937 to 1948, none of whom reoffended.

By way of summary it would appear that effects on sexual interest and functioning begin almost immediately in the majority of patients, but that some report the maintenance of sexual functioning for a long period of time, and that the effects of castration have great individual variability. However imperfect, this castration literature supports the assertion that castration has a profound effect on sexual functioning and on recidivism of sexual crime.

DESCRIPTION OF PROCEDURE,
MORBIDITY AND MORTALITY,
SIDE EFFECTS, AND THEIR
MANAGEMENT

Castration is a safe procedure that can be performed under local anesthesia as an outpatient. Anesthesia is injected into the inguinal cord. Sedation is often used. With the patient in a supine position bilateral incisions are made in the scrotum and the testicular artery, vein, and cord are ligated and then the testes are removed. Patients tolerate the procedure well. The procedure takes approximately half an hour to perform. As a rule, prostheses are not used. Morbidity includes bleeding, infection, and pain. Mortality is virtually nonexistant nowadays.

Hot flashes are commonly experienced with castration in medical patients. They usually require no treatment. However, estrogen, progesterone, or cyproterone acetate, each of which has its own risks and side effects, may ameliorate symptoms (Spetz, Zetterlund, Varenhorst, & Hammar, 2003). Clonidine and antidepressants can also be tried. However, this has not been reported to be a symptom that has been treated in the various studies of GNRH agonists with male sex offenders (Briken, Nika, & Berner, 2001; Krueger & Kaplan, 2001; Kruger & Kaplan, 2006; Rosler & Witztum, 1998; Saleh, Niel, & Fishman, 2004; Schober et al., 2005; Thibaut, Cordier, & Kuhn, 1993; 1996).

Osteoporosis is a significant side effect of patients with paraphilias treated with antiandrogen therapy (Grasswick & Bradford, 2003) and of men treated with medical or surgical castration for prostate cancer (Oefelein & Resnick, 2004). Oefelein and Resnick (2004) reported on the incidence and management of this side effect in patients treated for prostate cancer, indicating that this is a significant side effect and that vitamin D (800 IU/d), calcium supplementation (1200 mg/d), weight-bearing exercise, parenteral estrogen therapy, and bisphosphonate therapy can be used. For paraphiliacs or sex offenders treated with GNRH agonists, bisphosphonate therapy, such as alendronate, has been used in conjunction with calcium and vitamin D. This has, in the experience of one of the authors (Krueger, 2006, personal communication), resulted in no apparent decrease in bone density according to bone density scans performed at baseline and then yearly.

Another risk of androgen deprivation therapy is that castrated patients, if they develop prostate cancer, would have a much worse prognosis. Low serum free testosterone has been reported to be a marker for high grade prostate cancer (Hoffman, DeWolf, & Morgentaler, 2000) and a recent study comparing finasteride, an inhibitor of 5A-reducates that inhibits the conversion of testosterone to dihydrotestosterone, the primary androgen in the prostate, with placebo, suggested that this prevented or delayed the appearance of prostate cancer, there was an increased risk of high-grade prostate cancer. There is also a suggestion that the initiation of androgen suppressive therapy in men over 65 may be associated with increased cardiac events (D'Amico et al., 2007).

ETHICAL AND INFORMED CONSENT ISSUES

A comprehensive review of the legal and ethical issues inherent in orchiectomy is beyond the scope of this chapter. However, some discussion of these issues is provided. Although several states have passed legislation (Scott & Holmberg, 2003) mandating chemical or physical castration, as far as can be determined these laws have not been used. Orchiectomy is a surgical procedure and, as such, for its ethical application, requires informed consent. Basic elements of informed consent for a medical or surgical procedure are the capacity to understand the nature of the procedure and its risks and benefits, the provision of information, and that a decision be freely made. (Applebaum & Gutheil, 1991). Clearly, if an individual refuses to subject himself to such a procedure and/or to give his consent, then to proceed with castration would violate medical ethical guidelines and be considered unethical.

Some have pointed to the existence of a choice of prison or orchiectomy as being inherently coercive (Gaensbauer, 1973; Klerman, 1990). Indeed, within the United States criminal justice system, all of plea-bargaining could be said to be inherently coercive, requiring a choice of an admission of guilt or taking the risk of trial and a substantially longer prison sentence, yet this is considered legal and ethical. However, one can reason that sex offenders start from a different moral baseline than individuals who have not committed a sexual crime, in that they have victimized other individuals, and this fact mitigates against the coercive elements inherent in a choice of prison or castration (either medical or surgical) (Shajnfeld, 2008; Wertheimer, 1987).

Additionally, the choice of castration may be offered to an individual, and he may refuse it, but it cannot be forced onto a person. Accordingly, we would hold that presentation of a choice to an individual convicted of a sex offense and in need of such treatment as an alternative to incarceration is medically and morally ethical. Indeed, a case was recently reported of an individual with pedophilia who, faced

with 10 years of failure of cognitive behavioral therapy to stop him from repeatedly sexually acting out when released into the community, successfully sued to receive chemical castration (Krueger & Kaplan, 2006) He was then able to live in the community while treated with GNRH agonists without other sexual victims for the subsequent 10 years that he was treated. We would agree with Klerman, who emphasizes that prisoners should be allowed this option (Klerman, 1975).

COMPARISON OF ORCHIECTOMY WITH LONG-TERM GNRH SUPPRESSION

Orchiectomy has several advantages over medical castration. Cost is one evident factor with orchiectomy being undoubtedly less expensive than GNRH agonists, but not necessarily progesterone. However, GNRH agonists have a side effect profile which is substantially better than the more traditional androgen suppressing agents (estrogen, progesterone, cyproterone acetate, or flutamide) (Rosler & Witztum, 1998; Rösler & Witztum, 2000) and GNRH agonists would seem to be the most evident equivalent to surgical castration. Other authorities point out that there has been much greater experience with more traditional androgen suppressing agents with thousands of sex offenders in past or current treatment with such agents, and that such agents may cause less side effects related to androgen deprivation and are more capable of titration (Bradford, 2006, personal communication).

Many of the effects and side effects of orchiectomy and of GNRH agonist medication are related to the removal of testosterone, but there are some medication specific risks to the GNRH agonists as well as to the other antiandrogens, such as progesterone or cyproterone acetate that would not exist with orchiectomy. Any exogenous substance can cause an allergic or anaphylactic response, and such responses have been reported with GNRH agonists (Raj, Karadsheh, Guillot, Raj, & Kumar, 1996). Skin reactions have also been reported (Neely et al., 1992) (Labarthe, Bayle-Lebey, & Bazex, 1997; Monasco, Pescovitz, & Blizzard, 1993) although careful examination and consideration of injection technique, or a switch to another of the GNRH agonists with a different compound and different vehicle could resolve this. More serious side effects, such as pure red cell aplasia associated with leuprolide (Maeda et al., 1998) have been reported. The occurrence of these serious side effects could be avoided with different pharmacological agents or surgical castration. Some patients may prefer surgical to medical castration, choosing this to avoid injections or for other personal reasons.

Clearly, the obvious advantage of GNRH agonists is that they are reversible and they do not entail the psychologically adverse effects of castration. Additionally, GNRH agonists may be lowered in dosage or the time interval between injections may be extended, allowing for some titration to allow for an increase in testosterone and the facilitation of unproblematic sexual behavior, if it is determined that this is appropriate, although experience with this is limited, and current dosage packaging limits the flexibility of titration. Castration would not allow for this option. However, many individuals discussed in the aforementioned studies, although castrated, were able to retain some sexual functioning, and it is not certain that sexual functioning will completely disappear with surgical castration. Further, while "add-back" therapy with testosterone to castrated sex offenders is a possibility, one study (Hansen, 1991; Hansen & Lykke-Olesen, 1997) reported a relapse with this treatment. and it would be important to carefully consider and weigh the risks and benefits of such therapy before initiating it in this population.

TREATMENT AND MONITORING CONSIDERATIONS

It should be emphasized that castration by itself is not an exclusive or final treatment. Patients who are castrated can still function sexually, with erections, intromission and ejaculation, and perpetrators can victimize individuals without using a sexual organ. Rather, castration's main effect is to decrease or abolish the intensity of sexual cravings so as to allow a concomitant increase in volitional capacity to maintain self-control (Berlin, 2005). This implies that an individual has to be willing to acknowledge that his sexual behavior is a problem and to be motivated and to agree to make it a target of treatment. One has to form an alliance with the patient in this effort.

Additionally, continual monitoring of testosterone, monitoring for osteopenia or osteoporosis with bone density assessments, and periodic laboratory and physical examinations are all required to follow individuals treated with this modality. Treatment to prevent osteopenia and/or osteoporosis with bisphosphonates, calcium and vitamin D, are required medically as well as other treatments, including psychotherapy and sex offender specific therapy. Other modalities, such as ongoing monitoring by parole, housing, social services, and vocational rehabilitation, are important as well. Indeed, it may be that these other elements may contribute as much as or more than medical or surgical castration to reducing recidivism, and future research should configure study designs so as to assess the effects of sex offender therapy and other elements of a treatment plan, as well as medical or surgical castration, on recidivism of sexual crimes.

The largest open trial involving the use of a chemically castrating agent, tryptoreline, (Rosler & Witztum, 1998) relied on, among other measures, the self-report measure of the Bancroft Sexual Interest and Activity Scale (Bancroft, Tennent, Lougas, & Cass, 1974; Tennent, Bancroft, & Cass, 1974) and testosterone levels, both of which demonstrated change (a reduction in testosterone and in sexual interest and activity, as measured by a Likert scale and by asking the number of ejaculations a subject had experienced in the week before the questionnaire) related to GNRH treatment. These scales could be used to assess outcome and monitor a patient.

However, a recent study (Schober et al., 2005) reported on the use of leuprolide acetate to treat pedophiles, using testosterone levels, sexual interest preference by visual reaction time, penile tumescence, and polygraphs to assess the effects of leuprolide acetate. Subjects were noted to be deceptive regarding increased pedophilic urges and masturbatory frequency and it would be important to incorporate some of these objective modalities into treatment assessment and monitoring. Given the possibility of surreptitious anabolic steroids (Harris, Phoenix, Hanson, & Thornton, 2003, p. 65), it would also be important to screen for these in an ongoing way. Some in the United States have suggested that a urologist be involved in such treatment (Schober, Byrne, & Kuhn, 2006) and others that an internist or family doctor offers an initial medical assessment for clearance for such treatment.

Fundamentally, it cannot be said that castration is a be all and end all measure, and once castrated, society can be done with a sex offender. The marked individual variation in the effects of castration, with some individuals able to retain some sexual functioning, with a capacity for erections and ejaculation, and a motivation for sexual activity, even years after being castrated, suggest that it is critical to assess the actual effects of castration on the patient on whom it is performed. To this end, self-report scales, plethysmography, polygraphy, laboratory and clinical assessment, and observation should be utilized in an ongoing way.

CONCLUSION

Animal and human studies show that the main effect of orchiectomy is a substantial reduction in sexually motivated behavior, but this can have great individual variation. However, all studies on orchiectomy of sex offenders support its efficacy in reducing recidivism. Furthermore, it should be clear that orchiectomy is not a cure-all for sex offenders, nor is it something that can be utilized without a system of aftercare that would include extensive provisions for monitoring, treatment, and support.

Orchiectomy for the treatment of sex offenders has had a dark history, in many instances being performed on individuals against their will or who because of other reasons were unable to consent. Moreover, psychiatry has a history in the century past of utilizing treatments, such as frontal lobotomy or extremely high-dose neuroleptics, that were ultimately established as being extremely harmful and of limited or no therapeutic value. Use of orchiectomy to treat sex offenders in Europe has virtually disappeared and in the United States, although several states have passed laws mandating surgical (or medical) castration for a variety of sexual crimes, contemporary usage of surgical castration has also ceased.

However, orchiectomy's usage in the past century also antedated the modern era of biological treatment with much greater rigor in the classification of psychiatric disorders and research design and it can be anticipated that the future will bring better designed studies to objectively assess the effects of medical, if not surgical, castration, as well as the effects of other treatment modalities.

In spite of current pharmacological practice in the treatment of sex offenders, which includes serotonin-selective reuptake inhibitors and other androgen suppressing agents (see other chapters in this volume), as well as, more recently, GNRH agonists, cost considerations as well as medical ones suggest that orchiectomy could be a desirable alternative. Given the great number of sexual crimes and victims and the great expense sex offenders create for society, almost nothing is spent on research involving the biological treatment of sex offenders. This chapter should make clear that such treatments, including orchiectomy, have great promise and should be the subject of further consideration and investigation.

References

Alexander, M. (1993). Ethical considerations in using orchidectomy for social control. *British Medical Journal*, 307, 790.

Applebaum, P. S. & Gutheil T. G. (1991). Clinical handbook of psychiatry and the law. In P. S. Applebaum & T. G. Gutheil (Eds.), *Clinical Handbook of Psychiatry and the Law*. Baltimore, Maryland 21202: Williams & Wilkins.

Ayalon, D. (1999). *Eunuchs, Caliphs and Sultans. A study of power relationships*. Jerusalem, Israel: The Magnet Press, The Hebrew University.

Baltogiannis, D., Giannakopoulos, X., Charalabopoulos, K., & Sofikitis, N. (2004). Monotherapy in advanced prostate cancer: An overview. *Experimental Oncology*, 26(3), 185–191.

Bancroft, J., Tennent, G., Lougas, K., & Cass, J. (1974). The control of deviant sexual behaviour by drugs: 1. Behavioural changes following oestrogens and anti-androgens. *British Journal of Psychiatry*, 125, 310–315.

Bayoumi, A. M., Brown, A. D., & Garber, A. M. (2000). Cost-effectiveness of androgen suppression therapies in advanced prostate cancer. *Journal of the National Cancer Institute*, 92(21), 1731–1739.

Beach, F. A. (1970). Coital behavior in dogs. VI. Long term effects of castration upon mating in the male. *Journal of Comparative and Physiological Psychology Monograph*, 70, 1–32.

Beach, F. A. (1976). Cross-species comparisons and the human heritage. *Archives of Sexual Behavior*, 5(5), 469–485.

Berlin, F. S. (2005). Commentary: The impact of surgical castration on sexual recidivism risk among civilly committed sexual offenders. *The Journal of the American Academy of Psychiatry and the Law*, 33(1), 37–41.

Bingley, W. (1993). Surgical castration for sex offenders: An unlikely option. *British Medical Journal*, 307, 1141.

Bradford, J. M. W. (1985). Organic treatment for the male sexual offender. *Behavioral Sciences and the Law*, 3(4), 355–375.

Bremer, J. (1958). Part 1: Castration of men. In J. Bremer (Ed.), *Asexualization. A follow-up study of 224 cases*. Oslo, Norway: Oslo University Press.

Briken, P., Nika, E., & Berner, W. (2001). Treatment of paraphilia with luteinizing hormone-releasing hormone agonists. In R. T. Segraves (Ed.), *Journal of sex marital therapy*. London, UK: Taylor & Francis Ltd.

Bubley, G. J., Carducci, M., Dahut, W., Dawson, N., Daliani, D., Eisenberger, M., et al. (1999). Eligibility and response guidelines for phase II clinical trials in androgen-independent prostate cancer: Recommendations from the prostate-specific antigen working group. *Journal of Clinical Oncology*, 17(11), 3461–3467.

Bund, J. M. (1997). Did you say chemical castration? *University of Pittsburg Law Review*, 59, 157–192.

Cassileth, B. R., Soloway, M. S., Vogelzang, N. J., Schellhammer, P. F., Seidmon, E. J., Hait, H. I., et al. (1989). Patient's choice of treatment in stage D prostate cancer. *Supplement of Urology*, XXXIII (5), 57–62.

CBS News. (2004). Sex offender castrated voluntarily. In *CBS News*.

Chabner, B. A., Amrein, P. C., Druker, B. J., Michaelson, M. D., Mitsiades, C. S., Goss, P. E., et al. (2006). In L. L. Brunton, J.S. Lazo, & K.L. Parker (Eds.), *Goodman & Gilman's The Pharmacological Basis of Therapeutics. 11th Edition*. New York McGraw-Hill.

Chadwick, D. J., Gillatt, D. A., & Gingell, J. C. (1991). Medical or surgical orchiectomy: The patients' choice. *British Medical Journal*, 302, 572.

Cheney, V. T. (2004). The advantages of castration. In V. T. Cheney (Ed.), Vol. 1, *The American Focus on Castration*. P.O. Box 663, South Plainfield, NJ 07080–0663: USCCCNII/American Focus Publishing.

Cook, D. A. G. (1993). There is a place for surgical castration in the management of recidivist sex offenders. *British Medical Journal*, 307, 791–792.

Corbin, N. S. & Thompson, I. Jr. (2003). Urology and the Nobel Prize. *Urologic Oncology*, 21, 83–85.

Cornu, F. (1973). Katamnesen bei kastrierten. In F. Cornu (Ed.), *Katamnesen bei kkastrierten*. Verlag für Medizin und Naturwissenschaften, Basel: S. Karger AG.

D'Amico, A. U., Denham, T. W., Crooke, J., Chen, M. H., Goldhaber, S. F., Lamb, D. S.,et al. (2007). Influence of androgen suppression therapy for prostate cancer on the frequency and timing of fatal myocardial infarctions. *Journal of Clinical Oncology*, 25(17), 2420–2425.

Davidson, J. J., Stefanick, M. L., & Sachan, B. L. (1978). Role of androgen in sexual reflexes in the male rat. *Physiology & Behavior*, 21, 141–146.

Dixson, A. F. (1998). Primate sexuality. Comparative studies of the prosimians, monkeys, apes, and human beings. In A. F. Dixson (Ed.), *Primate sexuality. Comparative studies of the prosimians, monkeys, apes, and human beings*. New York, NY: Oxford University Press, Inc.

Eastman, N. (1993). Surgical castration for sex offenders: An unlikely option. *British Medical Journal*, 307, 1141.

Finch, J. (1993). The law is divided. *British Medical Journal*, 307, 792.

Freund, K. (1980). Therapeutic sex drive reduction. *Acta Psychiatrica Scandinavica*, 62, 3–38.

Gaensbauer, T. J. (1973). Castration in treatment of sex offenders: An appraisal. *Rocky Mountain Medical Journal*, 70, 23–28.

Gandhi, N., Purandare, N., & Lock, M. (1993). Surgical Castration for sex offenders. Boundaries between surgery and mutilation are blurred. *British Medical Journal*, 307, 1141.

Gijs, L. & Gooren, L. (1996). Hormonal and psychopharmacological interventions in the treatment of Paraphilias: An update. *The Journal of Sex Research*, 33(4), 273–290.

Grasswick, L. J. & Bradford, J. M. W. (2003). Osteoporosis associated with treatment of paraphilias: A clinical review of seven case reports. *Journal of Forensic Sciences*, 48(4), 849–855.

Greenstein, A., Plymate, S. R., & Katz, P. G. (1995). Visually stimulated erection in castrated men. *The Journal of Urology*, 153, 650–652.

Gugliotta, A. (1998). "Dr. Sharp with his little knife": Therapeutic and punitive origins of eugenic vasectomy—Indiana, 1892–1921. *Journal of the History of Medicine*, 53, 371–406.

Hansen, H. (1991). *Treatment of dangerous sex offenders*. Helsinki, Finland: Ministry of Justice, Government Printing Centre.

Hansen, H. & Lykke-Olesen, L. (1997). Treatment of dangerous sexual offenders in Denmark. *Journal of Forensic Psychiatry*, 8, 195–199.

Harris, A., Phoenix, A., Hanson, R. K, & Thornton, D. (2003). *Static-99 Coding Rules*. West Ottawa, Canada K1A 0P8.

Heim, N. (1981). Sexual behavior of castrated sex offenders. *Archives of Sexual Behavior*, 10(1), 11–19.

Heim, N. & Hursch, C. J. (1979). Castration for sex offenders, Treatment or punishment? A review and critique of recent European literature. *Archives of Sexual Behavior*, 8(3), 281–304.

Hellerstedt, B. A. & Pienta, K. J. (2003). The truth is out there: An overall perspective on androgen deprivation. *Urologic Oncology: Seminars and Original Investigations*, 21, 272–281.

Hensyl, W. R. (1990). Stedman's Medical Dictionary. In W. R. Hensyl (Ed.), *Stedman's Medical Dictionary*, 25th Edition Illustrated ed. Baltimore, Maryland: Williams & Wilkins.

Hicks, P. K. (1993). Castration of sexual offenders. *The Journal of Legal Medicine*, 14, 641–667.

Hoffman, M. A., DeWolf, W. C., & Morgentaler, A. (2000). Is low serum free testosterone a marker for high-grade prostate cancer? *The Journal of Urology*, 163, 824–827.

Huggins, C. & Hodges, C. V. (2002). Studies on prostatic cancer. i. the effect of castration, of estrogen and of androgen injection on serum phosphatases in metastic carcinoma of the prostate. *The Journal Of Urology*, 168, 12.

Icenogle, D. L. (1994). Sentencing male sex offenders to the use of biological treatments. *The Journal of Legal Medicine*, 15, 279–304.

Jones, R. H. & Vasey, P. A. (2003). Part I: Testicular cancer—management of early disease. *The Lancet Oncology*, 4, 730–737.

Jonker-Pool, G., Van de Wiel, H. B. M, Hoekstra, H. J, Sleijfer, D. Th, M. F., Van Driel, J. P., et al. (2001). Sexual functioning after treatment for testicular cancer—Review and meta-analysis of 36 empirical studies between 1975–2000. *Archives of Sexual Behavior*, 30(1), 55–74.

Joseph, P. (1993). Surgical castration for sex offenders. A ploy to deflect the blame. *British Medical Journal*, 307, 1142.

Kinsey, A. C., Pomeroy, W. B, Martin, C. E, & Gebhard, P. H. (1953). Sexual behavior in the human female. In A. C. Kinsey, W. B. Pomeroy, C. E. Martin, & P. H. Gebhard (Ed.), *Sexual Behavior in the Human Female*. Philadelphia: W.B. Saunders Company.

Klerman, G. (1975). Can convicts consent to castration? *Institute of Society, Ethics and the Life Sciences*, 17–18.

Klerman, G. L. (1990). The psychiatric patient's right to effective treatment implications of Osheroff v. Chestnut Lodge. *American Journal of Psychiatry*, 147(4), 409–418.

Krueger, R. B. & Kaplan, M. S. (2001). Depot-leuprolide acetate for treatment of paraphilias: A report of twelve cases. *Archives of Sexual Behavior*, 30(4), 409–422.

Krueger, R. B. & Kaplan, M. S. (2002). Behavioral and Psychopharmacological Treatment of the Paraphilic and Hypersexual Disorders. *Journal of Psychiatric Practice*, 8(1), 21–32.

Krueger, R. B. & Kaplan, M. S. (2006). "I want to try it. What else can I do?" Chemical Castration as a Treatment for Pedophilia. In R. Spitzer, J. Williams, & M. First (Eds.), *Case Book for DSM-IV-TR*, (pp. 309–334). Washington, DC: American Psychiatric Association Press. Chapter 24.

Labarthe, M. P., Bayle-Lebey, P., & Bazex, J. (1997). Cutaneous manifestations of relapsing polychondritis in a patient receiving goserelin for carcinoma of the prostate. *Dermatology*, 195, 391–394.

Langelüddeke, A. (1963). Die entmannung von sittlichkeitsverbrechern. In A. Langelüddeke (Ed.), *Die Entmannung von Sittlichkeitsverbrechern*. Berlin: Walter De Gruyter & Co.

Langeluddeke, A. (1963). Castration of sexual criminals. Berlin: W.De Gruyter.

Langelüddeke, A. (1968). Ergebnisse, Kasuistik und Diskussionen. Sur kastration von sitlichkeitsberbrechern; spate ruckfalle; entmannung aus 42b StGB Untergebrachter *Nervenarzt*, 39(8) 265–268.

Le Marie, L. (1956). Danish experiences regarding the castration of sexual offenders. *Journal of Criminal Law, Criminology, and Police Science*, 47, 295–310.

Lidberg, C. (1968). Sexual kriminalited efter kastration. *Nordisk Psykiatrisk tidssKrift J.* 22, 387.

Linsky, M. (1989). The most critical option: Sex offenses and castration in San Diego, 1938–1975. *The Journal of San Diego History*, 35(4), 1–13.

Loblaw, D. A., Mendelson, D. S, Talcott, J. A, Virgo, K. S, Somerfield, M. R, Ben-Josef, E., et al. (2004). American Society of Clinical Oncology Recommendations for the Initial Hormonal Management of Androgen-Sensitive Metastatic, Recurrent, or Progressive Prostate Cancer. *Journal of Clinical Oncology*, 22(14), 2927–2941.

Lösel, F. & Schmucker, M. (2005). The effectiveness of treatment for sexual offenders: A comprehensive meta-analysis. *Journal of Experimental Criminology*, 1, 117–146.

Loy, J. (1971). Estrous behavior of free-ranging rhesus monkeys (Macaca mulatta). *Primates*, 12, 1–31.

Maatman, T. J., Gupta, M. K., & Montie, J. E. (1985). Effectiveness of castration versus intravenous estrogen therapy in producing rapid endocrine control of metastatic cancer of the prostate. *The Journal of Urology*, 133, 620–621.

Maeda, H., Arai, Y., Aoki, Y., Okubo, K., Okada, T., & Ueda, Y. (1998). Leuprolide causes pure red cell aplasia. *The Journal of Urology*, 160, 501.

Maletzky, B. M., Tolan, A., & McFarland, B. (2006). The Oregon depo-Provera program: A five-year follow-up. *Sex Abuse*, 18, 303–316.

Marmon, S. (1995). *Eunuchs & sacred boundaries in islamic society*. 198 Madison Avenue, New York, NY 10016: Oxford University Press.

Mcleod, D. G. (2003). Hormonal therapy: Historical perspective to future directions. *Urology*, 61(Suppl. 2A), 3–7.

Meyer, W. J., III & Cole, C. M. (1997). Physical and chemical castration of sex offenders: A review. *Journal of Offender Rehabilitation*, 25(3/4), 1–18.

Miyamoto, H., Messing, E. M., & Chang, C. (2004). Androgen deprivation therapy for prostate cancer: Current status and future prospects. *The Prostate*, 61, 332–353.

Monasco, P. K., Pescovitz, O. H., & Blizzard, R. M. (1993). Local reactions to depot leuprolide therapy for central precocious puberty. *The Journal of Pediatrics*, 123(2), 334–335.

Neely, E. K., Hintz, R. L., Parker, B., Bachrach, L. K, Cohen, P., Olney, R., et al. (1992). Two-year results of treatment with depot leuprolide acetate for central precocious puberty. *Journal of Pediatry*, 121 (4), 634–640.

Oefelein, M. G., Feng, A., Scolieri, M. J., Ricchiutti, D., & Resnick, M. I. (2000). Reassessment of the definition of castrate levels of testosterone: Implications for clinical decision-making. *Urology*, 56(6), 1021–1024.

Oefelein, M. G. & Resnick, M. I. (2003). Effective testosterone suppression for patients with prostate cancer: Is there a best castration? *Urology*, 62(2), 207–213.

Oefelein, M. G. & Resnick, M. I. (2004). The impact of osteoporosis in men treated for prostate cancer. *Urologic Clinics of North America*, 31, 313–319.

Ortmann, J. (1980). The treatment of sexual offenders. *International Journal of Law and Psychiatry*, 3, 443–451.

Phoenix, C. H. (1980). Copulation, dominance, and plasma androgen levels in adult rhesus males born and reared in the laboratory. *Archives of Sexual Behavior*, 9(2).

Phoenix, C. H., Slob, A. K., & Goy, R. W. (1973). Effects of castration and replacement therapy on sexual behavior of adult male rhesuses. *Journal Of Comparative And Physiological Psychology*. 84, 472–481.

Potosky, A. L., Knopf, K., Clegg, L. X., Albertsen, P. C, Stanford, J. L, Hamilton, A. S, et al. (2001). Quality-of-life outcomes after primary androgen deprivation therapy: Results from the prostate cancer outcomes study. *Journal of Clinical Oncology*, 19(17), 3750–3757.

Raj, S. G., Karadsheh, A. J, Guillot, R. J., Raj, M. H. G, & Kumar, P. (1996). Case report: Systemic hypersensitivity reaction to goserelin acetate. *The American Journal of Medical Sciences*, 312(4), 187–190.

Ringrose, K. M. (2003). *The perfect servant. Eunuchs and the social construction of gender in Byzantium.* Chicago 60637: The University of Chicago Press.

Rosler, A. & Witztum, E. (1998). Treatment of men with paraphilia with a long-acting analogue of gonadotropin-releasing hormone. *The New England Journal of Medicine*, 338(7), 416–422.

Rösler, A. & Witztum, E. (2000). Pharmacotherapy of paraphilias in the next millennium. *Behavioral Sciences and the Law*, 18(1), 43–56.

Rousseau, L., Dupont A, Labrie F, & Couture M. (1988). Sexuality changes in prostate cancer patients receiving antihormonal therapy combining the antiandrogen flutamide with medical (LHRH Agonist) or surgical castration. *Archives of Sexual Behavior*, 17(1), 87–98.

Saleh, F. M., Niel T, & Fishman M. J. (2004). Treatment of paraphilia in young adults with leuprolide acetate: A preliminary case report series. *Journal of Forensic Sciences*, 49(6), 1–6.

Sand, K., Dickmeiss P, & Schwalbe-Hansen D. (1964). *Report on sterilization and castration.* 353 Copenhagen: Herstedvester Hospital Publication.

Sanford, E. J., Paulson, D. F., Rohner, T. J., Drago, J. R., Santen, R. J. & Bardin, C. W. (1977). The effects of castration on adrenal testosterone secretion in men with prostatic cancer. *Journal of Urology*, 118, 1019–1021.

Santen, R. (2003). Chapter 39. Endocrine-responsive cancer. In P. R. Larsen, H. M. Kronenberg, S. Melmed & K. S. Polonsky (Eds.), *Williams textbook of endocrinology.* The Curtis Center, Independence Square West, Philadelphia, PA 19106: Saunders.

Schober, J. M., Kuhn, P. J., Kovacs, P. G., Earle, J. H., Byrne, P. M., & Fries, R. A. (2005). Leuprolide acetate suppresses pedophilic urges and arousability. *Archives of Sexual Behavior*, 34(6), 691–705.

Schober, J. M., Byrne, P. M., & Kuhn, P. J. (2006). Leuprolide acetate is a familiar drug that may modify sex-offender behavior: the urologist's role. *British Journal of Urology*, 97, 684–686.

Scholz, P. O. (2001). *Eunuchs and Castrati. A Cultural History.* 231 Nassau Street, Princeton, NJ 08542: Markus Wiener Publishers.

Schroder, F. H. (1997). In R. S. Walsh & Vaughan (Eds.), *Campbell's urology.* Philadelphia: W.B. Saunders.

Scott, C. L. & Holmberg, T. (2003). Castration of sex offenders: Prisoner's rights versus public safety. *The Journal of the American Academy of Psychiatry and the Law*, 31(4), 502–509.

Shajnfeld, A. (2008). Sex offenders and informed consent to castration in the prison context. *Sex offender law report*, 9, 1, 1–11.

Sharifi, N., Gulley, J. L., & Dahut, W. L. (2005). Androgen deprivation therapy for prostate cancer. *Journal of the American Medical Association*, 294(2), 238–244.

Silcock, S. R. (1993). Surgical castration for sex offenders. *British Medical Journal*, 308, 613.

Simpson, J. A. & Weiner, E. S. C. (1989). *The Oxford English Dictionary.* In J. A. Simpson & E. S. C. Weiner (Eds.), *The Oxford English Dictionary 2nd Edition.* Oxford: Clarendon Press.

Spetz, A-C., Zetterlund, E-L., Varenhorst, E., & Hammar M. (2003). Incidence and management of hot flashes in prostate cancer. *The Journal of Supportive Oncology*, 1(4), 263–273.

Sturup, G. K. (1968a). *The mentally abnormal offender.* London.

Sturup, G. K. (1968b). Treatment of sexual offenders in Herstedvester, Denmark. *Acta Psychiatrica Scandinavica* 44, 1–64.

Sturup, G. K. (1972). Castration: The total treatment. In H. L. P. Resnik & M. E. Wolfgang (Eds.), *Treatment of the sex offender.* Boston: Little, Brown and Company.

Tancredi, L. R. & Weisstub, D. N. (1986). Technology assessment: Its role in forensic psychiatry and the case of chemical castration. *International Journal of Law and Psychiatry*, 8, 257–271.

Taus, L. & Susicka L. (1973). Five years long observation of five sexual deviants after therapeutic intervention. *Czechoslovakian Psychiatry*, 69(1), 51–55.

Taylor, G. (2000). *Castration. An abbreviated history of western manhood.* 29 West 35th Street, New York, NY 10001: Rutledge.

Taylor, P. J. (1993). An angry man let down by medical indifference. *British Medical Journal*, 307, 792.

Tennent, G., Bancroft, J., & Cass, J. (1974). The control of deviant sexual behavior by drugs: A double-blind controlled study of benperidol, chlorpromazine, and placebo. *Archives of Sexual Behavior*, 3(3), 261–271.

Thibaut, F., Cordier, B., & Kuhn, J-M. (1993). Effect of a long-lasting gonadotropin hormone-releasing hormone agonist in six cases of severe male paraphilia. *Acta Psychiatrica Scandinavica*, 87, 445–450.

Thibaut, F., Cordier, B., & Kuhn, J-M. (1996). Gonadotropin hormone releasing hormone agonist in cases of severe paraphilia: A lifetime treatment? *Psychoneuroendocrinology*, 21(4), 411–419.

Tougher, S. (2002). Eunuchs in antiquity and beyond. In S. Tougher (Ed.), *Eunuchs in antiquity and beyond*. P.O. Box 511, Oakville, CT 06779: The David Brown Book Co.

Tsai, S-S H. (1996). The Eunuchs in the Ming dynasty. In S. -S. H. Tsai (Ed.), *The eunuchs in the ming dynasty*, State University Plaza, Albany, NY.: State University of New York.

Van Basten, J. P. A., Van Driel, M. F., Hoekstra, H. J., Sleijfer, D. Th., Van De Wiel, H. B. M., Droste, J. H. J., et al. (1999). Objective and subjective effects of treatment for testicular cancer on sexual function. *BJU International*, 84, 671–678.

Wassersug, R. J. (2004). New age eunuchs: Motivation and rationale for voluntary castration. *Archives of Sexual Behavior*, 33(5), 433–442.

Weinberger, L. E., Sreenivasan, S., Garrick, T., & Osran, H. (2005). The impact of surgical castration on sexual recidivism risk among sexually violent predatory offenders. *The Journal of the American Academy of Psychiatry and the Law*, 33(1), 16–36.

Wertheimer, A. (1987). *Coercion*. Princeton, New Jersey 084540: Princeton University Press.

Wille, R. & Beier, K. M. (1989). Castration in Germany. *Annals of Sex Research*, 2, 103–133.

Winslade, W., Stone, T. H., Smith-Bell, M., Webb, D. M. (1998).Castrating pedophiles convicted of sex offenses against children: New treatment or old punishment? *Southern Methodist University Law Review*, 51, 349–412.

Young, J. B. & Landsberg, L. (2001). Synthesis, storage, and secretion of adrenal medullary hormones: Physiology and pathophysiology. In B. S. McEwen & Goodman, H. M. *Handbook of Physiology*. New York, NY: Oxford University Press, Inc.

Zverina, J., Zimanova, J., & Bartova D. (1991). Catamneses of a group of 84 castrated sexual offenders. *Ceskoslovenska Psychiatrie*, 87, 28–31.

Chapter 14

Pharmacological Treatment of Paraphilic Sex Offenders

Fabian M. Saleh

Sex offenders represent a heterogeneous population. A subgroup of sex offenders suffers from sexual disorders known in the sexological and psychiatric literature as paraphilias. According to the revised fourth edition of the *Diagnostic and Statistical Manual of Mental Disorders* (American Psychiatric Association, 2000) the "essential features of a paraphilia are recurrent, sexually arousing fantasies, sexual urges, or behaviors generally involving (1) nonhuman objects, (2) the suffering of oneself or one's partner, or (3) children or other nonconsenting persons that occur over a period of at least 6 months" (Criterion A). DSM-IV-TR also suggests that for some individuals "paraphilic fantasies or stimuli are obligatory for erotic arousal and are always included in sexual activity." For other individuals, paraphilic "preferences appear only episodically." Of the nine paraphilias listed in the DSM (see Table 14.1), pedophilia and exhibitionism are the most prevalent in outpatient settings (Abel, 1989). (Paraphilias are discussed in Chapter 2.)

Treatment of paraphilic sex offenders (i.e., sex offenders who suffer from one or more paraphilias) is multifaceted, and by present standards, encompasses psychologically, and where appropriate, biologically based therapies (Saleh & Guidry, 2003). This chapter will focus on the pharmacological treatment of paraphilic sex offenders. In particular, it will examine and review relevant data on the efficacy and safety of medications that reduce levels of androgens. Data on less established medications, such as the serotonergic antidepressants, will be reviewed briefly.

The following vignette describes the case of a paraphilic sex offender who improved in his overall level of functioning following treatment with leuprolide acetate (Saleh, 2005). This case presentation serves to frame some of the issues that will be discussed in this chapter.

CASE EXAMPLE

J.F., a 19-year-old, single male, was referred for a psychosexual and risk assessment after being convicted of several incidents of public masturbation and

TABLE 14.1 Paraphilic Disorders as Listed in DSM-IV-TR

Exhibitionism

Fetishism

Frotteurism

Pedophilia

Sexual masochism

Sexual sadism

Transvestic fetishism

Voyeurism

Paraphilia not otherwise specified

indecent exposure involving postpubertal teenage girls. Following a comprehensive psychiatric work-up, J.F. was diagnosed with a paraphilic disorder, best characterized as Paraphilia Not Otherwise Specified. He did not present with a comorbid mental illness or a substance abuse disorder. On mental status examination, J.F. endorsed deviant sexual fantasies and urges involving exhibitionistic and nonconsensual sexual acts. He also reported a 3-year history of heightened sexual drive, masturbating numerous times a day, up to 46 times a week, to age appropriate, and occasionally deviant, sexual fantasies. On penile plethysmograph testing, J.F. showed deviant sexual arousal to exhibitionistic and rape stimuli (see Figures 14.1 and Figure 14.2). (Penile plethysmography is discussed in Chapter 7.)

Because of his presentation, and following a pretreatment work-up (see following text for more details), J.F. was started on leuprolide acetate (7.5 mg per month) and flutamide. The latter medication was prescribed at a dose of 750 mg per day for 4 weeks. After about two weeks into the treatment, J.F. reported a decrease in the intensity and frequency of his paraphilic symptoms. His self-report of decreased sexual arousal was consistent with subsequent PPG findings, which showed no arousal to paraphilic stimuli (see Figure 14.3 and Figure 14.4).

By the third week, serum free testosterone level decreased from 140.40 to 31.6 pg/ml (J.F.'s hormone profile is shown in Table 14.2). Total sexual outlet, as measured in this instance by the frequency of orgasms per week, decreased after about 3 months to an average of two to three times a week. J.F. reported relief from intrusive sexual fantasies as well as superior work performance and improved interpersonal relationships.

To reduce the risk for medication-related side effects, leuprolide was eventually decreased to 3.75 mg per month. This was not associated with reoccurring paraphilic symptoms. Indeed, follow-up after 18 months revealed sustained improvement over time. To date, J.F. has remained symptom free. He has not reoffended sexually.

RATIONALE FOR PHARMACOLOGICAL TREATMENT AND DIAGNOSTIC WORK-UP

Not all sex offenders will benefit from testosterone-lowering medications. For example, offering an anti-androgen to a patient with schizophrenia or bipolar disorder would be inappropriate if the sexual offending behavior was a manifestation of a psychotic or manic episode. Antipsychotic medications or anticonvulsants (i.e., mood stabilizers) would be the treatment of choice in these cases (Smith & Taylor, 1999). Similarly, offering a testosterone-lowering medication to a developmentally delayed sex offender who offended because of a lack of understanding of, for example, the age of consent would be ill-advised. Counselling and psychosexual education would be the intervention of first choice in this latter case. On the other hand, failure to prescribe a testosterone-lowering medication to a symptomatic sex offender with paraphilic proclivities or an idiopathic paraphilic disorder could have devastating consequences for both the offender and the target of the offender's paraphilic interest (e.g., prepubescent children). Indeed, to mitigate a paraphilic sex offender's risk for sexual recidivism, testosterone-lowering medications should be made available to sex offenders who present with intense sexual urges or cravings for paraphilic activities. Suffice to say that any treatment decision should follow and be based on the results of a comprehensive diagnostic and medical work-up (Saleh & Guidry, 2003; Bradford, Boulet, & Pawlak, 1992).

Diagnostic Work-Up

Although the importance of a psychiatric and phenomenological interview cannot be overemphasized, a multimodal approach is recommended when evaluating sex offenders. This is particularly important given that sex offenders, with or without paraphilias, can be unreliable and self-serving reporters. As such,

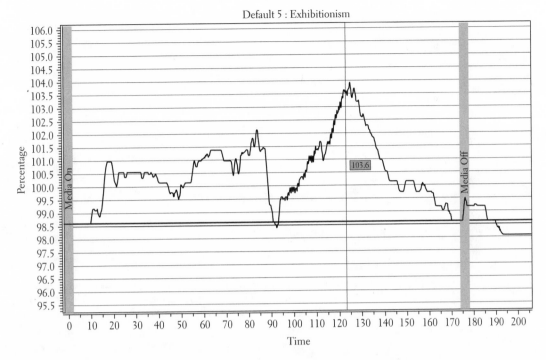

FIGURE 14.1 Pretreatment arousal response to a stimulus describing exhibitionistic activity.

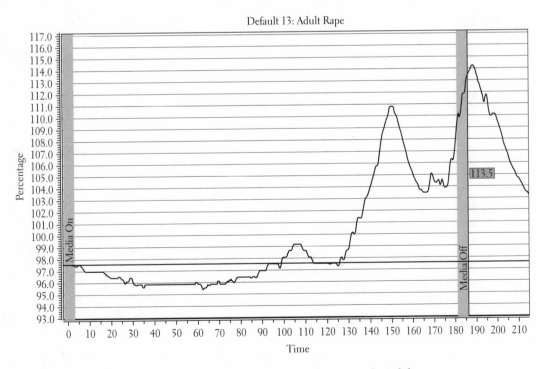

FIGURE 14.2 Pretreatment arousal response to a stimulus describing rape of an adult woman.

191

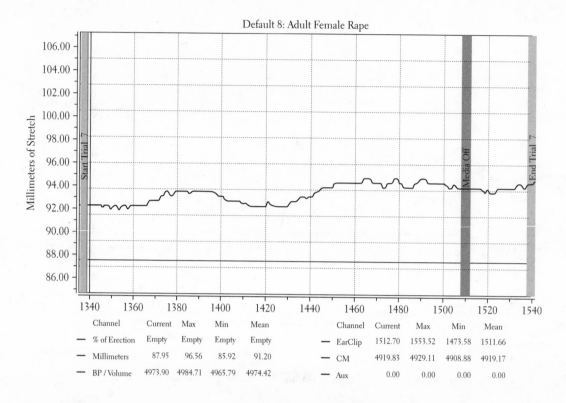

Default 8: Adult Female Rape

Channel	Current	Max	Min	Mean
— % of Erection	Empty	Empty	Empty	Empty
— Millimeters	87.95	96.56	85.92	91.20
— BP / Volume	4973.90	4984.71	4965.79	4974.42

Channel	Current	Max	Min	Mean
— EarClip	1512.70	1553.52	1473.58	1511.66
— CM	4919.83	4929.11	4908.88	4919.17
— Aux	0.00	0.00	0.00	0.00

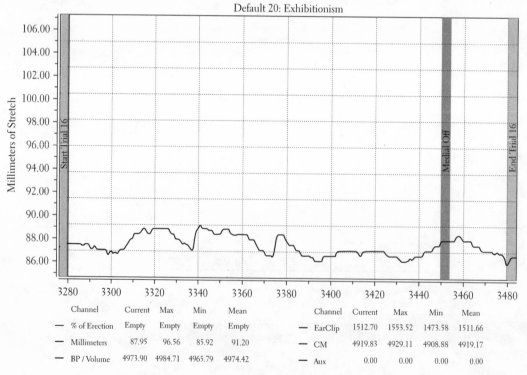

Default 20: Exhibitionism

Channel	Current	Max	Min	Mean
— % of Erection	Empty	Empty	Empty	Empty
— Millimeters	87.95	96.56	85.92	91.20
— BP / Volume	4973.90	4984.71	4965.79	4974.42

Channel	Current	Max	Min	Mean
— EarClip	1512.70	1553.52	1473.58	1511.66
— CM	4919.83	4929.11	4908.88	4919.17
— Aux	0.00	0.00	0.00	0.00

FIGURE 14.3 AND 14.4 Following treatment with leuprolide acetate and consistent with J.F.'s self-report of decreased arousal, J.F. did not show arousal to any of the paraphilic stimuli.

TABLE 14.2 Hormonal Profiles Prior to and During Leuprolide Acetate/Flutamide Therapy

Reference Range in Adult Males	Hormonal Levels in J.F.
Luteinizing hormone (LH): 1.5–9.3 mIU/mL	
Follicle stimulating hormone (FSH) 1.4–18.1 mIU/mL	
Testosterone (T): 241–827 ng/dL	
Free testosterone (Free T): 47–244 pg/mL	
Free testosterone concentration is derived from a mathematical expression based on constants for the binding of testosterone to sex hormone binding globulin	

Pretreatment

LH	2.71
FSH	<1.0
T	333.58
Free T	140.40

About 3 weeks into leuprolide therapy

LH	1.64
FSH	<1.0
T	110.26
Free T	31.6

4½ months into leuprolide therapy

LH	0.87
FSH	4.8
T	56.22
Free T	11.9

one should correlate, where possible, clinical data (self-report and clinician-administered measures—see Table 14.3) with collateral information, such as victim statements, police reports, prior mental health and medical records, juvenile and adult criminal records, and forensic reports. Along the same lines, treatment responses should be correlated with hormonal and penile plethysmography data (Saleh, 2005) (Violence risk assessment is discussed in Chapter 5).

Medical Work-Up

To exclude active medical conditions and minimize the risk for medication-induced side effects, patients considered for antiandrogen therapy should have a complete physical, and where indicated, neurological examination (Bradford, 2000; Saleh & Guidry, 2003). Baseline laboratory tests include the following:

- Complete blood count
- Serum electrolytes
- Calcium and phosphate
- Lipid profile
- Fasting glucose
- Liver function test: aspartate aminotransferase (AST), alanine aminotransferase (ALT), gamma-glutamyl transpeptidase (gamma-GT), alkanine phosphatase, albumin, and total protein
- BUN and creatinine
- Thyroid stimulating hormone (TSH)
- Parathyroid hormone (PTH)

Indices for the following hormones should also be obtained:

- Free and total serum testosterone (T)
- Progesterone
- Estradiol
- Follicle stimulating hormone (FSH)
- Luteinizing hormone (LH)
- Prolactin

Other tests that should be considered are urinalysis, urine toxicology, and a pregnancy test in women. Moreover, before starting treatment with one of the testosterone-lowering agents, patients should have a baseline bone densitometry evaluation (dual energy X-ray absorptiometry) and a baseline 12-lead electrocardiogram (with long rhythm strip). The foregoing tests should be repeated, at a minimum, at 6- to 12-month intervals to reduce for medication-related side effects. Likewise, vital signs (heart rate and blood pressure) and weight should be measured at baseline and then on a monthly basis.

Informed Consent

As with any other form of therapy, informed consent should be obtained before treatment (Berlin, 1989). First, a patient should be given adequate information with regard to the risks and benefits of the proposed treatment. Similarly, the risks and benefits of alternative treatments and of no treatment should be thoroughly reviewed. Equally important are the second and third element of the informed consent doctrine. In fact, for a consent to be valid it has to be given

TABLE 14.3 Selected Assessment Tools

Instrument	Content
Psychopathology-related measures	
Psychopathy Checklist–Revised (Hare, 2003)	The PCL-R is a clinical rating scale used to assess psychopathy. The PCL-R comprises 20 items scored on a 3-point scale (0 = item does not apply, 1 = item applies somewhat, 2 = item definitely applies). Total scores range from 0 to 40; Scores higher than 30 are considered diagnostic of psychopathy
The Michigan Alcohol Screening Test (Sletzer, et al., 1975)	The MAST is a self-report inventory used in the general population to identify incidence or behaviors indicative of alcohol abuse. This measure contains 25 "Yes–No" questions and yields an overall score ranging from 0 – 53
Montgomery-Asberg Depression Rating Scale (Montgomery & Asberg, 1979)	Montgomery-Asberg Depression Rating Scale measures overall severity of depressive symptoms. This measure is sensitive to change and uses a 10-item checklist, with items rated on a six point scale
The Hamilton Anxiety Rating Scale (Hamilton, 1959)	The Hamilton Anxiety Rating Scale is a measure of global anxiety, consists of 14 items that are rated on a 5-point scale, from 0 = no to 4 = severe, grossly disabling symptoms (Hamilton, 1959). Total scores range from 0 to 56, with scores greater than or equal to 14 indicating clinically significant anxiety (American Psychiatric Association, 2000)
The Yale Brown Obsessive Compulsive Scale (American Psychiatric Association, 2000)	The Y-BOCS is a clinician-administered scale that measures the severity of obsessive-compulsive symptoms. It is divided into two subscales: the Obsessions subscale and the Compulsions subscale
The Global Improvement Scale (Guy, 1976)	The Global Improvement Scale is a seven-point and rater-administered scale that measures general improvement. It ranges from a very much improved to very much worse
Measures of Sexual Functioning	
Bradford Sexual History Inventory	Bradford Sexual History Inventory is semistructured interview schedule that asks about a wide range of deviant and nondeviant sexual thoughts and activities commonly encountered in clinical and forensic settings
Greenberg Sexual Preference Visual Analogue Scale (Greenberg, 1991)	The GVAS is a self-report instrument that is used to assess the sexual preference of a sexual offender. The scale forces the sex offenders to choose between adult males, adult females, young girls, and young boys. It produces four scores indicating the degree of sexual preference for women, men, young girls, and young boys
Sexual Interest and Sexual Activity Rating Scale (Bancroft et al., 1974)	The Sexual Interest and Sexual Activity Scales record the degree of sexual interest and the frequency of sexual activity during the week preceding the assessment. The Sexual Activity Scale is a measure of sexual activity defined as the number of orgasms in the last 7 days. The Sexual Interest scale serves to rate the patient's general sexual interest on a five-point Likert scale
The Wilson Sex Fantasy Questionnaire (Baumgartner et al., 1988)	This is a self-report measure of sexual fantasies. The 40 sexual fantasy items are categorized into four fantasy subtypes consisting of 10 items each. They assess themes ranging "from the normal and innocuous to the deviant and potentially harmful."
Penile Plethysmograph (Blanchard et al., 2001)	The PPG is both a screening tool and an outcome tool. Penile tumescence is a good indicator of sexual arousal that is commonly used to identify individuals with deviant sexual arousal

voluntarily without undue influence or coercion. This is particularly important in this population given that the majority of prospective patients is either on probation or parole at the time of referral. Finally, a patient has to be *competent* to give informed consent. Indeed, if a patient does not possess the requisite abilities to give informed consent and is deemed incompetent (e.g., developmentally delayed and/or mentally ill paraphilic sex offender), informed consent needs to be obtained from a substituted decision maker (Cooper, 1986).

Testosterone-Lowering Treatments

Among the biologically based treatments one has to distinguish between orchiectomy (surgical removal of the testes) and pharmacotherapy (Stompe, 2007). It is important to point out here that data pertaining to orchiectomy provide the basis for our understanding of the mechanism and benefits of testosterone-lowering medications in paraphilic sex offenders. For example, Langelüddecke (1963) presented data on 1036 sex offenders who were offered orchiectomy. More than half of the cohort declined orchiectomy and served as the control group (N = 685). Recidivism rates declined to 2.3% for the orchiectomized offenders. That is, compared to 80% for the untreated group, only 24 out of 1036 reoffended following orchiectomy. Follow-up periods ranged from 6 weeks to 20 years. Fifty-eight offenders reported a complete cessation of their sexual drive. Fifteen reported a gradual decline in their sexual functioning, and 16 maintained erectile and orgasmic functioning despite having undergone orchiectomy. As reported by Sturup (1968), Sand et al. (1964) presented recidivism data on a cohort of 900 castrated sex offenders who were reexamined over a 30-year period. Follow-up inquiries approximated 4000. Similar to the data presented by Langelüddecke, recidivism rates were in the 2% range. These, and similar studies, show that orchiectomy causes a substantial decrease in sexual recidivism, with recidividism rates ranging from 1% to 3% for orchiectomized sex offenders versus a staggering 50% to 60 % for controls (i.e., nonorchiectomized sex offenders) (Orchiectomy is discussed in Chapter 13).

Although rather effective, the use of orchiectomy has become superfluous with the introduction of the below described hormonal treatments. Estrogens were among the first medications made available to this population. Although effective in ameliorating paraphilic symptoms, their use was limited because of their feminizing and carcinogenic properties (Foote, 1944; Golla & Hodge, 1949). Estrogen therapy was eventually superseded by the progesterone derivates, medroxyprogesterone and cyproterone acetate, respectively (Bancroft, Tennent, Loucas, & Cass, 1974; Money, 1968). Though less adverse effect prone than the estrogens, medication compliance remained a problem with the progesterone derivates. The pharmacological treatment of the paraphilias has changed during the last decade. In fact, the introduction of newer agents, especially the luteinizing hormone-releasing hormone agonists, has clinicians a new alternative in the treatment of paraphilic sex offenders (Briken, Nika, & Berner, 2001; Krueger & Kaplan, 2001; Rosler & Witztum, 1998).

The next section of this chapter will briefly review data on the selective serotonin-reuptake inhibitors (SSRIs). It will be followed by a more in depth discussion of the testosterone-lowering medications cyproterone acetate, medroxyprogesterone acetate, and the luteinizing hormone-releasing hormone agonists. (The neurochemistry and neurobiology of human sexual behavior is discussed in Chapter 4 and see Chapter 7 also.)

SELECTIVE SEROTONIN REUPTAKE INHIBITORS

While the role of serotonin (5-HT) in sexual behavior has been extensively studied in animals, research in humans has been relatively scant. Similarly, neurobiological data linking serotonin to the paraphilias is limited. Indeed, it remains to be seen whether serotonin plays a specific role in the pathophysiology of the paraphilias. On the other hand, a growing body pharmacological data suggest that increased serotonin levels in the central nervous system may adversely impact sexual behavior, causing various forms of sexual problems (i.e., sexual dysfunctions). Antidepressant-induced sexual side effects, specifically those related to SSRI use, range anywhere from 2.7% to 75% (Baldwin, Thomas, & Birtwistle, 1997; Patterson, 1993; Stark & Hardison, 1985), and include decreased libido, erectile difficulties, ejaculation failure, and delayed or absent orgasm (Rothschild, 2000).

Because of the foregoing, this class of antidepressants has been increasingly used to treat sex offenders presenting with paraphilic disorders. Although certainly intriguing, it is critical to take the following caveats into account when considering an SSRI for this subgroup of sex offenders:

1. Almost all SSRI-related sexual dysfunction data derive from studies involving male and female patients afflicted with depressive and anxiety disorders, and not paraphilias (Rothschild, 2000; Williams et al., 2006).

2. Sexual dysfunction, even in patients taking SSRIs, is a multifactorial phenomenon, and is caused or exacerbated by a myriad of conditions including but not limited to the psychiatric illness itself (depression or anxiety), co-occurring general medical illness (thyroid disease, diabetes mellitus, cardiovascular disease, atherosclerosis, etc.), concomitant medication use (antihypertensives, anticholinergics, antihistamines, anticonvulsants, etc.), drug of abuse and/or alcohol, psychological stress (recent involvement with the courts, interpersonal conflicts, etc), and finally halo effect (Baldwin, 2004; Keltner, McAfee, & Taylor, 2002; Lauman, Michael, & Gagnon, 1994). In other words, cause and effect between SSRIs and sexual dysfunction is not an explicit and unequivocal phenomenon (Williams et al., 2006).

3. The four phases of the normal human sexual response cycle (desire, excitement, orgasm, and resolution) are not equally affected by SSRIs. In males, ejaculatory dysfunction and delayed or absent orgasm are a more common occurrence than SSRI-emergent decreases in sexual desire (Ashton, Hamer, & Rosen, 1997; Keltner et al., 2002; Seidman, 2006; Williams et al., 2006).

4. SSRI-emergent sexual side effects are dose-dependent and reversible. With the exception of fluoxetine (an SSRI with a long half-life), sexual functioning improves within a few days following medication discontinuation (Rothschild, 1995; Zajecka, Mitchell, & Fawcett, 1997; Hirschfeld, 1999; Zajecka, 2001). Likewise, it is important to note that some patients develop tolerance to SSRI-induced sexual side effects (Zajecka, 2001).

5. Lastly, and probably most importantly, approximately 90% of surveyed patients discontinue or drop out of treatment because of SSRI-related sexual side effects (National Depression Manic-Depression Association, 2000). That is, SSRI-induced sexual side effects may contribute to poor treatment adherence and medication noncompliance (Keltner et al., 2002).

Although treatment of paraphilic sex offenders with SSRIs holds promise, and might be an option in carefully selected and highly reliable patients, the lack of placebo-controlled studies and unambiguous biological data, linking serotonin to the paraphilias, limits our ability to draw meaningful conclusions on the efficacy of these medications at this point in time. In fact, with the exception of a few open-label and retrospective studies (see subsequently), clinical trials assessing the efficacy of SSRIs in paraphilic sex offenders are nonexistent.

Selected Studies Pertaining to SSRIs and the Paraphilias

In an open-label trial of 3 months duration, Kafka and Prentky (1992) treated 20 patients, diagnosed with either paraphilia or "nonparaphilic sexual addictions," with fluoxetine (mean dose 39 mg per day). Paraphilic symptoms decreased after 4 weeks, yet conventional (normophilic) sexual behavior was maintained. Although the results of this trial are interesting, a placebo effect cannot be ruled out. In another open label study, Kafka (1994) treated a cohort of 24 men, diagnosed with paraphilia or paraphilia-related disorders, with sertraline (25 to 250 mg per day). Patients presented mostly with noncontact paraphilias, such as exhibitionism, fetishism, transvestic fetishism, telephone scatologia, and voyeurism. Mean duration of sertraline treatment ranged from 4 to 64 weeks. Partial responders (n = 4) received augmentation with lithium, methylphenidate, or trazodone. Sertraline non-responders (n = 9) were switched to fluoxetine with doses ranging from 10 to 80 mg per day. Three men on fluoxetine required methylphenidate augmentation. Of the cohort, 71% improved with either sertraline or fluoxetine. Side effects of sertraline included gastrointestinal distress, fatigue, "increased depression," sexual dysfunction, and headache. Side effects of fluoxetine and sexual recidivism rates were not reported. Limitations of this study included, among other things, the use of several agents with different pharmacodynamic properties and the lack of a control group.

In an open-label dose titrated study, Bradford et al. (1995) treated a homogeneous group of 18 pedophiles with sertraline using a mean daily dose of 131 mg.

Treatment response was based on patient self-report and penile plethysmograph data. Similar to the aforementioned study, deviant sexual arousal was reduced, whereas normophilic arousal was preserved, and even increased in two patients.

Cyproterone Acetate

Cyproterone acetate (CPA) is not available in the United States. CPA is an antiandrogen with both anti-androgenic and antigonadotropic properties (Gilman et al., 1990; Goldenberg et al., 1991). It has been used in the treatment of severe hirsutism, androgenetic alopecia, idiopathic precocious puberty, and prostate cancer (Jurzyk, Spielvogel, & Rose, 1992; O'Brien, Cooper, Murray, Seeman, Thomas, &. Jerums, 1991; Pavone-Macaluso et al., 1986). Since the mid- to late-1960s, CPA has also been used to treat hypersexual, sexually aggressive, and paraphilic patients. Similar to cimetidine, CPA exerts its antilibidinal effects by competitively blocking testosterone and dihydrotestosterone binding to peripheral and central androgen receptors. CPA also prevents binding of dihydrotestosterone to intracellular receptor sites and thus blocks the translocation of the androgen receptor complex into the cell nucleus (Brotherton, Burton, & Shuster, 1974; Goldenberg et al., 1988; Krogh, 1992; Reynolds, 1989).

CPA can be administered orally and intramuscularly. Oral dosages range from 50 to 200 mg per day, while intramuscular dosages range from 300 to 700 mg per injection. The latter has been given on a weekly or biweekly basis (Reilly, Delva, & Hudson, 2000).

With regard to its pharmacokinetic properties (see Table 14.4), oral CPA is slowly and poorly absorbed from the gastrointestinal tract (Jurzyk et al., 1992). After being metabolized in the liver to 15-β-hydroxycyproterone (its main metabolite), CPA is excreted via the urinary and gastrointestinal tract.

The side effects of CPA are dose dependent (Laschet & Laschet, 1975; Neuman et al., 1970) and include nausea, vomiting, diarrhea, constipation, breast tenderness, galactorrhea, decreased libido, thrombophlebitis, hypochromic anemia (rare), hypercalcemia, fatigue, lethargy, and weakness. Late or delayed side effects include gynecomastia, depression, benign nodular hyperplasia of the breast, and hypospermia (low semen volume). Elevated liver enzymes (AST, ALT, LDH), fatal hepatitis (Blake, Sawyerr, Dooley, Scheuer, & McIntyre, 1990; Levesque et al., 1989), decreased response to ACTH (with lowered cortisol levels), as well as carbohydrate metabolism dysregulations have also been reported with the use of CPA. Moreover, CPA treatment has been associated with lipid abnormalities, decreased spermatogenesis, headaches, weight gain, hot flashes, night sweats, and ophthalmologic abnormalities (Goldenberg & Bruchovsky, 1991; Jurzyk et al., 1992).

Selected Studies Pertaining to CPA

As reported by Bradford (2001), Laschet and Laschet (1971) treated a large cohort of 110 "sexually deviant men," diagnosed with pedophilia, exhibitionism, or sexual sadism, with either oral (100 mg per day) or intramuscular (300 mg every other week) CPA. About 50% of the cohort had histories of sexual offending behavior. Follow-up periods ranged from 6 to 50 months. Eighty percent of the patient population, receiving oral CPA, reported a substantial decrease in sexual drive, erections, and orgasm. Side effects included weight gain, depression, and feminization. Of note, in some cases, treatment response was maintained following medication discontinuation.

In a double-blind placebo crossover study, Bradford and Pawlak (1993a) treated a cohort of 19 sex offenders with either oral CPA or placebo. All subjects met DSM-III-R criteria for pedophilia. Pretreatment sexual recidivism rates were high, averaging 2.5 sexual offenses per subject. Subjects were randomly and double-blindly assigned to receive either CPA or placebo. Three subjects completed the full 13 months

TABLE 14.4 Pharmacokinetic Properties of CPA

Molecular Structure/ Chemical Name	Bioavailability	Maximum Plasma Half-Life	Metabolized	Main Metabolite
C24H29ClO4/ 6-Chloro-1α,2α-methylene-3, 20-dioxopregna-4, 6-dien-17-yl acetate	100% after oral administration	38 +/– 5 hours (oral CPA) 82 +/– 21 (intramuscular CPA)	Hepatically	15-β-hydroxycyproterone

trial period. Although not statistically significant, deviant sexual arousal, as measured by penile plethysmography and self-report, decreased in all subjects with active drug treatment.

In a follow-up study, Bradford and Pawlak (1993b) evaluated sexual arousal patterns of 17 pedophiles via penile plethysmography. Responses to pedophilic (mutually consenting and coercive) stimuli were significantly suppressed following treatment with CPA.

As indicated above, treatment with CPA decreases paraphilic symptoms and deviant sexual arousal within a relatively short period of time. And similar to what has been observed in orchiectomized patients, treatment with CPA substantially reduces recidivism rates (16% to 0% with treatment vs. 50% to 100% without treatment) (Appelt & Floru, 1974; Baron & Lenger, 1977; Davies, 1974; Fahndrich, 1974; Horn, 1972).

Medroxyprogesterone Acetate

Medroxyprogesterone acetate (MPA), the counterpart of CPA in the United States, is a potent synthetic progestational agent which has been used as a contraceptive in women of childbearing age (Depo-Provera). It has also been used to treat cancerous processes involving the endometrium, the breasts, and the kidneys (e.g., endometrial, renal cell carcinoma, hormonal-dependent carcinomas of the breast in postmenopausal women). Since the late-1960s, MPA has been used in the treatment of paraphilic sex offenders because of its testosterone-lowering properties—via induction of testosterone-A-reductase and dose-dependent inhibition of gonadotropin secretion (Albin, Vittek, & Gordon, 1973; Berlin & Schaerf, 1985; Camacho, Williams, & Montalvo, 1972).

MPA can be administered orally and parenterally. Dosages range from 60 to 100 mg per day (for the oral formulation) and 200 to 500 mg per week (for the intramuscular formulation), respectively (Berlin, 1983; Berlin, & Meinecke, 1981; Gagne, 1981; Hucker, Langevin, & Bain, 1988; Meyer, Collier, & Emory,

1992). The pharmacokinetic properties of MPA are shown in Table 14.5.

As true for all testosterone-lowering agents, MPA can cause a number of side effects, including but not limited to hypertension, thromboembolism, breast tenderness, galactorrhea, weight gain (Amatayakul, Sivasomboon, & Thanangkul, 1980), nightmares, hot flashes, acne, alopecia, hirsutism, hyperglycemia, diabetes mellitus, and hypogonadism. Cushing's syndrome (Dux, Bishara, Marom, Blum, & Pitlik, 1998; Shotliff & Nussey, 1997) and gallstones (Meyer, Walker, Emory, & Smith, 1985) have also been reported in patients taking MPA.

Selected Studies Pertaining to MPA

Berlin and Meinecke (1981) reported data on 20 male paraphilic patients treated with intramuscular MPA (150 mg every other week to 600 mg per week). Diagnoses included pedophilia, sexual masochism, sexual sadism, voyeurism, and exhibitionism. Although three patients relapsed during the MPA trial, 90% of the cohort reported a decrease in paraphilic symptomatology. One relapse was believed to be related to alcohol abuse. Recidivism rates were substantially higher for those patients who discontinued treatment against medical advice (10 out of 11 relapsed). Incidence of side effects was not reported.

In an open clinical trial, Gottesman and Schubert (1993) treated a heterogeneous cohort of seven male paraphilic patients with oral MPA, using dosages ranging between 60 to 80 mg per day for about 15.33 months. Patients were diagnosed with both "noncontact" (exhibitionism, voyeurism, telephone scatologia, transvestic fetishism, compulsive masturbation, and sexual masochism) and "contact" paraphilias (pedophilia, zoophilia, and sexual sadism). One patient was diagnosed with chronic paranoid schizophrenia. Testosterone levels and self-report ratings were the primary outcome measures (e.g., number of ejaculations per week, morning erections, frequency of paraphilic activities, preoccupation with

TABLE 14.5 Pharmacokinetic Properties of MPA

Molecular Structure/ Chemical Name	Bioavailability	Maximum Plasma Half-Life	Metabolized
Pregn-4-ene-3,20-dione, 17 (acetyloxy)-6-methyl-, 6 (α)	Orally and parenterally	Between 30–60 hours	Hepatically

paraphilic fantasies). A two-tailed sign test was used to compare pretreatment with posttreatment measures. Paraphilic symptoms decreased in all patients, with serum testosterone levels paralleling changes in patients' self-reports. None of the patients relapsed during this trial.

In a naturalistic follow-up study, Kravitz and colleagues (1995) treated a heterogeneous cohort of 29 paraphilic patients with intramuscular MPA. Dosages ranged from 300 to 900 mg per week. In addition to pharmacotherapy, patients attended weekly group psychotherapy sessions. Treatment response was measured via self-report ratings. All patients reported a decrease in paraphilic symptoms. Side effects included muscle cramps, weight gain, headaches, fatigue, drowsiness, sleepiness, and lethargy. Four patients experienced depressive and anxiety-related symptoms. Of note, one patient suffered a nonlethal episode of pulmonary embolism and another patient recidivated during the trial period.

In a retrospective study, Meyer et al. (1992) presented data on a heterogeneous cohort of 40 patients, presenting with pedophilia (n = 23), exhibitionism (n = 10) and "rape behavior" (n = 7). Treatment consisted of intramuscular MPA, sex offender group therapy, and individual psychotherapy. MPA was given for up to 12 years with dosages ranging from 400 mg to 800 mg per week. Thirty-two percent of the MPA treatment group presented with comorbid psychiatric disorders, primarily personality disorders. Twenty-one patients, presenting with similar clinical characteristics, but refusing MPA therapy, served as the control group. Eighteen percent reoffended while on MPA. Reoffense rates were higher for those who refused or discontinued MPA (58 vs. 35). MPA related side effects included: excessive weight gain (33%), malaise (3%), migraine headaches (3%), leg cramps (6%), hypertension (8%), gastrointestinal symptoms (6%), and gallbladder stone formation (10%). Three subjects (8%), suffering from obesity, developed diabetes mellitus.

Although MPA and CPA have somewhat different pharmacodynamic properties (see the preceding text), both agents seem to be equally effective in reducing paraphilic symptoms.

In a 28-week double-blind, placebo-controlled trial, Cooper et al. (1992) treated seven pedophilic men with MPA, CPA, or placebo. Six subjects presented with at least one comorbid paraphilia, including sexual sadism, sexual pyromania, exhibitionism,

fetishism, transvestic fetishism, or zoophilia. Treatment outcome was correlated to self-report, observed behavior, hormonal, and penile plethysmograph data. Both medications were equally effective in ameliorating paraphilic symptoms. Maximum treatment effects were reached by the eighth week. Clinically significant side effects were not reported. None of the subjects recidivated during the duration of the study.

Luteinizing Hormone-Releasing Hormone Agonists

Leuprolide acetate (leuprolide), a synthetic and potent nonapeptide analog of endogenous gonadotropin-releasing hormone (GnRH analogue), has been used to treat advanced prostate cancer, estrogen-dependent disorders (i.e., endometriosis and uterine fibroids), and central precocious puberty (Conn & Cowley, 1991; Smith, 1986; Williams et al., 1983). Given their testosterone-lowering properties, GnRH analogues have also been used to treat paraphilic sex offenders.

Luteinizing hormone-releasing hormone (LH-RH) agonists exert a kindling effect on the pituitary gland, which in turn causes an initial, but transient, increase in gonadotropin and hence testosterone and dihydrotestosterone secretion. This initial surge in sex hormone production can be attenuated or averted with the concurrent administration of an antiandrogen (MPA, CPA, flutamide). Continuous treatment with the LH-RH agonist eventually results in a down regulation of GnRH receptors and thus sex hormone production. In fact, testosterone and dihydrotestosterone (estrone and estradiol in premenopausal women) decline to prepubertal (postmenopausal) levels within 2 to 4 weeks (Briken, Hill, & Berner, 2003; Rich, & Ovsiew, 1994). Hormonal levels return to pretreatment levels following medication discontinuation. As an example for the LH-RH agonists, the pharmacokinetic properties of leuprolide acetate are described in Table 14.6.

In contrast to CPA and MPA, leuprolide lacks oral bioavailability and thus has to be given intramuscularly. Doses range from 3.75 to 7.5 mg per month or 11.25 to 22.5 mg every 3 months. Although LH-RH agonist therapy is less likely to cause steroid-induced side effects, a number of adverse effects have been described. These include but are not limited to hot flashes, headaches, peripheral edema, dizziness, anorexia, nausea, vomiting, diarrhea, constipation, muscle and bone pain, blurred vision, paresthesias,

TABLE 14.6 Pharmacokinetic Properties of Leuprolide Acetate

Chemical Name	Bioavailability	Elimination Half-Life	Metabolized	Metabolites
5-oxo-L-prolyl-histidyl-L-tryptophyl-L-seryl-L-tyrosyl-D-leucyl-L- leucyl-L-arginyl-N-ethyl-L-prolinamide acetate	Lacks oral bio-availability	3 hours	Hepatically by peptidase	Inactive Dipeptide, Tripeptides, and Pentapeptide

acne, rash, seborrhea, alopecia, breast tenderness, testicular atrophy, and urinary dysfunction. Serious, but less common side effects are hematological, cardiovascular, and metabolic in nature, and include leukopenia, pure red cell aplasia, pulmonary embolism, thrombosis, myocardial infarction, arrhythmias, gastrointestinal bleed, hypertriglyceridemia, hyperphosphatemia, and bone demineralization (see the following text). Erythema multiforme, gynecomastia, and anaphylaxis (Dickey, 1992) have also been reported. Because of its side effect profile, leuprolide should not be given to patients sufferings from congestive heart failure, gastrointestinal ulcers, and pituitary gland abnormalities (Morsi, Jamal, & Silverberg, 1996).

Osteopenia and osteoporosis

Long-term treatment with a GnRH analogue can cause hypoandrogenism, which in turn has been associated with a decrease in bone mineral content and/or bone mass (Dickey, 2002; Grasswick & Bradford, 2003; Krueger & Kaplan, 2001). Therefore, patients presenting with risk factors for osteoporosis (e.g., family history of osteoporosis, low body mass index, heavy abuse of alcohol or nicotine, chronic use of steroids, etc.) should be closely monitored for signs of osteopenia. Patients, who present with pretreatment osteopenia or osteoporosis, should be referred to an endocrinologist to determine the etiology of their metabolic abnormality.

Prophylactic treatment with calcium, vitamin D, and a biphosphonate agent, such as alendronate, should be considered in those patients who require long-term GnRH analogue therapy.

Selected Studies Pertaining to the Luteinizing Hormone-Releasing Hormone Agonists

Dickey (1992) described the case of a patient with pedophilia, voyeurism, exhibitionism, and fetishism.

Treatment with high dosages of intramuscular MPA (550 mg per week) and CPA (500 mg per week) had not shown satisfactory results. Consequently, leuprolide acetate was prescribed at a dose of 7.5 mg per month. Masturbation to deviant sexual fantasies decreased after about 2 weeks, and more importantly, deviant sexual activities ceased completely. Side effects were not reported.

Krueger and Kaplan (2001) treated a heterogeneous cohort of 12 sexually disordered men with leuprolide acetate, using a dose of either 3.75 or 7.5 mg per month for a period of 6 months to about 5 years. Psychiatric comorbidity was prevalent among the cohort (e.g., substance abuse, mood, and personality disorders). All subjects reported a decrease in paraphilic symptoms. Testosterone levels decreased to prepubertal levels. Side effects included erectile and ejaculatory dysfunction, gynecomastia, nausea, and depression. Three subjects, on long-term leuprolide therapy, showed a decline in their bone mineral density indices.

Briken et al. (2001) treated 11 paraphilic patients, diagnosed with pedophilia, sexual sadism, and "sexual impulsiveness," with leuprolide acetate (11.5 mg every 3 months). Personality and learning disorders were prevalent among the cohort. (Six patients were previously treated with CPA.) Frequency of sexual fantasies and sexual activity decreased with leuprolide acetate treatment. Side effects included but were not limited to weight gain, depression, and pain at the injection site. Sexual recidivism rates were zero.

In a case report series, Saleh et al. (2004) treated six treatment-resistant male paraphilic patients, ranging in age between 18 and 21 years, with monthly intramuscular injections of leuprolide acetate (7.5 mg/month). Patients met DSM-IV-TR diagnostic criteria for at least one paraphilic disorder. Comorbidity was prevalent and consisted of conduct disorder, attention-deficit/hyperactivity disorder, bipolar disorder, and Tourette's disorder. Three patients had histories of mild to moderate mental retardation, and one patient was diagnosed with Klinefelter's Syndrome (for a review on paraphilic patients with Klinefelter's Syndrome see Berlin, 1983). Treatment outcome was based on self-report data and staff observations. All patients, except for one, reported a substantial decrease in paraphilic symptoms. One patient required augmentation with MPA for residual pedophilic symptoms. Clinicians rated four patients as much improved and two as moderately improved. Clinically significant side effects were not reported.

Triptorelin, another long-acting LH-RH agonist, has also been shown to be effective in the treatment of the paraphilias (Rosler & Witztum, 1998; Thibaut, Cordier, & Kuhn, 1993). In an open label study, Thibaut et al. (1993) described the cases of six paraphilic subjects presenting with either pedophilia or exhibitionism. One subject was diagnosed with both exhibitionism and sexual sadism. Moreover, three subjects carried a diagnosis of mild to moderate mental retardation, two subjects were diagnosed with a personality disorder, and one subject was diagnosed with mixed bipolar disorder. Treatment consisted of monthly intramuscular injections of 3.75 mg triptorelin and monthly psychotherapy sessions. CPA at a mean dose of 200 mg per day (mean duration 4.5 months) was given in conjunction with triptorelin to counteract the initial surge in testosterone secretion. Frequency and intensity of deviant sexual fantasies and activities decreased with treatment. Follow-up periods ranged from 7 months to 3 years. Although usually well tolerated, a few patients developed hypoandrogenism-related side effects.

One patient relapsed within 10 weeks after withdrawing from treatment.

In an uncontrolled observational trial (the largest study to date), Rosler and Witztum (1998) treated 30 paraphilic men (mean age of 32 years) with monthly intramuscular injections of 3.75 mg triptorelin and supportive psychotherapy. Patients were treated for a period of 8 to 42 months. Twenty-five patients presented with "severe" pedophilia, whereas five patients had other paraphilias. Comorbidity was prevalent among the cohort and consisted of psychotic illnesses such as schizophrenia or schizoaffective disorder (n = 6), personality disorders (n = 9), and affective disorder (n = 2). Two patients had obsessive-compulsive disorder. Seven men had previous trials with CPA. Treatment outcome was based on self-reports, using questionnaires, such as the "Intensity of Sexual Desire and Symptoms Scale" as well as the "Three Main Complaints Questionnaire." Paraphilic symptoms decreased within a relatively short time period in all but one subject. Frequency of deviant sexual behavior decreased to zero. Testosterone levels decreased to prepubertal levels, paralleling the decrease in paraphilic symptomatology. Levels returned to baseline values within 2 months after discontinuation of triptorelin. Treatment effects persisted over time in patients receiving triptorelin for 12 or more months. Three men discontinued treatment because of side effects. Bone mineral density indices decreased in 11 men. Other side effects included progressive erectile failure (n = 21), unrelenting hot flashes (n = 6), decreased growth of facial and body hair (n = 3), as well as asthenia and muscle tenderness (n = 2).

In a placebo-controlled, blinded, 2-year study, Schober and colleagues (2005), treated five pedophiles with leuprolide acetate (22.5 mg every 3 months for a total of four injections). Subsequently, patients were given four consecutive placebo injections (normal saline injections every 3 months for 1 year). Outcome measures included self-report, penile plethysmograph, polygraph, and visual reaction time data. None of the patients reoffended and all favored treatment over placebo. During the placebo phase of the study, three patients had reoccurring pedophilic symptoms. Hot flashes and weight gain were the most common side effects; breast tenderness was a less common reported occurrence. None of the patients dropped-out off treatment. (Table 14.7)

CONCLUSION

In the era of evidence-based medicine, treatment decisions should be based on accurate diagnosis and unambiguous scientific and treatment data. This is particularly important when it comes to symptomatic paraphilic sex offenders. Prescribing a medication to a paraphilic sex offender that has little-to-no real impact on his or her underlying paraphilia could have devastating consequences for both the offender (e.g., sexual recidivism, civil commitment as a sexual predator, etc.) *and* the public at large. As described in this chapter, testosterone-lowering medications reduce the frequency, severity, and intensity of paraphilic symptoms within a short period of time. Similarly, and even more importantly, sexual recidivism rates in sex offenders treated with these agents parallel those of orchiectomized offenders (Berlin, & Meinecke, 1981; Berlin et al., 1991; Ortman, 1980).

TABLE 14.7 Studies from 1985 to 2005 Using Leuprolide Acetate or Triptorelin

Study (author & year of publication)	N	Paraphilia Diagnosis or Diagnoses	Type of LH-RH Treatment	Previous Testosterone-Lowering Medications	Duration of Follow-up Period	Pertinent Findings
Allolio et al., 1985	1	Pedophilia	Leuprolide	CPA	No follow-up	Greater efficacy than CPA
Rousseau et al., 1990	1	Exhibitionism	Triptorelin, flutamide	None	6 months	Sexual functioning maintained despite prepubertal testosterone levels. No significant side effects reported
Dickey, 1992	1	Exhibitionism, pedophilia, voyeurism, fetishism	Leuprolide	MPA 550 mg per week and CPA 500 mg per week	6 months	Paraphilic behaviors ceased No side effects reported
Marcus et al., 1993	1	Exhibitionism	Leuprolide	MPA	No follow-up	
Cooper & Cernowsky, 1994	1	Pedophilia	Leuprolide	CPA, placebo	4 years	Greater efficacy than CPA Outcome measure included penile plethysmograph
Thibaut et al., 1993, 1996	6	Pedophilia (4), exhibitionism (1), exhibitionism/sexual sadism (1)	Triptorelin	CPA (5)	17 years	Two patients relapsed following discontinuation of treatment
Gottesmann & Schubert, 1993	4	"Rape" (1), pedophilia (1), exhibitionism (1), fetishism(1)	Leuprolide	MPA (3)	10 months	Greater efficacy than MPA
Rösler & Witztum, 1998	30	Pedophilia (25), other (5)	Triptorelin	CPA (9), antidepressant (7), narcoleptics (9), lithium(2)	Up to 42 months	Greater efficacy than CPA SSRIs. Decrease in bone mineral indices in 11 patients. Two patients relapsed after switching to CPA

Study	N	Diagnosis	Medication	Other medications	Duration	Comments
Briken et al., 2001	11	Sexual sadism (4), pedophilia (4), "sexual impulsiveness" (3)	Leuprolide	CPA (6)	1 year	Personality and learning disorders prevalent. Greater efficacy than CPA. Sexual recidivism rates zero
Krueger & Kaplan, 2001	12	Pedophilia (6), mixed (6)	Leuprolide	MPA (2), antidepressant (9), other (7)	Up to 57 months	Psychiatric comorbidity prevalent. No relapses. Three patients, receiving long-term leuprolide therapy, developed osteopenia
Grasswick & Bradford, 2003	1	Sexual sadism, pedophilia	Leuprolide	CPA	4 years	Mild and reversible osteoporosis
Saleh et al., 2004	6	Pedophilia (5), Paraphilia NOS(1), sexual sadism (1), frotteurism (2)	Leuprolide	Antipsychotic (5) medications, mood stabilizing agents (3), lithium (1), antidepressants (3), MPA (1)	Up to 16 months	High comorbidity for psychiatric disorders. Hypoandrogenism-related side effects. One patient required augmentation with MPA. No relapses reported
Saleh, 2005	1	Paraphilia NOS and hypersexuality	Leuprolide	None	6 months	Outcome measure included penile plethysmograph. Serial hormonal profiles
Schober et al., 2005	5	Pedophilia	Leuprolide		12 months	Decrease in masturbation to pedophilic imagery and pedophilic urges Pedophilic interest as measured did not change

Adapted and updated from Briken, et al., 2003.

Notwithstanding the aforesaid, and despite the growing body of literature describing the beneficial effects of the testosterone-lowering medications, it is critical to point out that testosterone-lowering medications should not be considered a panacea for all sexual offending behavior. It is also important to bear in mind that these medications are not devoid of side effects. Quite to the contrary, not only is there a dearth of long-term safety data, but these medications can cause serious, and sometimes, irreversible side effects. As such, testosterone-lowering medications should be only used in carefully selected and closely monitored sex offenders suffering from genuine paraphilic disorders.

References

Abel, G. G. (1989). Paraphilias. In H. I. Kaplan & B. J. Sadock (Eds.), *Comprehensive textbook of psychiatry, 5th Edition* (Vol. 1, pp. 1069–1085). Baltimore: Williams & Wilkins.

Albin, J., Vittek, J., & Gordon, G. (1973). On themechanism of the antiandrogenic effect of medroxyprogesterone acetate. *Endocrinology*, 93, 417–422.

Allolio, B., Keffel, D., Deuß, U., & Winkelmann, W. (1985). Behandlung sexueller Verhaltensstörungen mit LH-RHSuperagonisten. *Deutsche Medizinische Wochenschrift*, 110 (50), 1952.

Amatayakul, K., Sivasomboon, B., & Thanangkul, O. (1980). Astudy of the mechanism of weight gain inmedroxyprogesterone acetate users. *Contraception*, 22(6), 605–622.

American Psychiatric Association. (2000). *Diagnostic andstatistical manual of mental disorders (text revision)* (p. 566).Washington, D.C: Author.

American Psychiatric Association. (2000). *Handbook of Psychiatric Measures*. Washington D.C.: Author.

Appelt, M. & Floru, L. (1974). Erfarung über die Beeinflussung der Sexualität durch cyproteron acetat (androcur, schering) [The effect on sexuality of cyproterone acetate]. *International Pharmacopsychiatry*, 9(2), 61–76.

Ashton, A. K., Hamer, R., & Rosen, R. C. (1997). Serotonin reuptake inhibitor-induced sexual dysfunction and its treatment. A large-scale reptrospective study of 596 psychiatric outpatients. *Journal of Sex & Marital Therapy*, 23, 165–175.

Baldwin, D. S. (2004). Sexual Dysfunction associated with antidepressant drugs. *Expert Opinion Drug Safety*, 3(5), 457–470.

Baldwin, D. S., Thomas, S. C., & Birtwistle, J. (1997). Effects of antidepressant drugs on sexual function. *International Journal of Psychiatry in Clincal Practice*, 1, 47–58.

Bancroft, J., Tennent, G., Loucas, K., & Cass, J. (1974). The control of deviant sexual behaviour by drugs. I. Behavioural changes following oestrogens and anti-androgens. *British Journal of Psychiatry*, 125(0), 310–315.

Baron, D. & Lenger, H. (1977). A clinical trial of cyproterone acetate for sexual deviancy. *New Zealand Medical Journal*, 85, 366–369.

Baumgartner, J. V., Scalora, M. J., & Huss, M. T. (2002). Assessment of the Wilson Sex Fantasy Questionnaire among child molesters and nonsexual forensic offenders. *Sexual Abuse: A Journal of Research and Treatment*, 14, 19–30.

Berlin, F. S. (1983). Sex offenders: A biomedical perspective and a status report on biomedical treatment. In J.B., Greer, & I.R. Stuart (Eds.), *The sexual aggressor: Current perspectives on treatment*, (pp. 83–123). New York: Van NOSTRAND Reinhold Co.

Berlin, F. S. (1989). The paraphilias and Depo-Provera: Some medical, ethical and legal considerations. *Bulletin American Academy of Psychiatry and the Law*, 17(3), 233–239.

Berlin, F. S. & Meinecke, C. F. (1981). Treatment of sex offenders with antiandrogenic medication: Conceptualization, review of treatment modalities, and preliminary findings. *The American Journal of Psychiatry*, 138(5), 601–607.

Berlin, F. S. & Schaerf, F. W. (1985). Laboratory assessment of the paraphilias and their treatment with antiandrogenic medication. In R.C.W. Hall, & T. P. Beresford (Eds.), *Handbook of psychiatric diagnostic procedures*, (pp. 273–305). New York: Spectrum Publications.

Berlin, F. S., Wayne, H. P., Martin, M. M., Dyer, A., Gregory, L. K., & Sharon, D. (1991). A five-year plus follow-up survey of criminal recidivism within a treated cohort of 406 pedophiles, 111 exhibitionists and 109 sexual aggressives:issues and outcome. *American Journal of ForensicPsychiatry*, 12(3), 5–28.

Blake, J. C., Sawyerr, A. M., Dooley, J. S., Scheuer, P. J., & McIntyre, N. (1990). Severe hepatitis caused by cyproteroneacetate. *Gut*, 31(5), 556–557.

Blanchard, R., Klassen, P., Dickey, R., Kuban, M. E., & Blak, T. (2001). Sensitivity and specificity of the phallometric test for pedophilia in nonadmitting sex offenders. *Psychological Assessment*, 13(1), 118–126.

Bradford, J. M. W. (2000). The treatment of sexual deviation using a pharmacological approach. *Journal of Sex Research*, 37(3), 248–257.

Bradford, J. M. W. (2001). The neurobiology, neuropharmacology, and pharmacological treatment of the paraphilias and compulsive sexual behaviour. *Canadian Journal of Psychiatry*, 46(1), 26–34.

Bradford, J. M. & Pawlak, A. (1993a). Double-blind placebo crossover study of cyproterone acetate in the treatment of the paraphilias. *Archives of Sexual Behavior*, 22(5), 383–402.

Bradford, J. M. W., Boulet, M. A., & Pawlak, A. (1992). The paraphilias: A multiplicity of deviant behaviours. *Canadian Journal of Psychiatry*, 37, 104–108.

Bradford, J. M. W. & Pawlak, A. (1993b). Effects of cyproterone acetate on sexual arousal patterns of pedophiles. *Archives of Sexual Behavior*, 22(6), 629–641.

Bradford, J. M. W., Greenberg, D., Gojer, J., Martindale, J. J., & Goldberg, M. (1995). Sertraline in the treatment of pedophilia: an open label study. New Research Program abstracts NR 441: American Psychiatric Association Meeting, May 1995; Miami, Florida.

Briken, M., Hill, A., & Berner, W. (2003). Pharmacotherapy of paraphilias with long-acting agonists of luteinizing hormone-releasing hormone: A systematic review. *The Journal of Clinical Psychiatry*, 64(8), 890–897.

Briken, P., Nika, E., & Berner, W. (2001). Treatment of paraphilia with luteinizing hormone-releasing hormone agonists. *Journal of Sex and Marital Therapy*, 27(1), 45–55.

Brotherton, J., Burton, J. L., & Shuster, S. (1974). Action of cyproterone acetate (letter). *Lancet*; 2, 176–177.

Camacho, A. M., Williams, L. D., & Montalvo, J. M. (1972). Alterations of testicular histology and chromosomes in patients with constitutional sexual precocity treated with medroxyprogesterone acetate. *Journal of Clinical Endocrinology Metabolism*, 34, 279–286.

Conn, M. P. & Cowley, W. F. (1991). Gonadtropin realeasing hormone and its analogues. *New England Journal of Medicine*, 324, 93–103.

Cooper, A. J. (1986). Progestogens in the treatment of male sex offenders: A review. *Canadian Journal of Psychiatry*, 31(1), 73–79.

Cooper, A. J., Sandhu, S., Losztyn, S., & Cernovsky, Z. (1992). A double-blind placebo controlled trial of medroxyprogesterone acetate and cyproterone acetate with seven pedophiles. *Canadian Journal of Psychiatry*, 37(10), 687–693.

Cooper, A. J. & Cernovsky, Z. Z. (1994). Comparison of cyproterone acetate (CPA) and leuprolide acetate (LHRH agonist) in a chronic pedophile: A clinical case study. *Biological Psychiatry*, 36, 269–271.

Davies, T. D. (1974). Cyproterone acetate for male hypersexuality. *Journal of International Medical Research*, 2, 159–163.

Dickey, R. (1992). The management of case of treatment-resistant paraphilia with a long-acting lhrh agonist. *Canadian Journal of Psychiatry*, 37(8), 567–569.

Dickey, R. (2002). Case report: the management of bone demineralization associated with long-term treatment of multiple paraphilias with long-acting LHRH agonists. *Journal of Sex & Marital Therapy*, 28(3), 207–210.

Dux, S., Bishara, J., Marom, D., Blum, I., & Pitlik, S. (1998). Medroxyprogesterone acetate-induced secondary adrenal insufficiency. *Annals of Pharmacotherapy*, 32(1), 134.

Fahndrich, E. (1974). Cyproteron acetat in the handling von sexual deviation [Cyproterone acetate in the treatment of sexual deviation in men (author's transl)] *Deutsche-Medizinische Wochenshrift*, 99(6), 234–248.

Foote, R. M. (1944). Diethylstilbestrol in the management of psychopathological states in male. *The Journal of Nervous and Mental Disease*, 99, 928–935.

Gagne, P. (1981). Treatment of sex offenders with medroxyprogesterone acetate. *American Journal of Psychiatry*, 138, 644–646.

Gilman, A. G., Rall, T. W., Nies, A. S., Taylor, P. (1990). (Eds): *Goodman and Gilman's The Pharmacological Basis of Therapeutics, 8th Edition*. New York, NY:Permagon Press.

Goldenberg, S. L., Bruchovsky, N., Rennie, P. S., et al. (1988). The combination of cyproterone acetate and diethylstilbestrol in the treatment of advanced prostatic carcinoma. *The Journal of Urology*, 190, 1460–1465.

Goldenberg, S. L. & Bruchovsky, N. (1991). Use of cyproterone acetate in prostate cancer. *Urologic Clinics of North America*, 18(1), 111–122.

Golla, F. L. & Hodge, S. R. (1949). Hormone treatment of sexual offenders. *Lancet*, 1949, 1:1006–1007.

Gottesman, H. G. & Schubert, D. S. P. (1993). Low-dose oral medroxyprogesterone acetate in the management of the paraphilias. *Journal of Clinical Psychiatry*, 54(5), 182–188.

Grasswick, L. J. & Bradford, J. M. (2003). Osteoporosis associated with the treatment of paraphilias: A clinical review of seven case reports. *Journal of Forensic Sciences*, 48, 849–855.

Greenberg, D. M. (1991). Greenberg's Sexual Preference Visual Analogue Scale (GSPVAS). Forensic Program, Royal Ottawa Hospital.

Guy, W. (1976). Clinical global impressions. In ECDEU assessment manual for psychopharmacology, revised (DHEW Publ No ADM 76–338). National Institute of Mental Health: Rockville, MD. 218–222.

Hamilton, M. (1959). The assessment of anxiety states by rating. *British Journal of Medical Psychology*, 32, 50–55.

Hare, R. D. (2003). *The Hare psychopathy checklist-revised, 2nd Edition*. Toronto, ON, Canada: Multi-Health Systems.

Hirschfeld, R. M. A. (1999). Management of sexual side effects of antidepressant therapy. *The Journal of Clinical Psychiatry*, 60, 27–30.

Horn, J. A. (1972). Die Behandlung von sexual delinqueten mit den antiandrogen cyproteron acetat (1971 bis 1975). *Der Informierte Arzt*, 3, 303–309.

Hucker, S., Langevin, R., & Bain, J. (1988). A double-blind trial of sex drive reducing medication in pedophiles. *Annals Review of Sex Research*, 1, 227–242.

Jurzyk, R. S., Spielvogel, R. L., & Rose, L. I. (1992). Antiandrogens in the treatment of acne and hirsutism. *American Family Physician*, 45(4), 1803–1806.

Kafka, M. P. (1994). Sertraline pharmacotherapy for paraphilias and paraphilia-related disorders: An Open Trial. *Annals Clinical Psychiatry*, 6(3), 189–195.

Kafka, M. P. (1997). A monoamine hypothesis for the pathophysiology of paraphilic disorders. *Archives of Sexual Behavior*, 26(4), 343–358.

Kafka, M. P. & Prentky, R. (1992). Fluoxetine treatment of non-paraphilic sexual addictions and paraphilias in men. *Journal of Clinical Psychiatry*, 53, 351–358.

Keltner, N. L., McAfee, K. M., & Taylor, C. L. (2002). Mechanisms and treatments of SSRI-induced sexual dysfunction. *Perspect Psychiatr Care*, 38(3), 111–116.

Kravitz, H. M., Haywood, T. W., Kelly, J., Wahlstrom, C., Liles, S., & Cavanaugh, J. L. (1995). Medroxyprogesterone treatment for paraphiliacs. *Bulletin American Academy of Psychiatry and the Law*, 23(1), 19–33.

Krogh, C. M. E. (Ed.). (1992). *Compendium of pharmaceuticals and specialties, 27th Edition*. (p. 64). Ottawa: Canadian Pharmaceutical Association.

Krueger, R. B. & Kaplan, M. S. (2001). Depot-leuprolide acetate for treatment of paraphilias: A report of twelve cases. *Archives of Sexual Behavior*, 30(4), 409–422.

Langelüddecke, A. (1963). Die Entmannung von Sittlichkeitsverbrechern in Deutchland. In A. Langelüddeke (Ed.), *Die entmannung von sittlichkeitsverbrechern in deutschland*. Berlin: Walter De Gruyter & Co.

Laschet, U. & Laschet, L. (1971). Psychopharmacotherapy of sex offenders with cyproterone acetate. *Pharmakopsychiatrie Neuropsychopharmakologic*, 4, 99–104.

Laschet, U. & Laschet, L. (1975). Antiandrogens in the treatment of sexual deviation of men. *Journal of Steroid Biochemistry*, 6, 821–826.

Lauman, E. O., Michael, R. T., & Gagnon, J. H. (1994). A political history of the national sex survey of adults. *Family Planning Perspectives*, 26, 34–38.

Levesque, H., Trivalle, C., Manchon, N. D., Vinel, J. P., Moore, N., Hemet, J., et al. (1989). Fulminant hepatitis due to cyproterone acetate. *Lancet*, 1(8631), 215–216.

Marcus, A. O, Fernandez, M .P, & De Kayser, L. (1993). Use of gonadotropin releasing hormone analogue in the treatment of exhibitionism (abstract). *Clinical Research*, 1, 107.

Meyer, W. J., 3rd, Walker, P. A., Emory, L. E., & Smith, E. R. (1985). Physical, metabolic, and hormonal effects on men of long-term therapy with medroxyprogesterone acetate. *Fertility and Sterility*, 43(1), 102–109.

Meyer, W. J., 3rd, Collier, C., & Emory, L. E. (1992). Depo provera treatment for sex offending behavior: An evaluation of outcome. *Bulletin of the American Academy of Psychiatry & the Law*, 20, 249–59.

Money, J. (1968). Discussion on hormonal inhibition of libido in male sex offers, In R. Michael (Ed.), *Endocrinology and Human Behavior*, (p. 169). London: Oxford University Press.

Montgomery, S. A. & Asberg, M. (1979). A new depression scale designed to be sensitive to change. *British Journal of Psychiatry*, 134, 382–389.

Morsi, A., Jamal, S., & Silverberg, J. D. H. (1996). Pituitary apoplexy after leuprolide administration for carcinoma of the prostate. *Clinical Endocrinology*, 44, 121–124.

National Depression Manic-Depression Association. (2000). Beyond diagnosis: A landmark survey of depression and treatment. Chicago, Ill: National Depression Manic-Depression Association.

Neuman, F., Von Berswordt-Wallrabe, R., Eiger, W., Seinbeck, H., Hahn, J., & Kramer, M. (1970). Aspects of androgen dependent events as studied by antiandrogens. *Recent Progress in Hormone Research*, 26, 227–342.

O'Brien, R. C., Cooper, M. E., Murray, R. M. L., Seeman, E., Thomas, A. K., &. Jerums, G. (1991). Comparison of sequential cyproterone acetate/estrogen versus spironolactone/oral contraceptive in the treatment of hirsutism. *The Journal of Clinical Endocrinology and Metabolism*, 72, 1008–1013.

Ortman, J. (1980). The treatment of sexual offenders. Castration and antihormone therapy. *International Journal of Law and Psychiatry*, 3, 443–451.

Patterson, W. M. (1993). Fluoxetine-induced sexual dysfunction [letter]. *The Journal of Clinical Psychiatry*, 54, 71.

Pavone-Macaluso, M., De Voogt, H. J., Viggiano, G., Barasolo, E., Lardennois, B., de Pauw, M., et al. (1986). Comparison of diethylstilbestrol, cyproterone acetate, and medroxyprogesterone acetate in the treatment of advanced prostate cancer: Final analysis of a randomized phase III trial of the European Organization for Research on Treatment of Cancer Urological Group. *The Journal of Urology*, 136, 624–631.

Reilly, D. R., Delva, N. J., & Hudson, R. W. (2000). Protocols for the use of cyproterone, medroxyprogesterone, and leuprolide in the treatment of paraphilia. *Canadian Journal of Psychiatry*, 45(6), 559–563.

Reynolds, J. E. F. (Ed.). (1989). *Martindale: The extra pharmacopoeia, 29th Edition*. (p. 1395). London: The Pharmaceutical Press.

Rich, S. S. & Ovsiew, F. (1994). Leuprolide acetate for exhibitionism in Huntington's Disease. *Movement Disorders*, 9, 353–357.

Rosler, A. & Witztum, E. (1998). Treatment of men with paraphilia with a long acting analogue of gonadotropin releasing hormone. *New England Journal of Medicine*, 338, 416–465.

Rothschild, A. J. (1995). Selective serotonin reuptake inhibitor-induced sexual dysfunction: Efficacy of drug holiday. *The American Journal of Psychiatry*, 152, 1514–1516.

Rothschild, A. J. (2000). Sexual side effects of antidepressants. *The Journal of Clinical Psychiatry*, 61, 28–36.

Rousseau, L. R., Couture, M., Dupont, A., Labrie, F., & Couture, N. (1990). Effect of combined androgen blockade with an LHRH agonist and flutamide in one severe case of male exhibitionism. *Canadian Journal of Psychiatry*, 35, 338–341.

Saleh, F. M. (2005). A hypersexual paraphilic patient treated with leuprolide acetate: A single case report. *Journal of Sex & Marital Therapy*, 31(5), 433–444.

Saleh, F. M. & Guidry, L. L. (2003). Psychosocial and biological treatment considerations for the paraphilic and nonparaphilic sex offender. *The Journal of the American Academy of Psychiatry and the Law*, 31, 486–493.

Saleh, F. M., Niel, T., & Fishman, M. (2004). Treatment of paraphilia in young adults with leuprolide acetate: A preliminary case report series. *The Journal of Forensic Sciences*, 49(6), 2–6 (Paper ID JFS 2003035).

Schober, J. M., Kuhn, P. J., Kovacs, P. G., Earle, J. H., Byrne, P. M., & Fries, R. A. (2005). Leuprolide acetate suppresses pedophilic urges and arousability. *Archives of Sexual Behavior*, 34(6), 691–705.

Seidman, S. (2006). Ejaculatory dysfunction and depression: pharmacological and psychobiological interactions. *International Journal of Impotence Research*. 18(Suppl. 1), S33–S38.

Shotliff, K. & Nussey, S. S. (1997). Medroxyprogesterone acetate induced Cushing's syndrome. *British Journal of Clinical Pharmacology*, 44(3), 304.

Sletzer, M. Vinokur, A., & van Rooijan, L. (1975). A self-administered Short Michigan Alcoholism Screening Test (S.M.A.S.T.). *Journal of Studies on Alcohol*, 36, 117–126.

Smith, J. A. (1986). Luteinizing hormone-releasing hormone (LH-RH) analogs in treatment of prostatic cancer. *Urology*, 27, 9–15.

Smith, A. D. & Taylor, P. J. (1999). Serious sex offending against women by men with schizophrenia: Relationship of illness and psychiatric symptoms to offending. *British Journal of Psychiatry*, 174:233–237.

Stark, P. & Hardison, C. D. (1985). A review of multicenter controlled studies of fluoxetine vs. imipramine and placebo in outpatients with major depressive disorder. *The Journal of Clinical Psychiatry*, 52, 66–68.

Stompe, T. (2007). Drug-therapy with sexual offenders. *Neuropsychiatrie*, 21(1), 12–7.

Sturup, G. K. (1968). Treatment of sexual offenders in Herstedvester Denmark: The rapist. *Acta Psychiatrica Scandinavica*, Suppl. 204.

Thibaut, F., Cordier, B., & Kuhn, J. M. (1993). Effect of a long-lasting gonadotropin hormone-releasing hormone agonist in sex cases of severe male paraphilia. *Acta Psychiatrica Scandinavica*, 87, 445–450.

Thibaut, B. Cordier, B., & Kuhn, J. M. (1996). Gonadotrophophin hormone releasing hormone agonists in cases of severe paraphilia: A lifetime treatment? *Psychoneuroendocrinology*, 21(4), 411–19.

Williams, G., Allen, J. M., O'Shea, J. P., Mashiter, K., Doble, A., & Bloom, S. R. (1983). Prostatic cancer: treatment with long-acting LHRH analogue. *British Journal of Urology*, 55(6), 743–746.

Williams, V. S., Baldwin, D. S., Hogue, S. L., Fehnel, S. E., Hollis, K. A., & Edin, H. M. (2006). Estimating the prevalence and impact of antidepressant-induced sexual dysfunction in 2 European countries: A cross-sectional patient survey, *Journal Clinical Psychiatry*, 67(2), 204–210.

Wilson, G. (1988). Measurement of sex fantasy. *Sexual and Marital Therapy*, 3, 45–55.

Zajecka, J. (2001). Strategies for the treatment of antidepressant-related sexual dysfunction. *The Journal of Clinical Psychiatry*, 62, 35–43.

Zajecka, J. Mitchell, S., & Fawcett, J. (1997). Treatment-emergent changes in sexual function with selective serotonin reuptake inhibitors as measured with the Rush Sexual Inventory. *Psychopharmacology Bulletin* 33, 755–760.

Part V

Juveniles

Chapter 15

Forensic Evaluations of Juvenile Sex Offenders

Charles Scott

Forensic expertise is often requested in situations involving a juvenile sex offender. But what does the term "forensic" actually mean and how does this evaluation process differ from the provision of clinical care? The American Academy of Psychiatry and the Law (AAPL) provides the following definition of forensic psychiatry in its Ethics Guidelines (American Academy of Psychiatry and the Law, 2005):

> Forensic Psychiatry is a subspecialty in which scientific and clinical expertise is applied in legal contexts involving civil, criminal, correctional, regulatory matters, and in specialized clinical consultation in areas such as risk assessment or employment.

Although clinical assessment skills are important when conducting a forensic examination of a juvenile sex offender, providers must be aware that having clinical expertise is vastly different than having the requisite skills to perform a forensic examination.

This chapter outlines important issues in conducting the forensic evaluation of a juvenile sex offender and special types of evaluations that may be requested when a juvenile is charged with a sexual offense in either a juvenile or an adult court.

CONDUCTING THE FORENSIC EVALUATION

Step One: Clarify the Request

The mental health professional must have a clear understanding of what they are being asked to do. In particular, is the requested evaluation for treatment purposes or for a legal purpose? Understanding this question in advance is necessary to avoid serving as both treatment provider and forensic expert, a concept known as dual agency or dual role. If the clinician has treated the youth before or following the alleged offense, he or she should generally avoid

providing an expert witness opinion on any forensic legal issue. The AAPL Ethics Guidelines for the
Practice of Forensic Psychiatry address this potential
conflict as follows (American Academy of Psychiatry
and the Law, 2005):

> Psychiatrists who take on a forensic role for
> patients they are treating may adversely affect
> the therapeutic relationship with them. Forensic
> evaluations usually require interviewing corrobo-
> rative sources, exposing information to public
> scrutiny, or subjecting evaluees and the treatment
> itself to potentially damaging cross-examination.
> The forensic evaluation and the credibility of the
> practitioner may also be undermined by conflicts
> inherent in the differing clinical and forensic
> roles. Treating psychiatrists should therefore gen-
> erally avoid acting as an expert witness for their
> patients or performing evaluations of their patients
> for legal purposes.

In situations where the mental health professional
is asked to provide an expert witness opinion, they
should evaluate if they have the appropriate expertise
in the area requested. One's expertise can be assessed
by evaluating their particular knowledge, training,
experience, skills, or education related to the referral
question. In addition, the evaluator must understand
the relevant legal standard, the skills to evaluate the
juvenile in relationship to this standard, the capacity to apply information to the legal construct, and
the capability to effectively translate and communicate their findings in the context of the legal system
(Grisso, 1998a).

The examiner should also carefully determine the
exact party requesting the evaluation. Is the evaluation being requested by the court, the defense attorney, the prosecutor, the family, or as a consultation
to a treatment team? One must also understand who
is responsible for paying for the evaluation and any
limitations on compensation. Finally, the evaluator
should inquire into any specific deadlines regarding
when the evaluation must be conducted, date any
written report must be submitted, and any proposed
trial dates for expert testimony.

Step Two: Understand the Juvenile's Legal Rights regarding the Interview

The mental health professional should determine
all parties that must be notified in advance of the
assessment and if any special approval or consent
is required before meeting with the juvenile. The
answer to this question is necessary so that the evaluator can adequately inform the youth, their legal
guardian, and their attorney regarding the parameters
of confidentiality. When appropriately informed, the
juvenile's attorney has the opportunity to educate his
client on the nature of the evaluation, the extent of
confidentiality, and the potential for self-incriminat-
ing statements. Some jurisdictions allow the attorney
to be present during certain types of evaluations.
In these situations, it is helpful to communicate in
advance to the attorney the general nature of the
interview and to explain that interference or disruptions may potentially contaminate the interview and
should be avoided.

In general, a juvenile's statements to mental health
professionals who are requested by the court and/or
the prosecutor to conduct a forensic evaluation are
not confidential. The practitioner may be asked
to prepare a report or testify in court regarding the
evaluation and any opinions. In addition to obtaining
an oral consent to the interview, the evaluator should
consider providing the youth, their parent, and their
attorney a written statement outlining the nature of
the evaluation, the reason for the evaluation, the parties who will likely have access to the evaluation, and
the parameters of confidentiality. In those situations
where the interview is either audio- or videotaped, the
consent process should also be recorded (Nye, 1992).

Failure to adequately inform the juvenile defendant regarding potential consequences of the interview may result in the court excluding statements
made by the defendant. For example, in the Canadian
case *R. v. MacDonald*, an adult defendant was interviewed by a psychiatrist retained by the prosecution
two days after the defendant had requested legal
counsel (*R. v. MacDonald*, 2000). The psychiatrist
later testified that he had informed the defendant that
he was hired by the police, that his statements were
not privileged or confidential, that the defendant was
not required to speak with him, and that he could contact his attorney for legal advice. Although the defendant was unable to reach his attorney by phone that
same day, he agreed to proceed with the interview.
The defense counsel challenged the use of statements
made by the defendant during the psychiatric evaluation emphasizing that the prosecution had used the
psychiatrist to obtain evidence regarding the defendant's mental state at the time of the offense without

notification of the defense counsel. On appeal, the Ontario Superior Court of Justice held that the psychiatrist had not adequately informed the defendant regarding the true purpose of the visit and the potential results of the interview. According to the Court, the defendant was deprived of a meaningful and free choice regarding his participation in the evaluation and statements he made to the psychiatrist were therefore not admissible. In addition, the Court noted that the defendant had not been allowed a reasonable opportunity to obtain legal advice regarding his rights related to the interview request.

To avoid any misconception about the forensic examination, the evaluator may wish to prepare in advance a statement regarding their role. The exact statement may vary depending on who has retained the expert. An example of a nonconfidentiality warning for a prosecution-or court-retained examination is as follows (Giorgi-Guarnieri et al., 2002):

I am a physician and psychiatrist who has been asked by [the court or the prosecuting attorney] to evaluate you in regards to _____. (The examiner should provide clear age appropriate language that details the exact nature of the referral question). Although I am a psychiatrist, I will not be treating you. My purpose is to provide an honest evaluation, which you, your parent (or guardian), or your attorney may or may not find helpful. You should know that anything you tell me is not confidential, as I may be requested to testify in court or to prepare a report that the judge, the prosecutor and your attorney will read. It is important that you be honest with me. You don't have to answer every question, but if you choose not to answer on, your refusal will be noted in my report. Do you have any questions? Do you agree to continue with the interview?

For those evaluators who are retained solely by the defense attorney, their findings are generally disclosed only when the defense attorney determines that this is in the best interest of their client. Therefore, the explanation provided to the juvenile in this circumstance differs. An example of a confidentiality warning in a jurisdiction where the defense evaluator is working under the attorney–client privilege reads (Giorgi-Guarnieri et al., 2002):

I am a physician and psychiatrist who has been asked by your defence attorney to evaluate you

in regards to _____. (The examiner should provide clear age appropriate language that details the exact nature of the referral question). Although I am a psychiatrist, I will not be treating you. My purpose is to provide an honest evaluation, which you, your parent (or guardian), or your attorney may or may not find helpful. If your attorney feels my opinion is helpful, what you tell me will be revealed in a report or in testimony in court. If your attorney feels my opinion is not helpful to your case, only you, your attorney and I will know what we discussed. It is important for you to be honest with me. You don't have to answer every question, but if you choose not to answer one, your refusal will be noted in my report. Do you have any questions? Do you agree to continue with the interview?

Even if a youth does not wish to have an attorney, one is appointed for her or him. Should a juvenile refuse legal counsel and demand to represent him or herself, then the evaluator must follow jurisdictional guidelines governing this extremely rare situation. Depending on the age of the juvenile, whether they are in adult versus juvenile court, and the legal standard governing competency to represent oneself, there is a remote possibility that an evaluator could be required to work with the juvenile acting as their own legal counsel.

The examiner must also communicate to the juvenile those situations that legally mandate sharing of specific information. For example, if the juvenile makes a threat to harm a third party, many jurisdictions require reporting this information so that the potential victim can either be warned or steps may be taken to protect the victim. Furthermore, if the youth is presently involved in other offenses, such as ongoing sexual abuse of a sibling or another youth, then notification of Child Protective Services or appropriate child welfare agencies is likely required. In most jurisdictions, there is no legal requirement to notify authorities regarding past crimes committed. However, if the juvenile communicates prior criminal behavior despite the nonconfidentiality warning, such statements could result in an investigation of potential additional charges.

If the examiner determines that the juvenile is so mentally ill that they cannot participate in the examination or that the examination would result in present harm, then the examiner may need to end the interview and notify appropriate parties of their concerns.

Furthermore, if the evaluator discovers that the youth is suicidal or homicidal at the time of the interview, then appropriate clinical interventions and notification of third parties are generally required even when the examination is for legal purposes.

Providers who treat a juvenile accused of a sexual offense should be aware of the distinct possibility that their treatment notes will be requested by a forensic evaluator. In particular, the juvenile may provide information relevant to a mental health defense that does not require mandatory disclosure to third parties. For instance, a juvenile may report that they were using drugs at the time of the offense or may fake psychiatric symptoms to help create a mental health defense. All of this information may be discoverable if a court orders the release records of the treatment provider. Providers who receive a subpoena for their treatment records should consider reviewing this request with their risk management office or legal counsel to determine the legality of the request. In addition, informing the legal guardian and juvenile's attorney (if they are not aware) of the request may assist in ensuring that the youth has not waived his or her privilege to confidentiality.

Step Three: Obtain Necessary Collateral Information

Collateral records and interviews are important when assessing the juvenile sex offender. When court appointed, juvenile court policies should outline the party responsible for obtaining consents from the court client when the evaluator requests records or permission to speak to third parties. Depending on the nature of the evaluation, state statute, court policy, and/or parental consent may determine the extent to which collateral information may be redisclosed. In situations where there is no governing policy, the evaluator should consider seeking a legal opinion from the court's legal officer or their own attorney in regards to obtaining and rereleasing collateral records and information from collateral informants (Nye, 1992).

Specific collateral records usually reviewed by the forensic examiner include police reports and witness statements regarding the alleged offense, the juvenile's legal history, prior psychiatric treatment, previous juvenile court interventions, medical records, academic performance, and occupational records. The evaluator may also need evaluations from other mental professionals before they are able to form a forensic opinion. Such information may include psychological testing, intelligence and educational testing, and medical consultation.

Step Four: Communicate Findings

In all situations involving a forensic evaluation, the examiner should preserve their interview notes and any audio or visual recordings related to the examination. When privately retained by defense counsel, the examiner typically provides a verbal consultation to the retaining attorney following their assessment. Depending on the results, the defense counsel may request a written report or may decide not to use the retained expert. When court appointed or retained by the prosecution, the examiner's findings are not confidential and the examiner may be required to either provide a written report or testify in a legal proceeding.

When preparing a written report, the examiner should clearly document all records and persons interviewed, examination dates, the juvenile's statements during the interview, any testing performed, and summarized information provided by collateral interviews. The opinion should clearly address the specific referral question/s with language that avoids psychiatric jargon in a manner easily understood by a lay person.

SPECIAL TYPES OF EVALUATIONS

Disposition Hearing

In juvenile court, the disposition hearing occurs after the adjudication phase and is the aspect of the juvenile court process that most closely symbolizes the rehabilitative intent of the juvenile justice system as it focuses on each youth's potential for positive change. In England, this hearing is referred to as "an order on such a finding." At the disposition hearing, the evaluator informs the court of their assessment findings and makes recommendations regarding appropriate placement. Assessment methods and factors associated with a juvenile's risk of future sexual offending are outlined in other chapters of this book.

The evaluator may be pressured to make placement recommendations based on what is available in the community rather than what is necessary to provide appropriate care. Despite the treatment limitations in the community, the mental health professional must state what the youth's actual treatment needs without making clinical comprises due to lack of financial resources. Second choice recommendations should be clearly defined as the best alternative among the available resources. Failure to provide honest recommendations exposes the forensic evaluator to a host of potential complaints to include accusations of unethical professional conduct, complaints to licensing boards, and a potential malpractice suit (Nye, 1992).

Waivers to Adult Court

In many countries, juveniles who are of a certain age and/or have committed a certain offense can be transferred, or "waived," to an adult court for their trial. If found guilty in adult court they can also face an adult sentence. In the United States, the most common mechanism for transferring a youth from juvenile court to adult court involves a judicial waiver (also known as a discretionary waiver, bind-over, certification, transfer, or remand hearing). In the 46 states with a judicial waiver mechanism, a juvenile court judge decides whether to transfer the youth to adult court for prosecution. Because this hearing required information about the youth and their background where information is presented to the judge, this particular hearing represents the waiver process most likely to involve input from a mental health professional. Before beginning the judicial waiver evaluation, the clinician should request a copy of his or her state's statute defining criteria for a judge to consider when determining if a youth should be tried as an adult. In general, most state statutes require the mental health clinician to evaluate two key areas: (1) the youth's risk of future dangerousness; and (2) the youth's amenability to treatment. Because a waiver hearing may result in the juvenile being tried in adult court, the report should address the juvenile's competency to stand trial in adult court if not specifically required by the examiner's jurisdiction (Benedek, 1985).

In some U.S. states, legislatures have passed statutes that automatically place youth of a certain minimal age who have committed a specified offense in the adult court system, a process known as legislative waiver. Although states vary in defining what offenses qualify for transfer, they generally involve violence, such as murder, manslaughter, and/or rape. No consideration of future dangerousness or amenability to treatment is considered in a legislative transfer as the transfer is automatic once predefined criteria are met (Scott, 2002).

In England and Wales, juveniles may be transferred from the jurisdiction of the juvenile system to that of the Crown Court (adult court) under section 53 of the Children and Young Persons Act 1933. Initially, this Act limited the offenses qualifying for transfer to murder, manslaughter, and wounding with intent to cause grievous bodily harm. However, in 1961 the range of offenses was extended by the Criminal Justice Act to include those offenses for which an adult could be sentenced for 14 years or more. This expansion allowed juveniles charged with robbery, arson, burglary, and some sexual offenses to be tried by the Crown Court (Morris & Gelsthorpe, 1993).

In contrast to the aforementioned trends in both the United States and Great Britain, Canada passed the *Youth Criminal Justice Act* (YCJA) in 2003, which eliminated the transfer hearing. Instead, a possible adult sentence can be imposed only after the youth has been found guilty in juvenile court. While the YCJA does lower the presumption of an adult sentence to youth 14 years of age or older, each province has the authority to set the age at 15 or 16 years should they so choose (Department of Justice, Canada, 2007).

Waiver of Miranda Rights

When police take a juvenile suspected of committing a sex offense into custody they are interested in obtaining a statement or confession from the youth regarding their involvement in the alleged offense. According to the U.S. Supreme Court holding in *Miranda v. Arizona*, suspects must be informed that they have a constitutional right to avoid self-incrimination and the right to an attorney during questioning. These rights have been extended to youth involved in juvenile court proceedings (*In re Gault*, 1967; *Kent v. United States* 1966). In some states, police officers must arrange for the youth to have contact with a parent, guardian, or other "interested adult" when the youth is advised regarding the waiver of his or her *Miranda* rights during police questioning. When determining if a constitutional right has been waived, the U.S. Supreme Court articulated in *Johnston v. Zerbst* (1938) that any such waiver must be done "voluntarily, knowingly, and intelligently."

The forensic evaluator may be requested to determine whether an alleged juvenile sex offender had the capacity to waive his or her *Miranda* rights when giving a statement or confession. If a youth is assessed as not having the requisite ability, his or her statements may ultimately be deemed inadmissible. Two key areas for the evaluator to consider in evaluating a juvenile's waiver of *Miranda* rights include (1) the circumstances under which the youth made the confession; and (2) characteristics of the particular youth's capacity to make a waiver. In examining the conditions of confinement when the youth waived his or her right, the evaluator should review the length of time the youth was detained without the opportunity to communicate with others, the physical conditions of the holding environment, any contact with other persons (particularly adults), access to food, water, and other basic necessities, and any behaviors by officers that may have resulted in fear or created an environment of coercion (Grisso, 1998b).

The second component of this forensic evaluation requires the evaluator to carefully examine the individual juvenile's capacity to waive his or her *Miranda* rights. Three important areas suggested by Grisso (1998b) to review when assessing this capacity include the "youth's ability to comprehend the Miranda warning, the ability to grasp the significance of rights in the context of the legal process, [and] the ability to process information in arriving at a decision about waiver." Comprehension of the *Miranda* warning addresses the youth's ability to understand the warning and to appreciate that they are not required to answer police questions. To understand the significance of the *Miranda* warning, the juvenile must not only recognize that he or she has a right to have an attorney present but also that the defense counsel serves as his or her advocate. The ability to process the warning requires some capacity for abstract reasoning as the youth must weigh short-term and long-term consequences of the decision to waive the right to self-incrimination.

Important collateral records in this assessment may include mental health evaluations, interviews with parents, delinquency records, police investigation reports, and audio and/or videotapes of the youth's questioning and confession. If the evaluator has concerns regarding the youth's cognitive abilities, cognitive measures of intellectual ability, and academic records may be indicated. Four standardized assessment tools to evaluate a youth's ability to comprehend and appreciate the *Miranda* rights have been developed by Dr. Thomas Grisso in collaboration

with the National Institute of Mental Health. These tools include the Comprehension of Miranda Rights, Comprehension of Miranda Rights—Recognition, Comprehension of Miranda Vocabulary, and the Function of Rights in Interrogation. Grisso recommends that in addition to information about the youth's psychosocial background information, the evaluator should include sections that specifically describe the juvenile's current ability to comprehend the *Miranda* warnings and their significance, an explanation of any discovered deficits and their relationship to the youth's capacity to waive the *Miranda* rights, a discussion addressing the possibility of dissimulation and malingering, and a description of those conditions involving the police encounter, disclosure of the *Miranda* rights, and the juvenile's response.

Competency to Stand Trial Evaluations

The substantive standard for competency to stand trial (CST) in the U.S. was established by the United States Supreme Court in *Dusky v. United States* (1960). The *Dusky* court defined the test of competency to stand trial as "whether the accused has sufficient present ability to consult with his lawyer with a reasonable degree of rational understanding and whether he has a rational as well as factual understanding of the proceedings against him" (*Dusky v. United States*, 1960). This standard focuses on two primary areas: (1) the individual's cognitive abilities to understand the trial process; and (2) the individual's ability to assist their attorney in their defense (Voigt, Heisel, & Benedek, 2002).

Although the *Dusky* standard did not specifically state that a mental disease or defect is necessary to find trial incompetency, the vast majority of state statutes require some type of mental disorder as the predicate basis for an incompetency to stand trial finding. The CST examination focuses on the presence of mental health symptoms at the time of the interview. The presence of a mental illness alone, however, does not automatically render a person incompetent to stand trial. The evaluator must illustrate the relationship of the mental illness to specific deficits in the defendant's understanding of the trial process or ability to cooperate with their attorney in their defense.

Numerous CST assessment instruments have been utilized in the adult population to assist the evaluator in assessing competency and these include the Georgia Court Competency Test (GCCT), the Competency Assessment Interview (CAI), the Interdisciplinary Fitness Interview (IFI), the Computer Assisted Competency Assessment Tool (CACAT), the MacArthur Competency Assessment Tool-Criminal Adjudication (MacCAT-CA), and the Competency Assessment for Standing Trial for Defendants with Mental Retardation (CAST-MR). McGarry et al. (1973) highlighted 13 areas to review when assessing trial competency.

Grisso et al. (1987) recommend that a juvenile's trial competence be questioned if any one of the following conditions are present: (1) age 12 or younger; (2) prior diagnosis/treatment for a mental illness or mental retardation; (3) borderline intellectual functioning or learning disability; and (4) observations that youth has deficits in memory, attention, or interpretation of reality. In a descriptive review of 136 juveniles aged 9 to 16 years who were referred for evaluation of trial competency in South Carolina, Cowden and McKee (1995) found that 80% of youth aged 9 to 12 years were incompetent to stand trial, nearly 50% of those aged 13 and 14 were trial incompetent, and approximately 25% of 15- to 17-year-olds were incompetent to stand trial. Cooper (1997), in another study of juvenile offenders in South Carolina, found that a majority of juvenile offenders of all ages had significant deficits in their competence-related abilities. Juveniles aged 13 and below and those with low average or below average IQ scores were particularly at risk. The significance of these findings is that an opinion that a given juvenile is incompetent to stand trial may be based solely on deficits due to developmental immaturity, rather than to a specific diagnosis or cluster of symptoms. In this case, the opinion will need to set forth, rather than a specific diagnosis, those specific abilities that are limited in a particular case.

Assessment of Insanity (Criminal Responsibility)

Insanity is a legal, but not psychiatric, term. The insanity evaluation determines whether a person is so mentally disordered that they are not blameworthy or criminally responsible for the behavior. In contrast to CST evaluations that focus on a defendant's present mental capacity as related to their understanding and participation in the legal process, an insanity evaluation involves a retrospective evaluation of a person's past mental state at the time of their alleged offense.

Because a juvenile court adjudication of delinquency was not traditionally considered a criminal conviction, raising the defense of insanity to excuse a juvenile's delinquent behavior is not a common practice in juvenile court. However, an understanding of the criminal responsibility evaluation remains important for two reasons: (1) Some jurisdictions now permit an insanity defense in juvenile court; and (2) juveniles who are transferred to adult court are eligible for the insanity defense when applicable.

The most common test of insanity in the United States is known as the M'Naghten standard that was developed in 1843 following the trial of Daniel M'Naghten. Mr. M'Naghten was found not guilty by reason of insanity after he attempted to assassinate the prime minister of Britain and instead shot his secretary Edward Drummond. Queen Victoria, angered by the legal outcome in this case, ordered her 15 Law Lords to draft a new standard of criminal responsibility. The new standard recommended by the Lords was as follows:

> To establish a defence on the ground of insanity, it must be clearly proved that at the time of the committing of the act, the party accused was labouring under such a defect of reason, from the disease of the mind, as not to know the nature and quality of the act he was doing, or if he did know it, that he did not know he was doing what was wrong. (Miller, 1994, p. 199; M'Naghten's Case, 1843).

This test is often referred to as the *right/wrong test* or *cognitive test* because of its emphasis on the defendant's ability to know, understand, or appreciate the nature and quality of their criminal behavior or the wrongfulness of their actions at the time of the crime.

Canada's insanity standard represents a more narrow version of the M'Naghten standard in that an analysis of the defendant's understanding of the nature and/or quality of their actions is not required. For purposes of finding a person insane, section 16 of the Canadian Criminal Code states that "the courts must determine whether the accused, because of a disease of the mind, was rendered incapable of knowing that the act committed was something that he ought not to have done" (*Criminal Code*, R.S.C., 1985). In reviewing whether the test should be restricted solely to a defendant's knowledge of the legal wrongfulness of their actions, the Canadian Supreme Court ruled that the insanity standard:

ought to be interpreted simply in sense of what one ought not to do, for whatever reason, legal or moral. In practice, this has the effect in most cases that where an accused is capable of knowing that his or her act is legally wrong, he or she will be held liable to the criminal process, regardless of what his or her moral appreciation may have been (R. v. Chaulk, 1990).

A second insanity test used in some jurisdictions is known as the *irresistible impulse* test. In essence, this test asks the evaluator to determine if the offender's mental disorder rendered them unable to refrain from their behavior, regardless if they knew the nature and quality of their act or could distinguish right from wrong. A major criticism of this test has been the broadness of its scope. In other words, because a defendant did not refrain from a particular criminal behavior, mental health clinicians could use this as evidence that they could not resist their impulse, thereby concluding that all criminal behavior not resisted equalled insanity. Despite its current unpopularity as a measure of criminal responsibility, this test survives, in part, as both Virginia and New Mexico combine the irresistible impulse test with the M'Naghten test (Giorgi-Guarnieri et al., 2002).

A third test used in only two jurisdictions in the United States is known as the *Durham rule* or *product test*. This insanity test derived from a D.C. Circuit case where Judge Bazelon allowed a finding of insanity if the defendant's unlawful act was a "product of a mental disease or defect." As with the irresistible impulse test, the product test expanded those eligible for a finding of insanity and rapidly fell out of favor. It is currently used in only two jurisdictions in the United States, New Hampshire and the Virgin Islands (Giorgi-Guarnieri et al., 2002).

A final test of insanity was developed in 1955 by the American Law Institute (ALI) when formulating the Model Penal Code. This test states,

A person is not responsible for criminal conduct if at the time of such conduct as a result of mental disease or defect he lacks substantial capacity either to appreciate the criminal of his conduct or to conform his conduct to the requirements of the law. (Giorgi-Guarnieri et al., 2002; ALI Model Penal Code, 1985).

This test involves both a cognitive arm ("appreciates the criminality of his conduct") and a volitional arm (ability to conform behavior).

A mental health professional requested to conduct an insanity evaluation of a juvenile sex offender should consider the following guidelines. First, the evaluator should request that the attorney or court provide them the exact language of the insanity statute as there are subtle yet important differences in the wording among the various states. Second, it is important to understand how mental disorders or defects are defined. The exact definitions of mental disease and mental defect are usually found in either case law and/or and statutes. The examiner should carefully review if any disorders are prohibited from consideration for the insanity defense. Diagnoses commonly excluded include voluntary intoxication with alcohol or other drugs, personality disorders, and adjustment disorders. Psychotic disorders, such as schizophrenia, schizoaffective disorder, or mood disorders with psychotic features are the most common diagnoses that qualify for an insanity defense. Although some youth in early adolescence may demonstrate premorbid symptoms of a significant thought disorder, they may not meet formal diagnostic criteria for a DSM-IV thought disorder, thereby making it difficult for them to meet the mental disorder requirement of an insanity defense.

Third, the examiner must closely review all of the defendant's statements regarding their alleged crime as well as available police reports and witness statements regarding the offense. Additional collateral records that may be important include prior mental health and medical records, academic records and any educational testing, and detailed social background history from family members and individuals who know the juvenile.

Even if the juvenile sex offender meets the jurisdictional criteria for a mental disorder or defect, having a mental disorder does not equate with the legal definition of insanity. Once the evaluator has determined if the juvenile meets the criteria for a qualifying mental disorder or defect, the evaluator must determine the relationship, if any, between the mental illness or defect and the alleged crime. Understanding the motivation behind the juvenile's actions is a critical component of the insanity evaluation. The evaluator should obtain the juvenile's account of the crime in great detail by asking the youth to describe their thoughts, feelings, and exact behaviors before, during, and after the alleged crime. It is important that the evaluator consider all rational, rather than psychotic, motives for the criminal offense. For example, if a juvenile commits an armed robbery to obtain money to buy drugs, the fact that they are depressed will unlikely establish a sufficient relationship between their mental state and their criminal behavior for purposes of the insanity defense. The final area the examiner must consider is whether the juvenile's mental state at the time of the crime meets the jurisdictional requirements for an insanity defense. As outlined earlier, there are various tests of insanity and it is feasible that youth may qualify for the insanity defense in one state but not in another.

In those jurisdictions that utilize some form of the M'Naghten test, the examiner should carefully review if the juvenile meets the criteria for each component of this test according to the precise governing language. In some states, the defendant must be so impaired from a mental illness that they are unable to know the nature and quality of their actions, or are unable to distinguish right from wrong. In general, an individual would have to be extremely impaired so as to not be aware of or know his or her actions. For a juvenile sex offender charged with the rape of a young child, even the presence of a significant mental illness would unlikely render the individual so impaired that he did not know that he was engaged in some type of sexual activity. Evidence indicating that the juvenile sex offender knew the nature of his or her actions would include statements telling the victim to undress or to get ready for sexual activity, wearing a condom, or bringing a weapon for the purpose of coercing the victim into sexual activity.

The more easily met component of the M'Naghten test involves whether the juvenile was able to know or distinguish right from wrong at the time of the offense. Evidence that the juvenile knew or understood the wrongfulness of his or her behavior would include wearing a disguise during the sexual offense to hide identity, taking the victim to a secluded or private area, attempting to hide or destroy evidence, threatening to harm the victim if they tell, having the victim shower in an attempt to remove any bodily fluid that could be used as evidence, lying to investigators regarding his or her actions, and fleeing from the scene so as not to be discovered.

The insanity standard in some jurisdictions requires an analysis of the individual's ability to refrain from his or her actions or to conform their conduct to the requirements of the law. This analysis focuses on how the juvenile's mental disorder or defect affected, if at all, his or her ability or capacity to control the behavior. In this context, the forensic examiner is evaluating if the juvenile had the ability to refrain from the behavior and chose not to. Evidence that the juvenile had the ability to refrain from unlawful sexual behavior would include delaying initiation of the sexual activity when learning that others are unexpectedly present or stopping sexual activity during a surprised interruption.

CONCLUSION

The forensic evaluation of a juvenile sex offender requires specialized knowledge and expertise by the examiner. The evaluator must possess a clear understanding of the exact nature of the interview, the legal standard governing the interview, parameters of confidentiality, and the scientific literature that supports any opinions and recommendations rendered. In contrast to a clinician's treatment relationship with his or her client, the forensic examiner's primary goal is to report objective information to the requesting party. In this manner, the forensic evaluator plays an invaluable role in helping the legal system determine how to best balance the safety needs of the community with the treatment needs of the juvenile offender.

References

ALI Model Penal Code, § 4.01 (1985).

American Academy of Psychiatry and the Law. (2007). *Ethical guidelines for the practice of forensic psychiatry.* [Online] Adopted May 2005. Available at: http://aapl.org/pdf/ETHICSGDLNS.pdf.

Benedek, E. P. (1985). Waiver of juveniles to adult court. In E. P. Benedek (Ed.). *Emerging issues in child psychiatry and the law,* (pp. 180–190). New York: Brunner/Mazel.

Cooper, D. K. (1997). Juveniles' understanding of trial-related information: "Are they competent defendants?" *Behavioral Science and the Law,* 15, 167–180.

Cowden, V. L. & McKee, G. R. (1995). Competency to stand trial in juvenile delinquency proceedings: cognitive maturity and the attorney-client relationship. *University of Louisville Journal of Family Law,* 33, 629–690.

Criminal Code, R. S. C., (1985), c.C-46.

Department of Justice, Canada. (2007). *Youth Criminal Justice Act.* [Online] Available at: http://www.justice. gc.ca/en/ps/yj/repository/2overvw/2010001a.html.

Grisso, T. (1998a). Preparing for evaluations in delinquency cases. In *Forensic evaluation of juveniles,* (pp. 1–35). Sarasota: Professional Resource Press.

Grisso, T. (1998b). Juveniles' waiver of Miranda rights, In *Forensic evaluation of juveniles,* (pp. 37–82). Sarasota: Professional Resource Press.

Grisso, T., Miller, M., & Sales, B. (1987). Competency to stand trial in juvenile court. *International Journal of Law and Psychiatry*, 10, 1–20.

Giorgi-Guarnieri, D. & Janofsky, J., Keram, E., Lawsky, S., Merideth, P., Mossman, D., et al., (2002). AAPL practice guideline for forensic psychiatric evaluation of defendants raising the insanity defence. *Journal of the American Academy of Psychiatry and the Law*, 30, S3–S40.

McGarry, A. L., Curran, W. J., Lipsett, P. D., Lelos, D., Schwitzgebel, R. K., Rosenberg, A. H., et al, (1973). Competency to stand trial and mental illness. Washington, D.C.: National Institute of Mental Health, Center for Studies for Crime and Delinquency. HEW Publication HSM 73–9105.

Miller, R. D. (1994). Criminal responsibility. In R. Rosner (Ed.), *Principles and practice of forensic psychiatry*, (pp. 198–215). New York: Chapman & Hall.

Morris, A. & Gelsthorpe, L. (1999). Juveniles-laws and facilities in the United Kingdom. In J. Gunn & P. J. Taylor (Ed.), Forensic Psychiatry-Clinical, Legal & Ethical Issues (pp. 210–251) (1993; reprint, Woburn, MA and Oxford: Butterworth Heinemann).

M'Naghten's Case 10 Cl. & F. 200, 8 Eng. Rep. 718 (H.L. 1843).

Nye, S. G. (1992). Professional concerns. In M. G. Kalogerakis (Ed.), *Handbooks of psychiatric practice in the juvenile court*, (pp. 131–136). Washington, D.C: American Psychiatric Association.

R. v Chaulk S.C.J. No. 139, p. 241. (1990).

R. v MacDonald O.J. No. 1833, Ontario Superior Court of Justice, 2000.

Scott, C. L. (2002). Juvenile Waivers to Adult Court. In D. H. Shetky & E. P. Benedek (Ed.), *Principles and Practice of Child and Adolescent Psychiatry*, (pp. 289–295). Washington, D.C.: American Psychiatry Association Press.

Dusky v. United States 362 U.S. 402 (1960).

Voigt, C. J., Heisel, D. E., & Benedek, E. P. (2002). State-of-mind assessments: competency and criminal responsibility, In D. H. Shetky & E. P. Benedek (Ed.), *Principles and practices of child and adolescent forensic psychiatry*, (pp. 297–305). Washington, D.C.: American Psychiatric Publishing.

Chapter 16

Juvenile Sexual Offenders: Epidemiology, Risk Assessment, and Treatment

Ernest Poortinga, Stewart S. Newman, Christine E. Negendank, and Elissa P. Benedek

In recent years more attention is being paid to juvenile sex offenders, even in the context of lower rates of violent crime committed by juveniles. The media portrayal of the juvenile sex offender has included children, adolescents, girls, boys, healthy children, and children with physical and emotional disabilities. The public's concern about juvenile sex offenders has waxed and waned in proportion to the number and heinousness of sex crimes reported during a given time period. The public's attitude toward the juvenile sex offender has vacillated between attempts to understand, treat, and rehabilitate the offender, to a wish to incarcerate and punish the youthful offender. In this chapter we explore the phenomena of the juvenile sex offender from three perspectives. We realize that this is but a limited picture of a multidimensional phenomenon and that there are other areas worthy of an in depth discussion. We have chosen to focus on the epidemiology of juvenile sex offenders, the recidivism potential of offenders, and the current available treatment models, as these areas of interest seem to

distinguish the juvenile offender from the adult. We leave the discussion of the developmental, biological, psychodynamic, and sociocultural factors that lead to juvenile sexual offending to others.

CASE EXAMPLES

Case 1—Ralph and Josh

Ralph is a 13-year-old male admitted to an acute adolescent inpatient psychiatric unit because of aggression toward other children in his foster care home. He was accused of bullying the younger children for lunch money. He showed little remorse or regret for this behavior. He was in foster care because his biological father had been convicted of Criminal Sexual Conduct for sexually assaulting Ralph when Ralph was 8 years old.

Josh is also 13 years old and a male. He was admitted to the same inpatient unit because of worsening aggression related to his pervasive developmental disorder. His outpatient psychiatrist told the treatment team that much of Josh's aggression seemed to be attention seeking in nature. On one of his weekend visits to his parents' home his father noticed that Josh perseverated on sexual terms such as, "Ralph made me kiss his penis." The more alarmed his father became, the more Josh perseverated. Soon, he would speak of little else. His father decided to file a medical malpractice suit against the hospital, alleging improper supervision of the adolescents.

Case 2—Jake

Jake, a 16-year-old, is convicted of criminal sexual conduct for performing fellatio on a 9-year-old boy while he and other young boys were in his bedroom playing a game of "Truth or Dare." Jake readily admitted to pulling the young boy's pants down and performing oral sex for "a few minutes." This was corroborated by other children who were in Jake's bedroom. Jake had a history of being sexually abused by his own father until the age of 7. He had been convicted 4 years earlier for fondling a young girl and had multiple episodes of past inappropriate sexual behavior. He had been placed on probation after the incident with the young girl. It was unclear if he had been provided with treatment but he and his mother had been instructed that he could not be left alone with young children during the course of his probation. Jake's probation had been completed 1 year before the most recent incident. Jake has multiple past psychiatric diagnoses including mild mental retardation, attention-deficit/hyperactivity disorder (ADHD), mood disorder, not otherwise specifiied, and pervasive developmental disorder. On interview he did not appear to understand the wrongfulness or illegality of performing fellatio on a young child despite his past conviction for fondling. He appeared immature and maintained an odd child-like affect throughout the course of the interview even when talking about possible consequences of his actions.

Case 3—Ronald

Ronald is an 8-year-old white male diagnosed with borderline intellectual functioning and learning disabilities, referred for an outpatient psychiatric evaluation due to behavioral problems in school. His special education teacher notes that Ronald has shown a decline in academics over the previous 12 months. He now has difficulty with following directions, attending to tasks, and respecting the personal space of peers. The content of his speech and drawings he makes in class are often violent themes. His special education teacher had previously worked as a receptionist in a psychologist's office, and was convinced the child was currently psychotic. The child came to the evaluation with his father, who described a long history of poor frustration tolerance, hyperactivity, and impulsivity. The father had not observed violent behaviors at home. The evaluation revealed no evidence of psychosis. There was no history of physical or sexual abuse. The symptoms at presentation were suggestive of pervasive developmental delay or ADHD as well as some cognitive limitations. After 3 days of the evaluation, the psychiatrist received a call from the child's school. The child had been inappropriately touching a younger peer during gym class, "goosing" this boy per the report of the gym teacher. The school requested an immediate reevaluation by the psychiatrist to assure the safety of other students in the school. The school official expressed fears of having a "sexual predator" at their school.

EPIDEMIOLOGY OF JUVENILE SEX OFFENDERS

Epidemiology is sometimes defined as the branch of medicine that investigates the causes and control of epidemics. Demography is the study of the vital statistics of human populations, as size, growth, density, and distribution. In this section of the chapter we discuss one system of classification of offenders in an attempt to isolate some of the factors leading to the epidemic nature of this societal problem. We examine the sex, gender of the offender, age of the victim, gender of the victim, relationship issues, use of violence, and psychiatric comorbidity. It may be possible to diminish the incidence of juvenile offenders by controlling some of these factors, in particular psychiatric comorbidity.

One out of every five sexual assaults involves an offender below the age of 18 (FBI, 2004). Persons below the age of 18 commit one-third to one-half of sexual assaults against children (Snyder & Sickmund, 1999) (Hunter, Figueredo, Malamuth, & Becker, 2003).

Compared to violent offenders, sexual offenders start offending at a younger age and are more likely to continue offending as they age (Caldwell, 2002). Juveniles who sexually offend are a heterogeneous group in terms of victim and offense characteristics, developmental histories, sexual experiences, cognitive functioning, and psychiatric illnesses (Knight & Prentky, 1993).

CLASSIFICATION OF JUVENILE SEX OFFENDERS

Several methods exist for classifying juvenile sex offenders:

By Age of Sex Offender

The average age of onset of offending by juvenile sex offenders is between 12 and 15 years with a median age of 14 to 15 years (CCJS, 1999; Ryan, 1991; Snyder & Sickmund, 1999; Utah Task Force of the Utah Network on Juveniles Offending, 1996). Rate of offending is highest between ages 13 to 16 years with a gradual decline in rate of offending through the mid thirties (CCJS, 1999; Snyder & Sickmund, 1999).

Children younger than 12 years may also sexually assault other children. Compared to older offenders, these youngsters are more likely to have been the victims of physical or sexual assault (Silovsky & Niec, 2002) and more likely to be female (Friedrich, Davies, Feher, & Wright, 2003). Thus, preteen sexually intrusive behaviors should be considered quite different than adolescent sexual offending.

By Gender of Offender

Ninety to 97% percent of juvenile sex offenders are male (Campbell & Lerew, 2002; Mathews, Hunter, Jr., & Vuz, 1997). Female juvenile sex offenders tend to have an earlier age of onset and more severe victimization histories (Mathews et al., 1997).

By Age of Victim

Classification by age of victim yields two main groups:

1. *Child Victims.* These sexual offenders prefer victims who are much younger than himself or herself, male, and well known or related to the offender. These offenders rarely display high levels of aggression. They also have greater deficits in psychosocial functioning than do offenders against peer or adult victims and are less likely to be under the influence of alcohol or drugs at the time of their offense (Hunter et al., 2003).
2. *Peer or Adult Victims.* This group prefers victims who are their own age or older, female, and often unacquainted. They tend to display high levels of aggression, with frequent use of weapons and frequent injury to victims.

By Gender of Victim

Female victims are far more prevalent (Hunter & Figueredo, 1999; Rasmussen, 1999) but some studies show male victims representing up to 25% of the sample (Rasmussen, 1999; Wieckowski, Hartsoe, Mayer, & Shortz, 1998).

By Relationship to Victim

Victims are often acquaintances or relatives (Rasmussen, 1999; Ryan, 1991; Wieckowski et al., 1998). The opportunity to offend may be provided by babysitting, and rarely are strangers assaulted (Fehrenbach & Smith, 1986; Smith & Monastersky, 1986).

By use of Violence

While juvenile sex offenders may force victim compliance with intimidation, threats of violence or physical force (Miranda & Corcoran, 2000), they tend to be physically violent less often than adult offenders (Knight & Prentky, 1993). A sample of 91 juveniles in Minnesota found that close to 40% used significant aggression in their sexual offenses (Miner & Siekert, 1997).

By Sexual Offense Characteristics

Acts perpetrated by juvenile sex offenders compose a wide range of behaviors. More than 50% of the acts in a study of Maine juveniles (Righthand & Hennings, 1989) involved oral–genital contact or attempted or actual vaginal or anal penetration. Miranda and Corcoran (2000) compared the offense characteristics of male juvenile and adult sexual offenders. They found that juveniles were more likely to participate in intrafamilial sexual abuse (67% vs. 21%) and used force more frequently than did adults. Juveniles were less likely to engage in penetration (13% vs. 41%).

By Psychiatric Comorbidity

Since paraphilias and sexual deviancy syndrome are believed to impact the behavior of adult sex offenders, (Saleh & Berlin, 2003) it stands to reason that the effects may be similar for juveniles who commit sexual offenses. Paraphilias are psychiatric disorders with deviant and culturally nonsanctioned sexual fantasies, thoughts and/or behaviors (DSM-IV). Data from recent studies suggest that the etiology of paraphilias may be biological (Quinsey, 2003).

Some of these juveniles may also suffer from symptoms of mental illness. Recent surveys (Becker, Kaplan, Tenke, & Tartaglini, 1991; Galli et al., 1999; Myers & Blashfield, 1997) found incidence rates for Major Depression of up to 42% in juvenile sex offenders. A recent Irish study reported high scores on the anxiety/depression and attention subscales of the Child Behavior Checklist for juveniles participating in sex offender treatment programs (O'Halloran & Carr, 2002). Impulsivity scores were not significantly different between the sex offender group and normal controls (O'Halloran & Carr, 2002).

Conduct disorder and substance abuse are commonly diagnosed in juvenile sex offenders but incidence rates may not differ significantly from other juvenile offenders (Kavoussi, Kaplan, & Becker, 1988; Lewis, Shankok, & Pincus, 1979; Lightfoot & Barbaree, 1993; Tarter, Hegedus, Alterman, & Katz-Garris, 1983).

According to Shaw, "there are essentially four kinds of juvenile sexual offenders." The classifications by Shaw are examples of the systems discussed earlier. His first three offender types (offenders with true paraphilias such as frotteurism, offenders with strong antisocial personality disorders, and offenders who are "compromised by a psychiatric or neurobiological disorder") are examples of classification by psychiatric comorbidity. Shaw's final category (2002), "youth with impaired social skills who turn to younger children for sexual gratification" is a combination of classification by victim characteristics and psychiatric comorbidity.

FACTORS ASSOCIATED WITH JUVENILE SEX OFFENDING

A number of nonpsychiatric factors have been found to be associated with juvenile sex offending. Chief among these factors is a history of being a victim of physical and/or sexual abuse. Incidence rates for sexual abuse victimization range from 47% to 66% (Johnson & Shrier, 1985; Longo, 1996). One study found that 19% of juvenile sex offenders had been physically abused before their own offense (Johnson & Shrier, 1985). The relationship between victimization and subsequent offending is more complex than simple cause and effect. Hunter and Figueredo (1999) found four variables that mediated this relationship: higher rates of the abusive incidents; lower level of perceived family support following disclosure of the abuse; long period of delay between abuse and disclosure of the abuse; and finally, younger age at the time of victimization. Moreover, juveniles who have been exposed to physical abuse by a father or stepfather had higher levels of anxiety and depression than juveniles who were not exposed to such abuse. The same high rates of anxiety and depression were present in juveniles who witnessed violence against females (Hunter et al., 2003).

To address the relationship between sexual victimization and subsequent sexual offending, Friedrich et al (2003) studied a group of 620 children aged 2 to 12 years who had a confirmed history of being sexually abused. They were compared to a control group of nearly 1700 preteen children with no abuse victimization history. With sexually intrusive behaviors as the dependant variable, sexual abuse was not the primary predictor. Rather, a model incorporating family adversity, modeling of coercive behavior, child behavior, and modeling of sexuality appeared to explain most of the variance in the sexually intrusive behavior.

Biological factors have been examined more extensively in adult rather than juvenile sex offenders. These factors have been reviewed elsewhere in this book.

Measures of neuropsychological functioning were compared between a group of 60 adolescent sex offenders and 60 nonsexual delinquent offenders. Both groups demonstrated a pattern of frontal executive dysfunction, scoring well below average on word association and trail-making tests but close to average on Tower of London and Wisconsin Card Sorting measures. Test scores did not correlate with IQ scores. The authors concluded that there is likely a subset of juvenile sex offenders who have latent neuropsychological dysfunction, manifest by increased impulsivity, poor planning, and poor verbal skills (Veneziano, Veneziano, Legrand, & Richards, 2004).

RECIDIVISM AND RISK ASSESSMENT OF JUVENILE SEXUAL OFFENDERS

An understanding of the rate of recidivism and the factors leading to recidivism is critical in prevention. No single test or interview question will predict the potential for recidivism. It is critical to understand factors associated with recidivism that influence the potential for repeat sexual offenses. In this section of the chapter we first present an overview of the known rates of recidivism. We also discuss the range of variables that can be used in an attempt to assess risk and predict recidivism, recognizing that risk assessment of juvenile sexual offenders is an imperfect science.

The Federal Bureau of Investigation's national incident-based reporting system indicate that approximately one out of every five sexual assaults and one-third of sexual assaults of children below the age of 12 years are perpetrated by an offender below the age of 18 years (Snyder & Sickmund, 1999). In addition, nearly one-half of adult sexual offenders report committing sexual offenses before the age of 18 years (Groth, Longo, & McFadin, 1982).

RATES OF RECIDIVISM

Studies of sexual and nonsexual recidivism of juvenile sex offenders range greatly depending on the study design. Variables in studies of recidivism include methodological design, type of referral offenses, length of the follow-up period, impact of clinical interventions, nature of the population being investigated and measures of recidivism (Sipe, Jensen, & Everett, 1998; Worling & Långström, 2003). The variability in the measurement of recidivism is dependent on the victim's willingness to report the crime, the ability of police and/or child protection agencies to investigate the complaint, the decision of police to press charges that reflect the sexual nature of the crime and the accurate and timely entry of the charge into a computerized database. Accurate recidivism data is also dependant on the sexual charges not being dropped or altered to a nonsexual charge through plea bargaining (Worling & Långström, 2003). Higher rates of sexual recidivism are generally associated with longer follow-up periods and stricter measures of recidivism (Nisbet, Wilson, & Smallbone, 2004).

Studies of juvenile sex offenders report sexual recidivism rates of 0% to 37%. Along with sexual recidivism data, multiple studies have also examined nonsexual offense recidivism rates which are consistently higher than sexual recidivism rates (32% to 65%). Mazur and Michael (1992) found a 0% recidivism rate after a short (6-month) follow-up using self-report data with 10 adolescents participating in community-based group treatment. Nisbet et al. (2004) studied 292 adolescent male sex offenders for which adult rearrest and reconviction data were obtained with a mean observation time of 7.3 years; 25% (75) of the adolescents received additional sexual convictions before their 18th birthday. As adults, 9% (14) of the sample was alleged to have sexually offended and 5% were reconvicted for sexual offenses. Of the 14 subjects reconvicted for sexual offenses, 11 (79%) also received new convictions for nonsexual offenses.

Sipe et al. (1998) examined adult arrest records of a group of adjudicated male sexual offenders. The sexual offender group included of 164 subjects ranging from age 11 to 18 years at the time of admittance into the study. Subjects were followed for 1 to 14 years after turning 18 with a mean age of 24 years at the time of data collection. Of the juvenile sex offenders 9.7% were arrested as adults for sexual offenses and 32.6% were arrested for nonsexual offenses. Smith and Monastersky (1986) studied 112 adolescent males who had been referred to a juvenile sex offender program. Length of follow-up ranged from 17 to 49 months with an average time of 28.9 months; 14% of subjects committed a sexual offense in the follow-up period according to juvenile justice system records.

Rasmussen (1999) followed 170 first-time juvenile sexual offenders for 5 years; 14.1% of the sample committed a sexual offense and 54.1% committed a new nonsexual offense. Långström and Grann (2000) studied 46 sex offenders aged 15 to 20 years old. Rates for sexual recidivism was 20% and general recidivism was were 65% with a mean time of risk being 5 years. Finally, Rubenstein et al. (1993) followed up 19 juvenile sexual offenders and 58 nonsexual offenders into adulthood. The follow-up period was 8 years after release from the juvenile justice system. Of the sample, 37% was found to have criminal records for sexual assaults as adults. The high rate of sexual recidivism in this study may have been related to the inclusion of juveniles in the study who were described as very assaultive.

Few studies have examined the impact of sexual offender treatment on recidivism rates. There is some controversy as to whether specialized treatment for juvenile sexual offenders affects recidivism rates, especially for nonsexual crimes (Berlinger, 1998; Milloy, 1998). However, as discussed by Worling & Curwen (2000), many early studies did not include a comparison group, had short follow-up times, and used conservative measures of recidivism. Two studies that used comparison groups and less conservative measures for recidivism report promising findings for specialized sexual offender treatment programs (Bourduin, Henggeler, Blake, & Stein, 1990; Worling & Curwen, 2000). Worling and Curwen collected data on 58 offenders participating in at least 12 months of treatment in a community-based specialized treatment program. The participants were compared to 90 adolescents who received only an assessment, refused treatment or dropped out of the program before 12 months. Follow-up time ranged from 2 to 10 years. Recidivism rates for the subjects who completed at least 12 months of treatment for sexual, violent nonsexual, and nonviolent offenses were approximately 5%, 19%, and 21% compared to 18%, 32%, and 50% for controls. There was a 72% reduction in sexual recidivism and a 41% reduction in nonsexual offense recidivism. These findings were comparable to those of Borduin et al. (1990) who found an 83% reduction in sexual assault recidivism and a 50% reduction in nonsexual recidivism after specialized treatment. Both of the treatment interventions in the earlier studies involved comprehensive treatment emphasizing offense-specific interventions and unique treatment approaches depending on the strengths and needs of the adolescent offenders and their families (Worling & Curwen, 2000).

FACTORS ASSOCIATED
WITH RECIDIVISM

Worling and Långström (2003) completed a comprehensive review of empirical and professional literature of factors associated with recidivism in adolescents who offend sexually. They divided risk factors for sexual reoffending into supported, promising, possible, and unlikely risk factors.

Supported risk factors were defined as risk factors with the most defensible empirical evidence. Supported risk factors included deviant sexual interest, prior criminal sanctions for sexual assaults, past sexual offenses against two or more victims, selection

of a stranger victim, lack of intimate peer relationships/social isolation, and incomplete offense-specific treatment.

Promising risk factors were described as factors that should be examined for risk assessment even though empirical support was limited. Promising risk factors included problematic parent–adolescent relationship/parental rejection and attitudes supportive of sexual offending. Possible risk factors were described as risk factors currently viewed by some researchers to be related to sexual recidivism in adolescents but were considered speculative secondary to lack of empirical support and opposing expert opinion. Caution was therefore advised when relying on these factors for risk assessment. Possible risk factors included a high-stress family environment, obsessive sexual interests/ sexual preoccupation, impulsivity, selection of a male victim, negative peer associations and influences, environment supporting an opportunity to reoffend, past sexual assault against a child, threats or use of excessive violence or weapons during sexual offense, indiscriminate choice of victims, unwillingness to alter deviant sexual interests/attitudes, interpersonal aggression, antisocial interpersonal orientation, and recent escalation in anger or negative affect.

Unlikely risk factors were described by the authors as risk factors that should not be used in risk assessment at present secondary to contradictory empirical evidence. Unlikely risk factors included denial of sexual offense, lack of victim empathy, history of nonsexual crimes, penetrative sexual assaults, and the offending adolescents own history of child sexual abuse. Worling and Curwen (2000) indicate that promising, possible, and unlikely risk factors may, in the future, be found to relate to adolescent sexual reoffending with further research and/or improved measurement techniques.

RISK ASSESSMENT

Assessments of adolescents who sexually offend are used to assist in various determinations at multiple decision points within the juvenile justice system (Prentky, Harris, Frizzell, & Righthand, 2000). These determinations include, but are not limited to, preadjudicatory diversion, potential prosecution of the adolescent, sentencing, dispositional and case planning, the level of treatment interventions and the decision if community notification is necessary (Worling &

Långström, 2003; Prentky et al., 2000). Many juris-dictions have amended community notification laws to exclude juvenile offenders. Other jurisdictions determine notification on a case by case basis and may go so far as to charge the juvenile as an adult. (DesLauriers & Gardner,1999). Two complicating factors in risk assessment of juvenile sex offenders are the heterogeneity of the population (Bourke & Donohue, 1996; Knight & Prentky, 1993) and the lack of empirically based studies on the development and validation of risk assessment measures (Prentky et al., 2000).

A comprehensive assessment of adolescents who offend sexually is a complicated and time-consuming task (Zonana & Abel, 1999) ideally performed by trained evaluators who are experienced in the assess-ment of adolescents who offend criminally and their families. Evaluators should have adequate knowledge of relevant sexual offender research regarding etiol-ogy, assessment, treatment, and recidivism and be aware of the static and dynamic factors which may contribute to sexual reoffending. Multiple methods of data collection should be used and should cover both sexual and biological domains of the adoles-cent's functioning (Worling & Långström, 2003). Proposed modalities of risk assessment include clin-ical interviews, collection of collateral information, psychological testing, empirically guided checklists, phallometry, visual reaction time (VRT) using the Abel Assessment for Sexual Interests, and polygraph testing (Abel, Jordan, Rouleau, Emerick, Barboza-Whitehead, & Osborn, 2004; Blanchette, 1996; Worling & Långström, 2003; Zonana & Abel, 1999).

STATIC VERSUS DYNAMIC FACTORS

Static risk factors are highly stable or historical fac-tors that do not change over time. Dynamic risk fac-tors are changeable characteristics that may affect an individual's recidivism risk or treatment plan (Hanson & Harris, 2000). Long-term recidivism in adult sexual offenders has been best predicated by static factors (i.e., early childhood experiences, offense history, personality characteristics, and dis-orders) and may indicate ongoing reoffense poten-tial (Hanson & Bussiere, 1998; Kenny, Keogh, & Seidler, 2001). However, static risk factors are not considered useful in directing therapy and therefore dynamic and potentially modifiable risk factors for

sexual recidivism are being studied. When dynamic risk factors such as criminal attitudes, denial of responsibility, rationalization, deviant sexual fanta-sies, cognitive and perceptual distortions, social skill and problem solving deficits, and coping style (Kenny et al., 2001) change they result in a corresponding increase or decrease in recidivism risk that is thought to be important for treatment planning and interven-tion (Hanson & Harris, 2000).

CLINICAL INTERVIEW

The clinical interview is the face-to-face interac-tion with the adolescent who has sexually offended. Although the clinical interview should not be used solely for risk assessment (Grove, Zald, Lebow, Snitz, & Nelson, 2000; Hanson & Bussiere, 1998) it is an important component of the evaluation (Blanchette, 1996). The clinical assessment should be performed by a specialized, well-trained, and expe-rienced evaluator with appropriate personal skills (Blanchette, 1996; Worling, 2004). The evaluator should also be culturally knowledgeable and sensitive to aide in the understanding of adolescents who have offended sexually, their families, and their communi-ties (Zonana & Abel, 1999). The clinical interview should ideally help to determine which dynamic fac-tors are present at the time of the evaluation and how these factors may increase or decrease the risk for recidivism. This will allow for further clarification of treatment approaches (Blanchette, 1996).

COLLATERAL INFORMATION

Collateral information is considered critical in the risk-assessment of juvenile sexual offenders. Obtain-ing collateral information allows for the genera-tion of a hypothesis which can then be explored during the clinical interview (Blanchette, 1996). The examination of collateral information can identify discrepancies between an adolescent's self-reporting and information obtained from other sources that will need further clarification and understanding (Zonana & Abel, 1999). Collateral information should include interviews with par-ents, family, and friends. These interviews should be combined with information contained from police reports, court transcripts, reports from the victim, presentence and postsentence disposition reports, psychological and psychiatric reports, case management documentation, and discussions with other mental health professionals familiar with the adolescent's case (Blanchette 1996; Worling & Långström, 2003).

PSYCHOLOGICAL TESTS

Psychological tests that have been used in risk assessment of the adolescent sexual offender include multiple self-report measures. These measures include the Adolescent Cognition Scale (Hunter et al., 1991) and the Adolescent Sexual Interest Card Sort (Becker & Kaplan, 1988). The Adolescent Cognition Scale is a true-false test developed to assess the presence of distorted cognitions regarding sexual behaviors (Hunter et al., 1991; Zonana & Abel, 1999). The Adolescent Sexual Interest Card Sort is used to detect deviant sexual interests. The test presents sexual vignettes during which the adolescent rates their level of sexual arousal. (Hunter, Becker, & Kaplan, 1995; Zonana & Abel, 1999; Rosner, 2003). General psychological assessment measures used in risk assessment of the adolescent sexual offender include the MMPI-A (Archer, 1997), Child Behavior Checklist (Achenbach, McConaughy, & Howell, 1987), Beck Depression Inventory (Beck & Ward, 1961), Matson Evaluation of Social Skills in Youngsters (Matson & Esveldt-Dawson 1983), and the Multiphasic Sex Inventory (Nichols & Molinder, 1984; Rosner, 2003).

EMPIRICALLY GUIDED CHECKLISTS

In addition to clinical judgment, actuarial methods are being developed to aide in risk assessment of juvenile sex offenders. Actuarial methods eliminate the disadvantages of subjective clinical judgment in assessing risk (Barbaree, Seto, Langton, & Peacock, 2001; Quinsey, Harris, Rice, & Cormier, 1998). Hanson and Bussiere (1998) found that unstructured clinical judgments were, on average, only modestly related to sexual recidivism. Berlin et al. (2003) have argued that actuarial methods represent a form of profiling that can be used only to identify a group of persons to be considered for possible civil commitment, and do not feel actuarial methods can be used to accurately predict the likelihood of future acts of sexual violence with respect to any specific individual within such a group. However, it is generally held that actuarial assessments are superior to unstructured clinical judgment when conducting risk assessments of individuals who sexually offend (Barbaree, et al., 2001; Grove et al., 2000; Hanson, 2000a; Worling, 2004). Specific structured assessments for juvenile sex offenders include the Juvenile Sex Offender Assessment Protocol-II (J-SOAP-II) (Prentky & Righthand, 2003) and The Estimate of Risk of Adolescent Sexual Offense Recidivism (ERASOR) (Worling & Curwen, 2001). The J-SOAP-II is a 28 item structured risk assessment measure involving 16 static and 12 dynamic items designed to assess the risk of sexual reoffense of males aged 12 to 18 years. The items are classified into four scales that include sexual drive/preoccupation, impulsive/antisocial behavior, intervention, and community stability/adjustment items. Authors of the J-SOAP-II stress that, at the present time, secondary to a lack of adequate data on sexual recidivism risk in large numbers of sexual reoffenders, the J-SOAP-II is not an actuarial scale but an "empirically informed guide." The authors also point out the importance of reassessing juvenile sexual offenders at a minimum of every 6 months secondary to rapid changes in cognitive development and life circumstances in adolescents (Prentky & Righthand, 2003).

The Estimate of Risk of Adolescent Sexual Offense Recidivism (ERASOR) was designed to assist evaluators to estimate the risk of sexual reoffense for individuals aged 12 to 18 years and contains 25 risk factors with 16 of the 25 factors being dynamic (Worling & Curwen, 2001). The 25 risk factors are classified into the categories of sexual interests, attitudes, and behaviors; historical sexual assaults, psychosocial functioning, family/environmental functioning; and treatment. Because the ERASOR contains multiple dynamic factors that need to be reassessed over time, the final risk estimate derived from using the ERASOR should be used for short-term risk (at most 1 year) and should not be used to predict long-term risk (Worling & Långström, 2003). Authors of both the J-SOAP-II and ERASOR emphasize that the earlier structured risk assessment measures should not be used as sole measures for reoffense risk but should be included as part of a comprehensive risk assessment involving case-specific risk factors (Prentky & Righthand, 2003; Worling & Långström 2003).

PHYSIOLOGIC TESTING

Physiologic testing of adolescent sex offenders has included plethysmography and the measurement of VRT by use of the Abel Assessment for Sexual Interests (AASI) (Abel et al., 2004). Plethysmography is the phallometric assessment of sexual arousal by measuring penile circumference (Zonana & Abel, 1999). VRT is the amount of time an individual looks at slides of potentially sexual stimuli and has been proposed as an alternative to plethysmography. The AASI examines VRTs of inappropriate sexual stimuli. In addition, the AASI records subjective ratings of sexual interests and obtains a sex offender specific questionnaire which includes the adolescent's sexual history and interests (Abel et al., 2004).

The use of VRT and plethysmography in adolescents is controversial secondary to exposure to nude photographs or sexually explicit audiotapes during the testing. In addition, there is a lack of empirical research regarding the reliability and validity of plethysmographic assessment in sexually offending adolescents (Abel et al., 2004). However, some studies of validation of plethysmography in sexually offending adolescents have been performed with promising results and suggest further research is indicated to assess the use of plethysmography in this population (Becker & Hunter, 1992; Seto, Lalumiere, & Blanchard, 2000). Standardized procedures for the use of phallometric equipment have been developed by the Association for the Treatment of Sexual Abusers (ATSA, 1997) and guidelines for the testing procedure have been proposed by the National Task Force on Juvenile Sexual Offending (NAPN, 1993). Zonana and Abel (1999) stressed the importance of following these guidelines and procedures for practitioners using phallometric assessment in the assessment of sexually offending adolescents.

VRT as measured by the Abel Assessment for sexual interest (AASI) and has been successfully compared to plethysmography in the assessment of adult child molesters (Abel, Huffman, Warberg, & Holland, 1998). Research has begun to support the use of VRT in adolescent male child molesters (Abel et al., 2004). Results of a study of 1704 adolescent males undergoing evaluation or treatment for sexual paraphilias indicated that the amount of time child molesters viewed slides was significantly longer than nonmolesters and viewing times of molesters was significantly correlated with the number of victims and the number of times they carried out acts of child molestation. An independent study has questioned the use of VRT in the assessment of adolescent sexual offenders secondary to the lack of independent studies supporting the reliability of VRT (Smith & Fischer, 1999). However, Smith and Fischer (1999) believe that these techniques may prove useful with further refinement and also point out strengths of the visual stimulus slides over plethysmography such as the use of clothed models and the absence of penile apparatus. Furthermore, these techniques are potentially useful in women.

TREATMENT OF JUVENILE SEXUAL OFFENDERS

As mental health professionals, one of our goals is the effective treatment of the mental health issues associated with the juvenile sexual offenses. There is much we do know as scientists and clinicians, and much that we still have to learn, with regard to balancing the community risks presented by the juvenile offender and the benefits of treatment. In this section we discuss available treatment options and the risks and benefits associated with those options, as well as the associated treatment outcomes. All juvenile offenders are not alike and the selection of appropriate treatment depends on an understanding of the offender, the factors which favor rehabilitation in a particular offender and those which suggest that treatment rehabilitation is not possible, and the need to protect the community.

There exists good evidence to support the treatment of juvenile sexual offenders. Studies have demonstrated that treatment is effective in ending the cycle of abusive sexual behaviors by offenders. Studies show a significant percentage of offenders will respond to treatment (Becker, 1994; Becker & Hunter, 1997; Bremer, 1992; Dwyer, 1997; Hall, 1995). Recidivism rates for untreated sexual offenders have been seen to be higher than those who complete a treatment program (Gallagher & Wilson, 1999; Hanson, 1998; Hanson, 2000; Hanson et al., 2002; Marshall & Barbaree, 1988; Rubenstein, Yeager, Goodstein, & Lewis, 1993). The economic burden to the community is decreased through treatment (Prentky & Burgess, 1990). Treatment programs are less expensive than residential or institutional placements (Farrell & O'Brien, 1988). Costs are also reduced through the prevention of further offenses. Garrett et al. (2003) also demonstrated that offenders report positive experiences of group treatment.

Treatment modalities for sexual offenders include psychotherapeutic modalities, including cognitive behavioral interventions such as psychoeducation, behavior modification, relapse prevention, and psychosocial therapies. Multiple studies have shown a combination of cognitive-behavioral approaches (Frost, 2004; Jennings & Sawyer, 2003; Laws, 1998; McGuire, 2000; Marshall, Fernandez, Hudson, & Ward, 1998; Pithers & Marques, 1983; Pithers, Kashima, Cumming, & Beal, 1988; Sawyer, 2000; Sawyer, 2002) and group therapy modalities to be the most effective interventions. Psychopharmacology may be utilized as an adjunct to treatment of some juvenile sexual offenders.

TREATMENT PLANNING

The primary task in the treatment of a juvenile sexual offender is the protection of the community (Shaw, 1999, 2001). Treatment is undertaken with the ultimate outcome of ending the offending behavior in the immediate sense, but also in doing so preventing these juveniles from becoming adult offenders in the future. The juvenile sexual offender population is not homogenous, but instead presents a wide variety of etiologies, comorbidities, and treatment needs. An integrated approach, addressing the emotional, behavioral, and developmental issues that a juvenile sexual offender presents, is the recommended approach for any treatment endeavor (Becker, 1994; Schwartz, 1992; Shaw, 1999). This reflects increasing evidence that sexually abusive behavior is not simply a disorder of sexual arousal or paraphilia in the strictest sense (Prentky et al., 2000; Schwartz, 1992; Weinrott, 1996). Treatment must also specifically addresses the unique needs and resources of the offender and be tailored to these needs. Shaw et al, (1999) reviewed relevant literature (Becker, 1994; Becker & Hunter, 1997; Hunter & Figueredo, 1999) to summarize a number of goals for the treatment of a juvenile sexual offender, as listed in Table 16.1. Inherent in treatment planning is also a decision regarding the level of care required, speaking directly to the need to protect the community.

In protecting the community, the clinician must weigh the potential for recidivism, and use this in determining recommendations for treatment. Recidivism encompasses both sexual and nonsexual criminal acts, as most juvenile sexual offenders

TABLE 16.1 Goals for the Treatment of the Juvenile Sexual Offender

Confronting the offender's denial

Decreasing deviant sexual arousal

Facilitating the development of nondeviant sexual interests

Promoting victim empathy

Enhancing social and interpersonal skills

Assisting with values clarification

Clarifying cognitive distortions

Teaching the juvenile to recognize the internal and external antecedents of the sexual offending behavior

Adapted (with permission) from The American Academy of Child and Adolescent Psychiatry Practice parameters for the assessment and treatment of children and adolescents who are sexually abusive of others, 1999.

are also at high risk for nonsexual crimes. Factors used in assessing recidivism risk include the frequency and diversity of the offenses, severity of aggressive-sadistic behavior, the premeditation versus impulsivity of the offenses, the level of psychological, neurological, and developmental disability, history of antisocial or violent behaviors, motivation for treatment, cognitive and emotional resources, and support systems (Hunter & Figueredo, 1999; Prentky et al., 2000; Rasmussen, 1999; Worling & Curwen, 2000).

Consideration for placement in a more restrictive environment should be on the basis of factors that might suggest a higher risk for recidivism or difficulty in complying with treatment. Offenders who display a consistent need to deny the offenses, demonstrate a lack of remorse or empathy for the victims, have severe comorbid psychopathology, or a high degree of sexual compulsivity or deviant arousal are candidates for a more restrictive treatment setting. Offenders who perpetrated frequent sexual offenses, perpetrated a diverse range of offenses, have multiple victims, or have a history of previous violent behaviors or previous arrests will also likely require placement in a more restrictive environment (Hunter & Figueredo, 1999; Rasmussen, 1999).

TREATABILITY OF JUVENILE SEXUAL OFFENDERS

Decisions about treatment for juvenile sexual offenders must take into account multiple factors unique to each individual. Factors that influence the treatability of the offender are summarized in Table 16.2. An assessment of these factors assists the clinician in making a reasoned decision regarding the level of care required, the optimal setting for the delivery of that care, and the resources required. This will also allow for stratification of priorities within treatment, such as aggressive treatment of psychiatric comorbidity before introducing the offender to a group therapy setting.

The heterogeneous nature of the juvenile sexual offender population is due in part to the fact that these offenders are still children. Being children, they continue to grow and learn, continue to internalize social experiences, and continue to develop in a cognitive and moral sense. The sexually abusive behaviors may be tied to the juvenile's continuing experimentation with sexual practices, and the lack of a firmly established pattern of normal sexual arousal. These attributes may contribute to better treatment outcomes on juveniles, and are summarized in Table 16.3.

PSYCHIATRIC COMORBIDITY

There have been multiple studies demonstrating the frequency and range of psychiatric comorbidity in the juvenile sexual offender population, as discussed earlier in this chapter. Frequency of both Axis I and Axis II disorders is high. Assessment of these factors and their contribution to the risk of recurrence for the

TABLE 16.2 Factors Influencing Treatability of Juvenile Sexual Offenders

The level of understanding of the seriousness of the offense

The motivation to discuss and understand the offense

The capacity for empathy and human relatedness

The severity of comorbid psychopathology

The entrenchment of deviant sexual arousal patterns

The type and frequency of the sexual offending behavior

The aggressiveness of the sexual offense

The degree of characterological impairment

The nature of the treatment program

Adapted (with permission) from The American Academy of Child and Adolescent Psychiatry Practice parameters for the assessment and treatment of children and adolescents who are sexually abusive of others, 1999.

TABLE 16.3 Why Adolescent Offenders May Be More Amenable to Treatment Than Adult Offenders

The adolescent offender's deviant pattern of sexual offending behavior is less deeply ingrained

The adolescent offender is still exploring alternative pathways to sexual gratification

The adolescent offender's central masturbatory fantasy is still evolving and is not fully consolidated

The adolescent offender is available for learning more effective interpersonal and social skills

Adapted (with permission) from The American Academy of Child and Adolescent Psychiatry Practice parameters for the assessment and treatment of children and adolescents who are sexually abusive of others, 1999.

juvenile is essential. The impact that these disorders may have on the juvenile's ability to successfully participate in and complete a treatment program must not be discounted. Treatment of the comorbid psychiatric disorders according to appropriate standards of care can improve the global level of function of the juvenile, and allow for treatment to then focus on the sexually abusive behaviors.

COGNITIVE BEHAVIORAL INTERVENTIONS

The therapeutic interventions seen to be most effective with juvenile sexual offenders can be broken down into three broad groups under the rubric of cognitive—behavioral interventions. Psychoeducational interventions focus on providing the offender with information that allows understanding of the maladaptive nature of the offenses and assist in correcting this. Behavioral interventions work to diminish or extinguish deviant sexual arousal patterns that have developed in the offenders. Relapse prevention interventions disrupt the sexual assault cycle, described by Ryan et al. (1987). Individualized treatment plans may draw on any combination of these interventions, dictated by the needs of the offender.

Psychoeducational interventions include didactic sessions in which relevant and accurate information is presented to the offender. Education on normal sexual development and practices allows for discussion of deviant sexual practices and the development of sexually aggressive behaviors. Cognitive restructuring corrects the cognitive distortions that support irrational beliefs that lead to sexually aggressive behaviors and clarify sexual values. This connects with efforts to teach empathy towards victims, and also explore the impact offending has on the individual. Offenders are provided with skills for coping with aggressive and sexual impulses, anger, and difficulty with socialization. Relaxation techniques, assertiveness training, and development of appropriate social skills provide means to negotiate appropriate sexual relationships (Becker & Hunter, 1997; Green, 1988).

Behavioral interventions are utilized to decrease or extinguish deviant patterns of sexual arousal in offenders. Various techniques have been used with varying level of success. Covert sensitization asks the offender to imagine a negative stimulus in an effort to extinguish the pleasurable response from specific preferred deviant stimuli (Cautela, 1966). Assisted covert sensitization incorporates the use of a noxious stimulus, such as an odor (Maletzky, 1974). Similarly, in olfactory conditioning a noxious odor is paired with a deviant stimulus to elicit a classical conditioned response. Imaginal desensitization uses relaxation techniques to disrupt the arousal cycle that a deviant stimulus might begin (McConaughy, Blaszczynski, Armstrong, & Kidson, 1989). Sexual arousal reconditioning pairs sexual arousal with appropriate, nondeviant sexual stimuli. Satiation techniques can be either verbal or masturbatory. The offender is asked to masturbate to ejaculation in response to appropriate sexual stimuli. After this experience the offenders is then asked to masturbate again to deviant sexual stimuli, or to dictate on audiotape deviant sexual imagery for at least 30 minutes. If the offender again becomes aroused, they are asked to return to the appropriate sexual stimuli. The technique assumes that the deviant stimuli become boring and are then abandoned (Schwartz, 1992).

The relapse prevention model, originally developed for substance abuse treatment, is based on an understanding that both immediate determinants and covert antecedents can contribute to relapse (Larimer, Palmer, & Marlatt, 1999). Relapse prevention has been adapted for use in sexual offender treatments (Mann & Thornton, 1998; Marques & Nelson, 2000). For sexual offenders, these factors can contribute to a relapse into the sexual assault cycle. Treatment focuses on interfering with the sexual assault cycle through the use of positive coping strategies and proactive avoidance of potential triggers or high-risk situations. Offenders are encouraged to identify high-risk situations or emotional states, and to modify life-style factors that contribute to the sexual assault cycle (Shaw, 1999).

PSYCHOSOCIAL INTERVENTIONS

Psychosocial interventions take an interpersonal approach to the treatment of the juvenile sexual offender, and are complementary to both cognitive-behavioral and psychopharmacological interventions. Offenders can be engaged in group therapy with other offenders, with family members in family therapy, or in more traditional individual therapy settings. Many of these modalities are used in concert with one another in various treatment programs.

Group therapy is one of the most common therapeutic settings for the treatment of juvenile sexual offenders. Groups are usually divided by age to provide some commonality in the social and developmental tasks and struggles of the group members. Divisions into early childhood, middle childhood, preadolescent, and adolescent groups is typical (Shaw, 1999). Groups are usually segregated by gender as well, as there is little advantage in mixing the sexes (Shaw, 1999). Participating in a group with other sexual offenders prevents minimization, denial, or rationalization of the sexual offenses. The group members, being offenders themselves, are less willing to tolerate such obfuscation and can more easily confront the peer. The group therapy process is often the setting in which psychoeducational interventions are presented and worked with. The group process serves as the milieu in which the offender can begin to develop positive peer relationships, practice social skills, and develop positive self regard. The participants can also develop a sense of trust within the group, allowing for the discussion of more difficult or threatening issues (Schwartz, 1988). The group leaders can model appropriate interactions for the members, and serve a source of authority for the offender to develop an appropriate relationship with.

Family therapy incorporates many of the same processes as group therapy, with the member of the group being drawn instead from the offender's own family. Focus of the therapeutic work is on the family dynamics that may contribute to the development or persistence of sexually abusive behaviors (Schwartz, 1988; Shaw, 1999). The majority of the experiences and information about gender roles, sexuality, and relationships come out of the family setting (Bischof, Smith, & Whitney, 1995). The therapy can also work to develop more positive communications styles and coping skills within the family unit. Stress is also placed on the family's role in supporting and assisting the offender to control the sexually abusive behaviors and prevent relapse. In cases where there is incest, and the offender will remain in the nuclear family, family therapy can be very effective (Shaw, 1999). It has been shown (NAPN, 1993) that treatment programs that involve family members are more likely to be effective than those which do not, thereby decreasing recidivism.

It has been noted that families vary in their motivation towards treatment of juvenile sex offenders and the degree to which they can assist in the process (Gray & Pithers, 1993). It has been recommended that parents be counselled to adopt the attitude of "knowledge is power" (Gray & Pithers, 1993). Families are given an opportunity to discuss the losses and feelings associated with learning of the juvenile's offenses, and their participation in the treatment process is actively facilitated. It is recommended that families are provided with a variety of resources regarding treatment of juvenile sex offenders. These should include written information on relapse prevention, cognitive distortions and the consequences of sexual abuse; educational videotapes of adolescent abusers discussing their relapse process and the need to be held responsible; literature on the recovery process of sexual abuse victims; referrals to treatment groups for adult sexual abuse survivors; opportunities to be included in sessions of the adolescent abuser groups; referrals to support groups of parents of abusive adolescents; and attention to the concerns of the offender's nonabusive siblings in the treatment process (Gray & Pithers, 1993).

Individual therapy is not a first line intervention in the treatment of juvenile sexual offenders. While the confidential therapeutic dyad can facilitate the development of trust in the therapist to explore individual psychodynamics, in this population several disadvantages develop. The therapist can be more easily manipulated, there is less confrontation and hence denial is less readily dismantled, and the secret nature of the sexual assaults is reinforced within the

treatment (Schwartz, 1988). Therapists must be on guard for efforts by the offender to manipulate, minimize, deny, or distort. Confrontation of erroneous information in a firm but nonjudgemental manner is essential. For offenders who may be acting out traumas from being sexually abused themselves, individual therapy is a valuable additional method for exploring and working through these feelings (Shaw, 1999).

PSYCHOPHARMACOLOGICAL INTERVENTIONS

The two predominant pharmacological treatment options for sexual offenders include serotonin modulating agents and hormonal modulating agents (Bradford, 1995). More recently, novel treatments including naltrexone and stimulant augmentation have also appeared. None of these agents are suitable as the sole treatment provided to a juvenile sexual offender. Instead, these agents may have a role in the comprehensive integrative treatment approach that includes the cognitive behavioral interventions discussed earlier.

Kafka has advanced the monoamine hypothesis of pathophysiology of paraphilic disorders (Kafka, 1997a; Kafka, 2003). It is based largely on the clinical observations that suggest that paraphilic behaviors and sexual offending can be best understood as disorders of sexual appetitive behavior disorders (Kafka, 1997). He notes that the monoamine neurotransmitters, including dopamine, serotonin, and norepinephrine, are key substances in the regulation of normal human and mammalian sexual behaviors (Kafka, 1997; Kafka, 2003; Owens & Nemeroff, 1999). Medications that affect these neurotransmitters can be seen to have significant sexual side effects, and can modulate sexual appetitive behaviors (Kafka, 1997; Kafka, 2003). Studies suggest that sexual offenders as a group display significant comorbidity of psychopathology which has monaminergic dysregulation as its etiology. Finally, studies have shown that agents that modulate the monoamine neurotransmitters can be effective in decreasing paraphilic symptoms and behaviors (Bradford, 1999).

Much of the current pharmacologic treatment evidence involves the use of selective serotonin reuptake inhibitor (SSRI) medications. The SSRIs were developed as antidepressant medications, but the approved indications and off-label usages have expanded their clinical applications. The SSRIs are used to treat obsessive compulsive behaviors, and are also recommended in the treatment of paraphilias and compulsive sexual behaviors (Bradford, 1999; Coleman & Cesnick, 1992; Greenberg & Bradford, 1997; Kafka, 1994; Stein et al., 1992). The SSRIs have also been shown to reduce sexual arousal, drive, and preoccupations. Impulsivity and aggressive behaviors have also been associated with serotonergic dysfunction in several studies. Fluoxetine is the most studied of these agents, and currently is also the only FDA approved antidepressant medication for use in children (Kafka & Prentky, 1992; Perilstein, Lipper, & Friedman, 1991). Yet a study by Greenberg et al. (1996) demonstrated no difference between fluoxetine, sertraline, and fluvoxamine. All were seen to be equally effective. A study utilizing nefazodone also demonstrated efficacy in adult males with non-paraphilic sexual compulsive behaviors (Coleman, Gratzer, Nesvacil, & Raymond, 2000). Nefazodone was also associated with a lower incidence of sexual side effects compared with SSRIs (Coleman et al., 2000). In this study, 11 of 14 adult men reported good control of or remission of their sexual obsessions and compulsions at doses of nefazodone averaging 200 mg daily (Coleman et al., 2000).

The addition of a stimulant medication, methylphenidate, has been shown to be effective in augmenting the action of the SSRIs for decreasing paraphilic behaviors (Kafka & Hennen, 2000). Twenty six men with paraphilias or paraphilia-related disorders were screened for a history of ADHD symptoms that persisted into adulthood. For these men, the addition of methylphenidate to SSRI pharmacotherapy had a statistically significant effect on the total sexual outlet and the time spent per day on paraphilic behaviors. While this study was done with adults, the vast majority of psychostimulant medications have proven safety for use in children. Stimulant augmentation may soon become a major therapeutic modality for the treatment of juvenile sexual offenders.

Hormonal modulating agents can be broadly classified into two groups, the antiandrogens and the luteinizing hormone-releasing hormone agonists (LHRH agonists). The antiandrogens include medroxyprogesterone acetate (MPA), Provera, and cyproterone acetate (CPA). MPA has become the more widely used agent in the treatment of sexual offenders in the US. It is a progestagen that induces testosterone reductase in the liver, thereby reducing circulating testosterone levels. It also appears to block the secretion of luteinizing hormone (LH) and follicle stimulating hormone (FSH). It can be given orally or intramuscularly. It has been shown to significantly reduce deviant sexual fantasies, urges, and behaviors at dosages of 200 to 400 mg IM (Reilly, Delva, & Hudson, 2000). All of the studies with MPA have been done with men, however. The use of MPA in adolescents is controversial due to the side effects of treatment, including disruption of normal pubertal development.

Though unavailable in the United States, CPA is the most widely studied of the hormonal modulating agents. Like MPA, it blocks the secretion of LH and FSH from the pituitary. Unlike MPA, CPA is considered a "true antiandrogen" as it is also a competitive inhibitor of testosterone and dihydrotestosterone receptors. Multiple studies in adult males have shown it to be effective in reducing sexual arousal, deviant sexual fantasies and urges, masturbation, and paraphilic behaviors (Reilly et al., 2000). Additionally, it has been noted that CPA seems to affect deviant sexual arousal differently than normophilic arousal, perhaps suggesting its superiority to MPA for treatment. As with MPA, the potential side effects make the use of CPA controversial with children.

The LHRH agonists include triptorelin and leuprolide, among others. These agents act by inducing secretion of GRH at the hypothalamus. This results in an initial rise in circulating gonadotropin-releasing hormone (GRH) levels, but then a subsequent reduction of GRH to nearly zero (Reilly et al., 2000). This causes a drop in testosterone and dihydroxytestosterone levels to those seen in castrated men (Bradford, 1995, 2000; Reilly et al., 2000). These agents have been studied in adult sexual offenders only, and use of these agents in adolescents is controversial due to the impact on sexual development these agents will have. Several studies have shown these agents to be effective in offenders where other agents have not shown benefit (Dickey, 1992; Rosler & Witztum, 1998; Rousseau, Couture, Duptont, Labrie, & Couture, 1990; Thibaut, Cordier, & Kuhn, 1993).

Naltrexone has also been shown to be effective in reducing paraphilic symptoms and behaviors in adolescent sexual offenders (Ryback, 2004). Naltrexone is a semisynthetic opiate antagonist used in the treatment of substance use disorders, obsessive compulsive disorder, impulse-control disorder, and bulimia nervosa. It has been suggested that the inhibition of dopamine release in the nucleus accumbens by naltrexone accounts for its efficacy in treating impulse-control disorders (Kim, 1998). In an adolescent male offender sample, 15 of 21 patients found naltrexone helpful for reducing arousal, masturbation, and fantasies. Effects were noted at dosages of 150 to 200 mg daily, and no benefit was seen with higher doses. When a subset of the patients had naltrexone discontinued, paraphilic symptoms and behaviors returned. Of the six patients who did not respond to naltrexone, five responded well to leuprolide. These offenders were noted as a group to have more victims, violent fantasies, thought process problems, adult and child victims, and were hospitalized longer compared to the offenders who responded to naltrexone (Ryback, 2004).

AFTERCARE

While treatment for sexually aggressive behaviors may be successful, the offender will never be cured. Ongoing care is a necessary requirement to prevent recidivism in the juvenile sexual offender population. As with treatment planning, an integrative approach meeting the unique needs of the individual is most appropriate. Continued care may include placement in a specialized setting, community-based outpatient treatment programs, and ongoing psychiatric and psychotherapeutic treatment.

CONCLUSION

The biological factors that have been examined in adult sex offenders should be studied in juveniles. With increasingly sophisticated tools for neuroimaging, such as functional magnetic resonance imaging and positron emission tomography scanning available to contemporary researchers, one can be optimistic that biological correlates for sex offending may be found. Of particular interest would be correlating the complicated statistical model of Friedrich (2003) with neuro-imaging studies to better characterize the relationship between victimization and future sex offending.

Risk assessment of sexually offending juveniles is a complicated and time-consuming process that should be performed by knowledgeable clinicians. Further research is needed to test the reliability and validity of recidivism risk factors and risk assessment measures. For the future of recidivism risk and treatment outcomes, researchers should focus on evidence-based outcomes. Does the use of structured instruments improve risk management and reduce recidivism in meaningful ways? Which risk factors provide the strongest evidence for recidivism? Are there qualitative aspects of juvenile sex offense recidivism that can improve the efficacy of treatment?

References

Abel, G. G., Huffman, J., Warberg, J., & Holland, C. L. (1998). Visual reaction time and plethysmography as measures of interest in child molesters. *Sexual Abuse: A Journal of Research and Treatment*, 10, 81–95.

Abel, G. G., Jordan, A., Rouleau, J., Emerick, R., Barboza-Whitehead, S., & Osborn, C. (2004). Use of visual reaction time to assess male adolescents who molest children. *Sexual Abuse: A Journal of Research and Treatment*, 16(3), 255–265.

Achenbach, T., McConaughy, S. H., & Howell C. T. (1987). Child and adolescent behavioral and emotional problems: Implications for cross informant correlations for situation specificity. *Psychological Bulletin*, 101, 213–232.

Archer, R. (1997). *MMPI-A: Assessing adolecents' psychopathology*. Mahwah, NJ: Lawrence Erlbaum Assoc.

ATSA. (1997). *Ethical standards and principles for the management of sexual abusers*. Beavertown, OR, Association for the Treatment of Sexual Abusers: 44–51.

Barbaree, H. E., Seto, M. C., Langton, C. M., & Peacock, E. J. (2001). Evaluating the predictive accuracy of six risk assessment instruments for adult sex offenders. *Criminal Justice and Behavior*, 28, 490–521.

Beck, A. T. & Ward, C. H. (1961). An inventory for measuring depression. *Archives of General Psychiatry*, 4, 561–571.

Becker, J. V. (1994). Offenders: Characteristics and treatment. *The Future of Children: Sexual Abuse of Children*, 4(2), 176–197.

Becker, J. & Kaplan, M. (1988). The assessment of adolescent sexual offenders. In R. J. Prinz (Ed.), *Advances in behavioral assessment of children and families*, (pp. 97–118). Greenwich, CT, JAI Press.

Becker, J., Kaplan M., Tenke, C. E, & Tartaglini, A. (1991). The incidence of depressive symptomology in juvenile sex offenders with a history of abuse. *Child Abuse and Neglect*, 15, 531–536.

Becker, J. & Hunter, J. A. (1992). Test-retest reliability of audio-taped phallometric stimuli with adolescent sex offenders. *Annals of Sex Research*, 5, 45–51.

Becker, J. V. & Hunter, J. A. (1997). understanding and treating child and adolescent sexual offenders.

In T. H. Ollendick & R. J. Prinz (Eds.), *Advances in Clinical Child Psychology*. NY, Plenum.

Berlin, F. S., Galbreath, N. W., Geary, B., & McGlone, G., et al. (2003). The use of actuarials at civil commitment hearings to predict the likelihood of future sexual violence. *Sexual Abuse: A Journal of Research and Treatment*, 15(4), 377–388.

Berlinger, L. (1998). juvenile sexual offenders: Should they be treated differently? *Journal of Interpersonal Violence*, 13(5), 645–646.

Bischof, G. P., Smith, S. M., & Whitney, M. L. (1995). Family environments of adolescent sex offenders and other juvenile delinquents. *Adolescence*, 30, 157–170.

Blanchette, K. (1996). Sex offender assessment, treatment and recidivism: A literature review. Canada: Research Branch Correctional Service of Canada, 1–34.

Borduin, C. M., Henggeler, S. W., Blake, D. M. & Stein, R. J. (1990). Multisystemic treatment of adolescent sexual offenders. *International Journal of Offender Therapy & Comparative Criminology*, 34, 105–113.

Bourke, M. L. & Donohue, B. (1996). Assessment and treatment of juvenile sex offenders: An empirical review. *Journal of Child Sexual Abuse*, 5(1), 47–70.

Bradford, J. M. (1995). Pharmacological treatment of the paraphilias. In J. M. Oldham & M. Riba (Eds.), *Review of Psychiatry*, (pp. 755–778). Washington, D.C: American Psychiatric Press.

Bradford, J. M. (1999). The paraphilias, obsessive compulsive spectrum disorder and the treatment of sexually deviant behavior. *Psychiatric Quarterly*, 70, 209–219.

Bradford, J. M. (2000). The treatment of sexual deviation using a pharmacological approach. *Journal of Sex Research*, 37, 248–257.

Bremer, J. F. (1992). Serious juvenile sex offenders: Treatment and long term follow-up. *Psychiatric Annals*, 22, 326–332.

Caldwell, M. F. (2002). What we do not know about juvenile sexual reoffense risk. *Child Maltreatment*, 7(4), 291–302.

Campbell, J. S. & Lerew, C. (2002). Juvenile sex offenders in diversion. *Sexual Abuse: A Journal of Research and Treatment*, 14(1), 1–17.

Cautela, J. R. (1966). Treatment of compulsive behavior by covert sensitization. *Psychological Record*, 16, 33–41.

CCJS. (1999). Sex offenders. Ottawa, Canada, Canadian Center for Justice Statistics.

Coleman, E. & Cesnick, J. (1992). An exploratory study of the role of psychotropic medications in the treatment of sex offenders. *Journal of Offender Rehabilitation*, 18, 75–88.

Coleman, E., Gratzer, T., Nesvacil, L., & Raymond, N. C. (2000). Nefazodone and the treatment of non-paraphilic compulsive sexual behavior: A retrospective study. *Journal of Clinical Psychiatry*, 61(4), 282–284.

DesLaurier, A. T. & Gardner, J. (1999). The sexual predator treatment program in Kansas. In A. Schlank & F. Cohen. (Eds.), *The sexual predator: Law, policy, evaluation and treatment*. Kingston, NJ: Civic Research Institute. Chapter 11.

Dickey, R. (1992). The management of a case of treatment-resistant paraphilia with a long-acting LHRH agonist. *Canadian Journal of Psychiatry*, 37, (567–569).

Dwyer, S. M. (1997). Treatment outcome study: Seventeen years after sexual offender treatment. *Sexual Abuse: A Journal of Research and Treatment*, 9, 149–160.

Farrell, J. K. & O'Brien, R. (1988). Sexual offense by youth in Michigan: Data implications and policy recommendations. Report to the Michigan Legislature. Detroit, Safer Society Resources of Michigan.

FBI. (2004). Crime in the United States, 2003. Washington, D.C: Government Printing Office.

Fehrenbach, P. A. & Smith, W. (1986). Adolescent sexual offenders: Offender and offense characteristics. *American Journal of Orthopsychiatry*, 56(2), 225–233.

Friedrich, W. N., Davies,W. H., Feher, E., & Wright, J. (2003). sexual behavior problems in preteen children: Developmental, Ecological, and behavioral correlates. *Annals New York Academy of Sciences*, 989, 95–104.

Frost, A. (2004). Therapeutic engagement styles of child sexual offenders in a group treatment program: A Grounded theory study. *Sexual Abuse: A Journal of Research and Treatment*, 16(3), 191–208.

Gallagher, C. A. & Wilson, D. B.(1999). A quantitative review of the effects of sex offender treatment of sexual reoffending. *Corrections Management Quarterly*, 3, 19–29.

Galli, V., McElroy, S. L., Soutullo, C. A., Kizer, D., Raute, N., Keck, P. E. Jr., et al. (1999). The psychiatric diagnoses of twenty-two adolescents who have sexually molested other children. *Comprehensive Psychiatry*, 40(2), 85–88.

Garrett, T., C. Oliver, C., Wilcox D. T., & Middleton, D. (2003). Who cares? The views of sexual offenders about the group treatment they receive. *Sexual Abuse: A Journal of Research and Treatment*, 15(4), 323–338.

Gray, A. S. & Pithers, W. D. (1993). Relapse prevention with sexually aggressive adolescents and children: Expanding treatment and supervision. In H. E. Barbaree, W. L. Marshall, & R. W. Hudson (Eds.), *The Juvenile Sex Offender*, (pp. 289–319). NY, Guilford Press.

Green, R. (1988). Psycho-educational modules. In B. K. Schwartz & H. Cellini (Eds.), *A Practitioner's guide to treating the incarcerated male sex offender*, (pp. 95–100). Washington, D.C: US Department of Justice, National Institute of Corrections.

Greenberg, D. M. & Bradford, J. M. (1996). A comparison of treatment of paraphilias with three serotonin reuptake inhibitors: A retrospective study. *Bulletin of the American Academy of Psychiatry & the Law*, 24(4), 525–532.

Greenberg, D. M. & Bradford, J. M. (1997). Treatment of the paraphilic disorders: A review of the role of selective serotonin reuptake inhibitors. *Sexual Abuse: Journal of Research and Treatment*, 9, 349–360.

Groth, N. A., Longo, R. E., & McFadin, J. B. (1982). Undetected recidivism among rapists and child molesters. *Crime and Delinquency*, 28(3), 450–458.

Grove, W. M., Zald, D. H., Lebow, B. S., Snitz, B. E., & Nelson, C. (2000). Clinical versus mechanical prediction: A meta-analysis. *Psychological Assessment*, 12, 19–30.

Hall, G. C. (1995). Sexual offender recidivism revisited: A meta-analysis of recent treatment studies. *Journal of Consulting and Clinical Psychology*, 63, 802–809.

Hanson, R. K. (1998). What do we know about sex offender risk assessment? *Psychology, Public Policy, and Law*, 4(1–2), 50–72.

Hanson, R. K. (2000b). *Risk assessment*. Beaverton, OR, Association for the Treatment of Sexual Abusers.

Hanson, R. K. (2000a). Treatment outcome and evaluation problems (and solutions). In D. R. Laws, S. M. Hudson, & T. Ward (Eds.), *Remaking relapse prevention with sex offenders: A sourcebook*. Thousand Oaks, CA, Sage.

Hanson, R. K. & M. T. Bussiere. (1998). Predicting relapse: A meta-analysis of sexual offender recidivism studies. *Journal of Consulting and Clinical Psychology*, 66(2), 348–362.

Hanson, R. K. & Harris, A. J. R. (2000). Where should we intervene? Dynamic predictors of sex offense recidivism. *Criminal Justice and Behavior*, 27, 6–35.

Hanson, R. K., Gordon, A., Harris, A. J., Marques, J. K., Murphy, W., Quinsey, V. L., et al. (2002). First report of the collaborative outcome data project on the effectiveness of psychological treatment for sex offenders. *Sexual Abuse: A Journal of Research and Treatment*, 14, 169–194.

Hunter, J. A. & Becker, J. V. (1991). The reliability and discriminative utility of the adolescent cognitions scale for juvenile offenders. *Annals of Sex Research*, 4, 281–286.

Hunter, J. A., Becker, J. V., & Kaplan, M. S. (1995). The adolescent sexual interest card-sort test: Test-retest reliability and concurrent validity in relationship to phallometric assessment. *Archives of Sexual Behavior*, 24, 555–561.

Hunter, J. A. & Figueredo, A. J. (1999). Factor associated with treatment compliance in a population of juvenile sexual offenders. *Sexual Abuse: A Journal of Research and Treatment*, 11(1), 49–67.

Hunter, J. A., Figueredo, A. J., Malamuth, N. M., & Becker, J. V. (2003). Juvenile sex offenders: Toward the development of a typology. *Sexual Abuse: Journal of Research and Treatment*, 15(1), 27–48.

Jennings, J. L. & Sawyer, S. (2003). Principles and techniques for maximizing the effectiveness of group therapy with sex offenders. *Sexual Abuse: A Journal of Research and Treatment*, 15(4), 251–267.

Johnson, R. & Shrier, D. (1985). Sexual victimization of boys: Experience at adolescent medical clinic. *Journal of Adolescent Health Care*, 6, 372–376.

Kafka, M. P. (1994). Sertraline pharmacotherapy for paraphilias and paraphilia-related disorders: An open trial. *Annals of Clinical Psychiatry*, 6, 189–195.

Kafka, M. P. (1997a). A monoamine hypothesis for the pathophysiology of paraphilic disorders. *Archives of Sexual Behavior*, 26, 337–352.

Kafka, M. P. (1997b). Hypersexual desire in males: An operational definition and clinical implications for men with paraphilias and paraphilia-related disorders. *Archives of Sexual Behavior*, 26, 505–526.

Kafka, M. P. (2003). The monoamine hypothesis for the pathophysiology of paraphilic disorders: An update. *Annals New York Academy of Sciences*, 989, 86–94.

Kafka, M. P. & Prentky, R. A. (1992). Fluoxetine treatment of nonparaphilic sexual addictions and paraphilias in men. *Journal of Clinical Psychiatry*, 53(10), 351–358.

Kafka, M. P. & Hennen, J. (2000). Psychostimulant augmentation during treatment with selective serotonin reuptake inhibitors in men with paraphilias and paraphilia-related disorders: A case series. *Journal of Clinical Psychiatry*, 61(9), 664–670.

Kavoussi, R. J., Kaplan, M., & Becker, J. V. (1988). Psychiatric diagnoses in adolescent sex offenders. *Journal of the American Academy of Child and Adolescent Psychiatry*, 27, 241–243.

Kenny, D. T., Keogh, T., & Seidler, K. (2001). Predictors of recidivism in australian juvenile sex offenders: Implications for treatment. *Sexual Abuse: A Journal of Research and Treatment*, 13(2), 131–148.

Kim, S. W. (1998). Opioid antagonists in the treatment of impulse-control disorder. *Journal of Clinical Psychiatry*, 59, 159–164.

Knight, R. A. & Prentky, R. A. (1993). Exploring characteristics for classifying juvenile sex offenders. In H. E. Barbaree, W. L. Marshall, & S. M. Hudson (Eds.), *The Juvenile Sex Offender*. New York, NY, Guilford Press.

Långström, N. & Grann, M. (2000). Risk for criminal recidivism among sex offenders. *Journal of Interpersonal Violence*, 15(8), 855–871.

Larimer, M. E., Palmer, R. S., & Marlatt G. A. (1999). Relapse prevention. An overview of marlatt's cognitive-behavioral model. *Alcohol Research & Health*, 23(2), 151–160.

Laws, D. R. (1998). Relapse prevention: The state of the art. *Journal of Interpersonal Violence*, 14(3), 285–302.

Lewis, A., Shankok, S., & Pincus, J. H. (1979). Juvenile male sexual assaulters. *American Journal of Psychiatry*, 136, 1194–1196.

Lightfoot, L. & Barbaree, H. (1993). The relationship between substance use and abuse and sexual offending in adolescents. In H. Barbaree, W. Marshall, & S. Hudson (Eds.), *The Juvenile Sex Offender*, (pp. 203–224). NY, Guilford Press.

Longo, S. (1996). Sexual learning and experiences among adolescent sexual offenders. *International Journal of Offender Therapy & Comparative Criminology*, 26, 235–241.

Maletzky, B. M. (1974). Assisted covert sensitization in the treatment of exhibitionism. *Journal of Consulting and Clinical Psychology*, 42, 34–40.

Mann, R. E. & Thornton, D. (1998). The evolution of a multi-site treatment program for sexual offenders. In W. L. Marshall, Y. M. Fernandez, S. M. Hudson, & T. Ward (Eds.), *Sourcebook of treatment programs for sexual offenders*, (pp. 47–58). NY, Plenum.

Marques, J. K. & Nelson, C. (2000). Preventing relapse in sex offenders: What we learned from SOTEP's experimental program. In D. R. Laws, S. M. Hudson, & T. Ward (Eds.), *Remaking relapse prevention with sex offenders*. Thousand Oaks, CA, Sage.

Marshall, W. L. & Barbaree, H. E. (1988). The long-term evaluation of a behavioral treatment program for child molesters. *Behavioural Research and Therapy*, 26, 499–511.

Marshall, W. L., Fernandez, Y. M., Hudson, S. M., & Ward, T. (Eds.). (1998). *Sourcebook of treatment for sexual offenders*. NY, Plenum.

Mathews, R., Hunter, Jr., J. A., & Vuz, J. (1997). Juvenile female sexual offenders: Clinical characteristics and treatment issues. *Sexual Abuse: A Journal of Research and Treatment*, 9(3), 187–200.

Matson, J. & Esveldt-Dawson, K. (1983). Validation of methods for assessing social skills in children. *Journal of Clinical Child Psychology*, 12, 174–180.

Mazur, T. & Michael, P. M. (1992). Outpatient treatment for adolescents with sexually inappropriate behavior: Program description and 6-month follow-up. *Journal of Offender Rehabilitation*, 18, 191–203.

McConaghy, N., Blaszczynski, A., Armstrong, M. S., & Kidson, W. (1989). Resistance to treatment of adolescent sex offenders. *Archives of Sexual Behavior*, 18, 97–107.

McGuire, J. (2000). Can the criminal law ever be therapeutic? *Behavioral Sciences and the Law*, 18, 413–426.

Milloy, C. D. (1998). Specialized treatment for juvenile sex offenders: A closer look. *Journal of Interpersonal Violence*, 13(5), 653–656.

Miner, M. H. & Siekert, G. P. (1997). Evaluation: Juvenile sex offender treatment program, Minnesota Correctional Facility-Saulk Center. Minneapolis, MN, University of Minnesota.

Miranda, A. O. & Corcoran, C. L. (2000). Comparison of perpetration characteristics between male juvenile and adult sexual offenders: Preliminary results. *Sexual Abuse: Journal of Research and Treatment*, 12(3), 179–188.

Myers, W. C. & Blashfield, R. (1997). Psychopathology and personality in juvenile sexual homicide offenders. *Journal of the American Academy of Psychiatry and the Law*, 25(4), 497–508.

NAPN. (1993). Revised report from the National Taskforce on Juvenile Sexual Offending. *Juvenile and Family Court Journal*, 44(4), 1–120.

Nichols, H. & Molinder, M. (1984). *Multiphasic sex inventory manual*. Tacoma, WA, Nichols and Molinder Assessments.

Nisbet, I. A., Wilson, P. H., & Smallbone, S. W. (2004). A prospective longitudinal study of sexual recidivism among adolescent sex offenders. *Sexual Abuse: A Journal of Research and Treatment*, 16(3), 223–234.

O'Halloran, M. & Carr, A. (2002). Psychological profiles of sexually abusive adolescents in Ireland. *Child Abuse & Neglect*, 26, 349–370.

Owens, M. & Nemeroff, C. (1999). Neuropeptides: Biology and regulation. In B. Sadock & V. Sadock (Eds.), *Comprehensive Textbook of Psychiatry*, (pp. 60–71). Philadelphia, Williams & Wilkins.

Perilstein, R., Lipper, S., & Friedman, L. J. (1991). Three cases of paraphilias responding to fluoxetine treatment. *Journal of Clinical Psychiatry*, 52, 169–170.

Pithers, W. D. & Marques, J. K. (1983). Relapse prevention with sexual aggressors: A self-controlled model of treatment and maintenance of change. In J. G. Greer & I. R. Stuart (Eds.), *The Sexual Aggressor: Current perspectives on treatment*, (pp. 214–239). NY, Van Nostrand Reinhold.

Pithers, W. D., Kashima, K. M., Cumming, G. F., & Beal L. S. (1988). Relapse prevention: A method of enhancing maintenance of change in sex offenders. In A. C. Salter (Ed.), *Treating Child Sex offenders and victims: A practical guide*, (pp. 131–170). Newbury Park, CA, Sage.

Prentky, R. A. & Burgess, A. W. (1990). Rehabilitation of child molesters: A cost-benefit analysis. *American Journal of Orthopsychiatry*, 60, 108–117.

Prentky, R. A., Harris, B., Frizzell, K., & Righthand, S. (2000). An actuarial procedure for assessing risk with juvenile sex offenders. *Sexual Abuse: A Journal of Research and Treatment*, 12(2), 71–93.

Prentky, R. A. & Righthand, S. (2003). Juvenile Sex Offender Assessment Protocol-II (J-SOAP-II): Manual. Published by United States Department of Justice. Washington, D.C. Available at http://www.csom.org/ref/juvwho.html

Quinsey, V. L. (2003). The etiology of anomalous sexual preferences in men. *New York Academy of Sciences*, 989, 105–117.

Quinsey, V. L., Harris, G. T., Rice, M., & Cormier, C. A. (1998). *Violent offenders: Appraising and managing risk*. Washington, D.C: American Psychological Association.

Rasmussen, L. A. (1999). Factors related to recidivism among juvenile sexual offenders. *Sexual Abuse: A Journal of Research and Treatment*, 11(1), 69–85.

Reilly, D. R., Delva, N. J., & Hudson, R. W. (2000). Protocols for the use of cyproterone, medroxyprogesterone, and leuprolide in the treatment of paraphilia. *Canadian Journal of Psychiatry*, 45, 559–563.

Righthand, S. & Hennings, R. (1989). *Young sex offenders in Maine.* Portland, ME, University of Southern Maine.

Rosler, A. & Witztum, E. (1998). Treatment of men with paraphilia with a long-acting analogue of gonadotropin-releasing hormone. *New England Journal of Medicine*, 338, 416–465.

Rosner, R. (2003). *Principles and practice of forensic psychiatry.* London, Oxford University Press.

Rousseau, L. R., Couture, M., Duptont, A., Labrie, F., & Couture, N. (1990). Effect of combined androgen blockade with an LHRH agonist and flutamide in one severe case of male exhibitionism. *Canadian Journal of Psychiatry*, 35, 338–341.

Rubenstein, M., Yeager, C., Goodstein, C., & Lewis, D. O. (1993). Sexually assaultive male juveniles: A follow-up. *American Journal of Psychiatry*, 150, 262–265.

Ryan, G. (1991). Juvenile sex offenders: Defining the population. In G. Ryan & S. Lane (Eds.), *Juvenile sex offending*, (pp. 3–8). Lexington, MA: Lexington Books.

Ryan, G., Lane, S., Davis, J., & Isaac, C. (1987). Juvenile sex offenders: Development and correction. *Child Abuse & Neglect*, 11(3), 385–395.

Ryback, R. S. (2004). Naltrexone in the treatment of adolescent sexual offenders. *Journal of Clinical Psychiatry*, 65(7), 982–986.

Saleh, F. M. & Berlin, F. S. (2003). Sexual deviancy: Diagnostic and neurobiological considerations. *Journal of Child Sexual Abuse*, 12, 53–76.

Sawyer, S. (2000). Some thoughts about why we believe group therapy is the preferred modality for treating sex offenders. *The ATSA Forum*, 12, 11–12.

Sawyer, S. (2002). Group therapy with adult sex offenders. In B. Schwartz & H. Cellini (Eds.), *The Sex Offender*, (p. 4). Kingston, NJ: Civic Research Institute.

Schwartz, B. K. (1988). Interpersonal techniques in treating sex offenders. In B. K. Schwartz & H. Cellini (Eds), *A Practitioner's Guide to Treating the Incarcerated Male Sex Offender.* (pp. 101–107). Washington, D.C: US Department of Justice, National Institute of Corrections.

Schwartz, B. K. (1992). Effective treatment techniques for sex offenders. *Psychiatric Annals*, 22, 315–319.

Seto, M. C., Lalumiere, M. L, & Blanchard, R. (2000). The discriminative validity of a phallometric test for pedophilic interests among adolescent sex offenders against children. *Psychological Assessment*, 12(3), 319–327.

Shaw, J. A. (1999). Practice parameters for the assessment and treatment of children and adolescents who are sexually abusive of others. *Journal of the American Academy of Child & Adolescent Psychiatry*, 30(Suppl. 12), 55S–76S.

Shaw, J. A. (2002). Juvenile sex offenders. In E. P. Benedek & D. H. Schetky (Eds.), *Principles and Practice of Child and Adolescent Forensic Psychiatry*, (pp. 504–506). Washington, D.C: American Psychiatric Publishing.

Silovsky, J. F. & Niec, L. (2002). Characteristics of young children with sexual behavior problems: A pilot study. *Child Maltreatment*, 7(3), 187–197.

Sipe, R., Jensen, E., & Everett, R. S. (1998). Adolescent sexual offenders grown up: Recidivism in young adulthood. *Criminal Justice and Behavior*, 13, 115–140.

Smith, W. R. & Monastersky, C. (1986). Assessing juvenile sexual offenders' risk for reoffending. *Criminal Justice and Behavior*, 13(2), 115–140.

Smith, G. & Fischer, L. (1999). Assessment of juvenile sexual offenders: Reliability and validity of the abel assessment for interest in paraphilias. *Sexual Abuse: A Journal of Research and Treatment*, 11(3), 207–216.

Snyder, H. & Sickmund, M. (1999). Juvenile sex offenders and victims: 1999 national report. Washington, D.C: Office of Juvenile Justice and Delinquency Prevention.

Stein, D., E. Hollander, E. Anthony, D. T., Schneier, F. R., Fallon, B. A., Liebowitz, M. R., et al. (1992). Serotonergic medications for sexual obsessions, sexual addictions, and paraphilias. *Journal of Clinical Psychiatry*, 53, 267–271.

Tarter, R., Hegedus, A., Alterman, A. L., & Katz-Garris, L. (1983). Cognitive capacities of juvenile, non-violent and sexual offenders. *Journal of Nervous and Mental Disorders*, 171, 564–567.

Thibaut, F., Cordier, B., & Kuhn, J. M. (1993). Effect of a long-lasting gonadotropin hormone-releasing hormone agonist in sex cases of severe male paraphilia. *Acta Psychiatrica Scandinavian*, 87, 445–450.

Utah Task Force of the Utah Network on Juveniles Offending Sexually. (1996). The Utah Report on juvenile sex offenders. Salt Lake City, Utah Task Force of the Utah Network on Juveniles Offending Sexually.

Veneziano, C., Veneziano, L., Legrand, S., & Richards, L. (2004). Neuropsychological executive functions of adolescent sex offenders and nonsex offenders. *Perceptual and Motor Skills*, 98, 661–674.

Weinrott, M. (1996). Juvenile sexual aggression: A critical review. Boulder, CO, University of Colorado, Institute for Behavioral Sciences, Center for the Study and Prevention of Violence.

Wieckowski, E., Hartsoe, P., Mayer, A., & Shortz, J. (1998). Deviant sexual behavior in children and young adolescents: Frequency and patterns. *Sexual Abuse: A Journal of Research and Treatment*, 10(4), 293–304.

Worling, J. R. (2004). The estimate of risk of adolescent sexual offense recidivism (ERASOR): Preliminary psychometric data. *Sexual Abuse: A Journal of Research and Treatment*, 16(3), 235–254.

Worling, J. R. & Curwen, T. (2000). Adolescent sexual offender recidivism: Success of specialized treatment and implications for risk prediction. *Child Abuse & Neglect*, 24(7), 965–982.

Worling, J. R. & Curwen, T. (2001). Estimate of risk of adolescent sexual offense recidivism (ERASOR; Version 2.0). In M. C. Calder (Ed.), *Juveniles and children who sexually abuse: Frameworks for assessment* (pp. 372–397). Dorset, England, Russell House Publishing.

Worling, J. R. & Långström, N. (2003). Assessment of criminal recidivism risk with adolescents who have offended sexually: A review. *Trauma, Violence and Abuse*, 4(4), 341–362.

Zonana, H., G. & Abel, G. (1999). Dangerous sex offenders: A task force report of the American Psychiatric Association, American Psychiatric Association.

Chapter 17

Juveniles Who Sexually Offend: Psychosocial Intervention and Treatment

Jeffrey L. Metzner, Scott Humphreys, and Gail Ryan

Juveniles perpetrate a significant percentage of all sexual violence and child sexual abuse in the United States and the United Kingdom. Juveniles account for 17% of arrests for sexual assault and for approximately 24% of sexual assault against victims aged 12 to 17 years (Federal Bureau of Investigation, 2001; Rich, 2003). More than half of male and 15% to 25% of female child sexual abuse victims were molested by a juvenile (Farber, Showers, Johnson, & Joseph, 1984). Criminal statistics from England and Wales indicated that during 2000, persons below the age of 21 years constituted approximately 18% of the total number (3943) of offenders found guilty of sexual offenses (Dent & Jowitt, 2003; Home Office, 2000). Of these 717 young offenders, 17.4% were between the ages of 10 and 15 years, 47.5% were between 15 and 18 years old, and 35% were between the ages of 18 and 21 years (Dent & Jowitt, 2003) The number of young people convicted of sexual offenses is just a subset of the total number of young persons who exhibit sexually abusive behaviors due to the underreporting of abusive acts and small arrest rates in this population.

Although there are similarities related to the nature of the sexual offenses committed, important distinctions exist that distinguish sexually abusive youths from adult sex offenders (Becker, 1998; Becker & Hicks, 2003; Masson & Hackett, 2003). In addition to juveniles who are known to have sexually offended exhibiting a lower frequency of sexually abusive acts, their developmental growth is less complete and more flexible than that of their adult counterparts. Research in this area suggests that the sexual interests and patterns of sexual arousal of juveniles are less fixated than those of older adult offenders (Veneziano & Veneziano, 2002). Reasonable arguments have been made to refer to these young people as children or adolescents who have been sexually abusive in contrast to the term *juvenile sex offenders*. This modification in descriptive language was an important change recommended in the National Task Force on Sexually Offending revised report in 1993 (National

Task Force on Juvenile Sexual Offending, 1993). The latter term can be construed to mean that such persons will always be sex offenders. Not only is this presumption not supported by data, the fact that juveniles are developmentally in the process of identity formation suggests that identifying them as "sex offenders" may be both inaccurate and counterproductive to the goal of preventing them from continuing to sexually offend. Therefore, children and adolescents who have committed sexual offenses or have been sexually abusive will be referred to as "sexually abusive youths" or "juveniles" throughout this chapter.

There is sparse and sometimes conflicting data regarding juveniles who commit sex offenses. Ryan et al. (1996) summarized information obtained from the National Adolescent Perpetration Network Uniform Data Collection System (UDCS), which contains data based on clinical interviews for over 1600 juveniles referred for evaluation and/or treatment to 90 sex-offender-specific programs in 30 states. In this sample youth ranged in age from 5 to 19 years with a modal age of 14 years. Approximately 25% reported earlier sexually abusive behavior before age 12. The juveniles were likely to be White and living with two paternal figures at the time of the offense. A prior adjudication for sexual assault was unlikely, although the identified assault usually did not represent the youth's first offense or first victim. Approximately one-third of the youth had been adjudicated for nonsexual delinquent behavior before their current identified sexual perpetration. The victim was generally not related to the juvenile (although siblings represented the largest victim pool) and the sexual behavior usually involved genital touching and often penetration.

These juveniles commonly have a history of having been a victim of sexual, physical, and/or emotional maltreatment and many have witnessed domestic violence (Ryan, 1997). However, the most common shared experiential variable in the Ryan et al. (1996) sample was "parental loss" via abandonment, termination of parental rights, or death of a parent. Childhood neglect was mentioned less often than abuse, but may be more prevalent than recorded. More recently, prospective studies of abused and neglected children have shown neglect as a more frequent precursor to sexual offending than either physical or sexual abuse (Widom & Williams, 1996).

Zolondek et al. (2001) administered a self-report survey to 485 males, aged 11 through 17, being evaluated for sex offenses. In their sample, the average age

of first offense was between 10 and 12 years. Sixty percent of the boys reported a history of molesting with an average of 4 victims and 11 acts. Rich (2003) summarizes the literature on sexually abusive youths' offenses in a concise manner. Statistically, the juvenile sexual offender is most likely to be a 14-year-old boy whose sexual abusive behaviors are directed against children and adolescents in contrast to adults. Most juvenile sexual offending is directed against girls and offenses against boys are directed mostly at children below the age of 7.

Although many adult sex offenders reported offending as adolescents, (Becker & Abel, 1985; National Task Force on Juvenile Sexual Offending, 1993) most sexually abusive youth do not become adult sex offenders. Because it is not clear which juveniles will continue offending and become adult sex offenders, it is clinically reasonable to consider children and adolescents who engage in sexually abusive behaviors to be "at risk" of becoming adult offenders. A comprehensive assessment and indicated treatment should be aggressively pursued. However, recidivism data indicate that most are at greater risk for nonsexual recidivism as delinquent youth and do not continue criminal behaviors as adults (Worling & Curwen, 2000).

Among adult sex offenders, "hands off" paraphilias, such as exhibitionism, have the highest prevalence (Abel, Becker, Mittelman, Cunningham-Rathner, Roleau, & Murphy, 1987). In contrast, molestation of significantly younger children is the sex offense most often reported in juveniles. This may be due to the possibility that other sexual offenses less often result in the arrest and/or adjudication of the juvenile. However, Ryan et al. (1996) found that 35% to 50% of the "hands off" juveniles had also sexually abused a child.

A literature review by Becker and Hicks (2003) reported that juveniles engaged in intrafamilial sexual abuse more frequently (67%) than adults (21%), although they were less likely to engage in penetration (13%) as compared to adults (41%), who also committed more sexually abusive acts as compared to the youths (Miranda & Corcoran, 2000).

Sexually abusive youths often have had previous consensual sexual experiences with similar age peers in addition to their offending behaviors (Becker, Kaplan, Cunningham-Rathner, & Kavoussi, 1986; Ryan, Miyoshi, Metzner, Krugman, & Fryer, 1996). There is only limited research relevant to the role of "deviant" sexual interest, preference and/or arousal among sexually abusive youths and there is no data regarding adolescent "norms." Similarly there are only limited studies relevant to the role of pornography among sexually abusive youths, although several studies reported that exposure to pornographic material at a young age among these juveniles was common (Hunter & Becker, 1994; Wieckowski et al., 1998).

Dent and Jowitt (2003) provide a summary of the literature relevant to children and adolescents who commit serious sexual offenses in the context of mental health problems. A significant prevalence of family dysfunction, learning difficulties, disordered behavior, posttraumatic stress, and substance abuse has been described in these populations. Clinicians in the field also report other comorbid conditions including, depression, bipolar disorder, and attention-deficit hyperactivity disorder. Becker et al. (1991) examined juveniles who had committed sex offenses and had a history of abuse themselves. They found that 42% of sex offenders experienced major depression as measured by the Beck Depression Inventory. These juveniles had a mean Beck score twice that of a random sample of adolescents.

Despite this statistical picture, the sexually abusive youth population is heterogeneous, with diverse characteristics and treatment needs. Hunter et al. (2003) described these youth in terms of age and gender of targeted victims, the level of violence displayed during the offense, and the social–ecological context of the offending behavior. They point out that some youths target only children, while others assault peers or adult females. Socialization patterns range from affiliation with the delinquent peers to significant social isolation (Righthand & Welch, 2001). Research consistently reports that a majority of juveniles with abusive sexual behaviors have significant deficits in social competence (Righthand & Welch, 2001).

As a whole, sexually abusive youths do not appear to differ significantly from juveniles who have committed other types of nonsexual delinquency (Becker & Hunter, 1997; Miner & Crimmins, 1995). Serious delinquency tends to occur most in dysfunctional families, and they are more likely to have been abused and to have received inadequate support and supervision. Poor verbal skills are often present, as are behavioral problems at school, lower academic achievement, and higher rates of learning disabilities. It appears that they also have higher rates of neuropsychological difficulties, particularly related

to planning and impulse control (Veneziano & Veneziano, 2002). However, there does appear to be some subgroups of juveniles who commit sex offenses, who do differ from juveniles, and who commit other offenses (Righthand & Welch, 2001).

There have been various attempts to classify sexually abusive youths according to their similarities and differences, although none have yet been empirically validated. O'Brien and Bera (1986) suggested a clinically derived classification scheme for sexually abusive youth, which was useful in identifying issues in treatment, as follows: (a) naive experimenters, (b) undersocialized child exploiters, (c) sexual aggressives, (d) sexual compulsives, (e) disturbed impulsives, (f) group influenced, and (g) pseudosocialized.

A meta-analysis by Graves et al. (1996) suggested three typologies: pedophilic, sexually assaultive, and undifferentiated. Pedophilic youths consistently molested young children. The sexual assault group generally assaulted peers or older females. The undifferentiated group committed a variety of offenses against victims, whose age ranged significantly. This latter group was characterized as being more antisocial and with the most severe social and psychological problems (Righthand & Welch, 2001).

Empirical research in progress supports the presence of identifiable subtypes of sexually abusive youths with distinct developmental trajectories and unique intervention needs (Hunter, Figueredo, Malamuth, & Becker, 2003). Comparative analysis of adolescent males who sexually offended against prepubescent children with those who targeted pubescent and postpubescent females reveals that the former group has greater deficits in psychosocial functioning, uses less aggression in their sexual offending, and are more likely to sexually abuse relatives. Their findings are consistent with prior reports that many of these youths have poor social skills and symptoms of depression and anxiety.

Sexually abusive youths have also been categorized by gender, age, and intellectual development. This chapter will not address issues related to sexually abusive behaviors by female youths, prepubescent children or juveniles with developmental disabilities. There is a sparse but growing literature relevant to these special populations (Bumby & Bumby, 1997; Gilby, Wolf, & Goldberg, 1989; Ryan, 1999).

The low rates of sexual recidivism in juveniles who have committed sexual offenses imply many of them will not go on to become adult sex offenders.

However, there is a subset that does continue sexual offending. This is another dimension of the heterogeneity of the population. Predictive factors for determining which juveniles will develop into adult sex offenders have been inconclusive. Static variables relevant to risk have been identified but accurate actuarial risk prediction is very difficult with youth due to the rapid changes of adolescence (Prentky, Harris, Frizell, & Righthand, 2000; Worling & Langstrom, 2003). The dynamics of juvenile offending are very changeable from day to day and over the course of development.

Conflicting findings concerning the rates of sexual recidivism for sexually abusive youths are present in the literature. Recidivism in terms of sexual offenses is not particularly high. Veneziano and Veneziano (2002) report recidivism rates for sexual offenses have ranged from 8% to greater than 30%, with most studies indicating ranges from 10% to 15% (Righthand & Welch, 2001). They describe higher recidivism rates for nonsexual offenses among this population, ranging from 16% (Sipe, Jensen, & Everett, 1998) to 54% (Rasmussen, 1999).

A number of factors appear to affect the estimate of recidivism among juveniles who have committed sex offenses. These include the length of follow-up period, the measurement of recidivism, the impact of clinical interventions, and the nature of the population under investigation (Worling & Langstrom, 2003). Mazur and Michael (1992) reported a 0% recidivism rate after a 6-month period, using self-report data following community-based group treatment with 10 adolescents. In contrast to the findings of Mazur and Michael (1992), Langstrom (2002) found that 30% of 117 young offenders referred for a psychiatric evaluation for the courts were reconvicted for a sexual assault following a mean follow-up period of 9.5 years (Langstrom, 2002). Worling and Curwen (2000) reported that, after a mean of 6.2 years, 5% of 58 adolescents who received treatment had subsequent sexual assaults charges compared to 18% of 90 adolescents who did not receive treatment. Gretton et al. (2001) found that 15% of 220 adolescents who had offended sexually received subsequent charges for sexual assaults following community-based treatment. Because many studies report very high sexual recidivism rates in juveniles (Awad & Saunders, 1991; Rubenstein, Yeager, Goodstein, & Lewis, 1993) and others identify low rates of sexual recidivism among juvenile populations (Prentky et al., 2000; Sipe

et al., 1998), Dent and Jowitt (2003) recommend recidivism research include follow-up periods significantly beyond 12 months. It will also be important to track whether recidivism occurs during adolescent years or later during adulthood.

Early "offense specific" treatment approaches for juveniles were largely modeled after adult sex offender treatment programs, on the basis of the implicit assumption that juvenile sexual offending would portend chronic and progressively more serious patterns of sexual perpetration (Hunter & Longo, 2004; Ryan, 1997). "Generic" juvenile offense-specific programming was typically offered in both institutional and community-based settings and included a focus on assessing and treating deviant sexual arousal and interests, improving impulse control and judgment, enhancing social skills and victim empathy, and correcting cognitions that support or justify sexual aggression (Freeman-Longo et al., 1995). Research support for this conceptual model for all or most juveniles who commit sexual offenses has not been demonstrated (Hunter & Longo, 2004) and randomized clinical trials have not been conducted to evaluate the effectiveness of this approach in deterring recidivism (Hunter & Becker, 1999).

With evidence supporting the heterogeneity of the population and clinical experience identifying a broad spectrum of diagnostic differences, current standards call for individualized and comprehensive evaluation and differential treatment plans (Colorado Sex Offender Management Board, Colorado Division of Criminal Justice, 2003). There is also clinical consensus that well-informed caregiver involvement benefits the supervision and treatment process.

ASSESSING THE RELATIONSHIP AND THE ACT

Identifying juveniles who commit sex offenses can be somewhat confusing. The problem stems from a general lack of understanding as to what constitutes an abusive or exploitive relationship between two children. Clear definition of what constitutes a sexual offense when the victim and the perpetrator are both children is imperative to be able to properly identify and treat juveniles who perpetrate sex offenses.

When an adult offends against a child, there is an inherent inequality of the relationship. In almost all societies, adult sexual contact with children and adolescents is prohibited by law and by societal norms. Societies and the law recognize that adults have much greater power than children and therefore true consent by the child to be sexual with an adult is not possible. As a result, adult–child sexual relationships are always illegal until the younger person is beyond a legally defined "age of consent." When a juvenile commits a sexual offense, it is often the case that the offender and the victim are relatively close in age. It is generally accepted to be abuse when an older adolescent has a sexual relationship with a significantly younger child. Defining abuse involving two children of similar ages is more difficult. When a juvenile is sexually involved with another juvenile, the nature of the relationship and interaction must be closely examined to determine whether it is abusive or not.

Such an evaluation is very challenging. We do not know enough about what constitutes "normal" childhood or adolescent sexuality and behavior. Research in this field was historically discouraged and it is difficult to obtain human subjects approval for any inquiry into child and adolescent subjects' sexuality. Historically, sexuality in childhood has been denied and repressed by the culture in the United States. Only recently have we begun to critically examine the characteristics of child and adolescent sexual relationships. Ryan (2000a) reviewed the literature regarding childhood sexuality and attempted to define normal from abnormal. Before the 1980s most research came from less repressive cultures. Subsequent studies have included surveys of adult recollection of childhood sexual experience, adult observations of the sexual behaviors of children, and interviews with juveniles who have perpetrated sexual offenses. Ryan (2000a) and Ryan et al. (1988) describe a range of prepubescent and postpubescent sexual behaviors as illustrated in Table 17.1.

Thinking of sexual behaviors along a continuum such as that summarized in Table 17.1 provides guidance to determine when a child's sexual behavior warrants closer investigation. However, the behavior itself is usually not sufficient to determine whether the behavior is problematic or not, and whether an interaction between two children is abusive or exploitive. In defining abusive behaviors, more information about the relationship and interaction of the two children should be gathered and analyzed.

Generally, an age difference of 5 years or more is assumed to be exploitive, the assumption being that

TABLE 17.1 Sexual Behaviors in Prepubescent and Postpubescent Children

Prepubescent Children

Normal/Developmentally Expected

Genital or reproductive conversations with peers or similar age siblings

Show me yours/I will show you mine with peers

Playing doctor

Occasional masturbation without penetration

Imitating seduction (i.e., kissing, flirting)

Dirty words or jokes within cultural or peer group norm

Requiring Adult Response

Preoccupation with sexual themes (especially sexually aggressive)

Attempting to expose other's genitals

Sexually explicit conversations with peers

Sexual graffiti (especially when chronic or impacting individuals)

Sexual innuendo/teasing/embarrassment of others

Precocious sexual knowledge

Single occurrences of peeping/exposing/obscenities/ pornographic interest/frottage

Preoccupation with masturbation

Mutual masturbation/group masturbation

Simulating foreplay with dolls or peers with clothing on (i.e., petting or French kissing)

Requiring Correction

Sexually explicit conversations with significant age difference

Touching genitals of others without permission

Degradation/humiliation of self or others with sexual themes

Inducing fear/threats of force

Sexually explicit proposals/threats including written notes

Repeated or chronic peeping/exposing/obscenities/ pornographic interests/frottage

Compulsive masturbation/task interruption to masturbate

Masturbation which includes vaginal or anal penetration

Simulating intercourse with dolls, peers, animals, with clothing on

Always Problematic; Requiring Intervention

Oral, vaginal, anal penetration of dolls, children, animals

Forced exposure of other's genitals

Simulating intercourse with peers with clothing off

Any genital injury or bleeding not explained by accidental cause

(continued)

TABLE 17.1 (Continued)

Postpubescent Children

Normal

Sexually explicit conversations with peers

Obscenities and jokes within cultural norm

Sexual innuendo, flirting and courtship

Interest in erotica

Solitary masturbation

Hugging, kissing, holding hands

Foreplay (petting, making out, fondling)

Mutual masturbation

Monogamous intercourse

Requiring Adult Response

Sexual preoccupation/anxiety (interfering with daily functioning)

Pornographic interest

Indiscriminate sexual contact with several partners in a short period of time

Sexually aggressive themes/obscenities

Sexual graffiti (especially when chronic or impacting individuals)

Embarrassment of others with sexual themes

Violation of other's body space

Single occurrences of peeping/exposing/frottage with friends of similar age

Mooning and obscene gestures

Requiring Correction

Compulsive masturbation

Degradation/humiliation of self or others with sexual themes

Attempting to expose other's genitals

Chronic preoccupation with sexually aggressive pornography

Sexually explicit conversations with significantly younger children

Touching genitals without permission (i.e., grabbing, goosing)

Sexually explicit threats (verbal or written)

Illegal Behaviors Defined by Law; Requiring Immediate Intervention

Obscene phone calls, voyeurism, exhibitionism, frottage, and sexual harassment

Sexual contact with significant age difference (child sexual abuse)

Forced sexual contact (sexual assault)

Forced penetration (rape)

Sexual contact with animals (bestiality)

Genital injury to others

Ryan, 2000.

the difference in ages and development is sufficient to give the older member control over the younger. This is a difficult measure to use when the children are closer in age. Also, it provides little guidance as to what constitutes exploitive behavior. By examining the dynamics between the two children, the evaluator can better determine whether a particular act is abusive or exploitive. When evaluating juveniles who are referred due to sexual behavior problems or adjudication for a sexual offense, it is important to first consider the relationship between the two juveniles.

Kempe (1980) defined sexual abuse as the involvement of dependent, developmentally immature children, or adolescents in sexual activities that they do not fully comprehend, to which they are unable to give informed consent, or that violate the social taboos or family roles. In evaluating sexual behavior that occurs between two juveniles, determination that an interaction has been abusive is based on three characteristics of the relationship: consent, equality, and coercion (National Task Force on Juvenile Sexual Offending, 1993; Ryan et al., 1996).

Consent

Consent, as a legal construct, is defined as beyond the competence of juveniles (Ryan, 1997). Juveniles process decisions differently than adults. It has been suggested that this difference in decision-making process is not due to intelligence or mental illness but due to emotional and intellectual immaturity. There is little data relating to the capacity of a child to consent to a relationship. However, we know juveniles frequently lack the capacity to proceed in court related matters. The MacArthur Juvenile Adjudicative Competence Study revealed that adolescents aged 11 to 13 years were three times more likely to be seriously impaired on evaluation of competence-related abilities than were young adults aged 18 to 24 years. Juveniles aged 14 to 15 years were twice as likely to be impaired. Adolescents younger than 15 years were less likely to recognize risks inherent in different choices and were less likely to think of the long-term consequences of their choices (Grisso, Steinberg, Woolard, Cauffman, Scott, & Graham, 2003).

When evaluating a sexual interaction between two juveniles, examination of the relationship and the interaction in question can suggest the presence or absence of consent. The elements of consent are generally defined as follows: an understanding of what is being proposed, knowledge of societal standards for what is being proposed, awareness of potential consequences, and assumption that either agreement or disagreement will be respected (National Task Force on Juvenile Sexual Offending, 1993). Notably, the perceived cooperation or compliance of the victim is not sufficient to determine consent because juveniles who offend typically use nonphysical methods to coerce their victims (Ryan et al., 1996). The determination of consent requires a thorough assessment of the elements of consent in the interaction of the two youths at the time of the act (Ryan, 1997). When the two juveniles' understanding of each element is similar, and both choose to participate without coercion, the interaction may be defined consensual, even though their decision may not be completely "informed" and the behavior may involve unknown risks/consequences for the children.

Equality

The assessment of equality focuses on power and control. Obviously, this may be defined by similarities or differences in age or size. But, the evaluation is more difficult when the two children are similar in age and size. Other factors should be considered including intelligence, emotional experience, popularity among peers, and whether the relationship is mutually respectful. Roles may play a large part in the balance of equality. When one juvenile who has been put in charge (e.g., to babysit a younger child), the imbalance of power and authority may have been created by their roles. When a child is designated as leader of his peer group, there is a shift of power toward that child (Ryan, Metzner, & Krugman, 1990).

Coercion

Coercion involves one person putting pressure on the other person to engage in sexual activity. Obviously, a child who is much larger or stronger may coerce the other in a physical way. But, coercion ranges from aggressive physical threats or actions to subtle, nonaggressive forms such as bribery or manipulation. Most sex offenses perpetrated by juveniles are verbally coercive (Ryan et al., 1996); however, threats may be implied rather than stated explicitly. Also, mental or physical tricks under the guise of a game may be used. Threats of loss of property, esteem, or relationship can be impressively coercive to a child. A threat

of loss of love, relationship, or esteem can be as coercive as the loss of privilege or threat of punishment (Ryan, 1997).

ASSESSMENT OF PERPETRATION

The assessment of a juvenile accused of a sexual offense is a complex process. A thorough clinical interview by a clinician knowledgeable in sexual perpetration issues is required and must be differentiated from interview for law enforcement or child protection purposes. The clinical assessment must address the patient's emotional make-up and behavior including the following: life story, history of sexual learning, experience, and behaviors, and other problematic behaviors such as interpersonal or self-destructive abusive behaviors and substance use, his cognitive abilities and personality traits, and the presence of a mental health disorder. The assessment should address treatment recommendations, placement decisions, types of treatment interventions, and levels of supervision. Amenability to treatment, community safety, potential to reoffend, and living arrangement options must each be considered.

In the mid-1980s, highly structured offense-specific assessment tools were developed. In response to the development of these offense-specific models, there was a tendency for clinicians to concentrate on "offense-specific" assessments and treatment. Unfortunately, the juvenile's psychosocial development and psychiatric needs were frequently overlooked while focusing exclusively on the offense behaviors.

Recently, more information has been gathered regarding offense patterns in these juveniles and the generality of their abusive behaviors has been illuminated. For many of these juveniles, there is a lack of specificity toward sexualized aggression. Focusing on the sexualized behavior exclusively puts the treating clinician at risk of missing the larger problem: the juvenile's pattern of abusive and dysfunctional responses in many different settings and the wider range of harmful behaviors. Research already referenced in this chapter has indicated the presence of comorbid psychiatric illness, other forms of delinquent law violations, and psychosocial problems that can be missed when focusing exclusively on the referring behavior.

Abusive youths may come to the attention of clinicians at several points through their legal process. The

National Task Force on Juvenile Sexual Offending (1993) has summarized differences in the purpose of each phase of involvement:

1. Pretrial (investigative)
2. Presentencing (dangerousness/risk; placement/prognosis; treatment issues/modes; levels of restriction/supervision)
3. Treatment needs (planning and progress in treatment)
4. Release/termination from treatment (community safety and successful application of treatment tools)
5. Monitoring and follow-up

The nature of the assessment depends on the referral question to be answered. This section will focus on pretrial and presentence evaluations. Referrals at this point are usually initiated by social services or the police. This is a good opportunity to gain the cooperation of the family because this is usually a time of crisis. When the juvenile or family is interviewed during this phase, they may be more likely to be open because of the imminent threat, real or perceived, of incarceration. However, the family may deny or minimize problems during this time, which would certainly affect the reliability of the information obtained from them (Ryan et al., 1990).

The charge of a sexual offense involves serious legal and socially stigmatizing consequences. This would be overwhelming for anyone, but particularly for someone immature. Through the process, the juvenile will experience a variety of complex emotions. Several common defenses used to relieve such stress can affect the integrity of the evaluation. For example, many juveniles have a tendency to deny or minimize their sexual offenses (Benda, Corwyn, & Toombs, 2001). This significantly complicates the interview. For this reason and many others, the use of multiple sources of information is critical to an accurate history in addition to multiple interviews with the juvenile. Interviews with the juvenile's parents are essential to the assessment process.

Collateral data can help provide information as to the juvenile's interest in treatment, degree of accepting responsibility, and range of denial and abusive behavior. With juveniles who have committed sex offenses, this collateral information should include police reports, victim statements, victim therapist reports, agency investigative summaries, and presentence investigation reports.

The assessment of the juvenile's home can provide invaluable information. The primary focus of the home assessment should be whether the environment provides adequate supervision of the juvenile to provide safety for others in the home and the community. Are both parents at home? How much time are they away during weekdays and weekends? Who is left in charge of the juvenile when they are away? Special attention should be paid to younger siblings or other children who may be at risk of being victimized (Center for Sex Offender Management, 1999). The juvenile's family resources should be evaluated. The amount of emotional support the juvenile can expect from his family will be important to his treatment. Out-of-home placement is frequently required when the victim or potential victims live in the same home or in close proximity to the juvenile.

The parents should be interviewed. As collateral informants, their perceptions of the juvenile's developmental history and current functioning can be important to formulation of the juvenile. In addition, the family attitude toward the offense needs to be assessed. Whether they are too lax or too punitive can have an effect on how the juvenile responds to treatment. It is also helpful to know how involved they plan to be in the juvenile's treatment (Ryan, 1997).

Forensic interviews with juveniles accused of sex offenses are often performed by adult psychiatry trained clinicians with little expertise in child psychiatry. The impact of subtle differences in interview style can have very dramatic, and often undesirable, effects when interviewing a juvenile. The tendency of the juvenile to shutdown and refuse to participate can be very frustrating to the interviewer. The clinician's tone through the interview is important. Ryan (1997) suggests an interactional style with a nonjudgmental approach that is respectful of the youth as an individual, while maintaining an awareness of the youth's motivation to manipulate the interview. A calm, straightforward, matter-of-fact style will yield more information than direct confrontation or poorly timed questions regarding why or whether the juvenile committed the offense in question. Providing information and language as a basis for talking about sexual issues must precede direct questions to avoid eliciting inaccurate statements that the youth is then committed to defend.

The evaluation should be conducted over multiple interviews, which allows the juvenile to become somewhat more comfortable with the interviewer. In general, the initial interview should be used for obtaining history from the juvenile that is not as emotionally charged as compared to the history relevant to the sexual perpetration.

The initial interview is often conducted without the parents being present. The juvenile may be embarrassed to talk about his/her behavior in the presence of parents. The juvenile may also fear additional punishment from the parents.

Joint interviews with the juvenile and his parents are also useful in obtaining more accurate history and a better understanding of psychodynamic issues. Discrepancies between the juvenile's report and information obtained from parents and other sources should be investigated and understood.

The assessment should be comprehensive and include the factors described in Table 17.2.

The setting of the assessment will usually be determined by the juvenile's clinical state and legal status. An inpatient psychiatric evaluation may facilitate completion of a comprehensive evaluation in a relatively brief period of time but is not cost-effective. A residential treatment setting may offer the advantages of an inpatient evaluation without the higher cost.

Culture is an important factor and should be considered in understanding sexually aggressive youths and their families and communities. The evaluator should keep in mind that cultural sensitivity does not equate to acceptance of abusive behavior (National Task Force on Juvenile Sexual Offending, 1993).

Assessments of these juveniles are complicated and time consuming. They are best performed over a longer period of time. A significant reason for this is the length of time it takes to develop a working relationship with the juvenile and family. Using multiple interviews to form an assessment also provides the evaluator with information relevant to coping skills and credibility issues.

PSYCHOLOGICAL TESTING

Psychological testing of those who sexually offend has been widely used and can be helpful in assessment, but is limited by the heterogeneous nature of these youth and their behaviors. The specific applicability of psychological testing in these juveniles is promising but no clear and consistent indication has been found. Researchers are trying to elucidate the role of

TABLE 17.2 Factors of a Comprehensive Assessment

Victim's statements

Background information (including family, educational, medical, psychosocial, developmental, and psychosexual histories)

Progression of sexually aggressive behavior over time

Dynamics/process of victim selection

Intensity of sexual arousal during and after the offense

Use of coercion, force, violence, and weapons

Spectrum of injury to the victim, (that is, violation of trust, fear, physical injury)

Sadistic elements

Ritualistic elements

Number of categories of deviant sexual interest

Reported use of sexually deviant fantasies

Deviant nonsexual interests

History of assaultive behaviors

Issues related to separation/loss

Sociopathic characteristics

Psychiatric diagnosis (i.e., affective disorders, personality disorders, attention deficit disorder, and posttraumatic stress disorder)

Presence of developmental disorders

Behavioral warning signs

Identifiable triggers

Irrational thinking

Locus of control

Attributions of responsibility

Degree of denial or minimization

Understanding of wrongfulness

Concern for injury to the victim

Quality of social, assertive, and empathic skills

Family's denial, minimization, and response

Effects of alcohol/drugs and pornography on deviant sexual behavior

History of sexual victimization, physical or psychological abuse

Family dysfunction

Reported ability to control deviant sexual interests

Mental status examination

Organicity/neuropsychological factors

Becker & Abel, 1985; National Task Force on Juvenile Sexual Offending 1993.

psychological testing more clearly. At present, psychological testing serves to add a norm-based reference of personality and behavioral traits to the general assessment of these juveniles.

Many psychological tests are commonly used with juveniles; however, because of the heterogeneity of juveniles who have committed sex offenses, there is no profile that distinguishes these juveniles from other juveniles who do not sexually offend (Bourke & Donohue, 1996). Although not predictive, psychological tests can be useful in assessing characteristics such as whether the juvenile tends to recognize and respond with socially desirable responses, or malingers. Information gained from a juvenile's personality profile may also allude to possible psychopathology. Identifying personality traits can be important in developing the optimal treatment strategy.

The psychological test most commonly used with juvenile sexual offenders is the Minnesota Multiphasic Personality Inventory—Adolescent (MMPI-A) (Butcher et al., 1992). Because of the heterogeneity of juveniles who have committed sex offenses, there is no MMPI or other psychological test profile that distinguishes these juveniles from juveniles who do not sexually offend (Bourke & Donohue, 1996). Although it is not predictive, the MMPI-A can be useful in assessing whether the juvenile is dishonest or malingering. The information gained from the juvenile's personality profile may allude to possible psychopathy. These traits can be important when developing the optimal treatment strategy.

The Multiphasic Sex Inventory (MSI) (Nichols & Molinder, 1984) is an assessment instrument used to evaluate sexual interests, knowledge, fantasies, and behaviors. It was designed for clinical and treatment purposes to assess the type and level of sexual deviance among juvenile sex offenders. The MSI can be helpful in providing clinical information by identifying psychosexual and personality characteristics (Sorensen & Johnson, 1996). In a study of 101 male offenders, aged 12 to 19 years, Butz and Spaccarelli (1999) examined the level of force as a possible characteristic to classify adolescents who commit sexual offenses. They divided the juveniles into three classes: rapists (those who use force), nonrapists, and deniers. They administered the MSI to the three groups. Rapists reported significantly more sexual assault fantasy/predatory behavior, greater preoccupation with children, and more paraphilias than did nonrapists and deniers.

Scales of psychopathy have emerged as an important factor in the study of adult criminal behavior including sexual offenses. Identification of psychopathy traits during adolescence is controversial and can

have unintended consequences in both legal dispositions and service provision. However, there may be an association between psychopathy traits and the level of violence used during sexual offense, as well as increased risk of adult criminality. In a chart review, Gretton et al. (2001) obtained psychopathy ratings for 220 males (age 12 to 18 years) who were treated in an offense-specific treatment program. Using charges and convictions, they compared the psychopathy scales to 5-year recidivism rates. They found adolescents with high psychopathy scores were three times more likely to commit a reoffense of any kind than those with a low psychopathy score. However, the study did not find high psychopathy scores to be significantly predictive of sexual offense recidivism.

A more promising and comprehensive approach may be the Multidimensional Assessment of Sex and Aggression (MASA) (Knight, Prentky, & Cerce, 1994). This is a computerized, self-report inventory that covers multiple domains, and a juvenile version has been validated. The questionnaire focuses on attitudes and behaviors in many areas of the individual's life, and includes methods for assessing response biases, random responding, and dissimilation. Given the juvenile version of this instrument is so new, very little information is available regarding its applicability for juveniles who commit sexual offenses (Righthand & Welch, 2001).

PENILE PLETHYSMOGRAPHY/ MEASUREMENT OF SEXUAL AROUSAL

Attempts to assess the sexual arousal of adolescents present a moral and ethical quagmire. Phallometric assessment (by penile plethysmography [PPG]) remains an area of controversy in the assessment of juveniles who have committed sex offenses.

Some investigators consider phallometric assessment the best means to assess individual's arousal patterns, (Weinrott, 1998); but controversy exists regarding the invasiveness of the testing, nature and variability of the stimuli used, and lack of comparison to any control group of juveniles who have not sexually perpetrated. With the lack of adequate studies, the role of phallometric assessment with juvenile populations is unclear. The lack of norms is a very complex problem due to the ethical complications of administering this testing to a control group. However, Weinrott (1998) points out that it may be possible to evaluate juveniles with stimuli that are less sexually explicit, since juveniles tend to have a low threshold of response to even mild sexual stimuli.

At this time, laboratory assessment of arousal may be most useful in individual cases, during treatment, as a means of evaluating the accuracy of the youth's self-awareness and their ability to suppress unwanted arousal using various strategies learned in treatment. Although adults often express concern that PPG assessments are too invasive, some youth report that the technology of a laboratory assessment is less intrusive than many of the verbal questions discussed in treatment sessions.

ASSESSING SEXUAL INTERESTS

Computerized assessment instruments are promising. The Abel Assessment for Interest in Paraphilias describes a pattern of the juvenile's sexual interest on the basis of visual reaction times (VRT) when viewing slides of potentially sexually evocative stimuli (Abel Screening, Inc., 1996). Computer assessments such as the Abel Assessment may have the advantage of being less invasive than phallometric assessment; however, there continue to be controversies regarding whether there is sufficient data to support the VRT as reliable and valid for juveniles (Smith & Fischer, 1999). Nonetheless, computer-aided assessments represent a relatively recent development, and as research continues, their place in the assessment of juveniles who commit sexual offenses may become more evident.

Polygraphy

Polygraph testing has been used with this population of juveniles to facilitate more complete disclosure of history and description of abusive behaviors. It can also be used to monitor compliance with conditions of probation and treatment contracts. Although the use of polygraph testing in juveniles who have sexually offended is relatively common in many jurisdictions, clear criteria for the circumstances under which a youth should be tested are not always clearly articulated. There are potential unintended consequences that must be considered when considering administration of a polygraph examination. For example, information regarding sexual or abusive behavior revealed in preparation or explanation of a polygraph

exam can lead to additional investigation and legal jeopardy.

The National Task Force on Juvenile Sexual Offending (1993) emphasizes that "it is critical that submissions to polygraph examinations be voluntary and with the full informed consent of the youth, parent, or legal guardian."

The purpose and use of information gleaned from the preparation and processing of results should be made clear as well as potential consequences associated with the outcome. The national task force also points out that some organizations' ethical codes restrict the use of instruments without empirical evidence of reliability and validity. Evidence supporting the reliability and validity of polygraph testing in juveniles who have committed sexual offenses is limited (Hunter & Lexier, 1998). Both false positives and false negatives appear with some regularity and the therapeutic consequences of these errors are unknown (Bonner et al., 1998). When polygraphs are ordered as a condition of probation, clinicians must be clear that the purpose is related to risk assessment and supervision, not a therapeutic intervention.

RISK ASSESSMENT

The criminal justice system is chiefly concerned with protecting the community. Most juveniles who commit sexual abuses come to the attention of treating clinicians as a result of their involvement with the courts. As a practical matter, it is important to understand the concerns the courts may have relating to these youths. As a result of their charge to protect the community, the courts are interested in the likelihood of reoffense. Within the criminal justice system, decisions relating to future care and containment are based upon perception of risk factors relating to recidivism. Expertise of clinicians can be helpful to the court in determining reasonable preadjudicatory planning and ongoing treatment recommendations.

As previously summarized, sexual assault recidivism rates vary widely throughout the literature. The recidivism rates for nonsexual offenses also vary widely with the literature reporting rates from 16% to 54% (Sipe et al., 1998).

Historically, decisions related to risk assessment have been based on subjective experience rather than objective data. This approach has provided suboptimal results. Using subjective factors to determine risk leads to inconsistency and bias (Hoge, 2002). Dependence on clinical experience rather than objective data is driven by the paucity of useful research findings in this area. A meta-analysis of follow-up studies of adolescents who have committed sexual abuses was done by Cottle et al. (2001). They found that only nine studies met the criteria for inclusion in the analysis and four of these studies were never informative for each of the risk factors examined. In the studies examined, associations between risk factors and recidivism were weak. However, research in the area of risk assessment for juveniles who have committed sex offenses is developing. Although much of the data remains inconclusive or conflicting, numerous promising risk factors are being identified and gaining empirical support.

History of assaults against more than one victim is one of the more consistently supported risk factors for recidivism. However, the literature examining this risk factor is relatively sparse. Rasmussen (1999) reported the number of female victims was significantly related to sexual offenses 5 years after release. In a 9-year postrelease follow-up of 126 adolescents aged 15 to 20 years, Langstrom (2002) found those who offended against two or more victims were two to three times more likely to recidivate than adolescents with one known victim.

Deviant sexual interest is one of the most strongly supported risk factors for reoffense. However, there is conflicting data in the literature, which makes it difficult to conclude this as a true risk factor for recidivism. In a follow-up study over an average 6-year period, Worling and Curwen (2000) found that self-reported sexual interest in children (including past or present sexual fantasies involving children, child–victim grooming behaviors, and intrusive sexual assault activities with children) was a significant risk factor for sexual reoffending. In a study comparing adolescents with a previous charge for sexual offending (sexual recidivists) to those charged for the first time, Kenny et al. (2001) found that sexual assault recidivists were significantly more likely to report deviant sexual fantasies that reflected force or young children. Schram et al. (1991) reported adolescents rated by clinicians as most likely to have deviant sexual interests were significantly more likely to reoffend sexually. Research relating to deviant sexual interest in youth that have sexually offended has been based largely on noninvasive data collection methods such as clinical interviews and rating scales.

There is very limited research regarding PPG measurements in this population. Gretton et al. (2001) administered PPGs to 186 adolescent males who had confessed to sex offenses. Her group reported that deviant sexual interest was not related to sexual assault recidivism. More research is needed before deviant sexual interest can be accepted or refuted as a predictive factor of recidivism.

Prior convictions for sexual assault represent another risk factor with predictive potential. There is limited research in this area. Schram et al. (1991) found that adolescents with at least one prior conviction for a sexual assault were significantly more likely to reoffend sexually. Langstrom (2002) also reported that a history of previous sexual offenses, including prior convictions, was related to sexual assault recidivism. However, although the data are suggestive that the presence of prior convictions may be promising as a potential risk factor, the extent of significance is inconclusive.

Selection of a stranger-victim as a risk factor is supported by limited, but consistent, data. Two studies found that the selection of stranger victims was moderately but significantly associated with sexual reoffending for adolescents (Langstrom, 2002; Smith & Monastersky, 1986).

A lack of peer relationships and lack of involvement in prosocial activities may be risk factors for sexual offending. The literature has supported a link between social isolation and general offending. In a meta-analysis of research with adolescents in the general population, as well as identified young offenders, Lipsey and Derzon (1998) noted that a lack of involvement in social activities was a robust risk factor for violent offending. There is increasing evidence for a link between social isolation and sexual offending. In a 5-year follow-up study of adolescents who had offended sexually, Langstrom and Grann (2000) reported adolescents with limited social contacts were at least three times more likely to be reconvicted for a sexual crime.

A number of other risk factors have been examined but the data collected is less promising than those risk factors already mentioned. Problematic parent–adolescent relationships and parental rejection have been shown to have a moderate relationship to recidivism Worling & Curwen (2000). Another concerning factor involves the adolescent having an attitude supportive of sexual offending. Characteristics of this type of attitude include blaming the victim or believing that the victim somehow "invited" the assault. High-stress family environment, impulsivity, sexual preoccupations, environments supportive of opportunity to reoffend, and the use of violence or excessive threats during the act should be considered to be potential factors related to risk of reoffense (Worling & Langstrom, 2003).

It is necessary to be aware of factors that likely contribute to recidivism. However, it is equally important to have knowledge of which factors suggested by empirical evidence are not related to an increased risk of reoffense. The most notable example of this is the abusive child denying the offense. Denial of sexual offense has long been accepted as a factor related to increased likelihood of recidivism. Notably, denial of sexual offense appears on most recidivism assessment guidelines. However, available studies indicate that a juvenile who denies his sexual offense is less likely to recidivate (Kahn & Chambers, 1991; Langstrom & Grann, 2000; Worling, 2002). A number of theories have been asserted to explain this, seemingly counterintuitive finding. One of the more widely accepted explanations suggests that juveniles who deny their offenses are more likely to have antisocial traits and therefore a tendency toward general criminal activity. So, their sex offense was more likely the result of an opportunistic criminal activity rather than deviant sexual interest. The lack of relationship between denial of the offense and recidivism has also been reported in the adult sex offender literature. (Hanson & Bussière, 1998). Other factors that appear to not be predictive of recidivism include a lack of victim empathy (Langstrom & Grann, 2000; Smith & Monastersky, 1986), sex assault involving penetration (Langstrom, 2002), history of nonsexual crimes (Kahn & Chambers, 1991; Lab, Shields, & Schondel, 1993; Langstrom, 2002), and the offending adolescent having a history of sexual abuse (Hagan & Cho, 1996; Rasmussen, 1999; Worling & Curwen, 2000).

Despite inconclusive data regarding risk factors, there are many promising possibilities that may develop into a definitive set of risks for recidivism. Importantly, many of the intuitive and subjective factors previously thought to be associated with recidivism have been shown to have little or no support based on empirical evidence. Some researchers have suggested that actuarial risk prediction for juveniles may never be validated due to the heterogeneity and rapid growth and change which are characteristic of adolescence.

TREATMENT

Understanding the complex nature of sexually deviant behavior requires an eclectic, multimodal approach. Intervention must include offense-specific interventions which have often been provided in a group setting (National Task Force on Juvenile Sexual Offending, 1993). However, offense-specific treatment is only part of a more comprehensive strategy that must be implemented to optimize outcomes and ultimately decrease the risk of recidivism. An effective treatment plan evolves from a comprehensive assessment of multiple influences affecting an adolescent's mental life. The presence of a mental disorder should be determined and treated. It is necessary to consider factors from the adolescent's life story with positive experiences being stressed and the effect of negative experiences managed. Cognitive abilities and personality traits shape the psychotherapeutic maneuvers that can be applied in various treatment settings. A comprehensive treatment plan must consider all aspects of the youth's functioning and environment using approaches from disease, personality, cognitive, and life story perspectives.

Models for treatment of juveniles who commit sexual offenses have evolved as our knowledge of the population has increased. Two main factors drive treatment protocols: (1) this is a heterogeneous population, and (2) the sexual offense is often the most obvious or referring symptom in a larger pattern of abuse. However, there are often many other symptoms of dysfunction which have gone unidentified or untreated, but which may be very relevant to both the initiation and maintenance of sexual and abusive behaviors. Every adolescent who presents for treatment needs to be considered as a unique individual, and treatment plans must address factors influencing the adolescent's current and future functioning, including patterns associated with all types of abusive behaviors and assets which support healthier, prosocial adaptation. Focusing exclusively on the history of past behaviors may have the unintended consequence of reinforcing the negative sense of self and fail to create a dissonance for abusive behaviors.

Static risk factors may be of critical importance in initial decision making regarding community safety, placement, and supervision, as well as the intensity and restrictiveness of the treatment setting, but it is the acute and chronic dynamic factors which are changeable over the course of treatment (Ryan, 2000).

CONFIDENTIALITY

Except in well-defined situations, traditional therapeutic relationships have usually guaranteed confidentiality to patients. Because sexual abuse occurs in secret and secrecy allows it to continue, executing a waiver of the right to confidentiality carries a strong therapeutic message to the youth and family regarding the need to give up the secrecy which has supported the abusive behavior. Many programs require a signed waiver of confidentiality, while others use extensive releases, before admission to enable the treatment provider to be in frequent open communication with all the systems and individuals who interact with the adolescent (Ryan et al., 1990). Such open communication is often a condition of court ordered treatment for youth on probation being provided in community-based settings.

MENTAL ILLNESS

There is little data regarding the prevalence of mental illness in this population, the effect of proper diagnoses and treatment of mental illness, and its relationship to recidivism in this population. However, intuitive presumption and clinical experience suggest that the symptoms of co-occurring disorders can affect an adolescent's behavior in a number of ways. For example, attention-deficit hyperactivity disorder (ADHD) and bipolar disorder can contribute to impulsivity and less resistance to abusive impulses. An adolescent with major depression may care less about himself and have less concern for the personal consequences resulting from his behaviors. He may also be more self absorbed and thus less aware or less caring of the impact of his behavior on others. Emotional reactivity or dissociation associated with anxiety of post-traumatic stress disorder (PTSD) may contribute to aggressive, hypersexual, and dysfunctional behaviors.

When sexual and/or abusive behaviors have been used as compensatory coping strategies to express or defuse untreated mental health issues or disorders, the effect on cognition may make it more difficult for the adolescent to recognize dysfunction or process alternative coping mechanisms. It is important to strive for correct diagnosis and effective treatment of co-occurring disorders which might impede successful participation in treatment. It is also important for the youth to come to understand diagnostic meaning and treatment interventions that prove helpful during treatment to address and support continued success in long-term relapse prevention plans. Failure to include necessary medical management of ongoing psychiatric disorders in aftercare plans may jeopardize treatment gains and contribute to the risk of relapse.

PHYSIOLOGICAL ASPECTS OF TREATING SEXUAL BEHAVIOR PROBLEMS

Although the sexual offenses committed by juveniles appear to be a product of dysfunctional coping, combined with a capacity to be abusive, more than physiological sexual deviance per se, there is a subset of youth who sexually offend who report problematic levels of arousal, in terms of frequency, intensity, or intrusive thoughts. Symptoms of hypersexual drive may be associated with numerous psychiatric diagnoses or may be a product of reinforcement and conditioning. For some youth it is difficult to engage and progress in treatment without first achieving some reduction of sexual arousal. Cognitive interventions and behavioral reconditioning strategies can be helpful for some, but are not always sufficient.

Drive-Reducing Medications and Selective Serotonin Reuptake Inhibitors

There is minimal data regarding the use of drive reducing medications in juveniles who have committed sexual offenses. There is still debate in the adult literature regarding who is most helped by these medications, but there is some consensus supporting the use of drive reducing medication for some paraphilic adults (Bradford, 1998). Only a subgroup of the juveniles who commit sexual offenses have hypersexual or deviant fixations, and there are significant ethical considerations in doing research with this population. For many youth, use of an antiandrogen medication is counterindicated because they have not reached their mature stature and bone growth might be affected. However, in some instances hormonal treatments may be useful, with close oversight from the prescribing physician. Saleh et al. (2004) examined the effect of Leuprolide Acetate in six young adults (aged 19 to 20 years) convicted of aggressive sexual offenses and been refractory to treatment.

These young adults subjectively reported a decrease in deviant sexual fantasy. Four of the subjects had no side effect while one suffered a loss of ejaculation and another experienced retrograde ejaculation. No clinically significant signs of osteopenia were evident on DEXA scan after 1 year.

Several characteristics may be considered indicators for consideration of drive-reducing treatment. Adolescents who may benefit from this pharmacotherapy might include those who have pathologically increased sexual drives, intrusive or abusive sexual interests, or who have impaired cognitive abilities that preclude appreciation of the consequences of their behavior for self and others and have a history of acting on deviant sexual impulses. Given the paucity of data regarding drive reduction in adolescents who sexually offend, it is not possible to make an evidence-based argument for which of these individuals will respond best to this treatment.

The presence of co-occurring mood disorders sometimes results in treatment of depressive symptoms with selective serotonin reuptake inhibitors (SSRIs) or tricyclics. The side effect of decreased sexual arousal which is sometimes associated with these medications can be a welcome relief for the hypersexual teen whose arousal has driven problematic behaviors. Although not normally prescribed as drive-reducing medications, there is a growing awareness of this potential for use in individual cases of treatment with juveniles who have sexually offended.

PSYCHOTHERAPY: RELATIONSHIP, EXPERIENCE, AND ENVIRONMENTAL CONSIDERATIONS

Neglect has often been ignored in understanding the behavior of adolescents. The commonly held belief that a history of being sexually abused is the major historical risk factor for sexual abuse perpetration draws attention away from other major risk factors. It is not just the bad things that happen that create risk, but also the absence of positive experiences and relationships. Widom and Williams (1996) demonstrated that childhood neglect and witnessing family violence may precede sexual offending even more often than physical abuse and sexual abuse. This has significant treatment implication because while it is not possible to undo past experiences, it is possible to create a more supportive environment for the adolescent.

Personality traits, cognitive abilities, prior experiences, and social situation will all have an impact on treatment. The goals of the treatment process are (1) to clearly define the abusive nature of past sexual behavior (i.e., lack of consent, inequality, use of coercion); (2) to aid the juvenile in understanding the process or context associated with the offending behaviors; (3) to develop skills and strategies for the juvenile to intervene in this process; (4) to motivate the juvenile to use these tools; and (5) to increase empathic foresight in future interactions. Achieving these goals will help the youth gain control over abusive impulses and will increase the safety of others in the community.

Lane (1991) describes five distinct phases of treatment in an offense-specific treatment unit: (1) penetrating denial concerning the sexually abusive behaviors, (2) identifying the adolescent's sexual abuse cycle, (3) helping the adolescent deal with unresolved emotional issues, (4) providing retraining in the areas of skill deficits, and (5) facilitating the adolescent's reentry into the community.

Although recent research suggests that denial may not be directly correlated with sexual recidivism, it is difficult to work on a problem that has not been named.

However, the focus in discussing past offenses has shifted from detailed disclosure of the sexually explicit details to more of the dynamic risks associated with future behaviors. The youth's ability to make accurate attributions of responsibility regarding their own and other's behaviors and to recognize the harm caused by abusive sexual behaviors is the necessary precursor to their being able to work on defining abuse, recognizing predictable precursors, and understanding empathic cues, even if they do not fully disclose every past behavior.

The offense-specific treatment of juveniles who have committed sexual offenses is often done in a group setting.

This is cost effective in that a lot of the group work provides education and skill building. One of the main advantages of the group setting is the effectiveness of the group dynamic to confront denial in other members with similar abuse patterns, while also providing the support that comes from knowing that they are not alone. Ideally, groups are led by cotherapists, both, male and female. Having both male and female therapists will manage the likelihood of transference issues being elicited by the therapists' gender.

The duration of treatment may range from a short-term, psychoeducational intervention to a very complex long-term process that may last from 1 to 3 years. The needs and issues for each youth are informed by the individualized assessment and there should be differential treatment plans for each youth. The focus, needs, and goals will not be the same for each individual in the group, but their exposure to those differences is congruent with their need to recognize that the needs and desires of others are not always congruent with their own. Nonetheless, a significant concern in bringing any group of delinquent youth together is the risk of "deviance training" or the negative influence of delinquent peers. Therapists must take responsibility for constantly assessing peer interactions within the group treatment setting to control for unintended reinforcement, and some youth will require individual therapy and/or family interventions before they become able to successfully function in a group with peers.

Issues to be addressed in the treatment of adolescents who have sexually offended include the following (National Task Force on Juvenile Sexual Offending, 1993):

1. Acceptance of responsibility for behavior
2. Identification of pattern or cycle of offense behavior
3. Effective interventions to interrupt the sexual abuse cycle
4. Victimization (e.g., sexual abuse) and issues for the offender
5. Capacity for empathy with others, especially past victims
6. Interpersonal power and control issues
7. Role of sexual arousal in offenses
8. Sexual identity
9. Consequences of offending
10. Family issues that support offending behaviors
11. Cognitive distortions related to offending behaviors
12. Expression of feelings
13. Skill deficits (social and academic)
14. Substance use/abuse
15. Relapse prevention
16. Management of concurrent psychiatric disorders

Effective treatment intervention requires intersystem cooperation and the support of the legal system. Clinicians generally agree that a mandatory treatment model is the most effective way to address the juvenile's reluctance to change and the need for external controls from the court, parents, or protective services system. The court's involvement requires that the juvenile take responsibility for behavior and demonstrate change. Mandated treatment can result from diversion programs, conditions of probation, or treatment plans related to dependency and neglect proceedings. Court-ordered treatment should be enforceable for at least 2 years because of the length of time required for adequate treatment and the frequency of premature termination of treatment when not mandated (Hunter & Figueredo, 1999).

THE CYCLE

The concept of an abuse cycle has been helpful for many adolescents as the cornerstone of the cognitive aspects of their treatment (Lane, 1991). Situational, affective, cognitive, and behavioral factors are considered to understand patterns associated with the individual's offending behaviors and to recognize predictable precursors which can then be handled differently.

Initially viewed specifically as a "sexual abuse cycle," the similarity of patterns associated with many dysfunctional behaviors illustrates habituation of behaviors which provide some immediate gratification, even when there are also negative consequences. The pattern is triggered by a situation that is perceived by the adolescent in a manner that causes emotional stress, feeling diminished, vulnerable, and unable to cope. This feeling in turn contributes to the adolescent expecting something bad to occur, which often results in him feeling threatened emotionally and/or physically. It is common for the youth to become reclusive during such times in an attempt to avoid the anticipated negative occurrence. During this isolation, projection, and externalizing cover the vulnerable feeling with anger and the adolescent fantasizes about retaliation (How can I get back—make others feel as bad as I do?) or compensation (How can I feel better?). These fantasies can become the basis for a plan which develops into the offense. When the motivation is retaliatory, the behaviors may be deliberately abusive, accompanied by a conscious desire to inflict pain, whereas the compensatory motive may simply disregard the victim's needs and fail to anticipate the abusive impact of the behaviors (Ryan, Lane, Davis, 1987).

It is helpful to think of the factors that contribute to abusive behaviors in terms of the possibility of them being altered through treatment. Ryan (2000b)

TABLE 17.3 Types of Factors That May
Contribute to Abusive Behaviors

Static *(Historical/Unchangeable)*

Condition at birth

Permanent disabilities

Family of origin

Early life experience

Stable *(Life Spanning/Less Changeable)*

Temperament

Intellectual potential

Physical attributes

Heritable neurological characteristics

Dynamic *(Change/Manage/Moderate)*

Situations

Thoughts

Feelings

Behaviors

suggests dividing these factors into static, stable, and dynamic categories (see Table 17.3).

Because we cannot change the past, the static and stable risk factors are difficult to modify. However, these factors may represent major obstacles for the adolescent to overcome as he/she progresses through the treatment process. These should be considered when assessing the adolescent's assets and weaknesses in the development of a comprehensive treatment plan. As in all therapeutic relationships, it is important to consider the patient's temperament when modifying a pattern of behavior.

Adolescents' personality and behavioral characteristics represent dynamic traits that are still malleable. Similarly, plethysmography evidence suggests that juvenile sexual offenses are not usually reflections of fixated interests or deviant sexual arousal. Much more than in the adult population, treatment of juveniles should concentrate on the more dynamic and changeable traits of these children. Prentky et al. (2000) describes the reduction of dynamic risks in terms of what might be observable in the treatment process: accepting responsibility, internal motivation to change, understanding the cycle, showing empathy and remorse, decreased cognitive distortions, anger management, stability in home and school, support systems, and quality peer relationships.

ASSESSMENT OF TREATMENT OUTCOMES

As treatment progresses, the adolescent should become proficient in defining all abuse and develop vigilance which makes it less likely that he may engage in, or be a victim of, abuse without defining it as such. The adolescent's knowledge and use of the abuse cycle is important in achievement of this goal. Through the use of the cycle, the adolescent will more readily identify when he or she is experiencing stress and immediately define fantasies about abuse, enabling them to interrupt the progression of these fantasies before they act on impulse.

The youth should begin to demonstrate the ability to be empathic during their daily interactions. They should be able to recognize the cues in self and others which indicate needs and emotions. The adolescent should take responsibility for his or her own behavior while not accepting responsibility beyond his or her control or trying to assume control of others.

Neglect and isolation are major risk factors for abusive behavior. A very important skill to counter these risks is the ability to create and maintain psychologically safe, empathic relationships. Prosocial relationship skills, and especially one's own ability to establish intimacy, closeness, and trustworthy relationships, demonstrates and supports a belief in the value of such relationships. A positive self-image is reliant on mastery of the developmental skills which enable individuals to be separate and independent, while a sense of personal competency supports personal responsibility.

Table 17.4 provides a treatment outcomes summary that is congruent with the outcomes required for successful completion of treatment under the Colorado State Standards (2003).

CONCLUSION

Juvenile sexual offenses cause tremendous harm to victims in the community, as well as legal jeopardy and social stigma for the youth. Awareness of the incidence and prevalence of juvenile offenses are recent phenomena, and community reactions are often harsh and punitive. It had been assumed that youth who sexually offended were expressing deviant sexual

TABLE 17.4 Observable Outcomes

Relevant to Decreased Risk

Consistently defines all abuse (self, others, property)

Acknowledges risk (foresight and safety planning)

Consistently recognizes and interrupts cycle no later than first thought of an abusive solution

Demonstrates new coping skills (when stressed)

Demonstrates empathy (sees cues of others and responds)

Accurate attributions of responsibility (takes responsibility for own behavior, does not try to control the behavior of others)

Rejects abusive thoughts as dissonant (incongruent with self-image)

Relevant to Increased Health

Prosocial relationship skills (closeness, trust, and trustworthiness)

Positive self-image (able to be separate, independent and competent)

Able to resolve conflicts and make decisions (able to be assertive, tolerant, forgiving, and cooperative. Able to compromise)

Celebrates good and experienced pleasure (able to relax and play)

Able to manage frustration and unfavorable events (anger management and self-protection)

Works/struggles to achieve delayed gratification (persistent pursuit of goals)

Able to think and communicate effectively (rational cognitive processing and adequate verbal skills)

Adaptive sense of purpose and future

---

preferences and would likely continue offending as adults. However, research has demonstrated that most are more like other delinquents than like adult sex offenders. This is good news, since most delinquents do not go on to a life of crime.

Sexual recidivism by juveniles is less than that of adults and even less after treatment. Nonetheless, these youth are often very troubled and troubling. Treatment requires patience and a nurturing environment to allow for the growth and development which will support more successful and prosocial functioning. At the same time, treatment must hold youth accountable for their behaviors and the harm they have caused, which they often resist acknowledging. A coordinated, multidisciplinary approach must be supported with the power of the juvenile court's order to achieve the best outcomes.

References

Abel, G. G., Becker, J. V., Mittelman, M., Cunningham-Rathner, J., Roleau, J. L., & Murphy, W. D. (1987). Self-reported sex crimes of non-incarcerated paraphiliacs. *Journal of Interpersonal Violence*, 2, 3–25.

Abel Screening, Inc. (1996). Abel assessment for sexual interest: Juvenile sex offenders: Therapist product information. Atlanta, GA: Brochure.

Awad, G. E. & Saunders, E. (1991). Male adolescent sexual assaulters, clinical observations. *Journal of Interpersonal Violence*, 6, 446–460.

Becker, J. V. (1998). What we know about the characteristics and treatment of adolescents who have committed sexual offenses. *Child Maltreatment*, 3, 317–329.

Becker, J. V. & Abel, G. (1985). Methodological and ethical issues in evaluating and treatment adolescent sex offenders. In E. M. Otey & G. D. Ryan (Eds.), *Adolescent sex offenders: Issues in research and treatment* (pp. 109–129). Rockville, MD, U.S.: Department of Health and Human Services.

Becker, J. V. & Hicks, S. J. (2003). Juvenile sex offenders: Characteristics, interventions and policy issues. *Annals Of NewYork Academy Of Science*, 989, 397–410.

Becker, J. V. & Hunter, J. A. (1997). Understanding and treating child and adolescent sexual offenders. In T. H. Ollendick & R. J. Prinz (Eds.), *Advances in clinical trials psychology* (vol.19, pp. 177–197). New York, NY: Plenum Press.

Becker, J. V., Kaplan, M. S., Cunningham-Rathner, J., & Kavoussi, R. (1986). Characteristics of adolescent incest sexual perpetrators: Preliminary findings. *Journal of Family Violence*, 1(1), 85–97.

Becker, J. V., Kaplan, M. S., Tenke, C. E., & Tarthelini, A. (1991). The incidence of depressive symptomatology in juvenile sex offenders with a history of abuse. *Child Abuse and Neglect: The International Journal*, 15, 531–536.

Benda, B. B, Corwyn, R. F., & Toombs, N. J. (2001). Recidivism among serious offenders: The prediction of entry into the correctional system for adults. *Criminal Justice and Behavior*, 28, 588–613.

Bonner, B., Marx, B. P., Thompson, J. M., & Michaelson, P. (1998). Assessment of adolescent sexual offenders. *Child Maltreatment*, 3(4), 374–383.

Bourke, M. L. & Donohue, B. (1996). Assessment and treatment of juvenile sex offenders: An empirical review. *Journal of Child Sexual Abuse*, 5(1), 47–70.

Bradford, J. M. W. (1998). Treatment of men with paraphilia. *New England Journal of Medicine*, 338, 464–465.

Bumby, K. M. & Bumby, N. H. (1997). Adolescent female sexual offenders. In B. K. Schwartz & H. R. Cellini (Eds.), *The sex offender: Vol. 2. New Insights, Treatment Innovations and Legal Developments* (pp. 10.1–10.16). Kingston, NJ: Civic Research Institute.

Butcher, J. N., Williams, C. L., Graham, J. R., Archer, R. P., Tellegen, A., Ben-Porath, Y. S., et al. (1992). *Minnesota Multiphasic Personality Inventory-Adolescent (MMPI-A): Manual for administration, scoring, and interpretation*. Minneapolis, MN: University of Minnesota Press.

Butz, C. & Spaccarelli, S. (1999). Use of physical force as an offense characteristic in subtyping juvenile sexual offenders. *Sexual Abuse: A Journal of Research and Treatment*, 11(3), 217–232.

Center for Sex Offender Management. (1999). *Understanding juvenile sexual offending behavior: Emerging research, treatment approaches and management practices*. Silver Spring, Maryland: US Department of Justice.

Colorado Sex Offender Management Board, Colorado Division of Criminal Justice. (2003). Standards for management and treatment of juveniles who commit sexual offenses, Available http://dcj.state.co.us/odvsom/Sex_Offender/SO_Pdfs/2003JUVENILESTANDARDS.pdf (March 2, 2005), 46–50.

Cottle, C. C., Lee, R. L., & Heilbrun, K. (2001). The prediction of criminal recidivism in juveniles: A meta-analysis. *Criminal Justice and Behavior*, 28, 367–394.

Dent, R. & Jeyarajah, J. S. (2003). Homicide and serious sexual offences committed by children and young people: Findings from the literature and a serious case review. *Journal of Sexual Aggression*, 9(2), 85–96.

Farber, E. D., Showers, J., Johnson, C. F., Joseph, J. A., & Oshins, L. (1984). The sexual abuse of children: A comparison of male and female victims. *Journal of Clinical Child Psychology*, 13(3), 294–297.

Federal Bureau of Investigation, Uniform Crime Report. (2001). United States Department of Justice. Available: http://www.fbi.gov/ucr/ucr.htm [February 13, 2005].

Freeman-Longo, R. E., Bird, S., Stevenson, W. F., & Fiske, J. A. (1995). 1994 *Nationwide survey of treatment programs & models: Serving abuse reactive children and adolescent & adult sexual offenders*. Brandon, VT: Safer Society Press.

Gilby, R., Wolf, L., & Goldberg, B. (1989). Mentally retarded adolescent sex offenders: A survey and pilot study. *Canadian Journal of Psychiatry*, 34, 542–548.

Graves, R. B., Openshaw, D. K., Ascione, F. R., & Ericksen, S. L. (1996). Demographic and parental characteristics of youthful sexual offenders. *International Journal of Offender Therapy and Comparative Criminology*, 40, 300–317.

Gretton, H. M., McBride, M., Hare, R. D., O'Shaughnessy, R., & Kumka, G. (2001). Psychopathy and recidivism in adolescent sex offenders. *Criminal Justice and Behavior*, 28, 427–449.

Grisso, S., Steinberg, L., Woolard, J., Cauffman, E., Scott, E., & Graham, S. (2003). Juveniles' competence to stand trial: A comparison of adolescents' and adults' capacities as trial defendants. *Law and Human Behavior*, 27, 333–363.

Hagan, M. P. & Cho, M. E. (1996). A comparison of treatment outcomes between adolescent rapists and child sexual offenders. *International Journal of Offender Therapy and Comparative Criminology*, 40, 113–122.

Hanson, R. K. & Bussière, M. T. (1998). Predicting relapse: A meta-analysis of sexual offender recidivism studies. *Journal of Consulting and Clinical Psychology*, 66, 348–362.

Hoge, R. D. (2002). Standardized instruments for assessing risk and need in youthful offenders. *Criminal Justice and Behavior*, 29, 380–396.

Home Office, Criminal Statistics England and Wales for the Year 2000, Supplementary Tables, Volumes 1 and 2 *(Proceedings in the Magistrates' Courts and the Crown Court)*. London: National Statistics.

Hunter, J. A., Jr. & Becker, J. V. (1994). The role of deviant sexual arousal in juvenile sexual offending: Etiology, evaluation, and treatment. *Criminal Justice and Behavior*, 21(1), 132–149.

Hunter, J. A. & Becker, J. V. (1999). Motivators of adolescent sex offenders and treatment perspectives. In J. Shaw (Ed.), *Sexual aggression* (pp. 214–234) Washington, D.C.: American Psychiatric Press.

Hunter, J. A. & Figueredo, A. J. (1999). Factors associated with treatment compliance in a population of juvenile sexual offenders. *Sexual Abuse: A Journal of Research and Treatment*, 11(1), 132–149.

Hunter, J. A., Figueredo, A. J. Malamuth, N. M., & Becker, J. V. (2003). Juvenile sex offenders: Toward the development of a typology. *Sexual Abuse: A Journal of Research and Treatment*, 15(1), 26–48.

Hunter, J. & Longo, R. E. (2004). Relapse prevention with juvenile sexual abusers: A holistic and integrated approach. In G. O'Reilly, W. Marshall, A. Carr, & R. C. Beckett (Eds.), *The handbook of clinical intervention with young people who sexually abuse*. New York, NY: Brunner-Routledge.

Hunter, J. A. & Lexier, L. J. (1998). Ethical and legal issues in the assessment and treatment of juvenile sex offenders. *Child Maltreatment*, 3(4), 339–348.

Kahn, T. J. & Chambers, H. J. (1991). Assessing reoffense risk with juvenile sexual offenders. *Child Welfare*, 70, 333–345.

Kempe, C. H. (1980). Incest and other forms of sexual abuse. In C. H. Kempe, R. E. Helfer (Eds.), *The battered child*, 3rd Edition (pp. 198–214). Chicago, IL: University of Chicago Press.

Kenny, D. T., Keogh, T., & Seidler, K. (2001). Predictors of recidivism in Australian juvenile sex offenders: Implications for treatment. *Sexual Abuse: A Journal of Research and Treatment*, 13, 131–148.

Knight, R. A., Prentky, R. A., & Cerce, D. D. (1994). The development, reliability, and validity of an inventory for the multidimensional assessment of sex and aggression. *Criminal Justice and Behavior,* 21(1), 72–94.

Lab, S. P., Shields, G., & Schondel, C. (1993). Research note: An evaluation of juvenile sexual offender treatment. *Crime & Delinquency,* 39, 543–553.

Lane, S. (1991). The sexual abuse cycle. In G. D. Ryan, S. L. Lane (Eds.), *Juvenile sexual offending* (pp. 103–142). Lexington, MA: Lexington Books.

Langstrom, N. (2002). Long-term follow-up of criminal recidivism in young sex offenders: Temporal patterns and risk factors. *Psychology, Crime and Law,* 8, 41–58.

Langstrom, N. & Grann, M. (2000). Risk for criminal recidivism among young sex offenders. *Journal of Interpersonal Violence,* 15, 855–871.

Lipsey, M. W. & Derzon, J. H. (1998). Predictors of violent or serious delinquency in adolescence and early adulthood: Asynthesis of longitudinal research. In R. Loeber & D. P. Farrington (Eds.), *Serious and violent juvenile offenders: Risk factors and successful interventions* (pp. 86–105). London: Sage.

Masson, H. & Hackett, S. (2003). A decade on from the NCH report (1992): Adolescent sexual aggression policy, practice and service delivery across the UK and Republic of Ireland. *Journal of Sexual Aggression,* 9, 109–124.

Mazur, T. & Michael, P. (1992). Outpatient treatment for adolescents with sexually inappropriate behaviour: Program description and 6-month follow-up. *Journal of Offender Rehabilitation,* 18, 191–203.

Miner, M. H. & Crimmins, C. L. S. (1995). Adolescent sex offenders: Issues of etiology and risk factors. In B. K. Schwartz & H. R. Cellini (Eds.), *The sex offender: Vol. I, corrections, treatment and legal practice* (pp. 9.1–9.15). Kingston, NJ: Civic Research Institute.

Miranda, A. O. & Corcoran, C. L. (2000). Comparison of perpetration characteristics between male juvenile and adult sexual offenders: Preliminary results. *Sexual Abuse: A Journal of Research and Treatment,* 12(3), 179–188.

National Task Force on Juvenile Sexual Offending. (1993). The revised report on juvenile sexual offending 1993 of the National Adolescent Perpetration Network. *Juvenile and Family Court Journal,* 44(4), 1–120.

Nichols, H. R. & Molinder, M. A. (1984). *Multiphasic Sex Inventory Manual,* (437 Bowes Drive, Tacoma, WA 98466) Nichols & Molinder Assessments.

O'Brien, M. J. & Bera, W. (1986). Adolescent sexual offenders: A descriptive typology. *Preventing Sexual Abuse,* 1(3), 1–4.

Prentky, R., Harris, B., Frizell, K., & Righthand, S. (2000). An actuarial procedure for assessing risk in juvenile sex offenders. *Sexual Abuse: A Journal of Research & Treatment,* 12, 71–93.

Rasmussen, L. A. (1999). Factors related to recidivism among juvenile sexual offenders. *Sexual Abuse: A Journal of Research and Treatment,* 11, 69–85.

Rich, P. (2003). *Understanding, assessing, and rehabilitating juvenile sexual offender* (pp. 23–31). Hoboken, NJ: John Wiley & Sons, Inc.

Righthand, S. & Welch C. (2001). Juveniles who have sexually offended: A review the professional literature. *Office of Juvenile Justice and Delinquency Prevention,* US Department of Justice, (March). 1–65.

Rubenstein, M., Yeager, C. A., Goodstein, C., & Lewis, D. O. (1993). Sexually assaulted male juveniles: A follow-up. *American Journal of Psychiatry,* 150, 262–265.

Ryan, G. (1997). Juvenile sex offenders: Defining the population. In G. Ryan & S. Lane (Eds.), *Juvenile sexual offending: Causes, consequences and corrections* (pp. 3–9). Lexington, MA: Lexington Books.

Ryan, G. (1999). Treatment of sexually abusive youth: The evolving consensus. *Journal of Interpersonal Violence,* 14, 422–436.

Ryan, G. (2000). Childhood sexuality: A decade of study. part I-research and curriculum development, *Child Abuse and Neglect,* 24, 33–48.

Ryan, G. (2000). Static, stable and dynamic risks and assets relevant to the prevention and treatment of abusive behaviour. Poster presentation at First National Sexual Violence Prevention Conference. Dallas, TX.

Ryan, G., Blum, J., Sandau-Christopher, D., Law, S. Weher, F., Sundine, C., et al. (1993). *Understanding and responding to sexual behavior of children. Trainers Manual.* Denver, Colorado: Kempe National Center, University of Colorado Health Sciences Center, 1988, revised.

Ryan, G. D., Lane, S., & Davis, J. (1987). Juvenile sex offenders: Development and correction. *Child Abuse and Neglect,* 11, 385–395.

Ryan, G. D., Metzner, J. L., & Krugman, R. D. (1990). When the abuser is a child. In R. Kim Oates (Ed.), *Understanding and managing child sexual abuse* (pp. 258–273). Philadelphia: W.B Saunders.

Ryan, G., Miyoshi, T. J. O., Metzner, J. L., Krugman, R. D., & Fryer, G. E. (1996). Trends in a national sample of sexually abusive youth. *Journal of the Academy of Child and Adolescent Psychiatry,* 35, 17–25.

Saleh, F. M., Niel, T. N., & Fishman, M. J. (2004). Treatment of paraphilia in young adults with leuprolide acetate: A preliminary case report series. *Journal of Forensic Science,* 49(6), 1–6.

Schram, D. D., Milloy, C. D., & Rowe, W. E. (1991). Juvenile sex offenders: A follow up study of reoffense behavior. Olympia, WA: Washington State Institute for Public Policy, Urban Policy Research and Cambie Group International.

Sipe, R., Jensen, E. L., & Everett, R. S. (1998). Adolescent sexual offenders grown up: Recidivism in young adulthood. *Criminal Justice and Behavior,* 25(1), 109–124.

Smith, G. & Fischer, L. (1999). Assessment of juvenile sexual offenders: Reliability and validity of the Abel Assessment for Interest in paraphilias. *Sexual*

Abuse: A Journal of Research and Treatment, 11(3), 207–216.

Smith, W. R. & Monastersky, C. (1986). Assessing juvenile sexual offenders' risk for reoffending. *Criminal Justice and Behavior*, 13, 115–140.

Sorensen, E. & Johnson, E. (1996). Subtypes of incarcerated delinquents constructed via cluster analysis. *Journal of Child Psychology and Psychiatry*, 37, 293–303.

Veneziano C. & Veneziano, L. (2002). Adolescent sex offenders: A review of the literature. *Trauma, Violence, & Abuse*, 3(4), 247–260.

Weinrott, M. (1998). Empirically based treatment interventions for juvenile sex offenders. Empirically-based treatment interventions for juvenile sex offenders. Presentation sponsored by the Child Abuse Action Network and the State Forensic Service, Augusta, ME.

Widom, C. S. & Williams, L. (1996). Cycle of sexual abuse. Research inconclusive about whether child victims become adult abusers. Report to House of Representatives, Committee of Judiciary, Subcommittee on Crime. General Accounting Office. Washington, DC.

Wieckowski, E., Hartsoe, P., Mayer, A., & Shortz, J. (1998). Deviant sexual behavior in children and young adolescents: Frequency and patterns. *Sexual Abuse: A Journal of Research and Treatment*, 10(4), 293–304.

Worling, J. R. (2002). Assessing risk of sexual assault recidivism with adolescent sexual offenders. In M. C. Calder (Ed.), *Young people who sexually abuse: Building the evidence base for your practice* (pp. 365–375). Lyme Regis, U.K.: Russell House Publishing.

Worling, J. R. & Curwen, T. (2000). Adolescent sexual offender recidivism: Success of specialized treatment and implications for risk prediction. *Child Abuse & Neglect*, 24, 965–982.

Worling, J. & Langstrom, N. (2003). Assessment of criminal recidivism risk with adolescents who have offended sexually—A review. *Trauma, Violence and Abuse*, 4(4), 341–362.

Zolondek, S. C., Abel, G. G., Northey, W. F., & Jordan, A. D. (2001). The self-reported behaviors of juvenile sexual offenders. *Journal of Interpersonal Violence*, 16(1), 73–85.

Part VI

Special Populations

Chapter 18

Substance Abuse and Sexual Offending

Peer Briken, Andreas Hill, and Wolfgang Berner

This chapter considers the effects of acute and chronic substance use on sexual offending. A significant proportion of sexual offenders suffer from substance use disorders. However, it remains unclear if sexual offenders differ in a characteristic way from other offender groups. Substance use seems to be more prevalent in rapists than in child molesters and more frequent in nonparaphilic than in paraphilic sexual offenders. The nature of the relationship between substance use and sexual offending is complex and confounded with several factors (dose, experience with the substance, social setting, personality factors, subjective expectancy of the substance effects, brain disorders etc.). Acute and long-term effects of alcohol probably play a contributive but not a primary causal role in sexual offending. The literature concerning drugs is reviewed but currently insufficient to draw conclusions. Substance abuse plays a significant role in risk assessment and relapse prevention and should be considered in treatment options more specifically.

Many pathways play a role in the development of sexual offending. This article, describes different aspects in which they are related to alcohol and drugs and will focus on the epidemiology, acute- and long-term effects as well as on therapy and risk assessment. Theoretical explanations of sexual offending consider both distal and proximal influences. When examining alcohol and drugs as distal factors, we will describe the relationship between long-term consumption as well as the influence of beliefs about the effects of the used substances (expectancies). Proximal models focus on characteristics of the specific situations in which the offense occurs, such as whether substance consumption played a role or not. Substance abuse and intoxication may also be used as an excuse for engaging in antisocial behavior, including sexual offenses. In addition, certain personality characteristics (e.g., impulsivity and antisocial behavior), neurobiological vulnerabilities, or neuropsychiatric disorders may increase the propensity to both substance abuse and sexual offending.

ASSESSMENT AND DIAGNOSIS

Assessment requires a thorough review of the psychiatric, medical, and criminal history. Most alcohol and drug abusers do not present themselves because of their substance-related problems. Shame and denial, but also using substance disorders—especially intoxications—as an excuse for sexual offending is common. Self-report questionnaires such as the Michigan Alcohol Screening Test (Selzer, 1971), semistructured interviews such as the Addiction Severity Index (McLellan et al., 1992), or structured interviews (such as the SCID-I-interview) can be used. Physical examination (e.g., to detect ascites or track marks of heroine use), laboratory testing (e.g., to test liver enzymes, MCV, CDT, hepatitis, urine, blood, or hair toxicology), and also neuropsychological examination can be useful.

The currently used definitions of intoxication, substance abuse and dependence are described in Table 18.1 (according to the *Diagnostic and Statistical Manual of Mental Disorders*, Fourth Edition, Text Revision, 2000, American Psychiatric Association).

TABLE 18.1 DSM-IV Criteria for Intoxication, Substance Abuse, and Dependence

Intoxication	Substance Abuse	Substance Dependence
Dysfunctional changes in physiological functioning, psychological functioning, mood state, cognitive process, or all of these, as a consequence of consumption of a psychoactive substance; usually disruptive, and often stemming from central nervous system impairment	(A) A maladaptive pattern of substance use leading to clinically significant impairment or distress, as manifested by one (or more) of the following, occurring within a 12-month period: (1) recurrent substance use resulting in a failure to fulfill major role obligations at work, school, or home (e.g., repeated absences or poor work performance related to substance use; substance-related absences, suspensions, or expulsions from school; neglect of children or household) (2) recurrent substance use in situations in which it is physically hazardous (e.g., driving an automobile or operating a machine when impaired by substance use) (3) recurrent substance-related legal problems (e.g., arrests for substance-related disorderly conduct) (4) continued substance use despite having persistent or recurrent social or interpersonal problems caused or exacerbated by the effects of the substance (e.g., arguments with spouse about consequences of intoxication, physical fights) (B) The symptoms have never met the criteria for substance dependence for this class of substance	(A) A maladaptive pattern of substance use, leading to clinically significant impairment or distress, as manifested by three (or more) of the following, occurring at any time in the same 12-month period: (1) tolerance, as defined by either of the following: (a) a need for markedly increased amounts of the substance to achieve intoxication or desired effect (b) markedly diminished effect with continued use of the same amount of the substance (2) withdrawal, as manifested by either of the following: (a) the characteristic withdrawal syndrome for the substance (refer to criteria (A) and (B) of the criteria sets for withdrawal from the specific substances) (b) the same (or a closely related) substance is taken to relieve or avoid withdrawal symptoms (3) the substance is often taken in larger amounts or over a longer period than was intended (4) there is a persistent desire or unsuccessful efforts to cut down or control substance use (5) a great deal of time is spent in activities necessary to obtain the substance (e.g., visiting multiple doctors or driving long distances), use the substance (e.g., chain-smoking), or recover from its effects (6) important social, occupational, or recreational activities are given up or reduced because of substance use (7) the substance use is continued despite knowledge of having a persistent or recurrent physical or psychological problem that is likely to have been caused or exacerbated by the substance (e.g., current cocaine use despite recognition of cocaine-induced depression, or continued drinking despite recognition that an ulcer was made worse by alcohol consumption)

METHODOLOGICAL ISSUES AND EPIDEMIOLOGY OF PSYCHOACTIVE SUBSTANCE ABUSE AND DEPENDENCE IN SEXUAL OFFENDER POPULATIONS

There are a lot of methodological issues to consider when interpreting the epidemiological data on psychoactive substance abuse and dependence in sexual offenders. These concern, first of all, the samples studied and the diagnostic measures used. Second, it is the question whether the offenses and offenders analyzed constitute representative samples. Intoxicated offenders may be overrepresented because of an increased likelihood to be arrested. Third, it has to be considered how many nonoffenders have alcohol or drug problems and do not commit sexual violence or how often substance abuse is associated with violent or nonviolent crime in general. It is questionable how often episodes of substance abuse occur without a sexual offense in investigated sexual offenders.

Another important factor that influences the interpretation of data are the consumption patterns of the victim. Approximately one-half of all sexual assault victims report that they were drinking alcohol at the time of the assault, with estimates ranging from 30% to 79% (Abbey, Ross, & McDuffie, 1994).

Recently a general population study in the United States (Stinson, Grant, Dawson, Ruan, Huang, & Saha, 2005) revealed prevalence rates of 7.4% for alcohol use disorders only, 0.9% for drug use disorder only, and 1.1% for comorbid alcohol and drug use disorders. In a representative sample of adults in the United States, Compton et al. (2005) found prevalence rates of 30.3% for alcohol use disorders and 10.3% for drug use disorders with a high comorbidity of substance disorders with antisocial syndromes. The prevalence rates in different prison populations ranged between 10% and 60% for alcohol and drug use disorders (Nika & Briken, 2004).

The rates of drinking by violent offenders during or immediately before commission of a violent crime are generally above 50% (Volavka, 2002). It is important to make a distinction between short effects of alcohol and the diagnosis of substance abuse or dependence. For example a major longitudinal prospective study of a New Zealand birth cohort (Arseneault, Moffitt, Caspi, Taylor, & Silva, 2000) could show that alcohol dependence marginally increased the risk for violent crime (odds ratio 1.9), but the increase was largely explained by actual alcohol use shortly before offending.

Depending on the sample studied and the measures used, the estimates for alcohol and drug abuse among sexual offenders have ranged from approximately 10% to about 60% (Allnut, Bradford, Greenberg, & Curry, 1996; Peugh & Belenko, 2001). Various studies estimate that between 40% to 90% of rapists and 30% to 40% of child sexual abusers were intoxicated at the time of the offense (Peugh & Belenko, 2001). In a nonclinical population 4.8% of male and 1.3% of female students (N = 71,594) (self-)reported a history of sexual violence perpetration (Borowsky, Hogan, & Ireland, 1997). Sexual aggression was associated with experiencing intrafamilial or extrafamilial sexual abuse, witnessing family violence, frequent use of illegal drugs, anabolic steroid use, daily alcohol use, gang membership, high levels of suicide risk behavior, and excessive time spent "hanging out." A survey of DSM-IV psychiatric disorders among criminal defendants referred for court-ordered forensic psychiatric evaluations in the United States (Cochrane, Grisso, & Frederick, 2001) suggested different prevalence rates among sexual offenders compared to other offender groups for diagnoses of mental retardation (11% vs. 2%), psychotic disorders (16% vs. 32%) but *not* for substance use disorders (42% vs. 48%).

Substance use disorders seem to be more common in rapists than in child abusers. Using the data from a national inmate prison survey by Peugh and Belenko (2001) relying on self-reports, among sexual offenders (N = 1273) two of three had a history of alcohol and drug use, abuse, or addiction. While rates of drug use were lower alcohol use was similar to that in other violent offenders (N = 4933). Drug and alcohol users stemmed more often from substance abusing family environments and had more often a history of childhood abuse, were more likely single, and previously involved in nonsexual crimes. Nonsubstance using perpetrators had more often victimized children. Some studies (Abracen et al., 2000; Langevin & Lang, 1990) used the Michigan Alcohol Screening Test (MAST; Selzer, 1971). With reference to the MAST scores Abracen et al. (2000) found severe levels of alcohol use in more than 40% of rapists and child molesters but only in approximately 4% of their comparison group of violent nonsexual offenders. Langström et al. (2004) investigated the psychiatric morbidity diagnosed during hospital admissions (using ICD-9/10 criteria) prior an index sexual offense from a nationwide, representative cohort in Sweden (N = 1215) with a retrospective follow-up design. Alcohol (2.7% within 1 year before the index offense; period prevalence 7.8%) and drug use (0.7% within 1 year before the index offense; period prevalence 2.8%) disorders were the most frequent diagnoses significantly more common in rapists than in child molesters (P<.001). In a recently published study Firestone et al. (2005) compared incest offenders whose victims were less than 6 years of age (N = 48) with incest offenders with adolescent victims (12 to 16 years; N = 71). The group with younger victims had a greater history of substance abuse and more current problems with alcohol, reported poorer sexual functioning, and was more psychiatrically disturbed than members of the other group.

In sexual homicide perpetrators prevalence rates range between 25% and 58% for alcohol use disorders (Hill, Habermann, Berner, & Briken, 2007; Langevin, 2003). Intoxications with alcohol at the time of the homicide are frequent (e.g., 39.8% in Hill et al., 2007); they are probably more frequently associated with the nonparaphilic offender types (Briken, Nika, & Berner, 2000; Briken, Habermann, Kafka, Berner, & Hill, 2006) and are less often found in those with neuropsychiatric abnormalities (Briken, Habermann, Berner, & Hill, 2005).

COMORBIDITY OF PSYCHOACTIVE SUBSTANCE ABUSE AND PARAPHILIAS

Raymond et al. (1999) investigated 45 male subjects with pedophilia who participated in residential or outpatient sex offender treatment programs using the Structured Clinical Interview for DSM-IV. The lifetime prevalence of psychoactive substance disorder was 60%. Kafka and Hennen (2002) clinically assessed 120 consecutively evaluated outpatient males with paraphilias (N = 88, including N = 60 sex offenders) and so-called paraphilia-related disorders (N = 32) according to DSM-IV diagnoses. In both groups psychoactive substance abuse (40%), especially alcohol abuse (30%), were commonly diagnosed. Cocaine abuse was statistically significantly associated with paraphilia, and paraphilic sex offenders were more likely to be diagnosed with alcohol and cocaine abuse. In a study by Dunsieth et al. (2004) 85% of the convicted sex offenders met the DSM-IV criteria for a psychoactive substance use disorder.

Nonparaphilic men had shown more substance abuse than paraphilic individuals.

Taking together the results from the different studies a significant proportion of sexual offenders or paraphilic patients suffer from substance use disorders. However, studies often lack appropriate comparison groups. As a conclusion at the moment it remains unclear, if and to what extend sexual offenders differ in a characteristic way from offenders in general or similar sociodemographical populations without sexual offending. Acute effects, that is, intoxications seem to be as common as in other offender groups. Substance use may be more prevalent in rapists than in child molesters and more prevalent in nonparaphilic than in paraphilic sexual offender groups.

PHARMACOLOGY

There are different ways to consume substances (ingestion, sniffing, inhalation, injection) that influence the pharmacodynamic and pharmacokinetic reactions and the resulting psychopathology. In addition, the consumers' physiology, psychology, and tolerance, the setting, and the expectations play a major role. The relevant substances can be differentiated into CNS depressants (e.g., alcohol, barbiturates, opiates, benzodiazepines), stimulants (cocaine, amphetamines, ecstasy), hallucinogens (marijuana, LSD, PCP), and finally anabolics. While the consumption of all drugs (except anabolics) leads via different pathways to a higher concentration of dopamine in brain circuits (e.g., 35-fold increase in cocaine, 2-fold increase in alcohol), the substances differ in their effect on other neurotransmitter systems (e.g., cocaine has a substantial influence on the serotonergic system). It is not within the scope of this article to discuss the specific neurobiological features of all substances in detail. We will focus on effects on aggression and sexuality. Table 18.2 gives an overview about factors and mechanisms that influence the effects of psychoactive substance use on aggressive and sexual behavior.

Alcohol

Alcohol has complex and variable effects on sexuality, aggression, and violent behavior depending on dose, personality, previous experience with the substance,

TABLE 18.2 Factors and Mechanisms Influencing the Effects of Psychoactive Substance Use on Aggressive and Sexual Behavior

Personality and intelligence

Brain disorder

Expectancy about the effect of the substance

Experience with the substance (i.e., tolerance, dependence)

Dose and bioavailability (blood and brain levels)

Effects of short-term or long-term administration

The affection of different neurotransmitter systems or hormones

The victims activity and factors in the setting

Modified from Volavka, 2002.

and factors such as behavior and intoxication of the victim (Volavka, 2002). Alcohol may increase aggression

- directly by anesthetizing the centers of the brain that normally inhibit aggressive responding (*physiological disinhibition explanation*);
- because people expect it (*expectancy explanation*); or
- by causing changes within the person that increases the probability of aggression (e.g., by reducing intellectual functioning; *indirect cause explanation*).

In a review by Bushman (1997) meta-analytic procedures were used to test the validity of these three explanations of alcohol-related aggression. The results were inconsistent with the physiological disinhibition and expectancy explanations, but were consistent with the indirect cause explanation. Experimental manipulations that increased aggression (e.g., provocations, frustrations, aggressive cues) had a stronger effect on intoxicated participants than on sober participants. Ito et al. (1996) conducted a meta-analysis of 49 studies to investigate two explanations of how alcohol increases aggression by decreasing sensitivity to cues that inhibit it. Both, the level of anxiety and inhibition conflict moderated the difference between the aggressive behavior of sober and intoxicated participants, but neither level adequately accounted for the variation in effect sizes. Additional analyses of three social psychological moderating variables—provocation, frustration, and self-focused attention—showed that the

aggressiveness of intoxicated participants relative to sober ones increased as a function of frustration but decreased as a function of provocation and self-focused attention.

The use of alcohol is believed to loosen sexual inhibitions and contribute to increased sexual activity. However, the actual direct and indirect effects of alcohol on sexual function are still not fully understood. In men, high alcohol doses generally reduce physiological sexual responding, whereas low and moderate alcohol doses increase subjective sexual arousal. Many studies have demonstrated that men who believe they have consumed alcohol experience greater physiological and subjective sexual arousal in response to erotic materials depicting consensual and forced sex than do men who believe they have consumed a nonalcoholic beverage, regardless of what they actually drank (Crowe & George, 1989). Barbaree et al. (1983) demonstrated that alcohol intoxication produced significantly more arousal to rape scenes in normal males than did a placebo condition. Furthermore, in laboratory studies, intoxicated men tend to retaliate strongly when they feel threatened, and once they begin behaving aggressively, they can only be stopped with great difficulty (Taylor & Chermack, 1993). Wormith et al. (1988) compared rapists and nonrapists who had been referred for a forensic evaluation by penile circumference responses (as a psychophysiological measurement of sexual arousal) and self-reported arousal to consenting sex, sexual assault, and physical assault. The assessments were repeated following instructions of the offenders to suppress their arousal and following the ingestion of alcohol. An alcohol-by-offender type interaction revealed that the lowering effect of alcohol on penile circumference response occurred only among the nonrapists. The suppression instruction paradoxically *increased* rapists' penile circumference response to rape and physical assault presentations relative to consenting sexual narrations. When the data were examined in relation to intelligence, low IQ-rapists displayed greater responses to rape than high-IQ rapists. Under the influence of alcohol, low-IQ rapists displayed greater arousal regardless of the stimulus, while high-IQ rapists showed no change, and nonrapists responded less than they did without alcohol. Abbey et al. (2003) in their study on 113 college men who reported that they had committed a sexual assault found that the quantity of alcohol the men consumed during the assault was linearly related to the level of aggression.

The anticipation of alcohol effects may especially facilitate sexual aggression in offenders with antisocial personality traits or disorders. Aromaki and Lindman (2001) compared rapists (N = 10) and child molesters (N = 10) with control subjects (N = 31). Cognitive expectancies related to alcohol use were explored by a standard questionnaire. Alcohol abuse was common in men convicted of both rape and child molesting and both sexual offender groups were the only groups to express significant alcohol-related cognitive expectancies linked to arousal and aggression. Expectancy patterns were linked to the antisocial personality characteristics. Since antisocial and dominance traits may be associated with higher testosterone levels and testosterone itself may enhance the effects on alcohol (Volavka, 2002, p. 39), there could exist biological interactions.

Discussing the long-term effects of alcohol abuse and addiction co-occurring factors have to be mentioned and to be controlled when trying to develop any explanation. For example, the Cloninger et al. (1981) typology revealed that type II alcohol abusers frequently show violence and antisocial personality disorders. Antisocial personality disorder may increase the propensity both to drink and to commit sexual violence. In addition, hormonal factors (e.g., long-term abuse of alcohol leads to a testosterone decrease), neurotransmitter interactions (e.g., a possible serotonergic dysfunction in type II alcohol abusers), and neurological symptoms (Briken et al., 2005) can interact with each other.

At the moment it can only be concluded with enough confidence that acute- and long-term effects of alcohol probably play a contributive but not a primary causal role in sexual offending (Peugh & Belenko, 2001).

Effects of Drugs

Evidence for a linkage between drug abuse and sexual offending varies depending on the drug. Not only pharmacological factors are important but also social, legal, and treatment factors (e.g., the availability of methadone treatment). While on one side there may be factors leading to an increased risk of sexual offending via an increase in aggression or libido, on the other side there may be drug abuse related factors that lead to a loss in libido or sexual dysfunctions. For example, Johnson et al. (2004) presented data about the prevalence of sexual dysfunctions

(DSM-III criteria) and their association with comorbid drug and alcohol use in a community epidemiologic sample (N = 3004). The prevalence of lifetime substance use among this population was 37%, with males meeting more drug and alcohol use criteria than females. After controlling for demographics, health status variables, and psychiatric comorbidity (depression, generalized anxiety disorder, and antisocial personality disorder), inhibited orgasm was associated with marijuana and alcohol use. Painful sex was associated with illicit drug use and marijuana use. Inhibited sexual excitement was more likely among illicit drug users. Decreased sexual desire was not associated with drug or alcohol use. Mentioning the role of substance abuse for sexual dysfunctions does not implicate that a sexual dysfunction is necessarily a protective factor *against* sexual offending. Sexual dysfunction in sexual offenders was rarely investigated but may be more frequent than one might expect (Hill et al., 2007).

On the other hand using a drug to enhance sexual experience is common. In a study on a nonclinical population by Foxman et al. (2006) the most commonly used substances were alcohol (83.7%), marijuana (34.7%), ecstasy, or "sextasy" (ecstasy combined with sildenafil; 8.2%), and sildenafil (7.5%).

Psychostimulants (Cocaine and Amphetamines)

In animals, effects of psychostimulants differ depending on species; social position in the group; and dose of the substance. In some species low doses may elicit aggression and sexual arousal while high doses may have an opposite effect (Volavka, 2002). Cocaine is used as hydrochloride salt (mostly intranasal or in a dissolved form intravenously) or as a free base ("crack"). Amphetamines were widely prescribed until the mid 1960s as stimulants and appetite suppressants, until the dependence potential was recognized. Amphetamine derivates are still prescribable for certain disorders (e.g., narcolepsy, attention-deficit hyperactivity disorders). The effects of amphetamines and cocaine are very similar, both affecting the same neurotransmitter systems. Amphetamines stimulate catecholamine release and cocaine reduces reuptake. "Ecstasy" (MDMA) and related drugs are amphetamine derivates that also have some of the pharmacological properties of hallucinogens. They have become popular in party scenes because they may enhance energy and sexual arousal.

Several studies reveal an association between chronic or heavy cocaine or amphetamine use and increased sexual activity and/or high-risk sexual behaviors, and use of both is considered a risk factor for HIV infection (for a review, Ross & Williams, 2001). However, none of these studies have resolved the question of whether psychostimulant consumption causes such behavior, or whether such behavior and drug use are both symptoms of an underlying risk-taking or sensation-seeking personality. Studies investigating the role of psychostimulants in sexual offenders specifically are missing. Clinical evidence however suggests that chronic stimulant users may be more likely to engage in sexual activity than users of other drugs (e.g., opiates). Cocaine and amphetamines can also cause intoxication and delusional disorders that may result in sexual aggressive behavior in special cases.

As a result of a small case control study Kafka and Hennen (2000) discuss the use of the psychostimulant methylphenidate for the *treatment* of paraphilic patients with a *comorbid diagnosis of attention-deficit hyperactivity disorder* in combination with SSRI antidepressants. With this combination effects on sexual arousal and aggression should be monitored cautiously.

Hallucinogens and Cannabis

To our knowledge there are no specific investigations about hallucinogens and sexual offending. Cannabis neither has a clear pharmacologic effect on neither an increased risk for aggression nor an increase in sexual arousability while dependence on cannabis may be associated with a higher risk for violent crimes (Volavka, 2002).

Opioids

Opioid use normally produces a decline in sexual functioning in men (loss of sexual interest, complete loss of sexual functioning, [Meston & Frohlich, 2000]) as well as a short-term antiaggressive effect. Opioids produce a decrease in sexual hormones like testosterone that might lead to sexual dysfunction. Withdrawal from opiate dependence on the other side can be characterized by an increased frequency of morning erections and spontaneous ejaculations

and also to dysphoria or aggression. However, to our knowledge there are no studies reporting specifically sexual offenses under opioid use.

Benzodiazepines

Benzodiazepines normally have sedative effects but can occasionally produce paradoxical increase of agitation. The benzodiazepine flunitrazepam is extensively prescribed to patients with insomnia in many countries, but has also become popular among alcohol and drug abusers. Some reports indicate that flunitrazepam is used as a "date rape" drug (Schwartz, Milteer, & LeBeau, 2000; Slaughter, 2000) and suggest that it could also precipitate violent behavior. It can be served to a prospective victim without her knowledge because it easily dissolves in water and is tasteless. Perpetrators choose these drugs because they act rapidly, produce disinhibition (particularly in combination with alcohol), muscle relaxation, and cause the victim to have lasting anterograde amnesia for events that occur under the influence of the drug.

Flunitrazepame is often used along with GHB (gamma-hydroxybutyrate, liquid ecstasy). GHB is a typical "date rape" agent as it is relatively easy to obtain, and it causes a rapid relaxing and disinhibitory effect. Moreover, since it is colorless and odor free, it is easily added to the potential victim's drink. GHB is difficult to identify in the urine as it is quickly eliminated from the body (Smith, 1999).

Anabolic Steroids

Anabolic–androgenic steroids (AAS) are synthetic derivatives of testosterone originally designed for therapeutic uses to provide enhanced anabolic potency with negligible androgenic effects. The effects on organs and the prevalence of altered behaviors in AAS abusers have been well documented in a number of studies (Trenton & Currier, 2005). Steroids may be used in oral or intramuscular preparations. Commonly, steroid users employ these agents at levels 10- to 100-fold in excess of therapeutic doses and use multiple substances simultaneously. Significant symptoms including aggression and violence, mania, and less frequently psychosis and suicide have been associated with steroid abuse. Long-term steroid abusers may develop symptoms of dependence and withdrawal on discontinuation of AAS. In a study by Borowsky et al. (1997), anabolic steroide use was a factor that differentiated between sexual aggressive and nonaggressive adolescents. Driessen et al. (1996) reported about a single case of child sexual abuse associated with anabolic androgenic steroid use.

"ADDICTIVE"-LIKE BEHAVIOR PATTERNS IN THE ETIOLOGY OF SEXUAL OFFENDING

The terminology for an "addictive" sexual behavior has a long tradition following the description by Richard von Krafft-Ebings (1886) of a so-called "Hyperesthesia sexualis" showing similarities to morphinism or alcoholism. Giese (1962)—a prominent German sex researcher—considered an *addictive course* as a diagnostic criterion of perversions (in that time synonymously used for paraphilias). The guidelines he used for his definition are similar to definitions for addiction:

- Decline in pure sensuality
- Increase in frequency accompagnied by a decrease in satisfaction
- Increasing promiscuity and anonymity of contacts
- Elaboration of fantasy, practice, and refinement
- Feeling compulsively addicted
- Periodicity of an urging restlessness

The terms sexual addiction (Carnes, 1983), compulsive sexual behavior (Coleman, Raymond, & McBean, 2003), and paraphilia-related disorder (Kafka & Hennen, 2002) were used to describe paraphilic and/or nonparaphilic sexual activities (compulsive masturbation, protracted promiscuity, dependency on pornography, or telephone sex). Some sex offenders themselves describe the escalating character of paraphilic activities as a form of addiction that absorbs them and seems to make it impossible for them to take into account the interests of other individuals.

Dysregulations of the dopamine system may cause individuals to have a high risk for addictive, impulsive, and compulsive behavioral propensities, such as drug-using behavior, attention-deficit hyperactivity disorder, antisocial traits, and also compulsive or "addictive"-like sexual behavior (Blum et al., 2000). All of the underlying psychopathological phenomena as well as normal repetitive and stimulating behavior may be connected to the mesolimbic dopamine system. However, much more research is necessary to clarify under what conditions a stimulus can activate and hijack this system and override other stimuli. The ability of individuals to invest in relationships may also enhance their ability to exchange needs and gratification of wishes with others and thus handle them with more control. Probably the feedback-loops, which connect this system with different parts of the prefrontal cortex (including the fronto-orbital cortex), influence the activity of the mesolimbic dopamine system in the "working-memory" (according to LeDoux, 2002, p. 245) and submit its activity under the influence of socially preformed judgment. Beauregard et al. (2001) demonstrated that in their impressive experiment on attempted inhibition of sexual arousal. In their study, brain activation was measured in normal men while they voluntarily attempted to inhibit the sexual arousal induced by viewing erotic stimuli. Their findings suggest that emotional self-regulation is normally implemented by a neural circuit including various prefrontal regions and subcortical limbic structures. Substance-induced frontal lobe dysfunction has been hypothesized to explain the impairment of self-control in addictions (Lyvers, 2000) but also in psychopathy (e.g., Yang, Raine, Lencz, Bihrle, LaCasse, & Colletti, 2005).

Looman et al. (2004) investigated and discussed Marshall's (1989) theory of intimacy deficits and insecure attachment patterns related to substance use disorders in sexual offenders and argue that these problems may act synergistically. The "self-medication hypothesis" by Khantzian (1997) describes that individuals predisposed by biological vulnerabilities consume substances in a more or less successful attempt to relieve psychological suffering with maybe some degree of substance specifity. From our viewpoint in a substantial subgroup of sexual offenders, not only alcohol and drugs but also paraphilic or nonparaphilic sexual activity may be used to cope with negative mood states such as depression, anxiety, loneliness, or boredom. The pathways may act synergistically but also alternating, and may be used to facilitate sexual arousal or aggression either as actively planned or as a more impulsive activity. Intimacy and attachment deficits may be underlying but unspecific roots that lead to moderating neurobiological associations (e.g., serotonergic dysregulation) and vice versa. Animal studies and observations lead to the suggestion that factors like attachment (Beech & Mitchell, 2005), social position (dominant or subordinate individuals), and temperament may moderate the individual effects of drugs into one or the other direction (inhibition or disinhibition). New experiences through the lifespan may change and moderate the balance between inhibition and disinhibition again.

Recidivism

The updated meta-analysis by Hanson and Morton-Bourgon (2004) again revealed that paraphilia and antisocial traits are the major risk factor for recidivism in sexual offenders. Substance abuse (31 studies with a total N = 9166) and substance intoxication (10 studies with a total N = 5276) during offense were significantly correlated to recidivism in sexual offenders but not sufficiently predictive to be used as a single factor for risk assessment. For example, in the follow-up study by Langström et al. (2004) a prior diagnosis of alcohol abuse or dependence more than doubled and a diagnosis of drug use disorder tripled the odds ratio for the index offense (while the odds ratio for personality disorders was 10.1). Evaluation of risk assessment needs to consider a variety of factors and in most currently used instruments alcohol and drug use disorders is one of them.

Treatment

Treatment programs for sexual offenders rarely focus on individual alcohol or drug problems. In the study by Peugh and Belenko (2001), only 34% of incarcerated sexual offenders with substance problems reported that they received a drug treatment and 21% participated in self-help groups. However, the relapse prevention model frequently used to treat sexual offenders was first employed as an approach to the treatment of substance dependent patients. It remains questionable to describe sexual offending or paraphilias as an analogue for addictions (see the aforementioned text). In addition, there is still little empirical evidence supporting that adoption of the relapse prevention model for sexual offenders alone reduces recidivism or prevents relapses. However, especially in patients with substance abuse disorders this model may be useful to explain and prevent both, substance abuse and the offense cycle. This cycle is initiated by so-called "seemingly unimportant decisions" (Eccles & Marshall, 1999). Such decisions may increase the probability for high-risk

situations. These situations themselves may have to do with substance abuse, consumption, or a failure to cope with problematic life situations. Looman et al. (2004) integrate the impact of substance abuse problems with reference to intimacy problems and help their clients to understand the way substance abuse may result in greater problems coping with anxiety and depression but also in the context of a criminal lifestyle (e.g., selling drugs). Participation in self-help groups can also be helpful.

Mandated addiction treatment can have as good outcome as voluntary treatment (Miller & Flaherty, 2000). Sentencing may involve requirements regarding treatment and sobriety (abstinence) as terms of probation and parole. Progress reports, treatment participation, and urine toxicological tests can be part of such requirements.

Pharmacotherapy can include medications for supporting abstinence, such as methadone for opiate dependence, antabuse for alcohol dependence, and also—hypothetically more specific—naltrexone (Kiefer et al., 2003; Ryback, 2004). Naltrexone is a long-acting opioid used in the treatment of alcoholism, drug abuse, obsessive-compulsive disorder, and impulse-control disorders. Ryback (2004) investigated whether naltrexone can also decrease sexual arousal in adolescent sexual offenders. In an open-ended prospective study, naltrexone was given to 21 adolescents participating in an inpatient adolescent sexual offenders program. Leuprolide was given if naltrexone was not sufficiently helpful. Fifteen of twenty-one patients were considered to have a positive result with decreased sexual fantasies and masturbation. Future research should focus on the question if naltrexone is an appropriate medication especially for sex offenders with substance use disorders and should then be considered in pharmacological treatment algorithms (Briken, Hill, & Berner, 2003).

References

Abbey, A., Ross, L. T., & McDuffie, D. (1994). Alcohol's role in sexual assault. In R. R. Watson (Ed.), *Drug and alcohol abuse reviews: Addictive behaviors in women* (Vol. 5, pp. 97–123). Totowa, NJ: Humana Press.

Abbey, A., Clinton-Sherrod, A. M., McAuslan, P., Zawacki, T., & Buck, P. O. (2003). The relationship between the quantity of alcohol consumed and the severity of sexual assaults committed by college men. *Journal of Interpersonal Violence, 18,* 813–833.

Abracen, J., Looman, J., & Anderson, D. (2000). Alcohol and drug abuse in sexual and nonsexual violent offenders. *Sexual Abuse: A Journal of Research and Treatment*, 12, 263–274.

Allnutt, S. H., Bradford, J. M., Greenberg, D. M., & Curry, S. (1996). Co-morbidity of alcoholism and the paraphilias. *Journal of Forensic Science*, 41, 234–239.

American Psychiatric Association. (2000). *Diagnostic and Statistical Manual of Mental Disorders, Forth Edition, Text Revision*. Washington, DC, American Psychiatric Association.

Aromaki, A. S. & Lindman, R. E. (2001). Alcohol expectancies in convicted rapists and child molesters. *Criminal Behavior and Mental Health*, 11, 94–101.

Arseneault, L., Moffitt, T. E., Caspi, A., Taylor, P. J., & Silva, P. A. (2000). Mental disorders and violence in a total birth cohort: Results from the Dunedin Study. *Archives of General Psychiatry*, 57, 979–986.

Barbaree, H. E., Marshall, W. L., Yates, E., & Lightfoot, L. O. (1983). Alcohol intoxication and deviant sexual arousal in male social drinkers. *Behaviour Research and Therapy*, 21, 365–373.

Beauregard, M., Levesque, J., & Bourgouin, P. (2001). Neural correlates of conscious self-regulation of emotion. *Journal of Neuroscience*, 21, RC165.

Beech, A. B. & Mitchell, I. J. (2005). A neurobiological perspective on attachment problems in sexual offenders and the role of selective serotonin re-uptake inhibitors in the treatment of such problems. *Clinical Psychology Review*, 25, 153–182.

Blum, K., Braverman, E. R., Holder, J. M., Lubar, J. F., Monastra, V. J., Miller, D., et al. (2000). Reward deficiency syndrome: A biogenetic model for the diagnosis and treatment of impulsive, addictive, and compulsive behaviors. *Journal of Psychoactive Drug*, 32(Suppl. 1), 112.

Borowsky, I. W., Hogan, M., & Ireland, M. (1997). Adolescent sexual aggression: Risk and protective factors. *Pediatrics*, 100, E7.

Briken, P., Nika, E., & Berner, W. (2000). Alkoholisierung und Alkoholprobleme im Zusammenhang mit sexuell motivierten Tötungsdelikten—eine thematische Übersicht und Ergebnisse aus 30 psychiatrischen Ggutachten. *Recht & Psychiatrie*, 18, 183–188.

Briken, P., Hill, A., & Berner, W. (2003). Pharmacotherapy of paraphilias with long-acting agonists of luteinizing hormone-releasing hormone: A systematic review. *Journal of Clinical Psychiatry*, 64, 890–897.

Briken, P., Habermann, N., Berner, W., & Hill A. (2005). The influence of brain abnormalities on psychosocial development, criminal history and paraphilias in sexual murderers. *Journal of Forensic Science*, 50, 1204–1208.

Briken, P., Habermann, N., Kafka, M. P., Berner, W., & Hill, A. (2006) The paraphilia-related disorders: An investigation of the relevance of the concept in sexual murderers. *Journal of Forensic Science*, 51, 683–688.

Bushman, B. J. (1997). Effects of alcohol on human aggression. Validity of proposed explanations. *Recent Developments in Alcoholism*, 13, 227–243.

Carnes, P. J. (1983). *Out of the shadows: Understanding sexual addiction*. Minneapolis, MN: CompCare Publications.

Cloninger, C. R., Bohman, M., & Sigvardsson, S. (1981). Inheritance of alcohol abuse. Cross-fostering analysis of adopted men. *Archives of General Psychiatry*, 38, 861–868.

Cochrane, R. E., Grisso, T., & Frederick, R. I. (2001). The relationship between criminal charges, diagnoses, and psycholegal opinions among federal pretrial defendants. *Behavioral Sciences and the Law*, 19, 565–582.

Coleman, E., Raymond, N., & McBean, A. (2003). Assessment and treatment of compulsive sexual behavior. *Minnesota Medicine*, 86, 42–47.

Compton, W. M., Conway, K. P., Stinson, F. S., Colliver, J. D., & Grant, B. F. (2005). Prevalence, correlates, and comorbidity of DSM-IV antisocial personality syndromes and alcohol and specific drug use disorders in the United States: Results from the national epidemiologic survey on alcohol and related conditions. *Journal of Clinical Psychiatry*, 66, 677–685.

Crowe, L. C. & George, W. H. (1989). Alcohol and human sexuality: Review and integration. *Psychological Bulletin*, 105, 374–386.

Driessen, M., Muessigbrodt, H., Dilling, H., & Driessen, B. (1996). Child sexual abuse associated with anabolic androgenic steroid use. *American Journal of Psychiatry*, 153, 1369.

Dunsieth, N. W. Jr, Nelson, E. B., Brusman-Lovins, L. A., Holcomb, J. L., Beckman, D., Welge, J. A., et al. (2004). Psychiatric and legal features of 113 men convicted of sexual offenses. *Journal of Clinical Psychiatry*, 65, 293–300.

Eccles, A. & Marshall W. L. (1999). *Relapse prevention*. In W. L. Marshall, D. Anderson, & Y. Fernandez (Ed.), *Cognitive behavioral treatment of sexual offenders* (pp. 127–146). Chichester: John Wiley & Sons, LTD.

Firestone, P., Dixon, K. L., Nunes, K. L., & Bradford, J. M. (2005). A comparison of incest offenders based on victim age. *Journal of the American Academy of Psychiatry and the Law*, 33, 223–232.

Foxman, B., Aral, S. O., & Holmes, K. K. (2006). Common use in the general population of sexual enrichment AIDS and drugs to enhance sexual experience. *Sexually Transmitted Diseases*, 33, 156–162.

Giese, H. (1962). Leitsymptome sexueller perversionen. In H. Giese (Ed.). *Psychopathologie der Sexualität* (pp. 420–465). Stuttgart: Enke.

Hanson R. K. & Morton-Bourgon A. (2004). Predictors of sexual offender recidivism: An updated meta-analysis. Canada: Public Works and Government Services.

Hill, A., Habermann, N., Berner, W., & Briken, P. (2007). Single and multiple sexual homicide. *Psychopathology*, 40, 22–28.

Ito, T. A., Miller, N., & Pollock, V. E. (1996). Alcohol and aggression: A meta-analysis on the moderating effects of inhibitory cues, triggering events, and self-focused attention. *Psychological Bulletin*, 120, 60–82.

Johnson, S. D., Phelps, D. L., & Cottler, L. B. (2004). The association of sexual dysfunction and substance use among a community epidemiological sample. *Archives of Sexual Behavior*, 33, 55–63.

Kafka, M. P. & Hennen, J. (2000). Psychostimulant augmentation during treatment with selective serotonin reuptake inhibitors in men with paraphilias and paraphilia-related disorders: A case series. *Journal of Clinical Psychiatry*, 2000, 61, 664–670.

Khantzian, E. J. (1997). The self-medication hypothesis of substance use disorders: A reconsideration and recent applications. *Harvard Review of Psychiatry*, 4, 231–244.

Kiefer, F., Jahn, H., Tarnaske, T., Helwig, H., Briken, P., Holzbach, R., et al. (2003). Comparing and combining naltrexone and acamprosate in relapse prevention of alcoholism: A double-blind, placebo-controlled study. *Archives of General Psychiatry*, 60, 92–99.

von Krafft-Ebing, R. (1886). *Psychopathia Sexualis. Eine klinisch-forensische Sstudie.* Stuttgart: Ferdinand Enke.

Langevin, R. & Lang, R. A. (1990). Substance abuse among sex offenders. Annals of Sex Research, 3, 397–424.

Langevin, R. (2003). A Study of the psychosexual characteristics of sex killers: can we identify them before it is too late? International Journal of Offender Therapy and Comparitive Criminology, 47, 366–382.

Langström, N., Sjostedt, G., & Grann, M. (2004). Psychiatric disorders and recidivism in sexual offenders. *Sexual Abuse: A Journal of Research and Treatment*, 16, 139–150.

LeDoux, J. (2002). *Synaptic self: How our brains become who we are.* London: Penguin Books.

Looman, J., Abracen, J., DiFazio, R., & Maillet, G. (2004). Alcohol and drug abuse among sexual and nonsexual offenders: Relationship to intimacy deficits and coping strategy. *Sexual Abuse: A Journal of Research and Treatment*, 16, 177–189.

Lyvers, M. (2000). "Loss of control" in alcoholism and drug addiction: A neuroscientific interpretation. *Experimental and Clinical Psychopharmacology*, 8, 225–249.

Marshall, W. L. (1989). Intimacy, loneliness and sexual offenders. *Behaviour, Research and Therapy*, 27, 491–503.

McLellan, A. T., Kushner, H., Metzger, D., Peters, R., Smith, I., Grissom, G., et al. (1992). The Fifth Edition of the Addiction Severity Index. *Journal of Substance Abuse and Treatment*, 9, 199–213.

Meston, C. M. & Frohlich, P. F. (2000). The neurobiology of sexual function. *Archives of General Psychiatry*, 57, 1012–1030.

Miller, N. S. & Flaherty, J. A. (2000). Effectiveness of coerced addiction treatment (alternative consequences): A review of the clinical research. *Journal of Substance Abuse*, 18, 9–16.

Nika, E. & Briken, P. (2004). Suchtbehandlung unter besonderen Bbedingungen. In M. Krausz & C. Haasen (Ed.), *Kompendium Ssucht.* Stuttgart (pp. 129–142). New York: Georg Thieme Verlag.

Peugh, J. & Belenko, S. (2001). Examining the substance use patterns and treatment needs of incarcerated sex offenders. *Sexual Abuse: A Journal of Research and Treatment*, 13, 179–195.

Raymond, N. C., Coleman, E., Ohlerking, F., Christenson, G. A., & Miner M. (1999). Psychiatric comorbidity in pedophilic sex offenders. *American Journal of Psychiatry*, 156, 786–788.

Ross, M. W. & Williams, M. L. (2001). Sexual behavior and illicit drug use. *Annual Review of Sex Research*, 12, 290–310.

Ryback, R. S. (2004). Naltrexone in the treatment of adolescent sexual offenders. *Journal of Clinical Psychiatry*, 65, 982–986.

Schwartz, R. H., Milteer, R., & LeBeau, M. A. (2000). Drug-facilitated sexual assault ('date rape'). *Southern Medical Journal*, 93, 558–561.

Selzer, M. L. (1971). The Michigan alcoholism screening test: the quest for a new diagnostic instrument. American Journal of Psychiatry, 127, 1653–1658.

Slaughter, L. (2000). Involvement of drugs in sexual assault. *Journal of Reproductive Medicine*, 45, 425–430.

Smith, K. M. (1999). Drugs used in acquaintance rape. *Journal of the American Pharmaceutical Association*, 39, 519–525.

Stinson, F. S., Grant, B. F., Dawson, D. A., Ruan, W. J., Huang, B., & Saha, T. (2005). Comorbidity between DSM-IV alcohol and specific drug use disorders in the United States: Results from the National Epidemiologic Survey on Alcohol and Related Conditions. *Drug and Alcohol Dependence*, 80, 105–116.

Taylor, S. P. & Chermack, S. T. (1993). Alcohol, drugs, and human physical aggression. *Journal of Studies on Alcohol*, 11, 78–88.

Trenton, A. J. & Currier, G. W. (2005). Behavioural manifestations of anabolic steroid use. CNS *Drugs*, 19, 571–595.

Volavka, J. (2002). *Neurobiology of violence. Second edition.* Inc. Washington DC, London England: American Psychiatric Publishing.

Wormith, J. S., Bradford, J. M., Pawlak, A., Borzecki, M., & Zohar, A. (1988). The assessment of deviant sexual arousal as a function of intelligence, instructional set and alcohol ingestion. *Canadian Journal of Psychiatry*, 33, 800–808.

Yang, Y., Raine, A., Lencz, T., Bihrle, S., LaCasse, L., & Colletti, P. (2005). Volume reduction in prefrontal gray matter in unsuccessful criminal psychopaths. *Biological Psychiatry*, 57, 1103–1108.

Chapter 19

Female Sexual Offenders

Wolfgang Berner, Peer Briken, and Andreas Hill

Approximately 1% of sentenced sexual offenders are female. Investigations on victims of child molestation reveal participation of female perpetrators in at least a quarter of cases of male victims and in 13% of female victims.

The spectrum of offenses of female offenders ranges from minor forms of indecency, exhibitionism, different forms of child molestation, and incest to all forms of aggressive acts including rape and murder. Male and female children are the most prominent victims. In a high percentage of offenses the female offender acts together with a male accomplice. Only in rare cases a diagnosis of paraphilia is reported, far more frequent are different forms of depression, alcohol and drug abuse, and personality disorders (borderline, antisocial, dependent). Most authors agree that a high percentage (over 50%) of female sexual offenders were themselves victims of sexual and/or physical abuse. Conflicts with the mother and resulting problems with women—especially mother identity—are reported by psychodynamically oriented authors.

Only few case reports exist on effective medical treatment with SSRI and antiandrogens. A carefully differentiated psychotherapeutic treatment program including group-, individual- and social-therapeutic strategies was developed especially in Minnesota.

Studies comparing the incidence of male and female sex offending mostly come to the result that one sentenced female sexual offender corresponds to approximately 100 male sexual offenders (Berner, Karlick-Bolton, & Fodor, 1987; Groth, 1979; O'Connor, 1987; Vandiver & Kercher, 2004). Therefore, it is understandable that most empirical studies on female sex offending are based on much smaller samples than studies on male sex offending, mostly with less than 30 female offenders. According to Finkelhor and Russel (1984) the extremely low "official" prevalence of female sex offending may be the result of underreporting, as women may have more possibilities to mask their inappropriate contact with children than men, their offenses often happening inside the family where reporting is rare and may be less physically injuring. Physical injury is correlated with higher rates of reporting, too. According to a study by Finkelhor and Russel (1984) on representative samples of female and male victims of sexual abuse; 24% of male victims and 13% of female victims had been abused by female perpetrators who either acted alone or with male partners. These figures do not allow a clear calculation of the prevalence of female sexual offenders who were not reported to the police. Nevertheless they corroborate the hypotheses that underreporting may play an important role in female offending.

Taking into account that not much is known about female sexual offending, the following chapter will focus on the differences between male and female sexual offending, as far as phenomenology, psychiatric diagnoses, treatment, and follow-up is concerned.

PHENOMENOLOGY

Some characteristics of female assaults simply may be explained by the fact that women have to consider men's superiority in physical strength while men as perpetrators may easily impress and threat their female victims. This can be demonstrated even in cases of "hands off" offenses like exhibitionism.

Exhibitionism

Only a few cases of female exhibitionism are described in the literature. Nevertheless the differences between these cases are exemplary. Female exhibitionism is much less stereotyped than male exhibitionism, and it is never known if it is related to direct sexual excitement or some other indirect form of psychologically experienced excitement or triumph (Zavitzianos, 1971). For instance, Hollender et al. (1977) described a case of female exhibitionism, which on the first glance seems very similar to male exhibitionism: "wearing only a raincoat she would stand in a doorway near the club, where she worked and flash (i.e., exhibit her breasts and genitals) before men she had seen or met previously" (p. 437). But according to the woman's explanation, she derived no sexual gratification from this behavior. She was neither seeking sexual liaisons nor soliciting customers for future shows. She stated that her motivation for flashing was solely attention seeking. The effort of this woman to draw attention to herself had a more desperate than aggressive quality, despite her profession of being a

glamorous dancer. Further she flashed before men she knew, while male exhibitionists nearly exclusively flash before women who are unknown to them. Nearly 10 years later Grob (1985) described a case of female exhibitionism with similar background but nevertheless differences in more than one aspect: A 43-year-old divorced female patient exhibited breasts and genitals to passing by truck-drivers on the highway while driving in her small car. It was not uncommon for her to spend as much as 30 minutes with a particular truck, playing an exhibitionistic cat-and-mouse teasing game, before suddenly turning off on an exit ramp where trucks could not follow. Contrary to the first case, this woman experienced high sexual arousal during the act and sometimes even orgasm. Similarities can be seen in the family background: both women have a dynamic of early deprivation of parental attention resulting in a profound inability to sustain deep personal relationships and a nearly addictive craving for a bodily experienced attention. In the second case, constant contact to an emotionally supporting therapist could reduce the tendency to exhibit and the attenuation of contact (for instance to a therapist) resulted in an increased craving for exhibitionistic activity.

Fear of being attacked by a stronger male may have been the reason why the first of the former described female exhibitionists only acted if she knew her male victims and the second choose a procedure where she easily could escape. But there may also exist a lot of other causes for differences in male and female sexual offending. For further exploration in this field we will examine a small sample of case histories from different clinical backgrounds:

Indecency

O'Connor (1987) reported on a representative sample of female sexual offenders who were committed to the main female remand prison for London and South East England between 1974 and 1985. Of these 19 women were charged with "Indecency" and 39 with "Indecent Assault" and "Indecency with Children." Only two of these cases were clear cases of "Indecent exposure," the term used for sentencing exhibitionism at court. One indecency consisted of urinating in public by a mentally handicapped woman who was drunk. In a case of "Outraging Public Decency" a 25-year-old single woman with a history of recurrent hypomanic episodes and several hospital admissions exposed her genitals in public inviting passers by to commit acts of indecency with her. Treatment of her hypomanic mood ended this episode immediately. In this study criminal recidivism was not reported.

Rape

Sarrel and Masters (1982) selected four cases where men were forced to sexual activities by physical constrains and life threatening from approximately 700 men who presented themselves to the Yale human sexuality program with a wide variety of problems and from over 3500 couples treated at the Masters and Johnson institute for sexual dysfunctions. In one case, a 27-year-old man was given a drink and afterward was tied to a bedstead, gagged, and blindfolded by a group of women. He was stimulated to erection and ejaculation, afterward restimulated until he was unable to function and then threatened with castration. In a second case two older men entrapped a 17-year-old boy, and three older women threatened to beat him up if he tried to get away. He was manually stimulated and fellated until ejaculation three times before the group let him free. In a third case, a 37-year-old man was accosted by two women who forced him to have intercourse and fellatio at gunpoint and only in the fourth case a single woman forced a 23-year-old medical student to have intercourse with her by threatening him with a scalpel. The first important finding in these cases is, that despite obviously experienced anxiety the men were able to react sexually, and the second, that in all four cases the victims developed severe sexual dysfunctions after the rape.

Struckman-Johnson (1988) reports that sexual victimization against men has increased since the 1970s. In a survey on male and female college students she found that 43 (16%) of the 268 men in her sample reported that they had been forced to engage in sexual intercourse on a date. Despite the fact that a similar proportion of females reported the same fact (22%) the experience of the type of coercion was quite different. While most women reported being physically forced (55%), the men reported coercion by psychological tactics such as verbal pressure to avoid guilt over disappointing their partners. In several cases men were blackmailed, but none of the male victims was actually physically unable to escape. The most severe examples of sexual victimization in this study were a few men who had unwanted sex while they were intoxicated.

Taking these two studies together we have to conclude that rape of a man by a female perpetrator is an extremely rare event and mostly happens as group rape, often with the help of men.

Sexual Serial Murderers

Some cases of female serial killers became very famous in the popular media. One of the best known in England is Myra Hindley (1942–2002) who tortured and murdered two girls and three boys aged between 10 and 17 years together with her partner Ian Brady between 1963 and 1966. She met Ian Brady when she was 18 and became dependent on him. He gave her Hitler's "*Mein Kampf*" and the works of Marquise de Sade and she was the person who contacted the later victims. The couple took audiotapes from their deadly torture scenes, which were played during the court procedures and shocked the nation (en/wikipedia/org).

Another case is the story of Rosemary West born in 1953 (en/wikipedia/org): She was convicted of murdering 10 teenage girls, including her own common law step-daughter, Charmaine, and also of a serious sexual assault on a woman. The police suspected she was also involved in further murders for which she has not been convicted. She killed Charmaine on her own, but her other murders were all believed to have been carried out with her husband and fellow serial killer Fred West.

Rosemary West was 15 years old when she met Fred West. She was West's second wife and West had murdered already before he met Rosemary. The couple developed a habit of picking up girls from bus stops in and around Gloucester, England, whom they would imprison in their home for several days before killing them. During the time of their imprisonment, the victims were sadistically tortured. Both appeared to be "addicted" to sexual sadism.

Rosemary West was brought up in a large family, many of her siblings were in public care, and all were abused. Rosemary West had a voracious sexual appetite and enjoyed extreme bondage and sadomasochistic sex, even more than her husband. She was bisexual, but preferred women, and it is likely that her victims (apart from Charmaine) were picked up mostly for her sexual pleasure. She also worked as a prostitute, often preferring black clients, and these clients fathered many of her children. The West's home was littered with hard-pornographic videos. To the neighbors, they were "motherly Rose" and "friendly Fred," a devoted couple who ran a cheap rooming house.

Also in this case, the strong relationship to a serial killing man is the prominent characteristic and therefore differs from most cases of male sexual murderers.

It is also important to mention that such extraordinary and extreme rare cases are not a phenomenon of the last century alone. Similar descriptions can be found in classical literature, for instance the case of a Hungarian aristocrat, Elisabeth Bathory (1560–1614), who killed female adolescents to take a bath in their blood (Farin, 1989). Without male servants assisting her she would not have been able to carry out her cruel deeds.

Berner (1991) reported about a female patient who tried to kill her female lover at the age of 16 years. The girlfriend became afraid of the patient after she enticed her in a "playful" mutual strangling to the point of loosing consciousness. When the girlfriend announced separation the patient began to act in a very strange and irrational way reminding of a psychotic state: First she strangled cats to death, then killed one cat with a knife, and shocked her girlfriend with her bloody hands. When the girl turned away to escape, the patient stabbed her in the back, injuring her very seriously. After a year of psychiatric hospitalization she had sadomasochistic relationships to men whom she regularly injured with razor blades. After giving birth to a female baby the patient repressed her sadistic impulses for years and lived a rather unhedonistic life with strong sexual inhibitions. Not long before menopause when she was 45 and her daughter left home, the patient restarted to kill animals and again developed urging impulses to kill a girl, which brought her back in psychotherapy (see the following text). In her childhood, war and flight experiences had left their marks. After the death of her mother due to breast cancer when she was 7 years old she was raised in different boarding schools. The patient's father beat her heavily for dating secretly with a boy and other disobediences.

Extra Familiar Child Molestation

Molestation of children needs much less physical strength and is carried out more often by women without the assistance of other persons. These cases seem to happen more frequently than rape (Vandiver & Kercher, 2004) but modern authors seem to agree that paraphilia in the sense of pedophilia is rather rare. This is in some contrast to Krafft-Ebing (1890) who first described "paedophilia erotica" as a disorder that can be found in women, too. Chow and Choy (2002) recently described one rather typical example of such a pedophilic woman: A 23-year-old single mother of two sons aged 6 and 7 years was charged for sexual assault and sexual interference when she performed oral sex on two 4-year-old girls on two different occasions during babysitting. The first incidence happened when she was 18; her first victim was the 4-year-old daughter of a friend. Earlier that evening, the woman watched a pornographic video together with her adult boyfriend, which aroused her sexually. While bathing the little girl later she became further aroused by touching her. After the bath she took the girl into the bedroom, spread her legs and licked the girl's vaginal area for a few minutes. This was sexually gratifying to her. Nevertheless, after that she went to her boyfriend who was still sitting in the living room to have intercourse with him. Five years later—while babysitting two 4- and 5-year-old girls of some other acquainted parents—the woman again molested during a bath. When the 4-year-old girl did not want to get dressed the patient felt sexually invited and teased by the child and chased after her. Finally she caught the 4-year-old in the bedroom, rubbed its genitals with her finger, and again licked the whole genital area as in the first case. Afterward she secretly masturbated in the bathroom. The woman revealed traumatic experiences and clinical characteristics similar to the other cases described earlier. Her parents divorced when she was an infant, during puberty she was sexually harassed by her mother's stepfather, her complaints about it being dismissed by the mother. She became pregnant from her first boyfriend at the age of 15, and after giving birth to her two sons she separated from her boyfriend, obviously just around the time of her first assault on a little girl. As a teenager she often broke dishes out of rage and later she complained about problems controlling her impulses—especially concerning money spending. She described herself as bisexual, more erotically interested in females than in men, and more in girls than in women, but her desire to have socially acceptable relationships meant that she only had ongoing relationships with adult men. She recalled interest in 3- to 4-year-old girls since an "early age as a child" and regularly masturbated to fantasies involving girls, although she also fantasized about adult women and men.

This case can be contrasted with another one from our outpatient clinic.

The now 30-year-old woman presented 5 years ago with heavy guilt feelings for having abused a little 5-year-old boy while babysitting him. She manipulated his penis while masturbating herself. Another symptom at that time was that she experienced an impulse to provoke old women traveling together with her in the bus or underground by insulting them with obscene and devaluating words or by openly masturbating in front of them. Another problem was, that she had recently fallen in love with one of the female therapists concerned with her former inpatient treatment. She grew up in a family of teachers and had three academic siblings, one older brother of her may have abused her, but her memory of this experience remained unclear. As a child she had severe dyslexia, which resulted in extended conflicts with her ambivalently loved and hated mother. Her sexual orientation was homosexual but only rarely she succeeded in establishing short relationships to beloved partners. Because of general impulsivity and relationship problems including suicidal acts she was diagnosed with borderline personality disorder and admitted to an institutional treatment for years. Five years after her first contact to our clinic she showed up again, now with another sexual impulse. She tended to make obscene telephone-calls, shocking randomly selected women by insulting them with a male-like voice, pretending she would masturbate like a man. After ending the call she felt guilty and decided she would never do it again, but only a short time later she again became obsessed with the idea to repeat the act. The paraphilic symptomatology of this patient is unspecific and cannot be classified as pedophilia or one of the other classic paraphilic disorders.

Sarrel and Master (1982) described victims of female babysitter perpetrators who needed treatment because of sexual dysfunctions. In one case a male patient reported that an "older woman" abused him when he was 10 years old. He remembered erections but no ejaculations. In his opinion the experiences were pleasurable as long as they remained secret, but when he informed his parents and was punished for keeping secretly for so long, conflicts and guilt feelings began, resulting in severe sexual inhibitions leading to treatment at special institutions.

In another example a patient was 11 years old when a 16-year-old female babysitter pulled off his pajamas and tried to put the patient's penis in her vagina. He had no previous sexual experiences and did not understand what happened to him. He became deeply inhibited from this time on and had no sexual experiences till he met his wife later. There was no premarital sexuality and later an unconsummated marriage brought both partners to sexual therapy. This patient related his difficulties directly to the experience of sexual abuse.

Mathews et al. (1989, 1991) developed a frequently used typology of child-molestation by women with five subcategories that may have some relevance in understanding the variation of motivation and differences in causation for these phenomena:

1. The so-called *teacher/lover* type of female offender consists of women who fall in love with teenage males and often remain naïve regarding the consequences and effect their action has on their victims.
2. The *exploration/exploitation* type in which a teenager fondles a younger child (during babysitting).
3. The *predisposed* type where a woman with a severe history of physical and sexual abuse molests closely related or known children.
4. The *psychologically disturbed* type which includes women with severe psychiatric impairment and/or substance abuse who are psychologically unstable at the time of the sexual abuse.
5. The *male-coerced* type consisting of dependent women participating in the molestation of children initiated by their husbands or boyfriends.

This typology is not very systematic and is based on a small number of cases seen by the authors, but it may have practical relevance because it is regularly cited in literature on female sexual offending (for instance: Correctional Service of Canada, www.csc-scc.gc.ca/text/pblct/sexoffender/female/female-02_e.shtml).

Incest

In a publication by Sarrel and Master (1982) one case of mother–son incest and one case of sister–brother incest are described. Both cases came to the attention of the authors because the male victims developed sexual dysfunctions later in their sexual lives. Both cases remained officially undetected, giving a hint that, especially in offenses that take place within the family reporting to the police and court procedures are extremely rare.

The mother–son incest started when the victim was 13 years of age and shortly after his first nocturnal emissions. The mother began playing with his genitals, in the following months progressed from manipulation to fellatio and even intercourse, which in the end took place two to three times weekly until the young man left college. Although the son never actively approached his mother, he always responded and enjoyed her pleasure more than his own. He felt strongly devoted to her and developed deep guilt feelings regarding her after his first dates with peers, which resulted in massive sexual dysfunctions and an ongoing sexual relationship to his mother until she died.

The case of sister–brother incest started when the brother was between 10 and 12 years and his sister 4 years older. When she stimulated him manually, orally, and by inserting his penis in her vagina he felt more frightened than stimulated. Later on she threatened him with a knife and he could not remember if he ejaculated or not. Both siblings needed psychiatric help. She was hospitalized and he entered psychotherapy because he was unable to consummate his marriage.

Faller (1987) reported that 72% of 40 female sexual offenders molested children in polyincestuous family situations involving at least two perpetrators and two or more victims, with the male offender usually initiating the sexual act.

EPIDEMIOLOGY

For example, in Austria 39 to 67 sexual offenses per 100,000 inhabitants are registered by the police within 1 year (Berner, Karlick-Bolton, & Fodor, 1987). But only 10 to 17 offenders per 100,000 inhabitants were sentenced by court within the same period. Between 1975 and 1980 only 0.6% to 2.6% of all sentenced sexual offenses involved a female perpetrator, i.e., the relation between male and female sex offenders is approximately 100 to 1. These figures are in agreement with data from other countries, for instance England (O'Connor, 1987) or the United States (Vandiver & Kercher, 2004). Nevertheless some authors suppose that most female sex offenders remain undetected by law enforcement agencies and the proportion of undetected offenses may be higher than in male offenders as female offending is often perceived as less serious. It has been found that females acting with male accomplices are often not reported (Vandiver & Kercher, 2004).

From the six cases found in the Austrian study (Berner, Karlick-Bolton, & Fodor 1987) concerned with sexual offending between 1975 and 1980 in a catchment area of 3.5 million inhabitants, one offense was incest on the 13-year-old son by his mother. The incest offense was committed repeatedly and sometimes by threatening the young boy with a knife. This female offender acted on her own. She had an alcohol problem and was without a male partner since the death of the victim's father 10 years ago. Two younger daughters of her were given to foster parents.

The second offense was committed by a 40-year-old divorced woman who tolerated and facilitated that her new sexual partner had intercourse with her 9- and 13-year-old daughters. She did not only support the man, but also laid herself down on the floor to offer the marital bed for the abuse of her children.

The third registered offense was an indecent exposure of a female offender, who was drunk and involved in obscene interactions with other men. The remaining three offenses consisted of assaults on other women together with male accomplices and in connection with prostitution.

The study by Vandiver and Kercher (2004) reported the number of all registered adult female sexual offenders in Texas as N = 471. In relation to all registered male sexual offenders (N = 29,376) this means that 1.6% of all sexual offenders were female. This figure is very similar to the percentage obtained in Austria. In Texas the term "registered" not only includes offenders sanctioned with imprisonment but also fines and probation orders. But the study by Vandiver and Kercher (2004) may teach us more than just this relation between male and female sexual offenders. In the great majority of offenses the victims were children: indecency and sexual contact with a child (N = 155, 33%), sexual assault on a child (N = 84, 18%), aggravated sexual assault on a child (N = 68, 14%), indecency and exposure with a child (N = 26, 6%). Using all the scanty data available on such a register, including data on the victims, a hierarchical model was calculated and an additional cluster analysis yielded six types of female sexual offenders:

1. **Heterosexual nurturers** consisted of 146 offenders and built the largest cluster. This group with an average age of 30 years, exclusively victimized boys with an average age of 12 years. The authors state that this type may coincide with the *teacher–lover* category proposed by

Mathews et al. (1989) but also include other forms of "mentorship" or caretaking roles. These females were the least likely to have an initial arrest for sexual assault.

2. *Noncriminal homosexual offenders* included 114 offenders who were the least likely to be subsequently arrested after their index offense, had the lowest average number of arrests and were the least likely to commit an assault. The average age was 32 years and the victims were nearly exclusively females with an average age of 13 years (the highest average age of all clusters). Unfortunately there was no information about accomplices in the files, but the authors presume a high proportion of male accomplices in this group.

3. *Female sexual predators* included 112 offenders who were the most likely to have a rearrest after their index offense. They were the second youngest (average age 29 years), had the most and relatively young victims (60% males, average age of 11 years) and showed the most similarities with female nonsexual offenders. Their sexual offending is interpreted as part of a general criminal disposition.

4. *Young adult child exploiters* consisted of 50 offenders with the fewest number of arrests; they were the youngest at the time of arrest (average of 28 years), most likely to commit sexual assault, and their victims were the youngest with an average age of 7 years. Since half of the victims were related to the offenders the authors presume that this group included mothers molesting their own children (one of the types of female offenders suggested as separate category by Mathews et al., 1989).

5. *Homosexual criminals* included 22 offenders who had a high average number of total arrests (10) and victimized partly older and partly younger victims. There were no sexual assaults in this group but a lot of forcing behavior and compelling to prostitution. These offenders seem more economically than sexually motivated and therefore represent the "normal criminal group" described by Wolfe (1985).

6. *Aggressive homosexual offenders* include only 17 offenders who were the oldest at the time of the offense, the most likely to commit a sexual assault, and to have the oldest victims (average age of 31 years).

This statistical typology cannot be translated directly in different types of psychological motivation or criminological characteristics. But it sheds some light on the variability of causes for female sexual offending and demonstrates that—beside the much lower frequency of female compared to male sexual offending—there are only few cases where sexual needs are obvious. Criminal exploitation, revenge, and compensation for lost intimacy play a great role. The most striking differences to male offending are the high amounts of offenses committed with accomplices and the fact that almost half of the victims are male.

DATA ON PSYCHIATRIC DISORDERS AND EARLY PSYCHOLOGICAL TRAUMA

According to most authors, the majority of female sex offenders do not receive a diagnosis of paraphilia according DSM-IV. But personality disorders, abuse of illegal drugs and alcohol, and depression are often diagnosed (Faller, 1987, 1995; Kaplan & Green, 1995; Lewis & Stanley, 2000; O'Connor, 1987; Rosencrans, 1997). Some authors think that "long standing psychiatric disorders" can be found in a substantial number of cases (Travin, Cullen, & Protter, 1990). O'Connor (1987) found depression, mental retardation, and sometimes schizophrenia, especially in the group of female offenders with charges for indecency. Since the reported studies are not representative for female sexual offenders, comparisons with samples of male sexual offenders (Kubik, Hecker, & Righthand, 2002) remain very hypothetical. The same is true for comparisons of female sexual offenders (N = 11) with female nonsexual offenders (N = 11, Green & Kaplan, 1994). The majority of subjects in both groups demonstrated major depression, alcohol/substance abuse and PTSD, but the sexual offenders demonstrated more psychiatric impairment on the Global Assessment and Functioning Scale. Both sexual and nonsexual female offenders described negative relationships with parents, care-takers, spouses, and boyfriends; however the sexual offenders perceived their parents as more abusive, the comparison women as more neglecting.

Kubik et al. (2002) compared 11 adolescent female sexual offenders with 11 female nonsexual offenders and found only some psychosocial differences: Nonsexual offenders had higher proportions of drug and alcohol abuse, more disruptive school behavior, and more truancy. In the same study a second comparison between male and female sexual offenders revealed even fewer differences. Only a history of physical (63% vs. 40%) and sexual victimization (63% vs. 50%) was more obvious in the female sexual offender group. Female sexual offenders experienced their own sexual abuse as more serious, happening more frequently, and involving more often more than one perpetrator and near relatives. It resulted more frequently in post-traumatic stress disorder (PTSD). In another study Tardif et al. (2005) compared 13 adult females (AF, ≥18 years at the time of the offense) with 15 juvenile females (JF, 12 to 17 years at the time of the offense) who sexually abused children and adolescents. This was the total number of evaluated cases of female perpetrators seen in the outpatient clinic of the Centre de Psychiatrie Legal of the Institut Philippe Pinel de Montreal during the period of 10 years (1992 and 2002): Data on family origin revealed that social and familial experiences were different in the two samples. The family structure was destabilized in 46.2% of the AF, caused by abandonment (23.1%) or death of the father (15.4%), and multiple hospitalizations of the mother (7.7%). AF reported a greater degree of deprivation and rejection related to the mother due to rejection (23.1%), lack of protection against their own sexual (23.1%) and physical abuse (7.7%). Of the total AF, 30.8% were affected by depressive episodes of the mother. The instability of the family had an impact on the JF subjects as well: 60% lived in a reconstituted family and 33% had half-siblings. More than half of the JF lived with their mothers (60%), the others either with their fathers (13.3%) or in a foster home (13.3%), and only 13.3% lived with both parents. Half of the JF experienced parental abandonment before the age of 4 years. Psychiatric diagnoses differed in both groups. For the AF sample the following DSM-IV diagnoses were reported: borderline personality disorder (30.8%), borderline personality disorder and dysthymic disorder (15.4%), depression and dependent personality disorder (30.8%), and dependant personality disorder alone (15.4%). All but two of the AF presented more than one type of substance abuse (61.5%), suicide attempts (38.5%), and self-mutilation (15.4%). In the group of JF, 86.7% had been followed by a health professional because of behavioral problems, academic difficulties, and adaptation problems, and 20% because of their deviant sexual behavior. The main diagnoses were learning disorder (80%), attention deficit/hyperactivity disorder (33.3%), dysthymic disorder (26.7%), conduct disorder (26.7%), and PTSD (20%). Nearly half (46.7%) of the JF had a history of both violence against others and drug consumption. The acting out after frustration is more directed against others in the JF group, whereas suicide attempts and self-mutilation are more prominent in the AF. In both samples a high percentage of physical (more than 40%) and sexual victimization (60%) was reported.

For the authors of this study the supposed common trunk of causation of female sexual offending is a primary disturbance of the mother–child relationship in both groups. As all but one AF had sexually abused her own children, Tardif et al. (2005) propose that a problematic development of maternal identity has occurred at least in the AF-cases, but probably in the JF cases, too:

> The childhood traumas and neglect might awaken the desire to repair the deprivations and injuries of the past, which sets up a powerful swaying mechanism between the desire to repair and the desire to inflict the same abuse on another child. (p. 163)

TREATMENT

The literature on treatment of female sexual offenders is even more limited than that on phenomenology or epidemiology. It is focused nearly exclusively on individual therapy, either cognitive-behavioral or psychodynamic (Travin, Cullen, & Protter, 1990).

So far, only two exceptions could be found: one case-report on cyproterone-acetate treatment for a female patient with "hypersexuality" (Mellor, Farid, & Craig, 1988) and one case-report on treatment with Sertraline (a selective serotonin-reuptake inhibitor) for a female pedophile patient (Chow & Choy, 2002). Both reports provide promising results of pharmacological treatment and suggest further research.

Psychotherapeutic strategies for female sexual offenders do not differ principally from those for male sexual offenders, primarily concentrating on reducing the risk of reoffending. Eldridge (1993) states that,

> if therapy is to be effective in achieving that end, than the offenders *motivation to offend* and the way in which she or he has *overcome internal and external inhibitors* needs to be examined. Therapy needs to address the offender as a *thinking, feeling* and *behaving* person and harness thoughts, feelings and behavior to prevent re-offending. (p. 93)

These are exactly the principles of modern cognitive-behavioral programs developed for incarcerated male sexual offenders like SOTP in England (Friendship, Mann, & Beech, 2003) or "Sex Offender Treatment and Evaluation Project" (SOTEP) in California (Marques, Wiederanders, Nelson, & Ommeren, 2005).

Reflecting the reported data about frequent problems of dependency on an accomplice partner in female sexual perpetrators, these problems (including dependent personality disorder) should receive particular attention in psychotherapy with these offenders.

A second special problem more prominent in female sexual offenders than in male is the victim-to-victimizer cycle, the tendency of the perpetrator to put a child in the same position as experienced in her own childhood. It should also play a more important role in treatment of female offenders than in therapy of male offenders.

According to an overview provided by the correctional services of Canada, the most prominent treatment programs for female sexual offenders are offered in Minnesota. The Minnesota Correctional Facility in Shacopee developed such programs since 1984, consisting of intensive group psychotherapy, additional couples and family therapy, and intensive two-day sexual learning seminars (Mathews, Mathews, & Speltz, 1991). Genesis II is an outpatient program for female sexual offenders in Minneapolis. Female patients are mainly referred by court but also by child protection social workers and private therapists. The duration of treatment is 15 months on average. The program consists of a comprehensive day treatment, which the women attend with their preschool aged children 6 hours a day, for a period of 8 to 12 months. The day program provides participants with additional individual and group therapy, independent living skills training, parenting education, adult education, sexuality education, and developmental day care (Mathews et al., 1991).

References

Berner, W., Karlick-Bolten, E., & Fodor, G. (1987). Zur Epidemiologie der weiblichen Sexualdelinquenz. Forensia, 8, 139–143.

Berner, W. (1991). Sadomasochismus bei einer Frau. Zeitschrift für Sexualforschung, 4, 45–57.

Chow, E. W. & Choy, A. L. (2002). Clinical characteristics and treatment response to SSRI in a female pedophile. Archives of Sexual Behavior, 31, 211–215.

Eldridge, H. (1993). Barbara's story—a mother who sexually abused. In M. Elliott (Ed.), Female sexual abuse of children: The ultimate taboo (pp. 79–95). Colchester, Essex: Longman.

Faller, K. C. (1987). Women who sexually abuse children. Violence and Victims, 2, 263–276.

Faller, K. C. (1995). A clinical sample of women who have sexually abused children. Journal of Child Sexual Abuse, 4, 13–29.

Farin, M. (1989). Heroine des Grauens. Wirken und Leben der Elisabeth Bathory. München: Kirchheim.

Finkelhor, D. & Russel, D. (1984). Women as perpetrators. In D. Finkelhor (Ed.), Child sexual abuse: New theory and research (pp. 171–185). New York, NY: Free Press.

Friendship, C., Mann, R. E., & Beech, A. R. (2003). Evaluation of a national prison-based treatment program for sexual offenders in England and Wales. Journal of Interpersonal Violence, 18, 744–759.

Green, A. H. & Kaplan, M. S. (1994). Psychiatric impairment and childhood victimization experiences in female child molesters. Journal of the American Academy of Child and Adolescent Psychiatry, 33, 954–961.

Grob, C. S. (1985). Female exhibitionism. The Journal of Nervous and Mental Diseases, 173, 253–256.

Groth, N. (1979). Men who rape. New York, NY: Plenum Press.

Hollender, M. H., Brown, C. W., & Roback, H. B. (1977). Genital exhibitionism in women. American Journal of Psychiatry, 134, 436–438.

Kaplan, M. S. & Green, A. (1995). Incarcerated female sexual offenders: A comparison of sexual histories with eleven female non sexual offenders. Sexual Abuse: A Journal of Research and Treatment, 7, 287–300.

Krafft-Ebing, R. V. (1890). Psychopathia sexualis, 5th Edition. Stuttgart: Ferdinand Enke.

Kubik, E. K., Hecker, J., & Righthand, S. (2002). Adolescent females who have sexually offended: Comparison with delinquent adolescent female offenders and adolescent males who sexually offend. Journal of Child Sexual Abuse, 11, 63–83.

Lewis, C. F. & Stanley, C. R. (2000). Women accused of sexual offenses. Behavioral Sciences and the Law, 18, 73–81.

Marques, J. K., Wiederanders, M., Day, D. M., Nelson C., & Ommeren, A. V. (2005). Effects of a relapse prevention program on sexual recidivism: Final results from California's sex offender treatment and evaluation project (SOTEP). Sexual Abuse: A Journal of Research and Treatment, 17, 79–107.

Mathews, J. K., Mathews, R., & Spelz, K. (1991). Female sexual offenders: A typology. In M. Q. Patton (Ed.), Family sexual abuse: Frontline research and evaluation (pp. 199–219). Thousand Oaks, CA, US: Saga Publications, Inc. viii, 246 pp.

Mathews, R., Mathews, J. K., & Spelz, K. (1989). *Female sexual offenders: An exploratory study*. Orwell, VT: The Safer Society Press.

Mellor, C. S., Farid, N. R., & Craig, D. F. (1988). Female hypersexuality treated with cyproterone-acetat. *American Journal of Psychiatry*, 145, 1037.

O'Connor, A. (1987). Female sex offenders. *British Journal of Psychiatry*, 150, 515–520.

Rosencrans, B. (1997). *The last secret: Daughters sexually abused by mothers*. Vermont: Safer Society Press.

Sarrel, P. M. & Masters, W. H. (1982). Sexual molestation of men by women. *Archives of Sexual Behavior*, 11, 117–131.

Struckman-Johnson, C. (1988). Forced sex on dates: It happens to men too. *Journal of Sex Research*, 24, 234–241.

Tardif, M., Auclair, N., Jacobs, M., & Carpentier, J. (2005). Sexual abuse perpetrated by adult and juvenile females: An ultimate attempt to resolve a conflict associated with maternal identity. *Child Abuse & Neglect*, 29, 153–167.

Travin, S., Cullen, K., & Protter, B. (1990). Female sex offenders: Severe victims and victimizers. *Journal of Forensic Sciences*, 35, 140–150.

Vandiver, D. M. & Kercher, G. (2004). Offender and victim characteristics of registered female sexual offenders in Texas: A proposed typology of female sexual offenders. *Sexual Abuse: A Journal of Research and Treatment*, 16, 121–137.

Wolfe, F. A. (1985). Twelve female sexual offenders. Presented at "Next steps in research on the assessment and treatment of sexually aggressive persons (Paraphiliacs)." March, 1985, St. Louis, MO.

Zavitzianos, G. (1971). Fetishism and exhibitionism in the female and their relationship to psychopathy and kleptomania. *International Journal of Psychoanalysis*, 52, 297–305.

Chapter 20

Professionals Who Are Accused of Sexual Boundary Violations

Stephen B. Levine and Candace B. Risen

A person can earn the label "sex offender" by engaging in a broad swath of socially unacceptable behaviors. When that person is a professional—a physician, mental health professional, lawyer, business executive, teacher, clergy person—these behaviors are looked at with particular shock, disbelief, and disappointment. When professionals' sex offenses are brought to the attention of officials, serious consequences ensue. Within their profession, the offenders may be punished by loss of license and job, public notoriety, and ostracization. The professional may or may not be given an opportunity for rehabilitation. If the professional's victim presses criminal charges, incarceration becomes a possibility. If the victim presses civil charges, the professional may be compelled to pay a monetary damage award. Recognition of professional sexual misconduct is always a life changing matter for the professional and his family. The consequences live on.

ABROGATION OF TWO ETHICAL PRINCIPLES

The offending behaviors contradict the ethical principle of beneficence, which is an injunction to strive to help. The law codifies the expectation of beneficence by using the term "fiduciary" to describe the responsibility of professionals to act in the best interest of the clients (or patients) under their guidance. The professionals' pursuit of gratification of their sexual needs is fundamental evidence that the clients' needs have been given short shrift. The law assumes that, at least in the long run, professional sexual misconduct also carries a large risk of actually harming the client—even when the sexual behavior was consensual. Damaging the client violates another fundamental ethical principle—nonmaleficence, which is an injunction to cause no harm.

Most of the attention to professional sexual misconduct has focused on physicians. The public's expectation of professional integrity among medical doctors is more widely understood than with other professions. The avoidance of sex with a patient, "free or slave" (rich or poor) has been articulated as an ethical principle since Hippocrates' days 2500 years ago (Markel, 2004). Society's current need to punish physician sex offenders is stronger than it was two decades ago. State medical boards are no longer responsive to the arguments that the patient consented, was obviously not harmed, or is an untrustworthy reporter because she or he has a psychotic or a borderline personality disorder. The boards assume that the patient brings to the doctor's office a childlike trust in the good intentions of the physician. By violating that trust the physician tarnishes the reputation of all doctors by making it more difficult for other patients to trust when they seek care. Ignorance of medical ethical principles is not an acceptable argument either. Years of immersion in the health-care culture should have made it obvious that it is always the doctor's responsibility to respect that trust by being dedicated to the patients' welfare. (For an excellent summary of ethical guidelines see Roberts & Dyer, 2004).

As society has clarified its views about the ethical violation represented by physician sexual misconduct, its expectations have also become clearer for other professional groups whose work necessitates a power differential between themselves and their clients or students. Professional behaviors in many disciplines are expected to consistently demonstrate integrity—that is, to be consistently based on clearly apparent, readily articulable values. Beneficence is imbedded in the social expectations of these professionals as well.

PROFESSIONAL SEXUAL MISCONDUCT BY MENTAL HEALTH PROFESSIONALS AND OTHERS

Much of the literature on professional sexual misconduct refers to the sexual violations of mental health professionals (MHPs) and is generated by forensic psychiatrists (Simon, 2004). This literature reflects the fact that forensic evaluations of MHPs who have had sex with patients/clients are increasingly common. Since forensic work only occurs after a professional has been reported to authorities, these discussions cannot describe the extent of the problem. In the 1980s an attempt was made to estimate the lifetime prevalence of professional misconduct among various professional groups. A questionnaire study of psychiatrists found that 16% of the anonymous responders acknowledged at least one sexual contact with a patient (Herman, Gartrell, Olarte, Feldstein, & Localio, 1987). Similarly studies found that the frequency of self-report of sexual misconduct ranged between 8% and 16%, a range that has also been found among most physician groups (Gartrell, Milliken, Goodson, Thiemann, & Lo, 1992). The response rate to these questionnaires is typically low. During the early 1990s, physicians in family medicine, obstetrics and gynecology, and psychiatry were the most commonly brought to board attention for sexual misconduct in Oregon (Erbom & Thomas, 1997). Both forensic and questionnaire data agree that approximately 90% of offending professionals are men.

In the 1980s the rash of accusations against MHPs led to four important social changes. Psychiatric malpractice insurance policies were redesigned to limit the coverage for defending a claim involving sexual involvement—even if the doctor claimed technical incompetence to manage the transference. Second, an extended debate about how long after the end of a professional relationship a therapist could begin a private relationship with the patient (Appelbaum & Jorgenson, 1991) was resolved toward "never." Third, most professional state boards rewrote their codes of ethics to strengthen the prohibition against forming sexual liaisons with clients/patients. Finally, state boards became harsher in response to sexual transgressions committed by MHPs than by physicians who deal with physical illness. They began to conceptualize policies to foster a zero tolerance.

Boards realize that patients in prolonged psychotherapies are more likely to experience intense erotic feelings toward their psychotherapists than are patients under care for physical abnormalities. Boards expect MHPs to have the skills necessary to manage their patients' feelings, ideally in a manner that benefits the patient. Incompetence is not an acceptable excuse.

Boards are official public policy agencies. They set and enforce standards. They are under scrutiny by the public through newspaper articles and television programs which monitor and editorially comment on the patterns of their decisions. In the 1980s, many boards were accused of not doing enough to ensure the public's safety from professional sexual misconduct. The strong political forces on Boards, however, have not yet translated into better education of MHPs to skillfully deal with erotic feelings.

There is a painful irony here. As paradigms in psychiatry have become more biological and psychotherapeutic interventions have become more short term, it is likely that the skills for handling a problematic erotic transference are diminishing among MHPs at the same time that expectations for it have increased. Nonetheless, Boards often critically point out that the professionals' behavior before their sexual misconduct was deficient (American Psychiatric Asociatio's Ethical Principles Committee, 2005) in that they did not

1. recognize the patient's erotic feelings as they emerged;
2. repeatedly discuss the problematic emotions as a transference from the patient's past within the therapy;
3. seek consultation;
4. if the problem cannot be resolved, transfer the patient to another therapist.

These solutions require doctors to admit being overwhelmed by their countertransference. Several increase the professional's expenses because consultation and supervision are not free (except for those in training). The final solution, when abruptly done, often amounts to abandoning the patient, which borders on malfeasance.

WHAT IS A BOUNDARY?

In recent years professional sexual violations, even those with consenting partners, have come to be known as boundary violations among diverse groups of professionals. Sexual boundary violations typically begin with

1. misuse of the psychological intimacy;
2. misuse of the physical examination;
3. misuse of spiritual or religious intimacies.

These can lead to nonconsensual sexual harassment, stalking, gross sexual imposition, as well as consensual sexual contact.

We think of a boundary as an edge, limit, a circle, or a frame within which the well intentioned work of the professional can proceed without the professional, the client, or society being concerned that fraudulence, advantage-taking, or harm is underway. When a professional acts within the socially constructed frame of appropriate behaviors, there is, of course, no guarantee that the patient's health will be improved. Adherence to proper boundaries only sets the stage to maximize the potential of the professional to create a lasting benefit for the patient in terms of symptom relief, world view, and the conduct of life.

Ten Guidelines for Mental Health Professionals

The boundaries are defined by relatively few rules for the conduct of professional life. While theoretically the rules equally apply to all health-care professionals, in actuality they do not. Specific boundaries vary with the type of professional work—a psychoanalyst and an addiction counselor use different rules, as do a pediatrician and an ophthalmologist. The rule, however, that is true for all health-care professionals is sexual avoidance. The other rules for professional life are largely intuitively understood by professionals and lay persons alike. Most of these guidelines cannot be stated in absolute terms (Roberts & Dyer, 2004). The following ten guidelines are our personal synthesis of the traditions of psychiatric ethics that can be found in numerous articles on the subject.

1. Beneficence—the use of one's expertise exclusively to help the ill: "I will act only for the benefit of the patient." Closely linked to beneficence is the concept of nonmaleficence, "First, do no harm."
2. Abstinence—there are to be no personal rewards for patient care other than the pleasures of the diagnostic and therapy processes and financial remuneration. There is to be a relative absence of physical expression of affection between the professional and patient.
3. Neutrality—the professional's work is to clarify the patient's options and explore the pros and cons of each behavioral course; it is not to cause the patient to make a choice that the professional feels is correct—for example, to influence whether a woman has an abortion. Neutrality is a means of fostering psychological independence or separateness in the patient. The professional's neutrality is a way of respecting and fostering patient self-determination. The professional is expected to highly value the patient's right to determine his or her own future.

4. Fiduciary agent—The mental health professional is expected to recognize the power imbalance between him or her and the patient. The power differential provides the professional with an opportunity to have too much influence over the patient, but this influence is expected by the law to always be in the patient's best interests.

5. Respect for patients' confidentiality—the professional has an obligation not to reveal patients' personal information without their explicit permission. Respect for confidentiality is an old time-honored tradition that forms the basis of the doctor–patient relationship.

6. Informed consent—patients must consent to the elements of their treatment. The professional is expected to be truthful in all ways with the patient. This expectation means that the professional must discuss the pros and cons of therapy options. For all procedures in medicine and in all forms of research, this means that an Informed Consent document must be signed. For informed consent to have taken place, the patient must be cognitively intact, relatively free of paralyzing psychological distress, and free of coercion.

7. Singularity of purpose to the professional relationship—professionals are expected to avoid dual relationships such as business partner and psychiatrist; employer and treating psychologist, friend and addiction counselor. This guideline means little to no other relationship before, during, or after therapy.

8. Professional work is to take place in the proper setting, its duration is defined (1/2 or 1 hour sessions), its costs are reasonable and clear.

9. Asymmetry of personal disclosure—a professional relationship is to be characterized by a one-way psychological intimacy (Levine, 2003): the patient speaks and the professional listens.

10. Patient's erotic fantasies are to be discussed with the purpose of understanding their meanings in terms of present and past life circumstances.

Professional sexual misconduct usually contradicts all of these rules. It is clearly unethical. Such boundary violations are typically preceded by boundary crossings.

What Is a Boundary Crossing?

Lesser departures of the therapeutic frame are referred to as boundary crossings (Epstein, Simon, & Kay, 1992). For the MHP, for example, making a friend of a patient by excessive personal exposure of the professional's personal life circumstances is a boundary crossing. Some boundary crossings are deliberate and therapeutic in intent (Frick, 1994). When a boundary crossing is recognized by the therapist as an error, the mistake can be discussed as an error without necessarily harming the relationship. Undiscussed crossings pose a danger to professional work when they increase in frequency and intensity over time. They are a "slippery slope" that is thought to increase the likelihood of a sexual boundary violation. This view of boundary crossings is based on cases that came to the attention of forensic psychiatrists (Simon, 1989). By retrospective analysis it was recurrently observed that sex between patient and professional was preceded by subtle forms of wordless negotiations that tested the receptivity, nerve, and daring of the dyad.

Many patients recognize the early boundary crossing explicitly or intuitively and leave the relationship. Their next therapist may learn about it. In this way, colleagues come to know the boundary crossings of others and occasionally the boundary violation patterns of others. Therapists do not generally report the colleague, however, even though the second section of the *Principles of Medical Ethics with Annotations Especially Applicable to Psychiatry* states that "a physician shall....strive to expose colleagues deficient in character or competence" (American Psychiatric Association [APA], 1993). Reporting a colleague without the patient's permission may violate confidentiality. (This does not apply when the patient is a minor or seriously mentally or physically handicapped. Most states have legal requirements that transcend the professional ethical guideline regarding confidentiality.) Reporting the colleague with the patient's permission may cause the patient unforeseen distress and harm and change the course of therapy. It is also dangerous because the patient's interpretation of the boundary crossing may be only one version of what transpired. The literature makes clear that the assessment of what is a serious boundary crossing short of sexual misconduct can be a complex matter (Martinez, 2000). Coworkers within the same institution are more likely to report to their mutual superior a colleague who seriously crosses boundaries with a client than to a state board. It then becomes the administrator's problem.

When sexual misconduct is revealed to a new therapist in private practice or in a different institution, he or she may rapidly recommend that the patient report the prior professional to the board.

The new therapist assumes that this course of action is necessary for the patient's recovery and for the good of the society. This stance requires a significant departure from therapeutic neutrality and, however well intentioned, may emotionally backfire and harm the patient. The patient is better served if the therapist is open to discussing the previous professional's sexual misconduct and maintains therapeutic neutrality about what "should" be done. Whatever the patient eventually decides to do, it will be his or her decision. These are typically very complex circumstances involving compromised mental health, past sexual abuse, and layers of patient guilt for acting out on erotic transferences. Dealing with them as though it were a simple matter of perpetrator and victim denies the patient his or her own experience of what took place. The simple assignment of culpability is the role of the board, not the psychotherapist.

A case in point: A middle-aged woman reports during her first session with a therapist that she had sexual activity with a previous therapist. At the end of this session, the new therapist urges her to report her previous doctor to the Board, a recommendation that her aggrieved husband had already been urging. After the second session, the new therapist wrote a letter of outrage to the Board recommending that the previous therapist's license be permanently revoked. As the adjudication processes went forward and the boundary crossing doctor suffered social, financial, and licensure losses, the patient became overwhelmed with guilt and began stalking the doctor to apologize and ask for his forgiveness, much in the same way she relentlessly pushed him to have sex with her for 2 years before his misconduct. Because of the adversarial relationship with her original therapist and the pressure of the new therapist, the patient found it impossible to effectively deal with her feelings about the entire matter.

THE PROGRAM FOR PROFESSIONALS

We began this program in 1991 with the assistance of a small foundation grant to learn more about professional sexual misconduct. The mission of the program was two-fold: to create a standard evaluation process that would routinely elicit an understanding of the circumstances and motivations for the professional's ethical breach and to formulate recommendations to the agency that ordered the professional to have the evaluation (Levine, Risen, & Althof, 1994).

Elements of the Evaluation

Our evaluation typically follows these steps over a 4- to 6-week period.

1. Discussion with referring agency about the reasons for evaluation and the specific questions that they would like us to address
2. Review of the documentation concerning the complaint and of any additional information that the agency possesses about the situation
3. Interviews conducted by a primary evaluator. One person on our team of three sees the person between 4 and 6 hours to determine the history of the problem from the perspective of the professional. This may sometimes include an interview with the spouse of the professional. It does not include an interview with the "victim" as that might create an emotional intensity in the victim for which we can take no professional responsibility. We do not wish to further traumatize the victim
4. Psychometric assessment with the MMPI-III and MCMI-2 Millon Multiaxial Personality Inventory. Two interpretations are available to us: one by the psychologist and one which is generated by the computerized scoring program
5. Case conference. The primary evaluator presents the case to the other two members of the team and our general staff, for a refinement of the unanswered questions and discussion of the apparent psychodynamics of the problematic situation
6. Interview conducted by a secondary evaluator for up to 2 hours. This interview provides another look at the professional while attempting to answer the questions raised at the case conference
7. Miniconference of the Program for Professional staff only to formulate conclusions and recommendations
8. Feedback session with the professional. The purpose is to reflect on the evaluation itself, obtain missing information, and to give the third member of the team an opportunity to observe the professional before and after the recommendations are conveyed
9. Report writing—the primary evaluator composes the report which is responded to and signed by all three team members

Sources of Referral

The Program for Professionals receives most of its referrals from one of four sources. It is rarely contacted by a professional seeking help to prevent or stop personal sexual misconduct.

1. State professional boards such as for medicine, psychology, social work, nursing, or education—having received and investigated a complaint against one of its licensees, the board seeks our opinions about the psychiatric diagnosis, motivations, public safety, and recommendations for future license restrictions. The referral is often mandated by the board through its Consent Agreement with the guilt-admitting professional.
2. Hospitals—usually the chief of staff or a department chairperson refers a problematic staff member for assistance in management, rehabilitation, and future conditions of employment.
3. Diocese—before the clergy abuse scandal in 2002, we received numerous referrals from Catholic institutions seeking guidance for priests, nuns, and deacons who had behaved inappropriately (Fones, Levine, Althof, & Risen, 1999). Of these referrals, 60% did not involve a minor.
4. Lawyers—professionals who have got into trouble in one state often seek legal assistance in relocating to another. The lawyer seeks our assessment of the situation so that he can represent his client more expertly in suggesting the conditions under which another state board might be reassured about public safety. Unlike the professionals who are referred as part of a Consent Agreement from their state board, our evaluations are done before the application for licensure to a new board.

The Easy Versus the Difficult Cases

Our experience within the Program for Professionals can be appreciated by grasping the differences between the easy and the difficult cases that we evaluate. What makes our evaluation easy is the professionals' willingness to tell us what happened in a relatively honest and reasonably complete fashion. Almost no one, however, can give us the full story, complete with all the relevant past and current aspects of the situation. Everyone is trying to salvage what is positive about their situation. While we accept practicing

damage control as normal evaluation behavior, it prevents us from completely understanding the situation. Our conclusions are presented with a caveat about the limitations of self-report. Nonetheless, the essence of the easy situation is, "Yes, I did engage in a sexual relationship with my client. Here is what I know about what happened and why."

The difficult case begins with the professional's position that he is innocent, did not do anything close to what he is accused of, is the victim of a misunderstanding or a malicious lie, or is in trouble because the accuser is seeking revenge for some other nonsexual matter of disagreement. It is certainly possible that a professional can be falsely labeled by malevolent dishonest accuser. In all cases we carefully note the personal style of the professional. Falsely accused people are usually eager to tell their stories, they give credible background accounts, speak knowledgably about what they did do wrong, and treat us with respect. There are those professionals, however, who demonstrate profound resistance to their evaluation and are disrespectful of our time and intentions to help. They present in an angry, confrontative, or insulting manner and provide sparse, incredible stories that assume no responsibility for any bad judgments.

When this happens, we try to address the dilemma the professional is in with us during the first session. This may enable him to become cooperative, respectful, and an "easy" case. If our emphatic and clarifying early intervention fails to elicit the professional's cooperation and his or her unpleasant unhelpful manner continues, our clinical experience has led us to more strongly suspect the person's guilt and speculate that he or she is character disordered as well. For instance, a 56-year-old physician was accused by four patients of fondling their breasts during physical examinations in his last job of 11 months. He had held jobs in 23 different settings. He claimed that he was never responsible for any of his previous contracts not being renewed—all were externally caused. He came to us knowing the evaluation fee was to be paid by the end of the evaluation. When we told him that we did not believe the likelihood that four women had independently misunderstood his innocent physical examination techniques and therefore could not recommend an immediate return to work, he refused to pay for his evaluation.

The Program for Professionals' process is not a legal finder of fact. If a professional maintains his or her absolute innocence during the evaluation, we explain this to the referral source. We cannot explain, interpret, or make recommendations about what did not happen. The Program for Professionals is best utilized for individuals who know that they have made a serious error in judgment and behavior. We attempt to help them explain the error to themselves and to the referring agency.

EXPECTATIONS FOR REASONABLE MORAL AND MENTAL HEALTH IN THE PUBLIC SPHERE

When a professional has sex with a patient, the act is considered egregious by various elements in society. The Program for Professionals responds by trying to determine the mind set of the professional, the number of prior patients he or she was involved with, and the factors that may have diminished the professional's judgment. We assess the rehabilitation potential and the future threat to public safety. Here is an example of a man we felt could not be allowed to practice medicine without a monitor present at all times: An internist with a stocking fetish had apparently disguised his sexual interest in women's undergarments and stockings throughout his career by providing calf and foot massages at the end of some of his physical examinations. A patient perceived that he had an orgasm during the massage after he placed a knee-high stocking on one of her legs without asking her permission. This physician had a highly compulsive paraphilia that spilled over into the conduct of his medical life.

The public expects that licensed professionals have a reasonable degree of moral and mental health in their personal lives. While most men with a paraphilia express their unique sexual patterns in privacy, some people are driven to public sexual behavior for their greater intensity of arousal. While they may be able to keep this pattern of behavior out of their professional work, their sexual proclivities become known within the community. This makes boards quite uneasy about the professional's ultimate judgment. They worry when, if ever, the problem will spill over to their professional life. Boards hold their professionals to a high standard of public morality and mental health. Conviction for felonies of any sort, for instance, often ultimately leads to a loss of license. Here are cases that caused state board's concern for the ultimate safety of the public: A family practitioner

surreptitiously video taped his girlfriend's teenage daughter in the bathroom; an anesthesiologist repeatedly watched his stepdaughter while she showered; a cancer surgeon was arrested in the park for soliciting homosexual sex; a gynecologist was arrested for exhibitionism at a mall. The Program for Professionals was asked in these cases whether the doctor was safe to practice medicine and what could be done to facilitate the permanent cessation of these uninspiring misdemeanors. The worry, of course, is that these episodes of sexual acting out will be a slippery slope that will lead to professional sexual misconduct.

A DIAGNOSIS IS NOT THE SAME AS THE DYNAMICS

In our reports to the referring sources, the Program for Professionals provides psychiatric diagnoses. Even a thorough five axis DSM-IV-R diagnosis, however, does not explain why the misconduct occurred. For example, a middle-aged psychologist claimed that a sheriff's agent raped her and was sexually abusing many of the prisoners at the women's division of the county jail. She provoked a costly investigation of the sheriff's department before her suicide attempt led to a psychiatric hospitalization where she was recognized as psychotic. She had been noncompliant with her medications and appointments and failed to explain to her psychiatrist what was going on in her life. The psychologist, who did not have sex with a patient but was preoccupied with other people's sexual misconduct, could not separate her patients' stories from her own perceptions. Classifying her inappropriate behavior about sex with the sheriff's deputy was easy once the diagnosis of psychosis was made. To consider rehabilitation, however, her evaluation focused on what precipitated her poor handling of her psychotic illness. After considerable confrontation, she was able to explain her humiliation over her recent marriage to a foreign-born man whose courtship behavior immediately changed into autocratic insistence on having his way in everything including sexual opportunities. "I was a fool—for the third time in my life!" Denial or minimization of a psychiatric illness does not generate confidence in a board's ability to protect the public's safety. However, state medical boards often allow individuals to practice when their mental illnesses are well-managed and they can serve their communities without incident.

Yes, We Can Categorize Professional Sexual Misconduct—But

After over 120 evaluations, we have learned that every case is unique and that categories, however, generally useful, do not take us very far in explaining ethical laxity. Most professionals are not conspicuously mentally ill, character disordered, sexually compulsive paraphilic addicts, facing death from a terminal illness, or grieving the acute loss of a spouse. Those who are, however, make dramatic case presentations. Many cases leave us in awe of the human capacity to give into temptation. Our best explanation then is, "We don't really know."

A 28-year-old virgin, first generation American, religiously sexually suppressed, a naïve believer in people's inherent goodness, lost his medical license because he gave too many opiods to a woman he did not recognized as a prostitute. She managed to entice him to trade more drugs for sex outside the hospital and became trapped in his error. When he refused to continue to provide drugs for her, she followed through on her threat to report him.

Our categories are for those psychiatric illnesses that we think served as a cofactor in generating misconduct. They are not for the reactive anxiety and depression reactions that often occur immediately after the misconduct and then inevitably with greater intensity when the misconduct is publicly identified. Numerous authors use slightly different categories (Norris, Gutheil, & Strasburger, 2003). We sometimes run into cases that fit more than one of these categories. Notice that substance abuse is not listed here. Sexual misconduct associated with substance abuse tends to be viewed as a symptom of addiction and is handled separately by most boards.

- *Brain disease*—a mental or brain illness, such as, schizophrenia, bipolar disorder, steroid psychosis, or Alzheimer's disease, may impair the judgment and impulse control of the professional
- *Depressive Life Processes*—a loss of an important person or job has created a sense of grief and despair that has motivated the professional to inappropriately reach out to a willing patient
- *Psychopathic Character*—usually refers to a narcissistic/psychopathic person with more than one professional sexual violation, an exploitative life pattern, and strong psychometric evidence of psychopathy. These people seem to lack restraint and evidence of struggle with

their conscience, and feel entitled to use the patient for their purposes
- *Sexual compulsivity with or without paraphilia*—while paraphilic problems are often evident from puberty, we have seen them arise with a compulsive intensity in young adulthood. The pressure of their sexual desires overwhelm their restraint mechanisms and cause the inappropriate behavior with their patients
- *Characterological Problems*—the most common diagnosis is mixed character disorder with a heavy use of externalization of blame. This perhaps just represents a strongly defensive posture that prevents us from finding out the more truthful version of the misconduct. Many of these individuals seem to be dysthymic
- *Absence of Pathology*—one might be tempted to assume that professional sexual misconduct never occurs without a significant recognizable pathological pattern, but our experience does not support this idea. We suspect that ethical breaches, even those involving sex (Gartrell et al., 1992), are more common than has been realized, and can result from ordinary human temptation to break the rules to satisfy some urgently felt personal need

CONCLUSION

The actual extent of professional sexual misconduct can not be ascertained with certainty for any professional group. When these egregious acts come to attention, however, the professional's personal and professional lives are inevitably profoundly altered. Social institutions such as state medical boards punish these cases severely in an attempt to diminish their incidence in others. The Program for Professionals systematically evaluates the accused and finds that most cases fall into one of five categories but a large minority of cases show no significant premorbid psychopathology.

References

American Psychiatric Association. (1993) *Principles of medical ethics with annotations especially applicable to psychiatry.* Washington, D.C.: American Psychiatric Association.

American Psychiatric Asociatio's Ethical Principles Committee. (2005). *Principles of ethics and professionalism in psychiatry* (pp. 1–27). Washington, D.C.: American Psychiatric Association.

Appelbaum, P. S. & Jorgenson, L. (1991). Psychotherapist-patient sexual contact after termination of treatment: An analysis and a proposal. *The American Journal of Psychiatry*, 148, 1466–1473.

Epstein, R. S., Simon, R. I., & Kay, C. G. (1992). Assessing boundary violations in psychotherapy: Survey results with the exploitation index: *Bulletin of Meninger Clinic*, 56, 150–166.

Erbom, J. A. & Thomas, C. D. (1997). Evaluation of sexual misconduct complaints: The Oregan Board of Medical Examiners, 1991–1995. *American Journal of Obstetrics and Gynecology*, 176(6), 1340–1346.

Fones, C. S., Levine, S. B., Althof, S. E., & Risen C. B. (1999). The sexual struggles of 23 clergymen: A follow-up study. *Journal of Sex & Marital Therapy*, 25(3), 183–195.

Frick, D. E. (1994). Nonsexual boundary violations in psychiatric treatment. In J. M. Oldham, & M. B. Riba (Eds.), *Review of psychiatry*. Washington, D.C.: American Psychiatric Press.

Gartrell, N. K., Milliken, N., Goodson, W. H. I., Thiemann, S., & Lo, B. (1992). Physician-patient sexual contact: Prevalence and problems. *The Western Journal of Medicine*, 157, 139–143.

Herman, J., Gartrell, N., Olarte, S., Feldstein, M., & Localio, R. (1987). Psychiatrist-patient sexual contact: Results of a national survey of psychiatrists' attitudes. *The American Journal of Psychiatry*, 144(1), 164–169.

Levine, S. B., Risen, C. B., & Althof, S. E. (1994). Professionals who sexually offend: Evaluation procedures and preliminary findings. *Journal of Sex & Marital Therapy*, 20(4), 288–302.

Levine, S. B. (2003). What patients mean by love, intimacy, and sexual desire, In Althof, S. E (Ed.), *The handbook of clinical sexuality for mental health professionals* (pp. 21–36). New York, NY: Brunner/Routledge.

Markel, H. (2004). Becoming a physician: "I Swear by Apollo"—On taking the Hippocratic oath. *New England Journal of Medicine*, 350(20), 2026–2028.

Martinez, R. (2000). A model for boundary dilemmas: Ethical decision making in the patient-professional relationship. *Ethical Human Sciences and Services*, 3(1), 43–61.

Norris, D. M., Gutheil, T. G., & Strasburger, L. H. (2003). This couldn't happen to me: Boundary problems and sexual misconduct in the psychotherapy relationship. *Psychiatric Services*, 54(4), 517–522.

Roberts, L. W. & Dyer, R. (2004). *Ethics in mental health*. Washington, D.C.: American Psychiatric Publications, Inc.

Simon, R. I. (1989). Sexual exploitation of patients: How it begins before it happens. *Psychiatric Annals*, 19, 104–112.

Simon, R. I. (2004) Maintaining treatment boundaries. *Psychiatric Times*, 11:14–17.

Chapter 21

Stalking

Ronnie B. Harmon

Stalking emerged in the national consciousness in the United States in the last decade of the twentieth century as a crime of passion and violence. A series of homicides, some involving celebrities and aggressive fans, some involving unstable individuals whose approaches to ordinary people were rejected, raised the awareness of the California legislature about what had, up to then, been a relatively overlooked phenomenon in criminal justice. To date, much research about stalking behavior has focused either on defining the problem, or on predicting which stalkers are more likely to become dangerous to their targets, and when such dangerous behavior might manifest itself. In many stalking cases, the only real guarantee of victim safety will come with the cessation of the stalking. Understanding which type of stalker will persist no matter what interventions are taken, versus which type of stalker can be encouraged to desist in their behavior, may facilitate the management of these difficult cases.

PROBLEMS OF DEFINITION

Initial attempts to clarify the nature of this phenomenon focused on the stalker as someone who was not well known (or not known at all) by the target of his attention (Dietz, Matthews, Martell, Stewart, Hrouda, & Warren, 1991a; Dietz et al., 1991b; Zona, Sharma, & Lane, 1993). By the mid-1990s, laws against stalking had evolved across the United States and around the world. Advocacy for victims of domestic violence had broadened the public's perception of stalking to include situations in which individuals who were trying to terminate former intimate relationships were relentlessly pursued by their former partners (Kurt, 1995; Meloy & Gothard, 1995). As awareness about stalking increased, the definition of the phenomenon broadened (Harmon, Rosner, & Owens, 1995, 1998; Mullen, Pathé, & Purcell, 2000). A stalker could be a former lover, an acquaintance, or a total stranger. The stalking could be done from a distance (by telephone or mail) or in person (through following and visiting). It could be accompanied by threats of violence, or protestations of undying love, or both.

The process of defining stalking has proceeded on two tracks: the legislative level and the behavioral level. Legislators were concerned with fashioning laws that would give local law enforcement the tools needed both to protect the public from perceived dangerous predators, and to prevent stalking behavior from escalating to violence. Behavioral scientists attempted to clarify the motives behind stalking activities, with the expectation that identifying the causes of the behavior might lead to an understanding of how to contain it.

Legislative Definitions

Purcell et al. (2004), in an extensive, international review of antistalking legislation, concluded that while there is no consistent, universal legal definition of stalking, most laws contain some combination of three elements: conduct requirements, intention, and the response of the victim.

Conduct requirements define stalking by the actions of the offender. In contrast to many other criminal offenses, such as robbery or homicide, with stalking there may be no single identifiable incident that marks the beginning, middle, or end of the crime. Stalking consists of a series of incidents occurring episodically. Some early antistalking legislation listed specific acts (i.e., following, telephoning, approaching, letter writing). When it became clear that it would not be feasible to list all actions that could be taken by a stalker, the legal phrase "course of conduct" was integrated into many antistalking laws. In New York State, judicial references to case law defining "course of conduct" date back to the English common law case of *Crepps v. Durden* (1777), in which the Court held that the sale of four loaves of bread on Sunday in violation of a statute forbidding such sale constituted one offense, not four. Case law decisions have resulted in the definition of "course of conduct" as "an intentional pattern of conduct encompassing a period of time, no matter how short, evidencing a continuity of purpose" (Rosenbaum, 2000). Generally speaking, a minimum of two specific actions have been considered to constitute a course of conduct.

Intention can be defined as the motivation behind the stalking behavior. Early anti-stalking laws required the perpetrator to have made a threat (Miller, 2003), and/or to intend to harm or frighten the victim. This was quickly recognized as being nonproductive in stalking cases where the pursuit was based on the desire to create and/or maintain a loving relationship, in which case the stalker could claim they had no intention of hurting anyone. In many jurisdictions, statutory requirements were amended so that the stalker only had to intend to commit the acts of which they were accused (i.e., making calls, mailing letters, sending gifts). Deliberate behavior, whether it was intended to cause fear or not, could be punished as stalking.

The response of the victim is an important element to the offense of stalking. In addition to the ongoing nature of the crime, the offense of stalking is also unusual in giving substantial weight to the impact of the offense on the victim. The stalking victim's perceptions, or the perceptions of an impartial "reasonable person," of the stalker's behavior as threatening or frightening, may determine whether a crime has been committed (U.S. Dept. of Justice, 1998). In many jurisdictions, if it can be demonstrated that the stalker knows or should know that his actions are causing fear in his target, then, regardless of his intent, he can be charged with stalking (Radosevich, 2000).

Behavioral Definitions

Behavioral definitions have focused on the development of classification systems, or typologies, intended to enable the understanding of stalking behavior and, through such understanding, to facilitate its management. Such classifications group stalkers according to such things as motivation, relationship with the targeted individual, and psychiatric disorder.

The United States' National Center for Victims of Crime has adopted a classification system that divided stalkers into two major categories, love obsessed and simple obsessed. This classification was developed by Dr. Michael Zona, a California-based forensic psychiatrist affiliated with American law enforcement's first organized antistalking unit, the Los Angeles Police Department's Threat Management Unit (Zona et al., 1993). Love obsessed stalkers are defined as being fixated on another individual with whom they have no relationship; simple obsessed stalkers have a history of a prior relationship with their targets. A third, much smaller category, erotomanics, is defined clinically in the *Diagnostic and Statistical Manual of Mental Disorders* (American Psychiatric Association, 2000). They constitute a specific subset of love-obsessed stalkers who believe that the object of their affection also loves them. The stalker believes that their targeted object is sending them coded, intimate messages, or, they may feel that the target has been unable to demonstrate their love because of outside interference, or shyness. The major problem with the Zona classification system is its failure to sufficiently distinguish among the many different types of "simple obsessed" stalkers who compose a large percentage of their sample population.

Mullen (2003) defined stalking as "[A] constellation of behaviors in which one individual persistently inflicts repeated, unwanted intrusions and communications on another." The typology developed by Mullen et al. (1999, 2000) under the auspices of Monash University and the Victorian Institute of Forensic Mental Health in Australia, incorporated these items in a multiaxial approach. Motive was divided into five types: the rejected may have been trying to reopen a terminated relationship, intimacy seekers were lonely individuals trying to create a relationship, resentful stalkers felt that they had been damaged in some way and sought justice, predatory stalkers included sexual predators who targeted specific victims, and the incompetent stalker also sought a relationship, but was incapable of using socially acceptable means to connect with a partner. Relationship categories included prior intimate partners, professional contacts, work-related contacts, casual acquaintances and friends, the famous, or strangers. Psychiatric disorder was classified as either psychotic or nonpsychotic. The system was intended for use in the development of predictions about the nature and course of the stalking, and the management of the behavior by treating mental health and law enforcement professionals.

Boon and Sheridan (2001) developed a four-part classification system from a sample of self-referred victims of serious stalking. Former intimate partners, especially when there was a history of domestic violence, were found to be at high risk for violence. Infatuated stalkers were a low-level risk for dangerous actions toward their targets, and might respond well to legal action. Stalkers who had a delusional fixation about their targets could be somewhat more dangerous; these individuals might have a history of psychiatric problems and/or of previously stalking other

victims, and were difficult to dissuade from their pursuits. This category includes individuals who can be diagnosed with the delusional mental disorder erotomania (American Psychiatric Association, 2000), in which the object of their affection is generally a person of higher status or reputation. Although they are strangers, the delusional individual firmly believes that there is an existing relationship between them. Because of this unshakable belief, all attempts to dissuade the stalker are viewed as either unwelcome interference from others (like security personnel or family members, who may consequently become at risk for harm), or as the stalking victim's roundabout means of communicating their love. Finally, sadistic stalkers (similar to the predatory stalkers discussed by Mullen et al. (1999, 2000)) see their targets as victims to be intimidated. The motive behind this type of stalking is the exertion of power and control over another individual, who is frequently a former intimate partner. This type can be very dangerous and capable of physical violence, and are considered the most difficult stalking cases to manage, from the point of view of law enforcement intervention.

For both legal and behavioral researchers of stalking, the most important objective was the development of a classification system that would serve as a workable resource for law enforcement officers attempting to predict the trajectory of stalking behavior and to respond accordingly to protect its victims from physical and emotional harm. Boon and Sheridan (2001) wanted to "serve the needs of law enforcement professionals" by identifying offenders according to "motivational orientation." Spitzberg (2002, p. 263), in his meta-analysis of studies of stalking behavior, notes that many attempts to define stalking have "the objective of managing risk to victim and society through risk prediction. This objective is illustrated by the attempt to identify characteristics of the perpetrator or the victim that distinguish the nature of victimization." Other studies (Palarea, Zona, Lane, & Langhinrichsen-Rohling, 1999; Roberts, 2002) looked at whether relationship behavior patterns could be used to predict post-breakup stalking, and also at when behavior can be considered to cross the line from normal courtship into obsession.

What is clear is that there is no one "profile" of a stalker or of stalking behavior. Different types of stalkers may share a common behavior pattern, but will react differently to attempts to control stalking behavior. Some will target one individual for a period of time, but will respond to an encounter with the criminal justice system by discontinuing their stalking behavior. Others will react by repeating the stalking, but against a different target. Finally, some will persist in their pursuit of a single victim regardless of all efforts to discourage them.

THE STALKING RECIDIVISM PROFILE

The following analysis is based on data collected for the studies of Harmon et al. (1995, 1998), reexamined in studies by Rosenfeld and Harmon (2002) and Rosenfeld (2003), and presented at national conferences (Ciric & Harmon, 2002; Harmon, 2001; Harmon, 2005).

Harmon et al. (1995, 1998) reported on a descriptive study of 174 stalkers referred for evaluation to the Forensic Psychiatry Clinic of the Criminal and Supreme Courts of New York, New York. The research resulted in a typology that theorized that stalking behavior was definable in two major dimensions (see Table 21.1). For the first dimension, a distinction was made between stalking which could be considered sexually motivated (amorous stalking, in which the focus was on situations in which the stalking behavior was related to a desire to either initiate or maintain an intimate relationship, or to punish the victim for terminating such a relationship) versus stalking which was in no way sexually motivated (persecutory, or vengeful stalking, in which the stalking behavior was related to a desire for revenge for a financial or situational wrong the victim was perceived as having committed against the stalker). Individuals may have been victimized because of either of these types of obsessions. The second axis of the typology grouped stalkers according to the relationship they had with

their victims before the stalking began. The initial grouping established six types of relationships: personal (including sexual partners and family members), professional (including professional individuals retained by the stalker), employment (supervisors, coworkers, and subordinates), media (celebrity stalking), and acquaintance (neighbors, former friends, casual dating relationships), and none (stranger stalking). In the 1998 paper of Harmon et al., these classifications were simplified to form three categories: "former intimates" included sexual partners and family members; "acquaintances" subsumed the professional, acquaintance, and employment classifications; and "no prior relationship," which included media or celebrity stalking and complete strangers. One of the goals of the classification system was to eliminate, as much as possible, overlap among the groups.

The research found that, for this specific population of criminally charged stalkers with suspected mental illness, the prestalking relationship between the parties was more important in predicting risk of harm than was the motivation behind the stalking. Threats to the target and the stalker's psychiatric diagnosis (particularly personality disorders and psychoactive substance use disorders) were also significantly more likely to predict aggressive behavior. For example, the woman whose neighbor stalks her because he believes she is the love of his life, and he wants to be united with her is likely to receive a different, less threatening type of attention from him than she gets from the ex-husband who can not accept the termination of their relationship. The lawyer whose former client has become hopelessly infatuated with him may receive the same level of attention as he does from the former client who is convinced that he cheated her out of her inheritance.

TABLE 21.1 Stalking Relationship Typology

Stalking Motive	Prior Relationship		
	Intimate/Former intimate	Acquaintance	None/Stranger
Amorous stalkers	Abusive ex-husband (domestic violence)	Infatuated employee (or neighbor, client)	Enamored fan (celebrity stalking)
Persecutory/vengeful stalkers	Estranged adult child seeking financial support	Disgruntled client neighbor, or employee	Angry constituent (victims)

Harmon, 2005.

Further analysis of this preliminary data set (Ciric & Harmon, 2002; Harmon, 2005) was initiated on the basis of the principle that researchers had been discovering that it was difficult to predict which stalkers might turn to physical violence in their pursuit patterns, and which stalking situations might remain psychologically stressful for the victim, but never escalate to dangerousness. If such prediction was not feasible, it was thought that it might be more fruitful to direct inquiries to the question of whether a stalker could be persuaded, either by legal or psychological means, to desist from the stalking behavior. A stalker who had abandoned his pursuit would, by default, no longer pose a risk to the victim.

The Stalking Recidivism Profile is based on the following definitions:

Single-incident stalking: A series of activities leading to an arrest either for stalking or for violating an initial order of protection. For this type of stalker, the behavior pattern is generally not repeated after the arrest/legal intervention. For example, a 51-year-old man was found incompetent to stand trial with a diagnosis of paranoid schizophrenia, on a charge of harassing a popular actress. He had sent numerous letters to her over a 5-year period, expressing his love and demanding money. Since this finding, and his consequent hospitalization in a State psychiatric facility, he has not returned to the attention of the Forensic Psychiatry Clinic, and there was no record of a further arrest at the time of the study data collection.

Persistent stalking: Multiple incidents of stalking behavior that do not cease subsequent to a legal intervention. This type of stalker does not appear to desist. All of the incidents of stalking in the arrest record relate to the same target or group of targeted individuals. For example, X. was a middle-aged white man charged with second-degree aggravated harassment on three occasions (August 1995, October 1995, and July 1996), and criminal contempt on three occasions (November 1995, March 1996, and July 1997). While in custody he continued to write letters to the complainant, a former acquaintance whom he had dated. Although these were the only charges reported in his New York State file, his Probation file indicated an arrest record dating back to 1958, in five other states, and on federal property. These offenses included weapons possession, drugs, assault, and robbery, and the sentences ranged from conditional discharge to as much as 4 years incarceration. This man would not be deterred by the legal system, and his harassing behavior toward the victim ceased only when he was killed in a motorcycle accident in 1999.

Serial stalking: Multiple incidents of stalking behavior in conjunction with legal action (arrest), where the targets of subsequent or simultaneous stalking are different, *unrelated* individuals or groups of individuals. It should be noted that Goldstein (2000) coined the term "serial stalking," which he defined as "the *sequential* stalking of discrete victims at different times" (emphasis in original), but does not consider the simultaneous stalking of multiple unrelated targets to be serial stalking. Thirteen percent of the stalkers in the current data set were serial stalkers. One of the more infamous of these was Ms. Y. Even before her first referral to the Forensic Psychiatry Clinic for evaluation, she had been accused of stalking a well-known local physician. At the time of her first referral to the Clinic, she had begun to stalk another physician from the staff of the same hospital facility. Ms. Y., a well-spoken, attractive woman in her late 30s, originally from a middle class background, believed that this doctor was her boyfriend. She was so convincing that she nearly persuaded the Court of the righteousness of her cause, until she began to stalk the (male) judge and prosecuting attorney assigned to her case. According to one evaluating psychiatrist's report:

> The Probation Department provided information that twenty individuals have taken out an order of protection against Ms.[Y., and] that four judges have taken themselves out of this case because of harassment or inappropriate behavior on the part of Ms....

Less dramatic, but still disturbing to the victims, was a homosexual woman diagnosed as a true erotomanic, who had multiple arrests over more than 10 years for assault, harassment, and violating orders of protection. She pursued a social worker who had been her counselor at a rehabilitation facility, and a second social worker with whom she claimed to have been sexually involved (the woman denied this). Another form of "concurrent" stalking can be related to celebrity stalking, where authorities have discovered that obsessed fans may stalk more than one star at a time. Robert Bardo, the stalker whose murder of actress Rebecca Schaeffer in 1989 made her the "poster child" for stalking in the United States, simultaneously stalked the then-popular singers Tiffany and Debbie Gibson (Gross, 1998).

The reexamination of the data explored whether there was any predictive significance for recidivism from a variety of independent variables, including the nature of the prior relationship, the categorization of the case as amorous versus persecutory, various demographic and clinical characteristics of the stalker, and various aspects of the criminal case (charges, dispositions, criminal history).

Three principal factors were identified that could assist victims, victim service providers, and law enforcement to determine if stalking might persist or desist.

1. **The previous relationship between the victim and the stalker:** Victims who were acquainted with their stalkers before the beginning of the harassment were more likely to be subjected to persistent stalking than victims for whom their stalkers had been strangers. Stalkers who had been intimately acquainted with their victims were most likely to continue their stalking behavior, in spite of efforts on all levels to control them.

2. **The violation of an order of protection by the stalker:** The violation of an order of protection is also an indication that the stalker will be persistent in his or her behavior. This is consistent with the first finding, since it is more likely that an order of protection can be obtained when the stalking is in the context of a previous domestic partnership. It is also true by definition, since the violation of the court order is, in effect, an additional incident of stalking behavior.

3. **Evidence of physical aggression by the stalker:** Stalkers who exhibit signs of physical aggression toward their victims are also more likely to be persistent in their approach. This is probably the most unsettling of the findings, and also the most important finding for law enforcement.

Another finding, not reaching the level of statistical significance, must be considered limited to this specific sample of mentally disordered stalkers. It appeared that the criminal disposition of the stalking cases in this small group of defendants did not affect recidivism. Whether a stalker was sentenced to incarceration or probation, or the length of the term of either sentence, did not have a significant impact on the recidivism profile. This suggests that some additional form of intervention, in addition to punishment by the criminal justice system, should be considered when mental illness is an issue in a stalking case.

It should be noted that the pilot study was based on a retrospective chart review of a small convenience sample of criminal offenders who had been referred for evaluation to a forensic psychiatry clinic in a major metropolitan area. The Court or the Department of Probation had some reason for suspecting that the assessment of psychiatric issues would be helpful for the disposition of these cases, and for most of the defendants, some psychiatric diagnosis was established. Because of confidentiality issues, some information regarding the criminal records of these defendants, both before and after the incidents, for which they were referred to the Forensic Psychiatry Clinic, could not be obtained, therefore, it is possible that their criminal history included other incidents of stalking either in New York City or other localities that could not be documented.

CONCLUSION

There is preliminary evidence that it may be possible to use the Recidivism Profile of a convicted stalker to evaluate the potential effectiveness of criminal justice system intervention on the duration of stalking behavior in mentally disordered stalkers. The principal factors to include in this profile are the prior relationship between the stalker and the targeted individual, any incidence of documented physical aggression during the course of the stalking, and whether the stalker violated an order of protection to obtain access to the victim. Law enforcement must pay particular attention to stalkers who have acted violently toward their victims or toward other individuals around their victims. These persons are among the most likely to persist in their stalking regardless of legal intervention. In such situations, the best defense against stalking may be keeping the victim safely separated from the stalker, either through incarceration or through hospitalization of the stalker, or through the careful relocation of the victim.

The author hopes that knowing whether a stalker may respond to the actions of the criminal justice system will provide some guidance in the management of these difficult cases.

References

American Psychiatric Association. (2000). Diagnostic and statistical manual of mental disorders (DSM-IV-TR). Washington, D.C.: American Psychiatric Publishing.

Boon, J. C. W. & Sheridan, L. (2001). Stalker typologies: A law enforcement perspective. *Journal of Threat Assessment*, 1(2), The Haworth Press, Inc.

Ciric, S. & Harmon, R. (2002). Serial stalking. Presentation at the annual meeting of the American Academy of Forensic Sciences, Atlanta, GA.

Crepps v. Durden [2 Cowp. 640, 98 Eng. Rep. 1283 (K. B. 1777)].

Dietz, P. E., Matthews, D. B., Martell, D. A., Stewart, T. M., Hrouda, D. R., & Warren, J. (1991a). Threatening and otherwise inappropriate letters to members of the United States Congress. *Journal of Forensic Sciences*, 36(5), 1445–1468.

Dietz, P. E., Matthews, D. B., Van Duyne, C., Martell, D. A., Parry, C. D. H., Stewart, T., et al. (1991b). Threatening and otherwise inappropriate letters to Hollywood celebrities. *Journal of Forensic Sciences*, 36(1), 185–209.

Goldstein, R. L. (2000). Serial stalkers: Recent clinical findings. In L. B. Schlesinger (Ed.), *Serial offenders: Current thought, recent findings* (pp. 167–185). Boca Raton, FL: CRC Press.

Gross, L. (1994). Understanding and surviving America's stalking epidemic: A special report. La Mesa, CA: Bear Publishing. http://www.ncjrs.gov/App/Publications/abstract.aspx?ID=177996.

Harmon, R. B. (2001). Criminal dispositions of mentally disordered stalkers. presented at the annual meeting of the Academy of Criminal Justice Sciences. Washington, D.C.

Harmon, R. B. (2005). The development of a typology of stalking behaviors to facilitate interventions. Presented at the annual meeting of the International Association of Forensic Mental Health Services. Melbourne, Australia.

Harmon, R. B., Rosner, R., & Owens, H. (1995). Obsessional harassment and erotomania in a Criminal Court Population. *Journal of Forensic Sciences*, 40, 188–196.

Harmon, R. B., Rosner, R., & Owens, H., (1998). Sex and violence in a forensic population of obsessional harassers. *Psychology, Public Policy and Law*, 4(1/2), 236–249.

Kurt, J. L. (1995). Stalking as a variant of domestic violence. *Bulletin of the American Academy of Psychiatry and the Law*, 23(2), 219–230.

Meloy, J. R. & Gothard, S. (1995). Demographic and clinical comparison of obsessional followers and offenders with mental disorders. *American Journal of Psychiatry*, 152, 258–23.

Miller, N. (2003). A law enforcement and prosecution perspective. National Institute of Justice to the Institute for Law and Justice (ILJ), grant no. 96-WT-NX-0007.

Mullen, P. E. (2003). Multiple classifications of stalkers and stalking behavior available to clinicians. *Psychiatric Annals*, 33(10), 651–656.

Mullen, P. E., Pathé, M., Purcell, R., & Stuart, G. W. (1999). Study of stalkers. *American Journal of Psychiatry*, 156, 1244–49.

Mullen, P. E., Pathé, M., & Purcell, R. (2000). *Stalkers and their victims*. Cambridge, UK: Cambridge University Press.

Palarea, R. E., Zona, M. A., Lane, J. C., & Langhinrichsen-Rohling, J. (1999). The dangerous nature of intimate relationship stalking: Threats, violence and associated risk factors. *Behavioral Sciences and the Law*, 17, 269–283.

Purcell, R., Pathé, M., & Mullen P. E. (2004). Stalking: Defining and prosecuting a new category of offending. *International Journal of Law and Psychiatry*, 27, 157–169.

Radosevich, A. C. (2000). Thwarting the stalker: Are anti-stalking measures keeping pace with today's stalker? U. Ill. L. Rev. 1371.

Roberts, K. A. (2002). Stalking following the breakup of romantic relationships: Characteristics of stalking former partners. *Journal of Forensic Sciences*, 47, 1070–1077.

Rosenbaum, D. J. (2000). What does "Course of Conduct" mean in the stalking law? http://www.correctionhistory.org/northcountry/html/knowlaw/courseofconduct3.htm, Prepared by the Domestic Violence Team of Albany County, March.

Rosenfeld, B. (2003). Recidivism in stalking and obsessional harassment. *Law & Human Behavior*, 27(3), 251–265.

Rosenfeld, B. & Harmon, R. (2002). Factors associated with violence in stalking and obsessional harassment cases. *Criminal Justice and Behavior*, 29(6), 671–691.

Spitzberg, B. H. (2002). The tactical topography of stalking victimization and management. *Trauma, Violence & Abuse*, 3(4), 261–288.

U.S. Department of Justice, Office of Justice Programs. (1998). *Stalking and domestic violence: The third annual report to congress under the violence against women act*. Washington, D.C.: Violence against Women Grants Office.

Zona, M. A., Sharma, K. K., & Lane, J. (1993). A comparative study of erotomanic and obsessional subjects in a forensic sample. *Journal of Forensic Sciences*, 38(4), 894–903.

Chapter 22

Child Pornography and the Internet

L. Alvin Malesky, Jr., Liam Ennis, and Carmen L. Z. Gress

INTRODUCTION

Although the Internet has experienced exponential growth since its inception, it has only been in existence for a relatively short time. The Internet as we know it today originated in the late 1960s when the Advanced Research Projects Agency (ARPA) of the United States Department of Defense funded the development of a communications system to be used in the event of an attack on the United States (Casey, 2004). By 1971, computers at 15 locations throughout the United States were connected via this system. In October of 1972, scientists showcased the ARPA network at the First International Conference on Computers and Communication by linking computers at 40 different locations (**http://www.let.leidenuniv.nl/history/ivh/frame_theorie.html**, accessed July 5, 2006). During this same year a new communication system that allowed direct person-to-person transition of electronic message (e-mail) became operational (**http://www.let.leidenuniv.nl/history/ivh/frame_theorie.html**, accessed July 5, 2006). Internet usages increased dramatically during the late 1980s and 1990s. By 2000, over 40% of U.S. households were connected to the Internet (U.S. Department of Commerce [USDOC], 2001). It is also estimated that over a billion people worldwide are currently using the Internet (**www.cia.gov/ciapublications/factbook/rankorder2153rank.html** accessed June 7, 2006).

Although the Internet has facilitated education and research, expedited communication and the flow of information, and assisted in commerce and business growth, the impact of this technology has not been entirely positive. Concerns about Internet usage include cyber addictions, in which individuals spend excessive amounts of time online, often at the expense of their family, friends, and job (Brody, 2000; Cooper, Delmonico, & Burg, 2000; Putnam & Maheu, 2000); its use in the advancement of extremist ideologies (Schafer, 2002); and its use in illegal activities (Casey, 2004; Conly, 1989). The use of the Internet to acquire and distribute child pornography in particular has received considerable attention from mental health clinicians, law enforcement personnel and the media (Cooper, 2001; Harrington, 2003; Thompson, 2002).

Irrespective of the increased focus of law enforcement or the extensive media coverage, the actual prevalence of this online behavior is unclear. A recent study by Wolak et al. (2005) estimated that there were approximately 1700 arrests in the United States for Internet-related child pornography possession in 2000. While this represents only 2.5% of roughly 65,000 arrests for all types of sexual assaults committed against minors during this time, it is uncertain as to how many individuals engage in this type of online behavior but do not come to the attention of law enforcement officers. The number of arrests and convictions is expected to grow with the increased use of the Internet coupled with law enforcement's improved knowledge and expertise in handling these types of cases (Wolak, Finkelhor, & Mitchell, 2005). However, at this time arrests and convictions for this online behavior remain relatively low compared to other types of child sexual exploitation.

Although child pornography on the Internet has received increased attention, understanding the complex issues surrounding the acquisition and distribution of online child pornography (e.g., etiology, treatment, and legal applications) is still in its infancy. This chapter addresses these issues by providing an extensive review of the legal and legislative issues pertaining to child pornography and the Internet in the United States, Canada, and Europe. The authors also draw upon developed bodies of research and established theoretical models from the fields of sociology, criminology, media psychology, and social psychology in offering an explanation as to why individuals use the Internet to collect and disseminate child pornography. Finally, assessment and treatment of individuals convicted for possession of child pornography is discussed.

DEFINING CHILD PORNOGRAPHY

The term child pornography is utilized in this chapter for purposes of consistency; however, it does not fully convey the nature and extent of abuse and exploitation that often occur with the production of this material (Wolak et al., 2005). The process associated with the creation of child pornography goes beyond commercial manufacturing typically associated with adult pornography and the adult entertainment industry. "Child abuse images" is a more appropriate descriptor of this material in that this phrase conveys the abuse that often occurs prior, during, and subsequent to the creation of pornographic images, audio, and video involving minors (Wolak et al., 2005). Furthermore, this phrase eliminates the commercial connotation associated with the term pornography (Lee, 2003). However, as previously stated "child pornography" will be used in this chapter to be consistent with the research literature as well as due to this term's widespread use in legal statute.

Legislative bodies that determine definitions, restrictions, and penalties for possession or distribution of child pornography share a common goal: the protection of children from sexual exploitation. However, definitions of what constitutes child pornography vary in accordance with the relevant legislation and legal precedents in each country or legal jurisdiction. This can provide advantages, such as the ability for local laws to reflect contemporary cultural and community standards. However, this lack of consistency also has distinct disadvantages, such as disagreement among cultures living within the same jurisdiction, and ambiguity in the law, which could make policing across jurisdictions difficult. The following section provides an overview of the American, Canadian, British, and European Union's legal definitions of child pornography.

Legal Definitions

The United States. Crimes involving child pornography are governed by federal or state law, depending on the specifics of the offense. For example, the federal statute oversees child pornography "where the producer or distributor knows or has reason to know, that the depiction was or will be transported in interstate commerce or was created using a camera, film, or other material that has traveled in interstate commerce" (Astrowsky & Peters, 2002, p. 1). When commerce does not cross state or national borders, or if the U.S. postal service was not used to receive and/or transport material associated with the crime, child pornography is prosecuted at the state level. Although guided by federal statute on child pornography, each state is able to augment or adapt their laws dealing with child pornography. Federal and state statutes concerning child pornography, sexual exploitation,

and child abuse and neglect can be reviewed at http://
www.ndaa.org/apri/programs/ncpca/ncpca_home.
html and http://www.childwelfare.gov respectively.

Currently, U.S. federal law defines child pornography as,

> ...any visual depiction, including any photo-
> graph, film, video, picture, or computer or com-
> puter-generated image or picture, whether made
> or produced by electronic, mechanical, or other
> means, of sexually explicit conduct, where
>
> 1. the production of such visual depiction
> involves the use of a minor engaging in sexually
> explicit conduct;
> 2. such visual depiction is a digital image,
> computer image, or computer-generated image
> (see discussion in this chapter on *Ashcroft v. Free
> Speech Coalition* and the PROTECT Act) that is,
> or is indistinguishable from, that of a minor engag-
> ing in sexually explicit conduct; or such visual
> depiction has been created, adapted, or modified
> to appear that an identifiable minor is engaging in
> sexually explicit conduct (18 U.S.C. § 2256[8]).

The term "sexually explicit" is defined by U.S.C. §
2256(2) as (1) graphic sexual intercourse, including
genital–genital, oral–genital, anal–genital, or oral–
anal, whether between persons of the same or opposite sex, or lascivious simulated sexual intercourse
where the genitals, breast, or pubic area of any person is exhibited; (2) graphic or lascivious simulated
(i) bestiality; (ii) masturbation; (3) sadistic or masochistic abuse; or (4) graphic or simulated lascivious exhi-
bition of the genitals or pubic area of any person.

In relation to child pornography, U.S. federal law
defines a minor as anyone below the age of 18. A
depiction is deemed to be "graphic" where, "a viewer
can observe any part of the genitals or pubic area of
any depicted person or animal during any part of
the time that the sexually explicit conduct is being
depicted" (U.S.C. § 2256[10]).

Defining lascivious behavior and determining lascivious intent represent an ongoing challenge in
the U.S. courts. These determinations are often
accomplished by comparing the visual depictions in
question to a nonexhaustive list of factors known as
the *Dost* criteria (Astrowsky & Peters, 2002; *United
States v. Dost*, 1986). In accordance with the Dost criteria lascivious behavior and intent are determined
on the basis of the following: (1) whether the genitals or pubic area are the focal point of the image;

(2) whether the setting of the image is sexually suggestive (i.e., a location generally associated with sexual activity); (3) whether the child is depicted in an
unnatural pose or inappropriate attire considering her
age; (4) whether the child is fully or partially clothed,
or nude; (5) whether the image suggests sexual coy-
ness or willingness to engage in sexual activity; and
(6) whether the image is intended or designed to elicit
a sexual response in the viewer.

Additionally, with the passing of the aforementioned sections, Congress augmented the definition
of child pornography to include "the scope of 'exhibi-
tion of the genitals or pubic area' in section 2256(2)
(E), in the definition of 'sexually explicit conduct'
is not limited to nude exhibitions or exhibitions in
which the outlines of those areas were discernible
through clothing." In other words, images that focus
on the genitals and pubic area can be considered lascivious even if the aforementioned areas are clothed,
a precedent set by *United States v. Knox* (1992).

To understand the current legislation, a review of
a few specific cases is required. In 1982, the Supreme
Court determined, in *New York v. Ferber*, that child
pornography was exempt from protection by the First
Amendment of the U.S. constitution (i.e., the right
to freedom of expression) because (1) the production
and dissemination of child pornography are related to
the sexual abuse of children, (2) the underlying activity (sexual molestation and exploitation) is illegal, and
(3) the societal and artistic value of child pornography
is "de minimus", or insignificant (New York v. Ferber,
1982; as cited in Bower, 2004, p. 239). In 1996, the
Child Pornography Prevention Act (CCPA, P.L.
104–208, 110 Stat. 3009–26) acknowledged the increasing role of technology in the production of child
pornography, including the production of computer-
generated images that are virtually indistinguishable
from real depictions of child sexual abuse. This Act
broadened the scope of what may be considered child
pornography to include not only depictions of actual
children, but also visual depictions that "*appears to
be*, of a minor engaging in sexually explicit conduct"
(emphasis added, Cohen, 2003). Subsequently, the
CCPA rekindled discussions about the limitations of
protection afforded by the First Amendment (Cohen,
2003).

In the case of *Ashcroft v. Free Speech Coalition*
(2002), the United States Supreme Court determined criminalization of fictitious or virtual (child)
pornography was unnecessary because (a) virtual

child pornography need not involve nor harm a real child in the production process and (b) virtual child pornography was not "intrinsically related" to child sexual abuse (*Ashcroft v. Free Speech Coalition*, 2002). Therefore, unlike "real" child pornography, the court granted virtual child pornography first amendment protection. Bower (2004) noted two important issues regarding this case: (a) the court did not address computer-modified images, which involves a real child and (b) the ruling provided an opening to present evidence that virtual child pornography is intrinsically related to child sexual abuse and exploitation and should not, therefore, receive First Amendment protection.

In 2003, the PROTECT Act (Prosecutorial Remedies and Other Tools to end the Exploitation of Children Today, the second major update to the initial Protection of Children Against Sexual Exploitation Act of 1977) amended the definition of child pornography to include "such visual depiction is a digital image, computer image, or computer generated image that is, or is indistinguishable from, that of a minor engaging in sexually explicit conduct" (pp. 108–21). This is a significant change because the inclusion of "…a digital image, computer image, or computer generated image that is indistinguishable" may be considered by some as unconstitutional under the Ashcroft decision (Cohen, 2003). At time of press, this has not yet been successfully challenged in court. Indistinguishable means "virtually indistinguishable" and does not apply to "drawings, cartoons, sculptures, or paintings" (18 U.S.C. § 2256[1], as added by the § 502(c) of the PROTECT Act).

Canada. Crimes involving child pornography are governed by federal law in Canada. The Criminal Code of Canada's definition of child pornography, last updated in 2005, is

(a) photographic, film, video or other visual representation, whether or not it was made by electronic or mechanical means,
    (i) that shows a person who is depicted as being under the age of eighteen years and is engaged in or is depicted as engaged in explicit sexual activity, or
    (ii) the dominant characteristic of which is the depiction, for a sexual purpose, of a sexual organ or the anal region of a person under the age of eighteen years;
(b) any written material, visual representation or audio recording that advocates or counsels sexual

activity with a person under the age of eighteen years that would be an offense under this Act;
(c) any written material whose dominant characteristic is the description, for a sexual purpose, of sexual activity with a person under the age of eighteen years that would be an offense under this Act; or
(d) any audio recording that has as its dominant characteristic the description, presentation or representation, for a sexual purpose, of sexual activity with a person under the age of 18 years that would be an offense under this Act (Criminal Code of Canada, Section 163.1 [1]).

Regina v. Sharpe (2001, 150 C.C.C. [3d] 321 [S.C.C.]) [Note: Criminal and civil cases taken (or defended) by a government in a Commonwealth country, such as Canada, the United Kingdom, and Australia, are undertaken in the name of the Commonwealth head of State (British Monarch) or Crown (aka Regina, Latin for Queen and Rex, Latin for King)] initiated a rewording of the child pornography legislation (reflected in the aforementioned definition and described further subsequently) and served as a legal precedent, providing two exemptions to the law on possession of child pornography, and reignited the defense of "artist merit" in Canada. In 1995, Robin Sharpe was charged with two counts of possession and two counts of distributing child pornography: the material in question were photographs, drawings, and 17 stories depicting sexual activity with minors (Grover, 2004). The defense argued that the charge of possession for the written material was unconstitutional because section 163.1(6) and (7) of the Canadian Criminal Code allowed a defense of "artistic merit or an educational, scientific or medical purpose" (Grover, 2004). After the British Columbia (BC) Supreme Court acquitted Sharpe of the charges and the BC Court of Appeal upheld the acquittal, the BC government appealed to the Supreme Court of Canada. The Supreme Court upheld the existing law but provided two exceptions: (a) the creator, and only the creator is a user of the material and (b) it did not involve minors (*Regina v. Sharpe*, 2001). As a result, Bill C-2, the latest in a series of proposals to amend the law regarding sexual offenders, made a number of changes significant to the definition of child pornography (represented in the current definition), including (a) audio as a possible source of child pornography and (b) a second category of written and audio material "whose dominant characteristic is the description, for a sexual purpose, of sexual activity with a person under the age of eighteen...."

A distinct difference between the U.S. and Canadian definitions of child pornography is Canada's ambiguity of what can be considered an image of child pornography and its inclusion of written and audio material. Written and/or audio child pornographic material is not included in the U.S. federal definition of child pornography and is, therefore, legal unless the material is deemed obscene by the court.

The United Kingdom and European Union. The United Kingdom consists of three separate legal jurisdictions: England and Wales, Scotland, and Northern Ireland. In England and Wales, child pornography is defined as an indecent photograph or pseudo-photography, such as a computer-modified image, of a child, including film, any form of video recording, and copies and/or negatives. Similar definitions are used in Northern Ireland and Scotland. A child, as related to child pornography, is a person below the age of 18 in all three of these jurisdictions. Like in the United States, these Acts only address photographic material. Other potential examples of child pornography, such as written work or audio recordings, are subject to general obscenity legislation (Gillespie, 2005). In addition, there are a series of exceptions as related to photographs of 16- and 17-year-olds, which if applicable, must be brought forth by the defense, rather than the police or crown. For example, in Scotland, exceptions include (1) photographs that are of a person aged 16 or over, or the accused reasonably believed that to be so; (2) the accused and the 16- or 17-year old subject of the photograph were either (a) married to or civil partners of each other or were partners in an established relationship at the time of the offense, or (b) at the time when the accused obtained the photograph, the subject of the photograph consented to being photographed, or (c) for the photograph to be in the possession of the accused (depending on which offense has been charged), or the accused reasonably believed this to be the case, or (d) that distribution was only to the 16- or 17-year-old subject of the photograph.

Indecency is not defined in any of the United Kingdom's Acts but is determined by a judge or jury as illustrated by cases such as *Regina v. Graham Kerr*, *Regina v. Smethurst*, and *Regina v. Murray* (Gillespie, 2005). The courts stated in *Regina v. Graham Kerr* (1988) and *Regina v. Smethurst* (2002) that

the decision as to what is indecent is an objective question for the jury to answer...this would mean, in contested cases, that the jury would be shown the images and asked to consider whether they believed they were an indecent image of a child (Gillespie, 2005, p. 438).

An interesting example of this was *Regina v. Murray* (2004). Murray recorded and modified a television medical documentary about a young male with a genital defect. His modifications included slowing the tape speed and focusing the image on the male's genitals. Defense argued that the images in question were decent because the video was decent and images were only clips from the video (Gillespie, 2005). The Court of Appeal rejected this argument stating the clips were images in their own right and the jury could decide if an image abstracted from a decent image was indecent.

In 2000, the EU-Framework Decision on Combating the Sexual Exploitations of Children and Child Pornography used the U.S. Criminal Code as a model for defining child pornography (Graupner, 2004). On the basis of the U.S. Criminal Code's definition of child pornography, the EU-Framework defines child pornography to include all visual depictions of explicit sexual conduct with a person below the age of 18 including fictitious depictions such as comic strips, drawings, paintings, and virtual imagery (Graupner, 2004). Consistent with the U.S. definition, the visual depictions need not be nude, nor does the EU-Framework require the establishment of the minor's true age.

USING THE INTERNET TO ACQUIRE AND DISTRIBUTE CHILD PORNOGRAPHY

Although there has been significant legislative activity, both in the United States and abroad, in crafting and/or revising laws dealing with child pornography fundamental questions still exist regarding the nature and function of the Internet in the dissemination and acquisition of these images. Specifically, (1) why is the Internet an attractive vehicle for engaging in this type of activity? (2) who is using the Internet for these purposes? (3) what effect, if any, do these online sexual behaviors have on the individuals who engage in them?

Why Do Individuals Use the Internet to Disseminate and Acquire Child Pornography?

Although child pornography predates the Internet, recent advances in technology have made digital cameras, home computers, and the Internet affordable and effective vehicles for the production, storage, dissemination, and acquisition of these images.

Cooper (1998) suggested that the accessibility, affordability, and perceived anonymity of the Internet make it an attractive tool for individuals interested in engaging in sexual activity. Cooper (1998) dubbed the accessibility, affordability, and anonymity provided by the Internet as the "Triple A Engine." Although Cooper did not introduce the "Triple A" framework to explain sexually exploitative online behavior specifically, his theory serves as a useful foundation in understanding why this technology is used for these purposes.

The Internet is extremely accessible. Millions of Americans have Internet access in their homes (USDOC, 2001). The Internet can also be accessed from public places such as libraries, coffee shops, and airports. In addition, cellular telephone users can now access the Internet, allowing one to get online from virtually anywhere at anytime.

Before the Internet, individuals interested in child pornography had to go to considerable lengths to indulge their interests. The Internet has created an omnipresent avenue by which people can access a limitless array of sexual preoccupations and interests. The National Center for Missing and Exploited Children (NCMEC) reported a 39% increase in reports of child pornography from 2003 to 2004. This was the seventh consecutive year that dramatic increases in reports of child pornography had been observed. This number has also increased in the United Kingdom. According to a National Children's Homes report, the number of individuals proceeded against by the police increased 1500% from 1988 to 2001 (Carr, 2004). Thus, not only is the Internet readily accessible but online child pornography is also accessible for the motivated and savvy Internet user.

In addition to being available, Internet access is relatively inexpensive. One can obtain a high-speed DSL or cable connection for approximately $40 a month and slower dial-up connections are even less expensive. One can also access the Internet from public places such as coffee shops or universities utilizing Wi-Fi or wireless technology for free. Once online, Internet users have access to an unlimited supply of sexually explicit material. Although pornography is a multibillion-dollar industry, tremendous amounts of sexually explicit material are available for minimal or no charge. Many adult websites offer free "samples" with the intention of enticing consumers to pay for access to a wider range of images and full-length movies. Furthermore, shareware websites facilitate the free exchange of pornographic images and video clips.

Although the online adult pornography industry generates billions of dollars in revenue each year, distribution of child pornography does not often appear to be a profit-driven venture (Taylor, 1999). In fact, some individuals distribute their "collection" of child pornography free of charge with the hope that others will reciprocate in the future (O'Connell & Taylor, 1998). Furthermore, individuals may disseminate images as a way to increase their social status and credibility in virtual pedophile communities (O'Connell & Taylor, 1998). The ease of copying and electrically sending these images also contributes to the "affordability" of acquiring, maintaining, and even distributing one's "collection" of child pornography. In summary, Internet access is inexpensive if not free. Once online, motivated individuals can acquire, reproduce, and disseminate child pornography at minimal expense.

Individuals typically keep their online sexual behaviors private (Cooper, Boies, Maheu, & Greenfield, 1999; Leiblum, 1997), particularly when the behavior is aberrant or illegal (Lanning, 1992). McKenna and Bargh (1998) stated, "In virtual groups, where people can be anonymous and do not deal in face-to-face interactions, individuals can admit to having marginalized, or nonmainstream, proclivities that they hid from the rest of the world" (p. 682). McGrath and Casey (2002) likened the Internet to "a mask that conceals more than just the face" (p. 85). The Internet affords one the ability to create e-mail addresses, screen names, and persona that not only prevent others online from knowing who they are, but also contribute to a sense of escapism and depersonalization. It has been argued that, by reducing social disincentives, the Internet blurs the boundaries between fantasy and reality, allowing the individual to explore and indulge their fantasies (McGrath & Casey, 2002).

In addition to the inherent anonymity of the Internet, extra precautions can be taken to further conceal the user's identity. Computer programs strip information from e-mails (remailers) that make it extremely difficult to detect who actually sent an e-mail. Encryption software and passwords can also be employed to conceal information transmitted electronically. Some online communities that advocate for adult/minor "relationships" actually post links to websites that offer free encryption and remailer software (Malesky, 2005), as well as discourage its members from using their actual names while posting on the group's bulletin board.

Although some individuals recognize the advantages of increased online security (i.e., encryption software) in avoiding detection by law enforcement it is clear that this realization is not universally shared (Malesky, 2005; Wolak et al., 2005). For example, Malesky (2002) found that only 17% of the incarcerated offenders in his study, who admitted using the Internet for sexually deviant and illegal purposes used encryption software or remailers to conceal sexual images of children. Wolak et al. (2005) found similar results with their study. One must be cautious, however, generalizing the results of these studies to all individuals exchanging child pornography over the Internet. The subjects in the research by Malesky (2002) and Wolak et al. (2005) comprised exclusively of individuals who were apprehended for sexual offenses, which, by definition, indicate that they were unsuccessful in their efforts to remain anonymous. It is possible that individuals who take greater precautions to maintain their anonymity in the course of their Internet activities are consequently more successful in avoiding detection, and are therefore underrepresented in correctional or forensic samples. Notably, when more than 100 members of an international network of child pornography collectors and distributors were arrested in 1998, hundreds of other members of this same network began to utilize encryption software and other tactics to conceal their identities, rather than discontinue their illegal online behavior (McGrath & Casey, 2002; Shannon, 1998). In summary, the Internet is readily available, affordable if not completely free, and relatively anonymous. This makes it an ideal vehicle for individuals interested in acquiring and disseminating child pornography.

In addition to Cooper's "Triple A" framework, media psychology can also be used to elucidate why individuals use the Internet to collect and distribute child pornography. Researchers in this field (Song, LaRose, Eastin, & Lin, 2004; Swanson, 1992) have identified two general motivations for using mass communication. The first content-oriented motivation refers to behavior that is engaged in for the purpose of acquiring information that can subsequently be used to obtain desired outcomes. With regard to the Internet, this could include learning where and how to access online child pornography and to avoid detection in doing so. Process-oriented motivations on the other hand, are actions that result in a pleasurable experience that is realized in the moment, while the media is being accessed (e.g., masturbation to online pornography). Cooper et al. (2004) found that men with online sexual behavior problems (broadly defined as the use of the Internet for any activity that involves sexuality and causes problems in off-line functioning) identified two motivational domains related to engagement in online sexual behaviors. The first reason men engaged in online sexual behavior was to advance their off-line sex lives, which is consistent with the content-oriented motivations identified in the media psychology research. The second reason men engaged in online sexual activities was as an alternative to off-line sexual relationships. This motivation appears to overlap with the concept of process-oriented media usage.

Although individuals manufacture, collect, and disseminate child pornography over the Internet for a variety of reasons, sexual interest appears to be the primary reason for engaging in these activities. A recent study using phallometric assessment of sexual arousal found that collecting child pornography was a stronger diagnostic indicator of pedophilia than actually sexually offending against a child (Seto, Cantor, & Blanchard, 2006). These authors stated, "people are likely to choose the kind of pornography that corresponds to their sexual interests, so relatively few nonpedophilic men would choose illegal child pornography given the abundance of legal pornography that depicts adults."

It should be noted that, although sexual gratification is likely the primary reason most individuals collect child pornography via the Internet, it may not be the sole motivation for engaging in this behavior (O'Connell & Taylor, 1998; Quayle & Taylor, 2002). Online pornographic images are often part of a larger collection or series. Some of these series have their own name (i.e., "Amy" or "Kevin"), supposedly named after the victim in the pictures (Lee, 2003). Individuals may collect images to complete a certain "set" or "series" much like an individual would collect baseball cards to complete a "set." Individuals may exchange electronic images of child pornography as a way to increase their social status and credibility in online pedophile communities (O'Connell & Taylor, 1998). Some of these individuals report collecting images they do not personally find sexually arousing with the intent of trading them with other collectors for more preferred images (O'Connell & Taylor, 1998). Wolak et al. (2005) also suggested that individuals may download child pornography because they are inquisitive about this type of sexual material and view these images to satisfy their curiosity. Finally, some individuals may also use these images as a way to "groom" potential victims by attempting to demonstrate, via these images, that there is nothing aberrant about adult/minors sexual contact. However, as previously stated sexual gratification is likely the primary reason most individuals collect child pornography.

Who Is Using the Internet to Collect and Disseminate Images of Child Sexual Abuse?

Before the advent of the Internet, the distribution and acquisition of child pornography required that the interested individual access a clandestine network of suppliers under significant risk of detection and arrest. It is logical to assume that these individuals had strong pedophilic interest as evidenced by their willingness to expend considerable effort and take substantial risks to acquire preferred pornographic materials (Taylor & Quayle, 2003; Quayle & Taylor, 2003). However, the Internet has removed many of the obstacles that previously would have deterred all but the highly motivated from procuring child pornography. Thus, it is likely that individuals convicted of Internet child pornography offenses represent a more heterogeneous group than samples that have historically been used in studies of child pornography possessors. The best descriptive information about child pornography offenders comes from the National Juvenile Online Victimiation Study (Wolak, Finkelhor, & Mitchel, 2005). Based on nearly 2000 arrests for Internet-related child pornography possession, Wolak et al. (2005) found that the vast majority of individuals arrested for possession of child pornography are male, Caucasian, over the age of 26 years, and have at least a high-school education. Most (62%) were unmarried, although many (42%) had biological children, and many (34%) were living with children at the time of the crime. Nearly half (46%)

had access to minors either as the result of their living arrangements or through work or organized youth activity. A significant minority in Wolak et al's sample had known substance abuse problems (18%) but few had been diagnosed with mental (5%) or sexual (3%) disorders. Twenty-two percent had prior nonsexual criminal histories, and prevalence of past violent and sexual offending was 11% and 22%, respectively. In a much smaller sample, Seto and Eke (2005) found higher rates of past offending, with 56% of their sample of 201 child pornography offenders having prior nonsexual criminal records, 24% and having prior sexual contact offenses. Fifteen percent of Seto and Eke's sample had prior charges for child pornography offenses.

The question of whether Internet child pornography offenders differ from contact sex offenders in terms of individual characteristics and behavioral motivations is an important one. At present, there has been little research comparing Internet child pornography offenders to individuals who have committed contact sex offences against children. On recent study that did compare child pornography offenders with child molesters (Webb, Craissati, & Keen, 2007) found more similarities than differences. Relatively high levels of self-reported psychopathology were evident in both groups, with 40% of the sample reporting serious and diffuse personality disorder. Both Internet offenders and child molesters were characterized by schizoid, avoidant, and dependent traits, suggesting a disordered attachment orientation that inclines them to fear rejection, withdraw from potentially threatening social situations and relationships, or an excessive reliance on others for assistance with coping. Internet offenders and child molesters were both characterized by problems with intimate relationships and general self-regulation, but Internet offenders were distinguished by greater problems with sexual self-regulation (i.e., sexual preoccupation, sex as coping, deviant sexual interests). In contrast, child molesters were rated as more psychopathic, had more problems with offence supportive attitudes, and greater problems with supervision noncompliance.

Although only minimal attention has been paid to comparing and contrasting the two groups, preliminary evidence suggests that Internet offenders generally resemble child molesters. The existing evidence, however, suggests that degree of nonsexual antisociality appears to be a factor that may have utility for distinguishing between those offenders who indulge their sexual proclivities through Internet pornography from those who directly victimize actual children for the same purpose. Ultimately, additional empirical attention needs to be paid to investigating similarities and differences between these groups, and to distinguishing between child pornography offenders who are content to indulge their sexual interests online and those for whom child pornography use is accompanied by hands-on offending.

Causes and Consequences of Collecting and Disseminating Child Pornography over the Internet

The question of whether viewing online child pornography contributes to the development of sexually exploitative tendencies or whether they simply reflect preexisting traits and interests has yet to be answered empirically. Research focusing on problematic Internet usage or Internet addiction suggests that the influence Internet use has on subjective well-being is dependent on the characteristics of the individual. For people who are more introverted, increased Internet usage has been linked with decreased well-being and self-esteem, and increased loneliness and negative affect. The opposite effects have been found for extroverts (Kraut, Kiesler, Boneva, Cummings, Helgeson, & Crawford, 2002). Davis (2001) proposed a cognitive behavioral model of Pathological Internet Use (PIU) that emphasized the etiological role of maladaptive cognitions that intensify or maintain the behavior. Cognitions associated with self-doubt, low self-efficacy and negative self-appraisal such as, "I can only get along with others in cyberspace," or "people treat me badly off-line" facilitate further use of the Internet to postpone or avoid anxiety provoking experiences. Avoidant behaviors, in turn, create significant problems with daily functioning and limit opportunities for corrective experiences.

Middleton et al. (2006) suggest that, "the focus of research on the effects of pornography should concentrate on the context and meaning of pornography for each individual user in meeting their sexual needs" (p. 3). Fisher and Barak (2001) proposed a model for understanding the antecedents and consequences of accessing sexually explicit materials on the Internet that, although developed to explain behavior around the acquisition of sexually explicit materials in general, is equally applicable to child pornography. In Fisher and Barak's (2001) model, erotic stimuli evoke cognitive responses that in turn interact with arousal and affective responses to initiate preparatory sexual behaviors. In the case of child pornography on the Internet, preparatory behaviors might include locking one's bedroom door, disrobing, and directing one's web browser to a favorite online source of child pornography. Successful engagement in preparatory behaviors increases the likelihood that overt sexual behaviors will occur. Sexual behaviors will result in outcomes that will be subjectively appraised as either positive or negative, and these outcomes feed back into the system to increase or decrease the likelihood that similar sexual behaviors will be repeated in the future. Which sexual behaviors an individual engages in is heavily influenced by three types of cognitive responses to sexually arousing stimuli: (1) informational responses (i.e., beliefs about sexual activity), (2) expectative responses (i.e., subjective probability estimates concerning outcomes of sexual activity), and (3) imaginative responses (i.e., scripts of sexual episodes that may be used to safely and privately experience behaviors that the individual would be reluctant to actually engage in).

Marshall & Barbaree, (1991) formulated an etiological theory of sexual abuse that provides a useful lens through which to view Internet based offending. Rooted in attachment theory (Bowlby, 1982), Marshall and Barbaree's (1991) theory describes the process by which children who fail to develop secure attachments with caregivers in early life subsequently fail to develop the emotional or behavioral capacity to successfully engage in intimate relationships. Moreover, they fear rejection and are afraid to look to others for assistance in meeting their needs. As these children approach and enter adolescence, the authors suggest that they are likely to resort to sexual self-stimulation to combat chronic feelings of emotional loneliness, and subsequently, the physical act of sex becomes associated with intimacy. Furthermore, because male self-esteem is at least partially based on the males' subjective sense of sexual competence (Schimel, 1974, as cited in Marshall, Hudson, & Hodkinson, 1993) insecurely attached young males will be attracted to cognitive sexual scripts that depict them as powerful, potent, and in control. Substantial increases in testosterone levels during pubescence likely make this a sensitive period during which adolescent males may be particularly responsive to whatever form of sexual imagery or fantasy they choose to indulge in (Smallbone, 2006). Through masturbatory conditioning, these coercive sexual scripts may develop in to engrained sexual preferences (Abel & Blanchard, 1974; Marshall & Eccles, 1993; Marshall et al., 1991).

It is most likely that the type of sexual material that individuals seek and find stimulating is related to preexisting vulnerabilities and other dispositional differences (Fisher & Barak, 2001; Morahan-Martin, 2005; Seto, Maric, & Barbaree, 2001; Seto et al., 2006). Marshall and colleagues (1993) surmised the appeal that coercive sexual fantasy and behavior has for emotionally isolated young males, noting that,

> having sex with a child requires none of the social skills that these boys have failed to acquire; it provides a rare opportunity in the lives of these young males to experience power and control, and to be relatively unconcerned with rejection; and it satisfies those needs that have become focused on physical gratification (p. 176).

The Internet provides a venue in which the insecurely attached youth in Marshall's model can seek sexual stimuli that reinforce the association between sex and intimacy, and fuel and shape sexual fantasies, and nurture the development of coercive sexual scripts. Engaging in online sexual behaviors may, in turn, serve to reinforce or shape the sexual and personal dispositions that motivated the individual to engage in online sexual behaviors in the first place (Fisher & Barak, 2001). Fisher and Barak (2001) noted that Internet users bring with them, a lifelong learning history including beliefs about sexuality, expectations about sexual outcomes, and emotional correlates of sexual arousal. Although online sexual behavior may interact with the individual factors to reinforce deviant sexual preferences or facilitate hands-on offending for some Internet users, most individuals with typical developmental learning experiences and nondeviant sexual preferences are inclined to avoid violent and pedophilic sexual stimuli (Bogaert, 2001; Fisher & Barak, 2001; Seto, Maric, & Barbaree, 2001). Thus, the evidence suggests that a reciprocal relationship exists in which self-motivated participation in online sexual behaviors reinforces and influences sexual attitudes and behaviors (Fisher & Barak, 2001; Malamuth, Addison, & Koss, 2001; Malamuth & Impett, 2001; Padgett, Brislen-Slutz, & Neal, 1989; Seto et al., 2001). Ultimately,

pornography use cannot be seen as a necessary or sole cause of contact sexual abuse, because many perpetrators have had little or no exposure to pornography, and many pornography users have not committed sexual offenses.

CHILD PORNOGRAPHY, SEXUAL CONTACT OFFENDING, AND RECIDIVISM

An important question is whether downloading child pornography is associated with risk for future offending, and if so, is risk restricted to further downloading of illegal pornography, or is there also increased likelihood of committing contact offenses. The available data suggest that a significant proportion of individuals arrested for possessing child pornography have committed "hands-on" sexual offences in the past. Data from the NCMEC (2005) indicated that 40% of men arrested for possession of child pornography had also sexually victimized children, and an additional 15% of offenders were "dual offenders" who tried to victimize children by soliciting undercover investigators who posed as minors online. Hernandez (2000) found that offenders convicted of possession of child pornography or crossing state lines to have sex with a minor reported having committed more contact sexual offenses than individuals arrested for contact sex offenses. Twenty-four percent of the 201 men in Seto and Eke's (2005) sample had a prior history of contact sexual offending at the time of their arrest for child porn possession. Thus, for many child pornography offenders, there is already a behaviorally demonstrated precedent for committing actual, as opposed to virtual, sexual abuse of a child.

There are few data to inform the issue of risk for future offending, be it in the form of accessing illegal pornography or the commission of contact offenses. Seto and Eke (2006) examined recidivism among 198 child pornography offenders over an average follow-up period of 3.6 years. Of the child pornography offenders, 13 (6.6%) committed a contact sexual offense during the follow-up period, whereas 14 (7.1%) committed another child pornography offense. The violent (including contact sexual offense) offense rate was 9%, and the overall rate for a new offense of any kind was 22%. Violent and sexual contact reoffending were predicted by variables related to violent offense history, and no significant predictors of child pornography recidivism were found. Seto and Eke (2006) recommended that variables associated with general antisocial tendencies, especially measures of psychopathy, appear to be useful tools for assessing and understanding recidivism among child pornography offenders.

Webb et al. (2007) compared Internet child pornography offenders and child molesters on measures of criminal recidivism and treatment compliance over a relatively short, 18 month follow up period. Overall findings indicated that child molesters were more likely than child pornography offenders to reoffend generally (8% vs. 1%), violently (3% vs. 0%), and to breach the conditions of community supervision (17% vs. 0%). Rates of sexual recidivism were similar for both groups, with 3% of child pornography offenders and 2% of child molesters incurring a new conviction for a sexual offence (Internet or contact). Child molesters were significantly more likely to be noncompliant with supervision, and were more likely to drop out of treatment (18%) compared to child pornography offenders (4%).

The available research suggests that at least a significant minority of child pornography offenders have committed hands-on sex offences in the past, and those rates would likely increase if undetected offending could be accounted for. However, little is known about the potential for child pornography use to escalate to actual, rather than virtual, sexual abuse of a child for offenders who have no prior history of contact offending. Calder (2004) suggested that accessing child pornography implies a desire for sexual contact with children, and others (Quayle & Taylor, 2002; Sullivan & Beech, 2003) have suggested that downloading illegal pornography can facilitate the commission of a contact offence through the pairing of sexual images, fantasy, masturbation, and cognitive distortions. Sullivan and Beech (2003) proposed a motivational typology based on variable degrees of pedophilic interest that implies corresponding variations in risk for committing a contact offence. Sullivan and Beech distinguish between individuals who access child pornography as part of a larger pattern of sexual offending (Type 1) from those who do so to nurture a developing sexual interest in children (Type 2), and those who are merely curious but not fixated (Type 3). Ultimately, links between downloading child pornography and the commission of hands-on sex offences are largely intuitive and theoretical at present.

RISK ASSESSMENT AND MANAGEMENT

An informed, comprehensive assessment of risk for reoffense is essential for the effective management of sex offenders. A good risk assessment should be both prescriptive and preventative; it should identify dispositional factors that made the offender vulnerable to committing the offense, and prioritize treatment interventions that serve to mitigate an offender's risk for sexual reoffense. The focus of risk assessment evaluations in these cases should be on understanding what the offender was trying to accomplish as a function of his or her Internet-related behavior. The evaluator's task is to formulate an opinion about how and why the offender chose to engage in the sexual behaviors that led to his charges, and to determine whether the factors that led to those behaviors might lead the offender to engage in similar behaviors in the future (Hart, Laws, & Kropp, 2003).

There have been considerable advances in the field of sex offender risk assessment over the past decade. These advances have led to the development of numerous scales and protocols for appraising recidivism risk (Epperson et al., 1998; Hanson, 1997; Quinsey, Harris, Rice, & Cormier, 1998). Unfortunately, these instruments were not developed with specific consideration of offenders who exploit children via the Internet. Thus, Internet offenders, including possessors of child pornography, are not specifically identified in the normative samples and the predictive utility of variables related to Internet usage was not investigated. Middleton et al. (2006) observed that, "it may be the case that current psychometric assessments, which have been developed and normed for use with contact sex offenders, are possibly not effective in highlighting the psychological vulnerabilities of this population" (p. 13). In lieu of data supporting the predictive validity of actuarial assessment instruments for cases involving Internet-related offending, the use of established norm-based estimates of sexual reoffense appears to be inappropriate, at least in cases where possession of child pornography is the sole sexual offense of record. Furthermore, these instruments observe the behavior of a whole population of test subjects. The utility concerning a specific individual is therefore limited to assessing how the individual's characteristics compare to members of a relevant sample population and how recidivism rates are distributed in a roughly similar population.

In addition to the aforementioned limitations, a more general limitation for most established sex offender risk assessment schemes is that they tend to be based exclusively on historical risk factors that are, by definition, not amenable to change (Hanson, Morton, & Harris, 2003; Ward & Beech, 2004). Consequently, these instruments are of limited utility for informing treatment planning and supervisory contingencies. In response to these limitations, recent approaches to risk assessment have increasingly emphasized a risk-need approach that focuses on the identification of dynamic or alterable risk factors in addition to static risk factors assessment (Bonta, 2002; Douglas & Skeem, 2005).

Dynamic Risk Assessment

Barbaree (2003) argued that static factors tell us which offenders are more likely to reoffend, whereas dynamic factors tell us when an offender is more likely to reoffend. To ensure public safety sex offenders must receive the appropriate level of service and supervision, and those decisions require the accurate identification and management of dynamic risk factors. Dynamic risk factors represent criminogenic needs that serve as treatment targets, and that, if successfully addressed correspond with changes in risk for reoffense (Andrews & Bonta, 2003; Andrews, Zinger, Hoge, Bonta, Gendreau, & Cullen, 1990; Bonta, 2002; Ward & Stewart, 2003). Dynamic risk factors can be divided into stable and acute factors (Hanson & Harris, 2000). Stable dynamic factors are those that are theoretically alterable but entrenched and slow to change (e.g., alcohol dependence). In contrast, acute dynamic factors are states that are subject to rapid fluctuations that may occur over periods of weeks, days, or even minutes (e.g., alcohol intoxication).

The authors have elected to discuss assessment and treatment within a risk-need framework, with a focus on stable dynamic factors for several reasons. First, as previously discussed, the predictive validity of established risk assessment instruments has not been established for Internet sex offenders, including those who download child pornography. Second, Ward and Beech (2004) proposed that stable dynamic factors represent individual vulnerabilities that have a causative relationship with sexual abusive behavior. Thus, discussion of stable dynamic factors affords the opportunity to discuss both evaluation and treatment considerations within a common model. Although there is growing empirical support for the consideration of dynamic risk factors in the assessment of sex offense risk (Hanson & Harris, 2000, 2001), the extent to which the established literature on sex offenders may be generalized to collectors of child pornography is not yet known. Moreover, there have been very few empirical studies of recidivism among offenders arrested for Internet-related sex crimes. Thus, the dynamic risk factors discussed in this chapter are presented not for their established predictive validity, but rather, for their theoretical and heuristic value, and for the purpose of generating discussion in the burgeoning area of Internet-related sexual abuse. The factors discussed in the remainder of this chapter are not mutually exclusive, and in fact it is likely that all five factors contribute to each occurrence of sexually exploitative behavior in varying degrees (Ward & Beech, 2004).

There are five stable dynamic risk factors of particular relevance for individuals who utilize the Internet to acquire or distribute images of child sexual abuse. Ward and Beech (2004) developed an etiological model of sex offense risk that incorporated four stable dynamic risk domains based on the work of Hanson and Harris (2001) and Thornton (2002). Those stable dynamic factors included (1) sexual self-regulation, (2) general self-regulation, (3) intimacy deficits/interpersonal functioning, and (4) offense supportive cognitions. The current authors also considered a fifth stable dynamic factor, negative social influences, on the basis of its established predictive utility in the nonsexual offender literature, its inclusion in current dynamic assessment schemes (Hanson & Harris, 2001), and its theoretical relevance for individuals who download images of child sexual abuse from the Internet.

Sexual Interests/Sexual Self-Regulation

This risk domain includes sexual preoccupation, use of sex for coping, affect regulation, and deviant sexual preferences. Quayle et al. (2006) likened sexual stimulation to a form of self-medication for some individuals; a tactic utilized to alleviate feelings of anxiety, loneliness, and depression. Contemporary theories of sexual deviance describe how, during childhood, some offenders become prematurely and inappropriately sexualized and develop a tendency to use sex as a mechanism for coping and affect regulation (Marshall & Barbaree, 1991; Marshall & Marshall, 2002; Ward, Hudson, Marshall, & Siegert, 1995; Ward & Sorbello, 2003). Masturbation is a reliable and pleasurable form of avoidant coping and therefore is a highly reinforcing and easily generalized behavior. Studies have shown that sexual offenders tend to utilize ineffective coping strategies in general, and are more likely to indulge in both coercive and consensual sexual fantasies when under stress (Cortoni & Marshall, 2001; Marshall, Serran, & Cortoni, 2000). These findings suggest that although the content of sexual fantasy may be a salient consideration for many sex offenders, the broader tendency to utilize sexual means of regulating one's affective state may be a more defining and etiologically significant characteristic for many offenders.

Quayle et al. (2006) described the Internet as a "perfect vehicle" for avoiding or altering negative mood states through sexual stimulation because it is readily available, immediate, and controllable. Cooper et al. (2004) found that over 80% of men identified as having noncriminal online sexual behavior problems engaged in online sexual activities as a form of distraction from their daily lives. An additional 56% of this same sample reported engaging in online sexual activities as a form of stress relief. Middleton et al. (2006) examined 43 men convicted of Internet-related sex offenses and found that 33% of them were characterized by the inability to identify and modulate mood states, and the tendency to self-soothe through sexual means. Quayle and Taylor (2002) stated,

> Through the Internet the unsatisfactory elements of life that were difficult to address or change could, for periods of time, be avoided and substituted for a world that was more controllable. Sexual satisfaction could be sought and gained, allowing the respondent to have perfect control (p. 349).

Recent data suggests that possession of images of child pornography may be a more valid indicator of pedophilia than actual history of contact offenses against children. Seto et al. (2006) found that men who had been convicted of possessing child pornography were three times more likely to be to be identified as pedophilic on the basis of results from phallometric testing than child molesters without charges related to child pornography. Although individuals who collect and/or disseminate these images likely do so as a result of preexisting traits and sexual interests, it has been argued that online sexual behaviors allow for the exploration, indulgence, and crystalization of sexual fantasies that otherwise would have self-extinguished (Cooper, Scherer, Boies, & Gordon, 1999). Empirical data and clinical intuition suggest that downloading child pornography is most frequently accompanied by sexual fantasizing and self-stimulation, and that users download specific images of child pornography on the basis of how well those images correspond with preexisting sexual fantasies (Quayle & Taylor, 2002; Seto et al., 2006). Moreover, Quayle and Taylor (2002) interviewed 13 men convicted of downloading child pornography and observed a pattern of escalating sensation seeking as individuals seek out increasingly extreme (e.g., depictions of younger children) sexually explicit materials. The authors opined that this pattern of escalation may be due to the rapidity with which individuals habituate to sexual stimuli delivered via the Internet, and their subsequent efforts acquire novel, provocative images.

Ward and Stewart (2003) suggested that the presence of deviant sexual interests signifies the absence or distortion of internal and external factors necessary for healthy, egalitarian relationships. Thus, a primary goal of therapy is the acquisition of additional skills to manage stress in life and to nurture healthy relationships. For offenders who have demonstrated a pattern of using masturbation or sexual fantasizing to regulate affect or distract from stressors, learning to effectively self-manage negative emotional states is a primary treatment goal. Interventions that contribute to the development of adaptive coping strategies, such as relaxation training and mindfulness exercises (see Linehan, Dimeff, & Koerner, 2007 for review of applicable cognitive behavioral techniques), aim to improve anxiety tolerance and encourage the use of more direct, effective strategies for coping and problem solving. By providing instruction in the use of adaptive coping skills early in treatment, offenders acquire functional skills that may serve in the stead of the maladaptive behaviors targeted by treatment. Daily diaries cataloguing the occurrence of emotionally provocative events, subjective ratings of emotional intensity, and ratings of the individual's confidence in his ability to tolerate the emotional experience, may serve as useful tools for treatment. Over the course of treatment offenders practice utilizing developing skills to manage anxiety that may be experienced before, during, and following therapy sessions, and therapy time is devoted to the discussion of successful and failed attempts to utilize new skills outside of treatment. By deconstructing his own offense process, each individual offender can learn to identify circumstances that are likely to elicit a strong emotional response, and to develop a plan to use alternative affect regulation strategies under such conditions. Treatment may also need to address off-line problems, such as family conflict or unemployment that the offender is attempting to avoid through sexual self-gratification. Some offenders, particularly those with avoidant attachment orientations, may experience difficulties in recognizing, labeling, and tolerating negative emotional states, and subsequently, interventions aimed at improving emotional self-awareness may be warranted early in the therapeutic process. Finally, although not universally effective for all offenders, behavioral procedures aimed at modifying deviant sexual arousal patterns may be beneficial for those with deviant preferences.

General Self-Regulation Problems

General self-regulation refers to the ability to plan, problem-solve, and regulate impulses to achieve long-term goals (Thornton, 2002). Problematic self-regulation as evidenced by lifestyle impulsivity and poor emotional control, is well correlated with general and violent offending (Lynam, Caspi, Moffitt, Raine, Loeber, & Stouthamer-Loeber, 2005; Pulkkinen, Virtanen, Klinteberg, & Magnusson, 2000; Seager, 2005; Zuckerman, 2002). Problems with behavioral self-regulation have also been associated with risk for sexual reoffending (Firestone, Bradford, McCoy, Greenberg, Larose, & Curry, 1999; Hanson & Bussiere, 1998; Prentky & Knight, 1991; Rice & Harris, 1997). Hanson and Harris (2001) found that, of all the items of the Sex Offender Need Assessment Rating (SONAR), general problems with self-regulation

demonstrated the strongest effect for discriminating between recidivists and nonrecidivists.

Impulsivity has been discussed in the literature as the inability to wait for delayed rewards and/or a tendency toward risk taking (Green & Myerson, 2004). Relapse prevention models of substance abuse and sexual offending have utilized the term Problems of Immediate Gratification (PIG) in reference to the principle that small, immediate rewards have greater subjective value than large, delayed rewards (Marlatt, 1989; Laws, Hudson, & Ward, 2000). Laws (2003) argued that the devaluation of delayed rewards "is almost certainly the behavioral mechanism by which certain precursors lead to impulsive sexual behaviors" (p. 77).

The Triple A Engine of the Internet has created the opportunity for near immediate gratification for anyone with an interest in child pornography. Sexual self-gratification may serve as a reliable, immediately available alternative to more prosocial behaviors and outcomes that are both uncertain and considerably delayed. Moreover, individuals may devalue the rewards of participating in appropriate egalitarian relationships or trying alternative coping strategies because they have no history of success in these realms and subsequently expect that future successes are improbable. For these individuals, masturbation fueled by sexually explicit images of children may represent the proverbial "bird in hand" that is preferred over the "two in the bush" represented by more adaptive, but less probabilistic behaviors. Temporal and probabilistic factors may also influence the appraisal of negative outcomes (e.g., criminal charges, public embarrassment, and loss of employment) that might otherwise serve as deterrents. Offenders may rightly believe that detection is improbable, and any negative consequences that are incurred will not be realized for weeks, months, or even years, contributing to the devaluation of long-term deterrents.

A fundamental aim of cognitive behavioral sex offender treatment is the enhancement of the offenders' self-management skills to maintain therapeutic gains achieved through treatment. Behavioral self-regulation is also relevant to the offender's willingness/ability to abide by supervisory restrictions, and to implement treatment recommendations in the community. Quayle et al. (2006) suggested that preference for immediate gratification interferes with the individual's ability to realize his personal goals and values. They further suggest that by getting the offender to examine and explicitly state their values, the treatment provider can assist the offender in examining how immediate gratification in general, and downloading child pornography in particular, may inhibit their ability to fulfill those values. Structured approaches to cost-benefit analyses, where values assigned to different behavioral outcomes are explored rationally, may be useful for this purpose.

Additionally, Laws (2003) emphasized importance of demonstrating the rewards of alternative behaviors early in treatment. Marlatt et al. (1997) stated, "Benefits from current treatment are far from certain, but if they were better defined, more probable, and occurred sooner, their value would be discounted less and treatment would be engaged in more" (p. 71). Consequently, behavioral goals should be clearly operationalized, systems of measurement should be instituted, and the offender should receive feedback, early and often, that highlights observable treatment gains. By formulating a functional analysis of the individual's interest in, and use of child pornography, the treatment provider can identify the purpose that downloading child pornography serves for the individual, as well as the contexts within which this behavior is likely to occur. It is important to recognize that offenders are being asked to relinquish behaviors that have reliably served a valuable purpose. Behavioral change is unlikely to occur or be maintained if the offender is not provided with alternative means by which to achieve the goals that were previously met through the target behavior. Thus, lack of behavioral control may be addressed by framing problems of immediate gratification as barriers to the achievement of personal goals, through participation in cost-benefit analyses, and by structuring treatment such that the individual will experience tangible benefits early in the treatment process.

Intimacy Deficits

Deficit models of sexual offending, whereby perpetrators choose inappropriate partners as a result of emotional loneliness and failed attempts to achieve intimacy with more suitable partners, have a long history in the sex offending literature (Marshall, 1993; Marshall, Hudson, & Hodkinson, 1993; Ward & Siegert, 2002). Research has shown that adult sexual offenders tend to feel inadequate and emotionally lonely in intimate relationships (Fisher & Howells,

1970; Marshall, 1989; Marshall, Payne, Barbaree, & Eccles, 1991; Pacht & Cowden, 1974), and anticipate that they will be rejected by intimate partners (Panton, 1978). Quinn and Forsyth (2005) commented that the Internet has "transformed vicarious sex into an increasingly viable and attractive substitute for interpersonal forms of sexual fulfillment" (p. 197).

The relationships that child pornography offenders experience online, including actual communications with other child pornography offenders as well as fantasy relationships the offender creates with children depicted in the pornographic images, may serve to compensate for unsatisfactory interpersonal relationships in the offender's off-line life. Middleton et al. (2006) examined the psychological profiles of 43 men convicted of Internet-related offenses within the context of pathways model by Ward and Siegert (2002) of sexual offending and found that 35% of the sample fell within the Intimacy Deficit pathway. Other authors have found that a disproportionate number of men arrested for possession or distribution of child pornography (33% to 80%) were not, and in many cases had never been, involved in an intimate romantic relationship (Frei, Erenay, Dittmann, & Graf, 2005; McLaughlin, 2006; Middleton, Elliott, Mandeville-Norden, & Beech, 2006). It should be noted, however, that Wolak and colleagues (2005) found that 37% of the child pornography offenders in their study were married or were living with a partner and 27% were separated, divorced, or widowed (indicating that they had at least been in a relationship at some point in time). Caplan (2002) observed that noncriminal problem Internet users demonstrate a preference for online, rather than in-person, interactions. Young (1997, as cited in Song et al., 2004) suggested that the anonymity of the Internet permits individuals to adopt new identities which may compensate for personal deficits that limit the individual's social comfort and success in their off-line lives. As noted by Middleton et al. (2006) many Internet offenders may find that, "images depicting children are less fearful and the child a more accepting partner, and they may use the Internet as a maladaptive strategy to avoid their perceived likelihood of failure in adult relationships" (p. 11).

Intimacy problems are frequently attributed to insecure attachment and subsequent difficulties in establishing satisfactory interpersonal relationships (Marshall, 1989; Ward, Hudson, & Marshall, 1996; Ward & Siegert, 2002). Attachment theory is based on the belief that early interpersonal experiences set the stage for predictable cognitive, affective, and relational behavior processes that guide personality and social behavior throughout the lifespan (Bowlby, 1982; Shaver & Mikulincer, 2002). Intimacy deficits can then be viewed as enduring traits that are unlikely to exhibit rapid therapeutic change. Because of the interpersonal nature of intimacy problems, the therapeutic process and quality of relationships between the offender and the therapist and/or therapy group are of particular importance (Serran, Fernandez, Marshall, & Mann, 2003). Individuals who substitute children for adult sexual partners will likely also present with distorted cognitions that frame sexual relationships with children in romantic, "adult-like" terms (Ward & Beech, 2004; Ward et al., 1996).

Thus, from a treatment perspective relationship, communication, and intimacy skill deficits need to be addressed. Couple counseling would also be appropriate for individuals who are already in relationships. Although the Internet is becoming an increasingly sociable acceptable mode of meeting potential dating and sexual partners via websites such as match.com and yahoo personals, for individuals with a history of using the Internet to engage in illegal behavior, this medium is not recommend to seek out potential relationships. This behavior might prove too tempting for some individuals in the early stages of treatment to fall back on maladaptive interaction patterns given the anonymity, accessibility, and affordability of the Internet.

Offense Supportive Cognitions

The concept of cognitive distortions has figured prominently in theories of sex offending etiology and treatment. Cognitive distortions are beliefs about sexuality and sexual behavior that individuals use to justify and disinhibit sexually abusive behaviors. Marshall et al. (1999) suggested that cognitive distortions may initially represent conscious efforts by the offender to overcome internal inhibitions deterring him from committing preferred sexual acts, and with repeated offending may become deeply engrained.

Exposure to child pornography may serve to reinforce the individual's self-justification for indulging their deviant sexual interests (Marshall, 2000). The very fact that these images are available on the Internet provides evidence for the downloader that others are engaged in similar or more egregious behaviors. This in turn may have a normalizing function for the individual. By focusing on the end product (i.e., child pornography) rather than the actual events that led to its production (i.e., sexual abuse of a child) the Internet user is able to create distance between his own behavior and the actual abuse of a child and may even start to view his behavior as a "victimless crime" thereby differentiating himself from those who have "direct involvement" in child sexual exploitation. Furthermore, child pornography that portrays children as compliant, willing, and even enthusiastic participants in sexual activities serves to reinforce the distortion that children can consent to engage in such behaviors, and that those behaviors are not harmful to the victim. Some child pornography offenders will justify their sexual behavior on the Internet by framing it as an outlet for sexual urges that allows them to refrain from committing contact offenses (Quayle & Taylor, 2002). There are no data to support or refute the contention that downloading these type images serves as an effective harm reduction strategy. At best, collecting and masturbating to child pornography appears to be a suboptimal tactic for managing inappropriate sexual urges. At worst, it perpetuates the abuse of children by creating a market for new images, reinforces cognitive distortions regarding the abuse of children, and may actually move the individuals closer to committing contact offenses against a child.

Bandura (1977) stated that so long as individuals "disregard the detrimental effects of their conduct, there is little likelihood that self-censuring reactions will be activated" (p. 157). Because cognitive distortions impede motivation and behavior change, they need to be identified and challenged early, and remain an ongoing treatment focus throughout therapy. Many offenders will embrace the notion that downloading child pornography is a victimless crime, or minimize severity of harm relative to more violent contact offenses. In these cases, the treating clinician will wish to explore and emphasize the experience of the child victim that led to the creation of pornographic images, and emphasize the permanence with which images of that abuse will persist in cyberspace.

NEGATIVE SOCIAL INFLUENCES

Association with people who have antisocial values and criminal tendencies has been identified as a robust predictor of nonsexual recidivism among juvenile and adult nonsexual offenders (Andrews & Bonta, 2003; Gendreau, Little, & Goggin, 1996). The role of social influences on the sex offending process has not, however, received much empirical attention, perhaps because sexual offenses are most frequently perpetrated by a lone offender.

The Internet provides a social forum for people to meet with others and exchange information (Quayle et al., 2006). McKenna and Bargh (1998) suggested that the Internet provides a venue where people who are socially isolated and/or have socially devalued traits can "reap the benefits of joining a group of similar others: feeling less isolated and different, disclosing a long secret part of oneself, sharing one's own experiences and learning from those of others, and gaining emotional and motivational support" (p. 682). Although McKenna and Bargh's (1998) comments were made in reference to the Internet as a positive influence on identity development, the Internet may also serve to plug isolated "sexually deviant" individuals into virtual social systems that promote deviant values and encourage enactment of sexually deviant or illegal inclinations.

Turkle (1995) argued that the Internet allows individuals to experiment with different personae under favorable conditions where the individual will not be punished or censured for expressing unpopular attitudes and behaviors. Research by McKenna and Bargh (1998) investigated the effects of Internet newsgroup membership on identity development for individuals with "concealable marginalized identities" (e.g., homosexuality; fetishism). The authors found that newsgroup involvement led to increased importance of the group identity, and that users "begin to feel that this aspect of themselves is more socially acceptable than they had thought. This reduces the inner conflict between the marginalized self aspect and cultural standards" (p. 692).

Ward and Hudson (2002) suggested that pedophilic offenders tend to gravitate toward individuals who share similar attitudes, beliefs, and preferences. Malesky and Ennis (2004) echoed this sentiment and speculated that individuals with pedophilic sexual preferences will be inclined to seek validation for their sexual proclivities from like-minded peers in virtual communities. An observational study of activity on a propedophilia Internet newsgroup found that although a substantial number of newsgroup postings included statements supportive of pedophilic

behaviors, and/or erotic images of young boys, the majority of newsgroup communications were unrelated to either sexuality or children (Malesky & Ennis, 2004). The majority of inter-user communications were conversational dialogues about current events, arts and entertainment, and other "nondeviant" topics. Malesky and Ennis (2004) proposed that through virtual communities,

> offenders and potential offenders may find a sense of membership and community that they lack in other aspects of their lives. The fact that the user is in contact with individuals who not only share their pedophilic interests, but also listen to similar music, read the same books, and have the same hobbies, may have a normalizing effect on one's perception of their deviant interests (p. 98).

In addition to providing a venue for social interactions, some online communities may serve as virtual "market places" where the acquisition and distribution of child pornography can be conducted freely, and where users can share information regarding where to find additional images, how to effectively conceal one's identity online, and disseminate information that would otherwise be difficult to access (e.g., membership information for propedophile organizations), and arrange in person meetings with other sex offenders (Durkin, 1996; Malesky, 2005). Durkin (1996) found that nearly one quarter of postings on a pedophilic Internet newsgroup represented efforts to orchestrate off-line contacts with other newsgroup users. Moreover, although illegal pornography can be accessed for free, many of the most content rich websites featuring child pornography are covert, and require knowledge (e.g., web address, passwords) that would only be available through "word of mouth," and virtual communities represent the most direct route by which to access this information.

Individuals who have been active traders of child pornography will likely have established communication networks with other traders. These traders may attempt to solicit further exchanges of pornography, regardless of whether the offender in treatment initiates contact. Furthermore, involvement in virtual communities that endorse sexually exploitative values and behaviors may serve to undermine treatment efforts aimed at creating dissonance between the offender's personal values and their sexually exploitative behavior.

Although some computer programs restrict adult material (pornographic websites) from being accessed over the Internet as well as monitor the user's online activity it is unrealistic to assume that these precautions (although helpful in some cases) would prevent all individuals from accessing online child pornography. Thus, other precautions can to be taken to reduce risk of reoffense. In extreme cases, Internet offenders employed in the fields of computer/Internet might need to pursue employment where they are not required to work on the Internet (especially if their work is largely unsupervised). In addition, high-risk Internet offenders should not be allowed to have computers in their homes. If this suggestion is unrealistic because of the presence of family members or roommates, then the offender should be closely monitored to ensure that he or she does not misuse the computer or the Internet. Finally, probation and parole officers working with this population should receive specialized training focusing on the strengths and weaknesses of filtering programs used to screen access to sexual material as well as on ways computer programs can be used to monitor one's online activity. Although these suggestions are not a panacea to prevent offenders from accessing child pornography over the Internet, they do make it more difficult for offenders to engage in illegal or sexually inappropriate online behavior. In addition to aforementioned suggestions, provisions prohibiting contact with potential trading partners or propedophilic online communities should be included in community supervision orders and treatment contracts. Furthermore, where polygraph examination represents a routine element of community management, examiner should question the examinee about his online communications and activities.

CONCLUSION

In summary, the Internet is ideally suited for individuals with sexual interests in children and has dramatically altered the behavioral economics that govern the acquisition of sexual goods, resulting in opportunities for near immediate gratification that were previously unavailable. However, technology is not solely responsible for changing the behavior of individuals who use it (McGrath & Casey, 2002). The Polaroid camera did not cause camera owners to develop an interest in creating pornographic images in their homes. Rather, it simply provided an avenue by which those with an interest in photographically documenting their sexual activities could create their own pornography in the home. Similarly, the Internet is primarily a catalyzing agent that allows individuals with particular psychological vulnerabilities to explore their sexual interests, indulge and operationalize their fantasy life, and avoid detection (McGrath & Casey, 2002).

Regardless of whether the offender's index offense involves use of the Internet, evaluators and treatment providers will be wise to determine whether Internet usage issues, be they indulgence in child pornography or an excessive involvement in online relationships at the expense of off-line relationships, play a role in the development or maintenance of the sexually abusive behavior. The evaluator should not only investigate the nature of the offender's Internet-related behaviors but also determine the function that online behaviors may serve for the offender. As suggested by Middleton (2004), "At the very least the treatment (of sex offenders) needs to be based on a specific assessment of the individual including the context in which the behavior was developed and sustained" (pp. 110).

References

Abel, G. G. & Blanchard, E. B. (1974). The role of fantasy in the treatment of sexual deviation. *Archives of General Psychiatry*, 30, 467–475.

Andrews, D. A. & Bonta, J. (2003). *The psychology of criminal conduct, 3rd edition.* Cincinnati, OH: Anderson.

Andrews, D. A., Zinger, I., Hoge, R. D., Bonta, J., Gendreau, P., & Cullen, F. T. (1990). Does correctional treatment work? A clinically relevant and psychologically informed meta-analysis. *Criminology*, 28, 369–404.

Ashcroft v. Free speech coalition, 535 U.S. 234, 250, 251 (2002).

Astrowsky, B. & Peters, J. (2002). Charging decisions and trial preparation in child pornography cases. Unpublished manuscript.

Bandura, A. (1977). *Social learning theory.* Englewood Cliffs, NJ: Cognitive Prentice-Hall.

Barbaree, H. (2003). Risk assessment: Discussion of the section. *Annals of the New York Academy of Science*, 989, 236–246.

Bogaert, A. F. (2001). Personality, individual differences, and preferences for the sexual media. *Archives of Sexual Behavior*, 30, 29–53.

Bonta, J. (2002). Offender risk assessment: Guidelines for selection and use. *Criminal Justice and Behavior*, 29, 355–379.

Bower, D. W. (2004). Holding virtual child pornography creators liable by judicial redress: An alternative approach to overcoming the obstacles presented in *Ashcroft v. Free speech coalition. BYU Journal of Public Law,* 19, 235.

Bowlby, J. (1982). *Attachment and loss: Vol. 1. Attachment* (Revised edition). New York, NY: Basic Books.

Brody, J. E. (2000, May 16). Cybersex gives birth to a psychological disorder. *New York Times.* (New York), 7, 12.

Calder, M. (2004). The internet: Potential, problems and pathways to hands-on sexual offending. In M. Calder (Ed.), *Child sexual abuse and the internet: Tackling the new frontier* (pp. 2–23). Dorset, UK: Russell House Publishing.

Caplan, S. E. (2002). Preference for online social interaction: A theory of problematic Internet use and psychosocial well-being. *Communication Research,* 30, 625–648.

Carr, J. (2004). Child abuse, child pornography and the Internet. Executive Report by NCH. Retrieved August 20, 2008 at http://www.nch.org.uk/information/index.php?i=94.

Cohen, H. (2003). Child pornography: Constitutional principles and federal statutes. In W. T. Holliday (Ed.), *Government principles and statutes on child pornography.* New York, NY: Nova Science Publishers.

Conly, C. H. (1989). Organizing for computer crime investigation and prosecution. Washington, DC: Government Printing Office, US Dept. of Justice.

Cooper, G. (2001). 100 Subscribers arrested in web child porn ring. *Washington Post.* A.11.

Cooper, A. (1998). Sexuality and the Internet: surfing into the new millennium. *Cyberpsychology and Behavior,* 1, 187–193.

Cooper, A., Boies, S., Maheu, M., & Greenfield, D. (1999). Sexuality and the Internet: The next sexual revolution. In F. Muscarella & L. Szuchman (Eds.), *The psychological science of sexuality: A research based approach* (pp. 519–545). New York, NY: Wiley Press.

Cooper, A., Delmonico, D. L., & Burg, R. (2000). Cybersex users, abusers, and compulsives: New findings and implications. *Sexual Addiction and Compulsivity,* 7, 5–29.

Cooper, A., Galbreath, N., & Becker, M. A. (2004). Sex on the Internet: Furthering our understanding of men with online sexual problems. *Psychology of Addictive Behaviors,* 18, 223–230.

Cooper, A., Scherer, C. R., Boies, S. C., & Gordon, B. L. (1999). Sexuality on the Internet: From sexual exploration to pathological expression. *Professional Psychology: Research and Practice,* 30, 154–164.

Cortoni, F. & Marshall, W. L. (2001). Sex as a coping strategy and its relationship to juveniles sexual history and intimacy in sexual offenders. *Sexual Abuse: A Journal of Research and Treatment,* 13, 27–43.

Criminal Code of Canada, R. S., 1985, c. C-46, s. 163; 1993, c. 46, s. 1. (1985). Retrieved April 7, 2006 at http://laws.justice.gc.ca/en/C-46/42053.html.

Davis, R. (2001). A cognitive-behavioural model of pathological Internet usage. *Computers and Human Behaviour,* 17, 187–195.

Douglas, K. S. & Skeem, J. L. (2005). Violence risk assessment: Getting specific about being dynamic. *Psychology, Public Policy, and Law,* 11, 347–383.

Durkin, K. F. (1996). *Accounts and sexual deviance in cyberspace: The case of pedophilia.* Unpublished doctoral dissertation. 73, 108. Virginia Polytechnic Institute and State University, Blacksburg, VA.

Epperson, D. L., Kaul, J. D., Huot, S. J., Hesselton, D., Alexander, W., & Goldman, R. (1998). *Minnesota Sex Offender Screening Tool—Revised (MnSOST-R).* St. Paul, MN: Minnesota Department of Corrections.

Firestone, P., Bradford, J. M., McCoy, M., Greenberg, D. M., Larose, M. R., & Curry, S. (1999). Prediction of recidivism in incest offenders. *Journal of Interpersonal Violence,* 14, 511–531.

Fisher, W. A. & Barak, A. (2001). Internet pornography: A social psychological perspective on Internet sexuality. *Journal of Sex Research,* 38, 312–323.

Fisher, G. & Howells, L. (1970). Psychological needs of homosexual pedophiliacs. *Diseases of the Nervous System,* 3, 623–650.

Frei, A., Erenay, N., Dittmann, V., & Graf, M. (2005). Paedophilia on the Internet—a study of 33 convicted offenders in the Canton of Lucerne. *Swiss Medical Weekly,* 135, 488–494.

Gendreau, P., Little, T., & Goggin, C. (1996). A meta-analysis of the predictors of adult offender recidivism: What works! *Criminology,* 34, 575–607.

Gillespie, A. A. (2005). Indecent images of children: The ever-changing law. *Child Abuse Review,* 14, 430.

Graupner, H. (2004). The 17-year-old child: An absurdity of the late 20th century. *Journal of Psychology & Human Sexuality,* 16(2), 7.

Green, L. & Myerson, J. (2004). A discounting framework for choice with delayed and probabilistic rewards. *Psychological Bulletin,* 130, 769–792.

Grover, S. (2004). Oppression of children intellectualized as free expression under the Canadian *Charter*: A reanalysis of the *Sharpe* possession of child pornography case. *International Journal of Children's Rights,* 11, 311.

Hanson, R. K. (1997). The development of a brief actuarial risk scale for sex offence recidivism. Ottawa, ON: Solicitor General of Canada. (HQ 71 H257 1997).

Hanson, R. K. & Bussiere, M. T. (1998). Predicting relapse: A meta-analysis of sexual offender recidivism studies. *Journal of Consulting and Clinical Psychology,* 66, 348–362.

Hanson, R. K. & Harris, A. J. R. (2000). The Sex Offender Need Assessment Rating (SONAR): A method for measuring change in risk levels. Ottawa, ON: Solicitor General of Canada. (HQ 71 H2573 2000).

Hanson, R. K. & Harris, A. J. R. (2001). A structured approach to evaluating change among sexual offenders. *Sexual Abuse: A Journal of Research and Treatment*, 13, 105–122.

Hanson, R. K., Morton-Borgon, K. E., & Harris, A. J. R. (2003). Sexual offender recidivism risk: What we know and what we need to know. *Annals of the New York Academy of Science*, 989, 154–166.

Harrington, R. (2003, January 14). Townshend arrested in porn sweep. *Washington Post*. C.01.

Hart, S. D., Laws, D. R., & Kropp, P. R. (2003). The promise and the peril of sex offender risk assessment. In T. Ward, D. R. Laws, & S. M. Hudson (Eds.), *Sexual deviance: Issues and controversies* (pp. 207–225). Thousand Oaks, CA: Sage.

Hernandez, A. E. (2000). Self-reported contact sexual offenses by participants in the Federal Bureau of Prisons' sex offender treatment program: Implications for Internet sex offenders. Poster session presented at: the 19th Annual Research and Treatment Conference of the Association for the Treatment of Sexual Abusers, November, San Diego, CA.

Kraut, R., Kiesler, S., Boneva, B., Cummings, J., Helgeson, V., & Crawford, A. (2002). Internet paradox revisited. *Journal of Social Issues*, 58, 49–74.

Lanning, K. V. (1992). *Child molesters: A behavioral analysis*. 3rd ed. Washington, DC: National Center for Missing & Exploited Children.

Laws, D. R. (2003). Behavioral economic approaches to the assessment and treatment of sexual deviation. In T. Ward, D. R. Laws, & S. M. Hudson (Eds.), *Sexual deviance: Issues and controversies* (pp. 65–81). Thousand Oaks, CA: Sage.

Laws, D. R., Hudson, S. H., & Ward, T. (2000). The original model of relapse prevention with sex offenders: Promises unfulfilled. In D. R. Laws, S. H. Hudson, & T. Ward (Eds.), *Remaking relapse prevention with sex offenders: A sourcebook* (pp. 3–24). Thousand Oaks, CA: Sage.

Lee, J. (2003). High tech helps child pornographers and their pursuers. *New York Times* [electronic version]. Accessed February 9, from http://www.nytimes.com/2003/02/09technology/09PORN.html.

Leiblum, S. R. (1997). Sex and the net: Clinical implications. *Journal of Sexual Education and Therapy*, 22, 21–27.

Linehan, M. M., Dimeff, L. A., & Koerner, K. (2007). *Dialectical behaviour therapy in clinical practice: Applications across disorders and settings*. New York, NY: Guilford.

Lynam, D. R., Caspi, A., Moffitt, T. E., Raine, A., Loeber, R., & Stouthamer-Loeber, M. (2005). Adolescent psychopathy and the Big Five: Results from two samples. *Journal of Abnormal Child Psychology*, 33, 431–443.

Malamuth, N. M., Addison, T., & Koss, M. (2001). Pornography and sexual aggression: Are there reliable effects? *Annual Review of Sex Research*, 11, 26–91.

Malamuth, N. M. & Impett, E. A. (2001). Research on sex in the media: What do we know about effects on children and adolescents? In D. G. Singer, & J. L. Singer (Eds.), *Handbook of children and the media* (pp. 269–287). Thousand Oaks, CA: Sage.

Malesky, L. A. (2002). Sexually deviant Internet usage by child sex offenders. Unpublished doctoral dissertation. Memphis, TN: University of Memphis.

Malesky, L. A. (2005). The use of the Internet for child sexual exploitation. In S. Cooper, A. P. Giadino, V. Vieth, & D. Kellogg (Eds.), *Medical and legal aspects of child sexual exploitation: A comprehensive review of child pornography, child prostitution, and Internet crimes against children*. Saint Louis, Missouri: GW Medical Publishing.

Malesky, L. A. & Ennis, L. (2004). Supportive distortions: An analysis of postings on a pedophile Internet message board. *Journal of Addiction and Offender Counselling*, 24, 92–100.

Marlatt, G. (1989). Feeding the PIG: The problem of immediate gratification. In D. R. Laws (Ed.), *Relapse prevention with sex offenders* (pp. 56–62). New York, NY: Guilford.

Marlatt, G. A., Tucker, J. A., Donovan, D. M., & Vuchinich, R. E. (1997). Help-seeking by substance abusers: The role of harm reduction and behavioral economic approaches to facilitate treatment entry and retention. In L. S. Onken, J. D. Blaine, & J. J. Boren (Eds.), *Beyond the therapeutic alliance: Keeping the drug-dependent individual in treatment* (National Institute on Drug Abuse Research Monograph Number 165, pp. 44–84). Rockville, MD: U.S. Department of Health and Human Services, Public Health Service, National Institutes of Health.

Marshall, W. L. (1989). Invited essay: Intimacy, loneliness and sexual offenders. *Behaviour Research and Therapy*, 27, 491–503.

Marshall, W. L. (2000). Revisiting the use of pornography by sexual offenders: Implications for theory and practice. *Journal of Sexual Aggression*, 6, 67–78.

Marshall, W. L., Anderson, D., & Fernandez, Y. M. (1999). *Cognitive behavioural treatment for sex offenders*. London: John Wiley.

Marshall, W. L. & Barbaree, H. E. (1991). An integrated theory of the etiology of sexual offending. In W. L. Marshall, D. R. Laws, & H. E. Barbaree (Eds.), *Handbook of sexual assault: Issues, theories, and treatment of the offender* (pp. 257–275). New York, NY: Plenum.

Marshall, W. L. & Eccles, A. (1993). Pavlovian conditioning processes in adolescent sex offenders. In H. E. Barbaree, W. L. Marshall, & S. M. Hudson (Eds.), *The juvenile sex offender* (pp. 118–142). New York, NY: Guilford.

Marshall, W. L., Hudson, S. M., & Hodkinson, S. (1993). The importance of attachment bonds in the development of sexual offending. In H. E. Barbaree, W. L. Marshall, & S. M. Hudson (Eds.), *The juvenile sex offender* (pp. 164–181). New York, NY: Guilford.

Marshall, W. L. & Marshall, L. E. (2000). The origins of sexual offending. *Trauma, Violence, & Abuse*, 1, 250–263.

Marshall, W. L., Payne, K., Barbaree, H. E., & Eccles, A. (1991). Exhibitionists: Sexual preferences for exposing. *Behaviour Research and Therapy*, 29, 37–40.

Marshall, W. L., Seran, G. A., & Cortoni, F. A. (2000). Childhood attachments, sexual abuse, and their relationship to adult coping in child molesters. *Sexual Abuse: A Journal of Research and Treatment*, 12, 17–26.

McGrath, M. G. & Casey, E. (2002). Forensic psychiatry and the Internet: Practical perspectives on sexual predators and obsessional harassers in cyberspace. *Journal of the American Academy of Psychiatry and Law*, 30, 81–94.

McKenna, K. Y. A. & Bargh, J. A. (1998). Coming out in the age of the Internet: Identity "demarginalization" through virtual group participation. *Journal of Personality and Social Psychology*, 75, 681–694.

Middleton, D., Elliott, I. A., Mandeville-Norden, R., & Beech, A. R. (2006). An investigation into the applicability of the Ward and Siegert Pathways Model of child sexual abuse with Internet offenders. *Psychology, Crime & Law*, 12, 589–603.

Morahan-Martin, J. (2005). Internet abuse. Addiction? Disorder? Symptom? Alternative explanations? *Social Science Computer Review*, 23, 39–48.

National Center for Missing and Exploited Children. (2005). Reports of child pornography to The National Center for Missing and Exploited Children continue to rise. Press release issued January 27. Retrieved from http://www.missingkids.com/missingkids/servlet/NewsEventServlet?LanguageCountry=en_US&PageId=1865 on May 17, 2006.

New York v. Ferber, 458 U.S. 747 (1982).

O'Connell, R. & Taylor, M. (1998). Paedophile networks on the Internet: the evidential implications of paedophile picture posting on the Internet. Paper presented at the Combating Paedophile Information Networks in Europe (COPINE) Project Conference, January. Dublin Castle: Ireland.

Pacht, A. R. & Cowden, J. E. (1974). An exploratory study of five hundred sex offenders. *Criminal Justice and Behavior*, 1, 13–20.

Padgett, V. R., Brislen-Slutz, J. A., & Neal, J. A. (1989). Pornography, erotica, and attitudes towards women: The effects of repeated exposure. *The Journal of Sex Research*, 26, 479–491.

Panton, J. H. (1978). Personality differences appearing between rapists of adults, rapists of children, and nonviolent sexual molesters of children. *Research in Communications, Psychology, Psychiatry, and Behavior*, 3, 385–393.

Pulkkinen, L., Virtanen, T., Klinteberg, B. A., & Magnusson, D. (2000). Child behavior and adult personality: Comparisons between criminality groups in Finland and Sweden. *Criminal Behaviour and Mental Health*, 10, 155–169.

Putnam, D. E. & Maheu, M. M. (2000). Online sexual addiction and compulsivity: integrating web resources and behavioral telehealth in treatment. *Sexual Addiction and Compulsivity*, 7, 91–112.

Prentky, R. A. & Knight, R. A. (1991). Identifying critical dimensions for discriminating among rapists. *Journal of Consulting and Clinical Psychology*, 59, 643–666.

Quayle, E. & Taylor, M. (2002). Child pornography and the Internet: Perpetuating a cycle of abuse. *Deviant Behavior: An Interdisciplinary Journal*, 23, 331–361.

Quayle, E. & Taylor, M. (2003). Model of problematic Internet use in people with sexual interest in children. *Cyberpsychology & Behavior*, 6, 93–106.

Quayle, E., Vaughan, M., & Taylor, M. (2006). Sex offenders, Internet child abuse images and emotional avoidance: The importance of values. *Aggression and Violent Behavior.*

Quinn, J. F. & Forsyth, C. J. (2005). Describing sexual behavior in the era of the Internet: A typology for empirical research. *Deviant Behavior*, 26, 191–207.

Quinsey, V. L., Harris, G. T., Rice, M. E., & Cormier, C. A. (1998). *Violent offenders: Appraising and managing risk.* Washington, D.C.: American Psychological Association.

Regina v. Sharpe, (1 S.C.R. 45 2001).

Rice, M. E. & Harris, G. T. (1997). Cross-validation and extension of the Violence Risk Appraisal Guide for child molesters and rapists. *Law and Human Behavior*, 21, 231–241.

Schafer, J. A. (2002). Spinning the web of hate: Web-based hate propagation by extremist organizations. *Journal of Criminal Justice and Popular Culture*, 9, 69–88.

Seager, J. A. (2005). Violent men: The importance of impulsivity and cognitive schema. *Criminal Justice and Behavior*, 32, 26–49.

Serran, G. A., Fernandez, Y. M., Marshall, W. L., & Mann, R. E. (2003). Process issues in treatment: Applications to sexual offender programs. *Professional Psychology: Research and Practice*, 34, 368–374.

Seto, M. C., Cantor, J. M., & Blanchard, R. (2006). Child pornography offenses are a valid diagnostic indicator of pedophilia. *Journal of Abnormal Psychology*, 115, 610–615.

Seto, M. C. & Eke, A. W. (2005). The criminal histories and later offending of child pornography offenders. *Sexual Abuse: A Journal of Research and Treatment*, 17, 201–210.

Seto, M. C. & Eke, A. W. (2006). Extending the follow-up of child pornography offenders reported by Seto and Eke (2005). Paper accepted for presentation at the Annual Research and Treatment Conference of the Association for the Treatment of Sexual Abusers. Chicago, IL.

Seto, M. C., Maric, A., & Barbaree, H. E. (2001). The role of pornography in the etiology of sexual aggression. *Aggression and Violent Behavior*, 6, 35–53.

Shaver, P. R. & Mikulincer, M. (2002). Attachment-related psychodynamics. *Attachment & Human Development*, 4, 133–161.

Shannon, E. (1998, September 14). Main street monsters. *Time Magazine*. p. 11 (available at http://www.time.com/time/magazine/article/0,9171,989082–1,00.html).

Smallbone, S. W. (2006). Social and psychological factors in the development of delinquency and sexual deviance. In H. E. Barbaree, & W. L. Marshall (Eds.), *The juvenile sex offender, Second Edition* (pp. 105–127). New York, NY: The Guilford Press.

Song, I. S., LaRose, R., Eastin, M. S., & Lin, C. A. (2004). Internet gratifications and Internet addiction: On the uses and abuses on new media. *Cyber Psychology & Behavior*, 7, 384–394.

Sullivan, J. & Beech, A. (2004). Assessing internet offenders. In M. Calder (Ed.) *Child sexual abuse and the internet: Tackling the new frontier* (pp. 69–83). Dorset, UK: Russell House Publishing.

Swanson, D. L. (1992). Understanding audiences: Continuing contributions of gratifications research. *Poetics*, 21, 305–328.

Taylor, M. (1999). Congress introductory paper: The nature and dimensions of child pornography on the Internet. Presented at the International conference Combating child pornography on the Internet. Vienna, Austria. Accessed July 16, 2006 at http://www.ipce.info/library_3/files/nat_dims_kp.htm

Taylor, M. & Quayle, E. (2003). *Child pornography: An Internet crime*. Brighton, UK: Routledge.

Thompson, C. W. (2002, March 19). FBI cracks child porn ring based on Internet. *Washington Post*. A2.

Thornton, D. (2002). Constructing and testing a framework for dynamic risk assessment. *Sexual Abuse: A Journal of Research and Treatment*, 14, 139–153.

Turkle, S. (1995). *Life on the screen: Identity in the age of the Internet*. New York, NY: Simon & Schuster.

United States v. Dost, 636 F. Supp. 828 (S.D.C.A. 1986).

United States v. Knox, 977 F.2d 815, 820–821 (3d Cir. 1992).

U.S. Department of Commerce. (2001). *Home computers and Internet use in the United States: August 2000*. Washington, DC: Government Printing Office; September. P23–207.

Ward, T. & Beech, A. R. (2004). The etiology of risk: A preliminary model. *Sexual Abuse: A Journal of Research and Treatment*, 16, 271–284.

Ward, T., Hudson, S. M., & Marshall, W. L. (1996). Attachment style in sex offenders: A preliminary study. *The Journal of Sex Research*, 33, 17–26.

Ward, T., Hudson, S. M., Marshall, W. L., & Siegert, R. (1995). Attachment style and intimacy deficits in sex offenders: A theoretical framework. *Sexual Abuse: A Journal of Research and Treatment*, 7, 317–335.

Ward, T. & Siegert, R. J. (2002). Toward a comprehensive theory of child sexual abuse: A theory knitting perspective. *Psychology, Crime, & Law*, 8, 319–351.

Ward, T. & Sorbello, L. (2003). Explaining child sexual abuse: Integration and elaboration. In T. Ward, D. R. Laws, & S. M. Hudson (Eds.), *Sexual deviance: Issues and controversies* (pp. 3–20). Thousand Oaks, CA: Sage.

Ward, T. & Stewart, C. A. (2003). The treatment of sex offenders: Risk management and good lives. *Professional Psychology: Research and Practice*, 34, 353–360.

Webb, L., Craissati, J., & Keen, S. (2007). Characteristics of Internet child pornography offenders: A comparison with child molesters. *Sex Abuse*, 19, 449–465.

Wolak, J., Finkelhor, D., & Mitchell, K. J. (2005). *Child-pornography possessors arrested in Internet-related crimes: Finding from the national juvenile online victimization study*. Alexandria, VA: National Center for Missing & Exploited Children.

Zuckerman, M. (2002). Personality and psychopathy: Shared behavioral and biological traits. In J. Glicksohn (Ed.), *The neurobiology of criminal behavior* (pp. 27–49). Dordrecht, Netherlands: Kluwer Academic Publishers.

Chapter 23

Sexual Abuse by Clergy

Graham Glancy and Michael Saini

Sexual abuse by clergy receives a great deal of media attention and generates immense public outcry toward the perpetrators (Saradjian & Nobus, 2003). Plante and Daniels (2004) suggest there are several factors that account for this attention. First, the Roman Catholic Church is an intriguing organization with perceived secrecies and inner workings, which make the incidents of clergy abuse fascinating and of great interest to the media and general population (Wills, 2000). Clergy are often placed on a spiritual, moral, and ethical pinnacle, which leads to an expectation of the highest level of behavior: "When they error, sin, and fall from grace, it is a much bigger drop for them" (Plante & Daniels, 2004). As well, Catholic clergy take a vow of celibacy prohibiting sexual contact of any kind, thereby creating an expectation of complete abstinence from their sexual behaviors. Plante (1996) further suggests that much of the media has cast the Roman Catholic Church as being unable or unwilling to deal with clergy abuse within the Church.

Given the American media attention to clergy abuse, it is not surprising that most literature found in this area is focused on clergy of the Roman Catholic Church in the United States. Perpetrators of child sexual abuse, however, can be found among clergy of various denominations and in various countries (Saradjian & Nobus, 2003). Furthermore, based on the review by Wolfe et al. (2003), allegations of child sexual abuse have been made in almost every type of community institution serving children, including schools, nursery schools, sports, and voluntary organizations. This has led to revelations and inquiries into the issue of childhood abuse in various institutions (Law Commission of Canada, 2000).

Although child abuse by family members has received considerable scientific and professional attention, we know less about the etiologies, typologies, and treatment options for members of community organizations and institutions who abuse children (Wolfe et al. 2003). Plante (1996), for example, notes the plethora of commentary on clergy abuse but the dearth of empirical information on those who are accused of committing these acts. Songy (2003) highlights that several scholars have suggested examining the etiology and treatment of sex offenders within a broader comprehensive model of offending. However, others like Marshall (1997) and Songy (2003) argue that developing a general framework for sex offenders oversimplifies the complexity of sexual abuse in various settings and circumstances. Consistent with this view, Songy states, "Given the complexities of etiology, it is essential that a treatment program thoroughly evaluate all possible factors leading to the sexual offenses of a particular client." In other words, special attention is needed to examine the available empirical information of clergy abuse in order to screen, prevent, and treat those clergy who sexually abuse children.

The current limited empirical evidence of clergy abuse is partly due to the lack of access to priests and a general lack of data on them (Connors, 1992). Much of the literature consists of either anecdotal descriptions or impassioned arguments detailing the characterization of the Church's response to clergy abuse (Terry & Terry, 2005). In reviewing the modest sample of empirical literature on clergy abuse, it should further be noted that many of these studies suffer from methodological flaws, including small sample sizes, lack of comparison groups, and the employment of study designs that lack scientific rigor. Keeping these limitations in mind, we reviewed the existing compilation of empirical studies on clergy abuse toward children to begin developing a framework to improve our understanding of this phenomenon.

In this chapter, we focus on etiological factors comprising of intrapersonal, interpersonal, and systemic levels of analysis and present current clergy offender typologies that have attained general acceptance within the scientific community. In the anticipation of understanding the etiological factors of these offenders, we have initiated a scholarly discourse of their characteristics within the context of their institutions. In the review of literature concerning sexual abuse by clergy, we will go on to make some suggestions regarding prevention, training, and treatment.

At the outset of this chapter, it is important to emphasize that we are not seeking to excuse this behavior, but rather, to understand it better to be able to make some suggestions for preventing the repetition of a scandal that has caused so much public discontent, as well as private pain and suffering. Although some statements may be considered controversial, it is important to present all of the empirical data to ensure that the review remains comprehensive and scientifically objective in its presentation.

Much of the inquiry in this field relates to the Catholic Church. However, we have broadened our field of inquiry to include other religious denominations when the data is available.

BACKGROUND

According to Doyle (2003), sexual abuse by clergy is not a new issue for the Church. It has existed throughout the history of the Roman Catholic Church, as well as other religious groups. He amasses evidence to suggest that the abuse of minors was considered a heinous crime worthy of significant punishment over the course of some centuries. The 1917 Code of Canon Law, for example, specifically articulated sexual contact with a minor by a cleric as being an ecclesiastical crime. Doyle further argues that, contrary to the suggestion of many authors, the Church has officially acknowledged sexual abuse as a problem for centuries.

Doyle notes that at the end of the Second Vatican Council in 1965, the Church underwent significant changes, including a demythologizing of the Church, its rituals, and clergy. Although a decline in clergy reverence has occurred, Doyle suggests that the Church has not diminished the feelings of elitism among its clergy. Furthermore, the hierarchical system of the Church remains largely intact. Doyle also points to the power of "clericalism" within the Church as being a contributing factor to clergy abuse. He describes "clericalism" as the Church's policy of maintaining or increasing the power of the Church, thereby creating power imbalance between individual clerics and their parishioners. Doyle suggests that this unequal distribution of power fosters an atmosphere that facilitates sexual abuse by the clergy against the more vulnerable parishioners.

When sexual abuse by clergy occurs, research indicates that the survivors can experience a significant array of harm including depression, self-harm, suicide, self-blame, posttraumatic responses, and major life derailments (Bera, 1996; Fortune, 1989; Harris, 1990).

Qualitative accounts from survivors suggest that children who are sexually abused by clergy can typically be divided into two groups: those whose families are deeply involved in the Church community, therefore have deep faith in both clergy and religion, and those from troubled families (Bera, 1996).

On the basis of a large number of media articles reporting cases of sexual abuse by clergy across the United States, Canada, and Europe, Doyle (2003) suggests that incidents of sexual abuse by clergy have certain common facets:

- The victims are generally from families closely involved in the life of the Church.
- Abuse takes place many times over a prolonged period of time.
- Disclosures are initially met with disbelief by parents and others.
- Church leaders first try to silence the victims to avoid a scandal.
- Disclosures are often not made until the victim reaches adulthood.
- Many victims experience trauma and dysfunction following the abuse.

Notwithstanding the long history of sexual abuse within the Church context and the known negative consequences for children who fall victim of clerical abuse, less is known about the characteristics of clergy who abuse these children.

PREVALENCE

Very few systematic, well-controlled studies have been conducted to determine actual prevalence of clergy abuse (see Kelly, 1998; Saradjian & Nobus, 2003). McGlone (2001) notes the unreliability of any estimated figures due to the inherent problems of relying on victim disclosure or perpetrator's reports. It is noteworthy that he did not have an easy task when attempting to simply find actual numbers of Roman Catholic brothers and priests in the United States. This bespeaks the uncertain and complicated structure of the Church. McGlone estimates that there are 53,000 Roman Catholic brothers and priests in the United States. On reviewing the professional and lay media, he estimates that between 0.2% and an upper limit of 4% of Roman Catholic brothers and priests have committed sexual abuse. This suggests that there are between 100 and 2,000

priest perpetrators in the United States. Loftus and Camargo note that among 1,322 male Roman Catholic clerics who had been treated at a treatment center for troubled clerics, 2.7% of these were pedophiles, 8.4% were viewed as hebephiles, and 27.8% incidentally were sexually active. Out of the 111 priests who were perpetrators of sexual misconduct with children, 98 had perpetrated against boys (Loftus & Camargo 1993). Goodstein (2003) further estimates a prevalence rate of 1.8% based on stories in the American national press.

In reviewing the various studies, Plante (2003) concludes that approximately 2% of Roman Catholic priests have sexually exploited minors. He asserts that sexual abuse by clergy is found among male clergy members at about the same percentage in most faiths. He also makes the point that men who work in a variety of occupations, which bring them into close contact with children, such as Boy Scout leaders, sports coaches, school bus drivers, and teachers have the same proportion of sexual perpetrators as the clergy. He concludes that the Catholic priests are not more likely to sexually abuse children than clergy in other faiths, people whose jobs bring them into close contact with children, or adult males in the general population.

Plante also goes on to note that the vast majority of priests who sexually abuse children choose adolescent boys rather than latency—aged children or young girls. A further study by McGlone (2001) compared a group of pedophile clergy offenders to hebephiles and found that 68% were male-to-male abusers, 20% male-to-female abusers and 12% abused both men and women.

ETIOLOGICAL FACTORS

Songy (2003) argues that few scholars have offered enough information to describe clearly the nature and etiological factors of sexual abuse by clergy. In response, we have searched the professional literature for empirical investigations of clergy abuse and have summarized the etiological factors leading to the sexual offense against children. In our review, we have uncovered three levels of analysis in the study of clergy abuse: intrapersonal, interpersonal, and systemic. Each level will be presented, followed by our proposed model to connect the levels into a working model of sexual abuse by clergy.

Intrapersonal Factors

Langevin and Watson (1996) reviewed the general etiologic factors that predispose individuals to sexually offend. They highlight sexual deviance as the primary factor and note that the majority of sex offenders are motivated by the presence of a sexual disorder. This is often accompanied by a number of disinhibiting factors such as substance abuse, antisocial personality disorders, psychotic mental illness, criminality, neuropsychological impairment, and endocrine disorders. Of these disinhibiting factors, alcohol intoxication and alcohol abuse are found to be significant contributors to sexual offenses. For example, 52% of sex offenders in Langevin and Watson's study were alcoholics and 52% of all sex offenses were carried out under the influence of alcohol. Drug abuse, in contrast, is found in only 3% of sex offences (Langevin, Curnoe, & Bain, 2000).

Researchers have claimed that clergy offenders are unique in comparison to other offenders within the general population (Terry & Terry, 2005). To examine these potential differences, Langevin et al. (2000) compared 24 male clerics accused of sexual offenses with 24 sex offender controls and matched them by offense type, age, education, and marital status and then compared to a control sample of 2125 sex offenders matched only according to offense type. They found that clerics in the study were, as a group, statistically older, more educated, and predominantly single as compared to the groups. They found that all groups suffered from sexual disorders and most disorders were predominantly homosexual pedophilia. In Langevin and Watson's (1996) in-depth study of clerics, they found that 70% reacted most strongly to male children physiologically, representing a lifelong preference to male minors over adults.

Not surprisingly, Langevin et al. (2000) found that clerics reported a prosocial history, mental stability, and the absence of antisocial personality disorders in contrast with the general population of sexual offenders. However, clerics also reported more endocrine disorders. These disorders, "such as diabetes and thyroid disorders may mimic the symptoms of major mental disorders and are associated with mood swings, depression, aggressiveness, and cognitive dysfunction." Also noteworthy, a third of all groups were alcoholics. These observations are similar to results found by Loftus and Camargo (1993) (Table 23.1) In one of the most scientific studies, Loftus and

TABLE 23.1 Etiological Factors—Individual

Paraphilic
Neuropsychological impairment
Endocrine abnormalities
Alcohol abuse
Personal history of having been sexually abused
Immaturity/intrapsychic problems

Camargo (1993) examined 158 clerical clergy priests in a treatment center using a control group of nonoffending priests by employing the Millon Multiaxial Personality Inventory (MMPI)-III and the Rorschach inkblot method. Loftus and Camargo found high levels of dependency and schizoid features in pedophile priests. Surprisingly, they did not find higher levels of narcissism or differences in sexual knowledge compared with national norms for men. Gerard Jobs, Cimbolic, Ritzbbler, and Montana (2003) noted pathological responses in a variety of Rorschach Scales in a group of cleric sex offenders who were hebephilic. In another study using the Rorschach Scales, hebephile Catholic priests were found to demonstrate significant pathological responses.

In a retrospective study of 1322 male clergy in a residential treatment centre, Camargo (1997) found that molesters of youth had distinctly unique neuropsychological variables compared to other sexually active clergy. This is consistent with the findings of Langevin et al. (1987) on pedophiles in the general population and Langevin and Watson's (1996) study on clerics who commit sexual offences, as well as on sexually offending physicians (Langevin, Graham Glancy, Curnoe, & Bain, 1999). Studies have revealed that substance abuse, endocrine disorders, and neuropsychological factors may be disinhibiting factors in those whose sexual preference is deviant, resulting in the acting out of fantasies (Langevin et al., 1999).

Haywood et al. (1996) suggest that cleric child molesters are more likely to have been sexually abused in childhood. They conclude that being sexually abused in childhood is associated with child molestation in adulthood but is no different when comparing clerics and nonclerics. In general, their rates of child abuse among child molesters were significantly higher than in most other reports (see Marshall & Barbaree, 1990). Bryant (1999) found that 66% of his small cohort of clergy who had sexually abused had been sexually abused themselves. However, Langevin et al.

(1999) dismiss this as an etiological factor. Similarly, Ruzicjka (1997) found no incidences of sexual assault in 10 convicted clergy.

While acknowledging the complexity of sexual offending, Lothstein (1999) cites increasing evidence of the association between frontotemporal pathology and clergy sex abuse. This is construed by electroencephalogram (EEG) abnormalities supported by neuropsychological testing. Lothstein argues, however, that these studies suffer from methodological flaws, which preclude generalizing a causal link between brain dysfunction and child sexual abuse by clergy. He also notes that the possible link is further complicated by the presence and unknown effects of substance abuse by clergy who offend. Lothstein recommends that when assessing clergy for brain abnormalities, those who have a history of hard neurological signs, such as head trauma and seizures, should be considered to be at high risk for sexual disinhibition and those with a history of soft neurological signs, such as impulsivity, should be considered to be at lower risk, but still in need of a comprehensive evaluation to determine actual risk.

Rossetti and Anthony (1996) compared 100 same-sex priests who had abused adolescents with the purpose of constructing and validating an MMPI-II scale. Rossetti constructed a 23-item scale and was able to statistically differentiate the same-sex hebephiles from controlled groups who were being evaluated for nonsexual psychiatric disorders as well as a normative sample. Plante (1996) could also differentiate priests who sexually abuse minors from nonabusing controls on the overcontrolled hostility scale of the MMPI and by using verbal intelligence quotient (IQ), which approached statistical significance.

Falkenhain (1998) examined the MMPI-II profiles of 97 Roman Catholic priests and compared them to a population of secular childhood sexual abusers. By using a method to delineate clusters, Falkenhain found a sexually and emotionally underdeveloped cluster, a significantly psychiatrically disturbed cluster, a defended characterological cluster, and an undefended characterological cluster.

The findings noted used sensitive phallometric testing administered by an experienced expert and/or standardized measurements for data collection, but it is interesting to note the self-reported sexual preferences of priests. For instance, a study often cited (Staff, 1999) notes that 83% of priests consider themselves heterosexual and 17% consider themselves

homosexual. McGlone (2001), in a study of 80 priest volunteers, notes that 60% considered themselves homosexual, 31% heterosexual, and 9% bisexual. According to Scheper-Hugues and Devine (2003), the majority of priests who assault young boys are not homosexual in orientation or preference, but rather, they are more likely "sexual immature, regressed, or sexually adolescent males" (p. 27). Although this article is filled with polemic and invective, the authors fail to provide real scientific information to back claims being offered.

Interpersonal Factors

Plante and Daniels (2004) report that there is no evidence to suggest that Catholic priests are more likely to sexually offend against children than clergy from other religious traditions or men in general. Based on these findings, they argue that allowing clergy to marry or engage in sexual relationships with consenting adults would not significantly reduce clergy abuse. Fones et al. (1999), however, studied the sexual struggles of 19 clergy and found that these men wanted to be known by others beyond their role of clergy and that they felt isolated from others and had feelings of loneliness (Table 23.2).

Scholars have also reported that a combination of loneliness and social isolation were common complaints among the clerics in their studies (Cowan 2002; Langevin et al. 1999). This data, supported by empirical research conducted on sex offenders within the general population, finds sex offenders scoring lower on measures of intimacy and higher on measures of loneliness than nonoffending males in community comparison groups (Garlick, Marshall, & Thornton, 1996; Seidman, William, & Stephen, 1994). Markham and Mikail (2004) suggest that these empirical results match their clinical experiences as they find that the majority of clergy child sex offenders have a high prevalence of loneliness, lack

TABLE 23.2 Etiological Factors—Interpersonal

Wish to be known beyond their role to others

Few friends of their own age

Loneliness

Relationships with youth

Power-over in relationships

Lack of boundaries in relationships

rewarding close adult relationships, and often have an overidentification with the clerical role.

In Kennedy's (1992) study, 57% of clergy were considered to be emotionally underdeveloped. From an attachment perspective, when strong emotional bonds are not established, individuals experiencing some loss or emotional distress are more likely to act out as a result of loneliness and isolation (Markham & Mikail, 2004). Cowan, for example, notes that in a study of three Protestant male clergy who had offended against adult females, these men reported maternal and paternal abandonment and a lack of childhood play (Cowan, 2002).

Extensive empirical research has demonstrated that child sex offenders exhibit a compromised capacity to form intimate relationships (Markham & Mikail, 2004). Marshall (1989), for example, found that men who abuse children often have not developed the social skills and self-confidence necessary for them to form effective intimate relationships with peers. Kennedy (1992) reports that clergy in the sample were more comfortable with relationships with teenagers, had fewer friends their own age, and used intellectualization as a coping device in relationships. Based on a qualitative analysis, Bryant (1999) found that the majority of clergy sex offenders in the study claimed they were heterosexual rather than homosexual in orientation and that these clergy cited a variety of circumstances to explain choosing male victims, including access to teen boys, discomfort with women, and fear of pregnancy. Bumby and Hansen (1997) also found that child sex offenders expressed higher levels of fear of intimacy than other sex offenders.

Systemic Factors

Lack of openness in Church: McGlone (2003) reports on the many writers who have chronicled sexual abuse by clergy within the Church and has noted a history of unintentional and intentional neglect and ignorance on the part of the Church leaders to confront the problem of sexual abuse (Table 23.3). Jenkins (1996) states that the problem of sexual abuse has been obscured by the divergent political agendas of the Church leaders who want to bury the problem instead of taking proactive steps in trying to screen, prevent, and deal with cases of abuse. Plante and Daniels (2004) further note that the Catholic Church has had a history of acting in a highly defensive manner regarding sexual abuse by clergy. They note that

TABLE 23.3 Etiological Factors—Systemic

Lack of openness in Church
"Clericalism"
Seminary training
  Insularity
  Lack of training in boundaries and sexuality
Lack of clear ethical codes
Lack of supervision
Celibacy

the Catholic Church has not always treated victims and their families with understanding and compassion. In addition, the Catholic Church has been unwilling or unable to sponsor and lead genuine research in the area of sexual abuse (Loftus, 1999; Plante, 1999). Sipe (1999) argues that the Church's history of secrecy concerning sexual matters is intertwined with the Church's lack of information about sexual abuse against children. He contends that this combination of missing information and secrecy has contributed to the Church's failed attempts to manage sexual abuse by using methods that were counterproductive to healing, which included (1) the reassignment of priests; (2) sending them on a retreat to repent for their sins; or (3) sending them to a psychiatric institution run by the Church (Table 23.3).

Clericalism: Doyle (2003) explains that "clericalism" represents a policy of maintaining or increasing the power of the Church. This policy has contributed to a power imbalance between individual clerics and their parishioners. When these hierarchical relationships exist, whether perceived or real, the potential for abuse of power is present (Robison, 2004). The notion of clericalism is especially important to the study of sexual abuse by clergy, given that clergy lack ethical codes or guidelines that guide behaviors protecting against abuses caused by power differentiations.

Seminary training: Carnes and Delmonico (1994) notes the inadequacy of the seminary model of training in critical areas of sexuality, which then heightens the possibility of future sexual misconduct. Irons and Laaser (1994), for example, studied 25 clergy who had been referred for sexual misconduct and found that they had little insight into the areas of abuse, did not appreciate how their own history of trauma might affect their professional life and had a lack of training in the issue of transference and countertransference.

They further found that clergy had little training or education regarding sexual abuse, domestic violence, addictive diseases, and healthy professional boundaries.

Norris (2003) discusses the role of forensic psychiatrists in developing preventative training programs and consulting with the Church, which is consistent with Plante's (1996) plea that mental health professionals become involved in this issue. It is important for any program therefore, to include training on boundaries, healthy sexuality, and learning about individual coping mechanisms as well as spirituality. These programs should address primary prevention of clergy sexual abuse if delivered to receptive vessels. Receptivity of the seminary students can be increased with greater accuracy by careful screening of applicants.

Lack of clear ethical codes: Sipe (1999) notes the absence of clear ethical codes for the clergy. Although he acknowledges that the Canon Code is quite explicit, this has never been translated into a clear ethical code that could become a guiding document and then taught and discussed in seminary training. Robison (2004) also highlights the lack of written rules to govern clergy conduct and behaviors and suggests that this lack of codes has been a contributing factor in the misuse of power in religious institutions. Robison observes that the role of clergy within the Church is set up for dual relationships between clergy and parishioners. For example, clergy must ensure professional distance while also being expected to participate and engage in social activities with the parishioners. Given the lack of clear relationship definitions and the feelings of loneliness expressed by many clergy, they are particularly vulnerable to boundary violations when seeking emotional support from their parishioners. Calling for the need of clearly defined ethical codes, Lebacqz and Barton (1991) note that notions of mutuality are missing in the clergy–parishioner relationship given that parishioners share deeply personal information with the clergy but this sharing is not reciprocal, thereby creating power imbalances.

Lack of supervision: Sexual addiction has been linked to high demanding jobs with little structure or supervision (Carnes, Delmonico, Griffin, & Moriarty, 2001). According to Saradjian and Nobus (2003), the most pervasive systemic problem of sexual abuse within the Church is reflected in the Catholic Church's inadequate response in dealing

with the clergy who abuse children and in the lack of supervision of the clergy to prevent abuse. They report of clergy simply being moved from a parish when accused of sex abuse, thereby exacerbating the problem by providing them with further opportunities to offend against more unsuspecting victims and their families. They report that the Catholic Church in the Unites States, Canada, and Europe has since acknowledged these problems.

To demonstrate the impact of this systemic problem, Saradjian and Nobus (2003) used a grounded theory approach to investigate cognitive distortions in self-report statements of 14 clergy who had sexually abused children and found that the Church's inadequate dealings of the accused clergy offenders (Plante, 1996) contributed to the offender's perception of an approval of higher allegiances (Thomson, Joseph, & David, 1998). Saradjian and Nobus (2003) found that offenders' attributions related to not getting caught, which only served to increase the likelihood of subsequent offenses and to provide the clergy with accessto more unsuspecting children. Plante and Daniels (2004) emphasize that not all church jurisdictions have dealt with clergy abuse in the same manner, but these experiences have been true for many.

Vow of Celibacy: Gregoire (2003) argues that it is not the task of therapists to debate the relevance of clergy celibacy, but rather to increase the therapist's sensitivity to the culture of celibacy so as to implement better informed treatment strategies for celibates when dealing with issues of sexuality. Adams (2003) suggests that mental health professionals have historically failed to address issues of celibacy in treatment with clergy because of its connection with the Church. He argues that celibacy should be explored on an individual level to determine whether its potential implications for abuse and whether celibacy itself has causative or aggravating factors related to the offense. Adam further suggests that the issue of celibacy is a critical point of treatment for clergy given their internal struggles between coming to consciousness regarding their sexual feelings and behaviors and the violation of their vows of celibacy by exploring healthy forms of sexual expressions.

Gregoire (2003) gives a readable explanation regarding the history and meaning of celibacy and points out that celibacy is practiced by different religious and nonreligious groups. In the religious context, celibacy is believed to help in the advancement toward spiritual enlightenment and salvation. However, the definition of celibacy is imprecise. Some regard celibacy as a commitment to remain unmarried and others regard celibacy as a voluntary renunciation of genital sex. Sipe (1995) argues that it is this imprecision that leads to ambiguity, a lack of a clear definition of clergy abuse and subjective interpretations of what it means to be celibate.

For many clergy, vows of celibacy are no easier to keep than vows of faithfulness and loyalty among the married (Rossetti & Lothstein 1990; Thoburn & Balswick 1994; Young, Eric, Al, O'Mara, & Buchanan, 2000). Sipe (1999), for example, found that only 2% of his cohorts of about 1300 Catholic clergy were genuinely celibate, another 20% desperately tried to maintain celibacy, and about 80% of the clergy in the sample were not celibate. Gregoire (2003) also notes that 50% of vowed celibates are involved in long- or short-term relationships.

Relating the issue of celibacy and sexual abuse by clergy, Adams (2003) poses a bipartheid question. Firstly, "Do individuals with vulnerable sexual problems choose the priesthood as a refuge?" The second question is "Does celibacy lead to sexual abuse?" He argues that the answer is "yes" to both questions. He believes that young men chose priesthood before conscious acceptance of their own sexuality. Sexuality is not integrated into a priest's identity. As such, the expression of sexuality is disassociated from the value system of the moral governing self. Sexual feelings generate feelings of loss and result in resentment and entitlement. Lothstein (1999) reports on the belief system of a number of priests who did not view sex with men or boys as violating their vow of celibacy.

Langevin et al. (1999) suggest that many offending clergy have a sexual preference for minors, which is presumed to have started in adolescence. This supports the theory that is borne out of personal experiences where many priests enter the clergy to seek a refuge from anomalous sexual urges. They believe that celibacy has a magical way of protecting them from acting out their fantasies. However, when certain disinhibiting factors such as neuropsychological damage, endocrine disorders, or substance abuse collide with loose boundaries and opportunity, the stage is set for sexual abuse. In some individuals, however, celibacy may contribute to offending and it is perhaps timely for the Church to examine this issue.

Toward an Etiology Model of Clergy Abuse

The literature review has demonstrated that the path that leads clergy to sexually offend against children can vary considerably and the propensity of clergy abuse can be explained by the interrelationships between intrapersonal, interpersonal, and systemic factors. As stated previously, empirical research is limited and many of the studies suffer from methodological flaws. Therefore, it would be premature to speculate whether certain factors have more predictive value than others in determining the likelihood of clergy committing abuse. More scientific studies are needed before such claims can be made. Within the current state of empirical knowledge, we propose an overarching etiology model that focuses on the intersection of intrapersonal, interpersonal, and systemic for the assessment and analysis of clergy abuse. Within this multilevel framework, each level encompasses major variables located within the available empirical research.

The model (Figure 23.1) subscribes to the notion that clergy abuse is caused by a full complexity of factors. Arrows in the model move from both directions to indicate that it is both the individual characteristics and the clergy's experiences with environmental factors that will determine whether abuse is more likely to occur. All factors are considered to interact with the others and the model provides an etiological factor analysis that addresses the complexities in the field. No single individual factor alone can determine the likelihood of clergy committing a sexual offense against a child and there remains considerable debate in the field about the potential impact on many of the factors. For example, much debate continues on whether being a previous victim of sexual abuse increases the risk of clergy abuse. Some studies found no association between previous abuse and clergy abuse (Langevin et al., 1999; Ruzicjka, 1997) while others have found an association between the two (Bryant, 1999). In this proposed model, we suggest noting past sexual abuse as a possible factor, but only in combination with other factors at all three levels. Therefore, we put forth this model as a "guidepost approach" to help practitioners and researchers consider the full complexity of the intersection between these etiological factors. We further propose that prevention, screening, and treatment are best achieved by considering the combination of variables impacting clergy abuse.

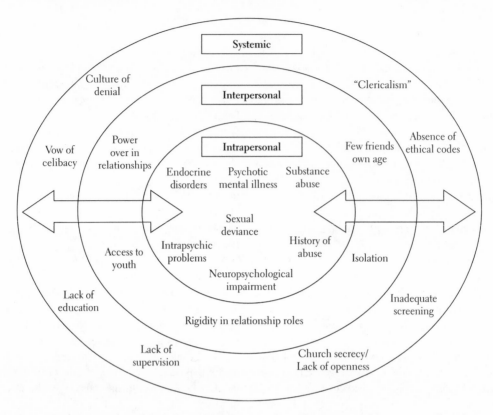

FIGURE 23.1 An etiological model of clergy abuse: Intersections of intrapersonal, interpersonal, and systemic factors.

Within this framework, we propose that improvements to the intrapersonal level of functioning (e.g., substance abuse treatment, counseling for past abuse, treatment for personality problems, etc.) will have a stronger effect if these changes are complimented with changes to both the interpersonal level (e.g., improved social supports, increased flexibility in relationships, etc.) and the systemic level (e.g., ongoing supervision, increased educational opportunities, a move toward more openness within the Church culture, etc.). These targeted areas for prevention and treatment will be examined in further detail within the chapter.

Typology

Gonsiorek (1999) proposes a typology based on the observations at a walk-in counseling center in Minneapolis for cases of various types of sexual misconduct.

Gonsiorek points out that within the first group of "naïve offenders," clergy are inadequately trained regarding ethics, professional conduct, and sexual information, which sets the stage for poor negotiation of gray areas in boundary management. By the nature of the work, clergy are often thrown into positions where these areas may be difficult. At-risk situations often occur when the clergy is involved in activities with adolescent parishioners. These activities often take place outside of Church and may involve volunteer work, attending people's houses, or recreational activities such as camping and trips. One of the particular pitfalls we have seen in our practice is when clergy begin to form a relationship with an adolescent male to introduce him to priesthood with the hope that he will enter priesthood. This type of behavior may involve dinners at the subject's house and then weekend or camping trips. These boundary crossings set the stage for the slippery slope that sometimes leads to a more serious boundary violation, such as sexual misconduct (Table 23.4). In the second group of the "normal to mildly neurotic," the clergyman is often at a crisis in his own life and feels depressed and isolated. Lacking proper social support, he uses the parishioner to satisfy his own needs as a person

TABLE 23.4 A Typology of Sexual Misconduct

Naive

Normal and/or mildly neurotic

Severely neurotic and/or socially isolated

Impulsive character disorders

Sociopathic or narcissistic character disorders

Psychotics

Classic sex offenders

Medically disabled

Masochistic/self-defeating

who listens and helps him. This can proceed to a romantic relationship. Gabbard (2001) uses the term love sick when describing physicians in this role. This appears to be one of the commonest groups of sexually exploitative clergy and generally the prognosis for rehabilitation is said to be good.

The third group, "the severely neurotic," has chronic moral problems of low self-esteem, personal inadequacy, and social isolation. Often, they are particularly involved in their work since they have little else in their lives. Gonsiorek (1999) states that this behavior tends to be repeated every decade or so, as their basic character structure is chronically impaired. Like other professionals who are involved in sexual misconduct, they are often known as particularly hardworking, well-liked professionals, known for their stellar work, dedication, and open-door policies. It is a regretful paradox that often these most dedicated professionals, in their zeal to help, allow boundary crossings to become boundary violations and end up damaging parishioners instead of helping them.

In the next group, "the impulsive character disorders," clergymen generally have legal or interpersonal difficulties in their histories. This group is rare since it is unusual for a person with this type of character to complete the training and dedication needed to become a clergyman. However, some scrape through and once they do, their behavior may be out of control in a number of contexts. They are differentiated from the next group, the "sociopathic or narcissistic character disorders," in that the latter group's behavior tends to be more deliberated and planned. The sociopathic character disorders are described as calculating and lacking in empathy. They may select parishioners who are the most vulnerable and therefore less likely to complain and be believed.

Another rare group is the "psychotic group." They suffer from a serious mental disorder. Once treated, they generally demonstrate an understanding and feel remorse. Their prognosis is dependent on the treatment of the underlying condition.

Another group is the "classic sex offender" group, in other words, those suffering from a paraphilia. A study by Langevin et al. (1999) suggests that paraphilias, mainly, homosexual pedophilia, or hebephilia is common among clergy who sexually abuse their parishioners. As part of any reasonable relapse prevention plan, they should only be allowed back into the profession if they are not allowed access to their preferred object, most commonly, adolescent boys. Therefore, they should only be allowed to work in administration or other positions. Supervision should be built in for a long period of time, as it is not uncommon for them to slip back into frontline positions if they are not supervized.

The final group is the "masochistic/self-defeating" group. These are people who are unable to resist the demands of a small group of parishioners and, therefore, their boundaries are eroded. Not uncommonly, they attempt counseling with parishioners who have severe personality disorders, which occasionally leads to romantic and sexual contact with resulting mayhem. They often display other types of self-defeating behavior such as not collecting their salary and not taking care of themselves in other areas in their life. This group represents a high proportion of sexual offenders.

PREVENTION AND SCREENING

Davis (1998) notes two factors that need to be addressed in what he refers to as clergy sexual addiction. These are the environment in which the clergy are required to work and the demands made on them as individuals.

Regarding the environment, he stresses the clergy's unclear boundaries that are repeatedly alluded to in this chapter. This results in role confusion. The clergy have little structure and supervision, yet the expectations placed upon them are unrealistically high. First of all, they act as caregivers, a fact that makes it difficult for them to ask for or receive care. Secondly, they are expected to be both perfect and godly and live their lives effectively in a goldfish bowl scrutinized by the whole community. Davis asserts that as a result, they cannot be truly themselves. They become personally and professionally isolated and cannot deal with their inner shame. He advocates that early boundary violations should not be swept under the carpet but should be addressed in the climate of openness. Priests should be educated at an early stage, presumably in the seminary, to explore sexual issues and connection with others, thereby breaking their feelings of shame and humiliation.

Once in practice, their emotional and physical isolation should not be allowed to fester. Davis advocates for support groups after graduation, which encourages openness and accountability. Likewise, Delmonico (2003) calls for openness within the Church, formal training on professional and sexual boundaries, and avenues for help, guidance, and self-care for the clergy.

In a chapter on the prevention of clergy sexual abuse, Sipe (1999) complains of the lack of methods in screening out possible sex offenders from candidates to the priesthood. Glancy and Langevin (2002) in a proposal that was eventually put before the Canadian Conference of Bishops argue that there are well-established tests that can be used for screening, and would be no more expensive than methods used thus far. Evidence suggests that the MMPI can not only be used to identify a significant number of those that sexually abuse but is also useful for identifying serious psychopathology and personality disorders and for screening those who are likely not ideally suited for such a responsible profession. In addition, the Wechsler Adult Intelligence Scale (WAIS) would point to neuropsychological factors that in association with other pathology might raise some red flags (Camargo, 1997). Most particularly, we advocate the use of the Abel Screen (Johnson & Listiak, 1999). This is a computer-based test that measures reaction time to a variety of stimuli. It has been demonstrated to have acceptable psychometric properties and due to the fact that no sexually explicit images are used, it is something that does not cause any moral dilemmas. We would also advocate the use of a questionnaire that looks at the presence of sexual deviation and sexual functioning such as the Sexual History Questionnaire (Paitich, Langevin, Freeman, Mann, & Handy, 1977) as well as screening for substance abuse. This screening would be associated with criminal background checks, reference checks, and a personal interview. A further safeguard would be to ensure close supervision and support for all new clergy admitted to the seminary.

Davis (1998) argues for an in-depth examination of professional ethics. Sipe (1999) decries the lack of professional ethical standards available to priests. Many professional bodies (Law Commission of Canada, 2000) have set out clear ethical standards and procedures for their professions that delineate clear boundaries, openness, and accountability. We would argue that the Church needs to parallel such developments even at the expense of limiting the type of work the clergy are able to do and the circumstances in which they can complete their work. Traditionally, priests have been expected to enter into the community and practice in all sorts of settings. This may not be appropriate, given the crisis in which the Church finds itself.

TREATMENT PROGRAMS

Marshall (1999) advocates the establishment of treatment centers for offending clergy. His model incorporates a standard relapse prevention model with some of the components noted that are specific to clergy. He also discusses the importance of ongoing supervision and follow-up of clergy offenders. It is our experience that clergy can respond to a relapse prevention approach similar to that used in other sexual offenders. This is the only method of treatment that is evidence based (Marshall, 1999) for offenders and is widely used across the world. These programs are based on cognitive behavioral therapies and are generally delivered as part of a multimodal problem. Cognitive behavioral programs lend themselves to adjunctive treatment such as the use of sex drive–reducing medications (Bradford, 2000). In addition, empathy training is generally included as a type of victim sensitization (Regehr & Glancy, 2001) (Table 23.5).

TABLE 23.5 Ongoing Training

1. Ongoing supervision and training in boundaries

2. Ongoing dialogue regarding healthy general and individual sexuality

3. Ongoing availability of support regarding intrapsychic issues

4. Ongoing supervision and dialogue regarding spirituality

Bryant (1999) describes a program called *Victim Sensitive Offender Therapy* that comprises many of the elements in a multimodal relapse prevention program. He emphasizes the perpetrator accepting responsibility for his actions and the harm that it caused to his victims. Following victim sensitization, the offender learns to understand his offence cycle and prepares a relapse prevention plan. Echoing many others in the field, Bryant advocates the long-term execution of such a program to reflect the chronic nature of a paraphilia.

Another facet of the program works on addressing cognitive distortions, which is common in thinking about sex offenders in general and clergy in particular (Sheldon & Parent, 2002). These disturbances may be a function of a lack of sexual knowledge, social knowledge, or education and discussion of sexual matters.

Laaser (Laaser & Gregoire, 2003) advocates a similar model to any sexually addictive client involving inpatient or intensive outpatient treatment as well as individual and family therapy. He quotes Carne's model of recovery, which contains educational, behavioral, and psychodynamic components as the most effective form of treatment. He discusses the issue of whether the group should be homogeneous for clergy or a mixed group (Laaser, 1991).

Nunez (2003) takes homogeneity a step further in describing an outpatient group, based on a 12-step recovery program, comprising of clergy hebephiles only. Laaser and Gregoire (2003) discusses countertransference issues that can sabotage therapy unless addressed. He also stresses vocational guidance since many offenders will be voluntarily or involuntarily leaving the clergy and venturing into the secular world. Like others before him (Hudson, 1997), he stresses spiritual direction and counseling. He also notes the emotional abandonment felt by many of these people, urging maximal long-term support in conjunction with ongoing monitoring and surveillance.

Adams (2003) suggests that one facet of treatment should be to increase awareness of issues within the perpetrators' background so that they can understand their own individual personality and sexual problems. He also advocates exploring the role of celibacy within their lives as well as the meaning of this concept. Alvarez (2003), in discussing clergy who have had problems with what he describes as sexual addiction, not necessarily sexual molestation

of minors, urges addressing issues of theology and values when working with clergy who are at a stage where they are yet to assault anybody. In this way, he suggests that an understanding of healthy sexuality, as discussed in his article, will help clergy resolve many of their early sexual issues (Alvarez, 2003). It is possible that if this is affected either in training or early in a career, this can prevent future and more serious sexual misconduct.

Gregoire (2003) makes the extremely important point that early indicators or anomalous sexual preference should lead to the decision to remove the clergyman from the ministry and moved into a more appropriate career that does not involve any contact with or power over minors. This is particularly important, as we have discussed earlier, in that some clergy believe that a celibate life will miraculously solve their sexual problems or alter their sexual orientation. *The Charter for the Protection of Children and Young People* by the United States Conference of Catholic Bishops (2005), mandate that the goals of treatment when dealing with Catholic priests can no longer include a return to the ministry. Therefore, Songy (2003) urges the consideration of alternative goals, presumably together with vocational guidance. He urges treatment programs to consider reclaiming the sacrament of priesthood. He argues that as priests reclaim their pastoral sensitivity they will devote more of their prayer to the mental and spiritual health of their victims and the healing of the Church. However, it is argued that relapse prevention programs should address the particular sexual misconduct and this can be affected in conjunction with other therapists who address spiritual issues.

Irons and Laaser (1994), based on a large clinical experience, assert that restoration is possible. They advocate 2 to 3 years of treatment plus ongoing monitoring. However, they do not state that a career change may be necessary. It would be our opinion, that, based on the principles of relapse prevention, it is likely not possible for a clergyman to be restored to his previous position wherein he has power and control over minors. He should be moved to a clerical position. It should be noted, however, that there have been instances in our experience where this has led to "slippage," whereby the priest starts doing occasional work with the community that exposes minors to him and, therefore, puts the community at risk. Repeated monitoring should carefully safeguard against this.

FUTURE DIRECTIONS

Plante (1999) and colleagues suggest eight directions, which have been outlined by Plante and Daniels (2004). We present these eight directions and add our own emphasis to better address sexual abuse by clergy.

1. *Accept and understand the facts.* Plante (1999) and colleagues state that we must deal with clergy abuse guided by reason and compassion rather than bias and hysteria. We must collect all of the available data and let the facts inform our thinking in order to deal more effectively with the prevention and treatment of sexual abuse by clergy.
2. *Treat offending clergy.* We have reviewed presented existing treatment available for clergy who sexually abuse. It is important that clergy are given the opportunity to attend treatment and that they are supported through this process.
3. *Collaborate between mental health and church professionals.* We have alluded to this earlier. Mental health and church professionals should come together with a clear mandate to protect and prevent future clergy abuse by ensuring that all clergy receive adequate training and support. Furthermore, offenders or those who are at high risk of offending should be effectively diagnosed and treated.
4. *Treat victims.* Victims and their families need both validation and treatment. Victims should be offered counseling and support.
5. *Share Data.* Data obtained by the Church and treatment facilities should be made available to each other and to researchers to develop a more comprehensive understanding of clergy abuse. Plante and Daniels (2004) point out that far too many researchers have been unable to study these problems because of a general lack of cooperation from the Church.
6. *Develop clear policies for intervention.* Sipe (1999) notes the absence of clear ethical codes that could form guiding policies. Plante and Daniels (2004) suggest that national and international standards could be developed and issued by the Church in collaboration with appropriate mental health and legal professionals.
7. *Train and support clergy.* Delmonico (2003) notes the inadequacy of the seminary model of training in critical areas, which prepares the ground for sexual misconduct. Clergy need training and supervision to ensure health; personal and professional boundaries are both understood and maintained. Clergy also need ongoing support regarding issues related to sexuality, sexual expression, and celibacy.
8. *Practice what you teach.* Plante and Daniels (2004) call for common sense and compassion instead of the recent hysteria and demonization of the clergy in the media.

CONCLUSION

We believe that further empirical studies are needed to address current gaps in the knowledge base of sexual abuse by clergy. We agree with McGlone (2003) that the collection of both preliminary and descriptive data is essential to advance our basic understanding of clergy abuse. We have also proposed a model that includes etiological factors found within existing scholarly work. Future research should test the proposed model by conducting multivariate analysis to determine whether a hierarchy of variables can be used to better screen and assess the risk of clergy abuse.

We agree with the pleas from Plante and Daniels (2004) that mental health professionals should become more involved with the prevention, screening, and treatment of clergy who sexually abuse. As they point out, many of the experts of sexual offences toward minors are psychologists and other mental health professionals (Daw, 2002; Rossetti, 1996). Therefore, psychologists and counselors have the "interest and skill to help consult and manage these issues working closely with Church officials, offending clergy, the media, child protective services, law enforcement, abuse victims and victim groups and the Catholic laity" (Plante & Daniels, 2004).

We also suggest that scholarly clinical researchers are required to become more involved in the study of clergy abuse and should take on a more predominant role in these research activities. Future research to advance current knowledge on the etiological factors, preventions, and treatments of sexual abuses by clergy should utilize generally accepted scientific procedures and standardized methodologies to eliminate potential bias. Although important in all fields of study, researchers need to be aware of the political, religious, and social implications of their work and should guard against these forces to ensure that future work remains uncontaminated.

Given the current crisis in the Roman Catholic Church and other denominations, Church leaders ought to inspire themselves and others to become active participants in the process of scientific discovery to ensure the cultivation of reliable information to help and treat the clergy who abuse. Religious leaders could facilitate a culture of openness, thereby breaking down current barriers for sample recruitment strategies, as an example. Becoming more open to scientific research has many benefits for the Church and its clergy. First, a move toward openness would demonstrate a genuine eagerness to address the Church's current crisis. Second, by participating in research, validity and reliability of data collection would be improved because the data would become more representative of the clergy population. Third, empirical results can demystify current inaccurate portrayals of clergy in the general public, such as all clergy are "pedophilic priest" (Jenkins, 1996). Lastly, by increasing openness and involvement, Church leaders position themselves as active players in the search of effective solutions to prevent abuse and develop evidence-based interventions to treat those clergy who commit sexual abuse against children.

References

Adams, K. M. (2003). Clergy sex abuse: A commentary on celibacy. *Sexual Addiction & Compulsivity,* 10(2–3), 91–2.

Alvarez, M. L. (2003). Issues of values: Clergy and treatment. *Sexual Addiction & Compulsivity,* 10, 151–66.

Bera, W. H. (1996). Clergy sexual abuse and male survivors: A study of stress and coping among 25 men abused by the same minister during their adolescence. *Dissertation Abstracts International: Section B: The Sciences and Engineering,* 56(10-B), 5758.

Bradford, J. M. W. (2000). The treatment of sexual deviation using a pharmacological approach. *Journal of Sexual Research,* 37, 237–45.

Bryant, C. (1999). Psychological treatment of priest sex offenders. In T. G. Plante (Ed.), *Bless Me Father for I Have Sinned: Perspectives on Sexual Abuse Committed By Roman Catholic Priests* (pp. 87–110). Westport, CT: Praeger Publisher.

Bumby, K. M. & David J. H. (1997). Intimacy deficits, fear of intimacy, and loneliness among sexual offenders. *Criminal Justice and Behavior,* 24(3), 315–31.

Camargo, R. J. (1997). Factor, cluster, and discriminant analyses of data on sexually active clergy: Erratum. *American Journal of Forensic Psychology,* 15(3), 64.

Carnes, P. J. & Delmonico, D. L. (1994). Sexual dependency inventory. Wickenburg, AZ: The Meadows Institute.

Carnes, P., Delmonico, D. L., Griffin, E., & Moriarty, J. (2001). *In the Shadows of the Net: Breaking Free of Compulsive Online Behavior.* Hazelden Centre City, Minnesota, MN: Hazelden Educational Materials.

Connors, C. (1992). Priests and pedophilia: A silence that needs breaking? *America,* 166, 400–1.

Cowan, E. G., Jr. (2002). Understanding Protestant pastors who have had sexual relationships with women in their congregations: A multiple-case study. *Dissertation Abstracts International: Section B: The Sciences and Engineering,* 62(8-B), 3837.

Davis, M. (1998). Clergy a sexual malfeasance: Restoration, ethics and process. *Journal of Psychology and Theology,* 26(4), 333–339.

Daw, J. (2002). Can psychological help a church in crisis? *Monitoring on Psychology,* 33, 24–6.

Delmonico, D. L. (2003). There but for the grace of God... *Sexual Addiction & Compulsivity,* 10(2–3), 89–90.

Doyle, T. P. (2003). Roman Catholic clericalism, religious duress, and clergy sexual abuse. *Pastoral Psychology,* 51(3), 189–231.

Falkenhain, M. A. (1998). Child sexual abusers among Roman Catholic priests and brothers: A cluster analytic study. *Dissertation Abstracts International: Section B: The Sciences and Engineering,* 58(8-B), 4444.

Fones, C. S. L., Stephen B. L., Stanley E. A., & Candace B. R. (1999). The sexual struggles of 23 clergymen: A follow-up study. *Journal of Sex & Marital Therapy,* 25(3), 183–95.

Fortune, M. (1989). *Is Nothing Sacred?* San Francisco, CA: Harper.

Gabbard, G. O. (2001) *Treatments of Psychiatric Disorders, 2nd edition.* Washington, D.C.: American Psychiatric Association.

Garlick, Y., Marshall, W. L., & Thornton D. (1996). Intimacy deficits and attribution of blame among sexual offenders. *Legal & Criminological Psychology,* 1(2), 251–258.

Gerard, S. M., Jobes, D., Cimbolic, P., Ritzler, B. A., & Montana S. (2003). A Rorschach study of interpersonal disturbance in priest child molesters. *Sexual Addiction & Compulsivity,* 10(1), 53–56.

Glancy, G. & Langevin, R. (2002). Proposal to the Archdiocese of London for Screening Novitiates. Toronto, Canada.

Gonsiorek, J. C. Forensic psychological evaluations in clergy abuse. (1999). In T. G. Plante (Ed.), *Bless Me Father for I Have Sinned: Perspectives On Sexual Abuse Committed By Roman Catholic Priests,* (pp. 27–57), Westport, CT: Praeger/Greenwood.

Goodstein, L. (2003, January 12). Trail of pain in Church crises leads to nearly every diocese. *New York Times* (New York), 1–6.

Gregoire, J. (2003). Understanding the culture of celibacy for the treatment of priests and religious. *Sexual Addiction & Compulsivity,* 10, 167–77.

Harris, M. (1990). *Unholy Order: Tragedy at Mount Cashel.* Toronto, Ontario: Viking Press.

Haywood, T. W., Kravitz H. M., Wasyliw O. E., Goldberg J., & Cavanaugh J. L. Jr. (1996). Cycle of abuse and psychopathology in cleric and noncleric molesters of children and adolescents. *Child Abuse and Neglect*, 20(12), 1233–43.

Hudson, P. E. (1997). Spirituality as a component in a treatment program for sexually addicted Roman Catholic clergy. *Counseling and Values*, 41(2), 174–82.

Irons, R., & Laaser M. (1994). The abduction of fidelity: Sexual exploitation by clergy—experience with inpatient assessment. *Sexual Addiction & Compulsivity*, 1(2), 119–29.

Jenkins, P. (1996). *Pedophiles and Priests: Anatomy of A Contemporary Crisis*. New York, NY: Oxford University Press.

Johnson, M. & Listiak, A. (1999). The measurement of sexual preference-A preliminary comparison of phallometry and the Abel assessment. In B. Schwartz (Ed.), *The Sex Offender* (pp. 26.1–26.19). Kingston, New Jersey, NJ: Civic Research Institute.

Kelly, A. F. (1998). Clergy offenders. In W. L. Marshall, Y. M. Fernandez, S. M. Hudson and T. Ward (Eds.), *Sourcebook of Treatment Programs for Sexual Offenders. Applied clinical psychology*, (pp. 303–18) New York: Plenum. Kennedy, E. (1992). The Catholic priest in the United States: Psychological investigations. Paper presented at the Catholic Conference, Washington, D.C.

Laaser, M. & Gregoire L. (2003). Pastors and cybersex addiction. *Sexual & Relationship Therapy. Special Cybersex*, 18(3), 395–406.

Laaser, M. R. (1991). Sexual addiction and clergy. *Pastoral Psychology*, 39(4), 213–35.

Langevin, R., Curnoe S., & Bain J. (2000). A study of clerics who commit sexual offenses: Are they different from other sex offenders? *Child Abuse and Neglect*, 24(4), 535–45.

Langevin, R., Mark B.-A., Wortzman G., Dickey R., et al. (1987). Brain damage, diagnosis, and substance abuse among violent offenders. *Behavioral Sciences & the Law. Special Issue: Homicidal behavior*, 5(1), 77–94.

Langevin, R., Graham, D. Glancy, S. C., & Bain J. (1999). Physicians who commit sexual offenses: Are they different from other sex offenders?" *Canadian Journal of Psychiatry*, 44(8), 775–86.

Langevin, R. & Watson R. J. (1996). Major factors in the assessment of paraphilics and sex offenders. *Journal of Offender Rehabilitation*, 23, 39–70.

Law Commission of Canada. (2000). Restoring dignity: Responding to child abuse in Canadian institutions, Ottawa: Minister of Public Works and Government Services.

Lebacqz, K. & Barton, R. G. (1991). *Sex in the Parish*. Louisville, KY: Westminster Press.

Loftus, J. A. (1999). Sexuality in priesthood: Noli me tangre. In T. G. Plante (Ed.), *Bless me Father for I Have Sinned: Perspectives On Sexual Abuse Committed by Roman Catholic Priests*, (pp. 7–19). Westport, CT: Praeger/Greenwood.

Loftus, J. A. & Robert J. C. (1993). Treating the clergy. *Annals of Sex Research*, 6(4), 287–303.

Lothstein, L. (1999). Neuropsychological findings in clergy who sexually abuse. In T. G. Plante (Ed.), *Bless me Father for I Have Sinned: Perspectives on Sexual Abuse Committed by Roman Catholic Priests*, (pp. 59–85) Westport, CT: Praeger/Greenwood.

Markham, D. J., & Samuel F. M. (2004). Perpetrators of clergy abuse: insights from attachment theory. *Studies in Gender and Sexuality*, 5(2), 197–212.

Marshall, W. L. (1999). Current status of North American assessment and treatment programs for sexual offenders. *Journal of Interpersonal Violence*, 14, 221–39.

Marshall, W. L.(1989). Intimacy, loneliness and sexual offenders. *Research Therapy*, 27, 491–503.

Marshall, W. L. (1997). Pedophilia: Psychopathology and theory. In D. R. Laws & W. T. O'Donohue (Eds.), *Sexual Deviance: Theory, Assessment, and Treatment*, (pp. 152–174). New York, Guilford Press.

Marshall, W. L. & Barbaree H. E. (1990). An integrated theory of the etiology of sexual offending. In W. L. Marshall, D. R. Laws, & H. E. Barbaree, (Eds.), *Handbook of Sexual Assault: Issues, Theories, and Treatment of the Offender. Applied Clinical Psychology* (pp. 257–275). New York, NY: Plenum Press.

McGlone, G. J. (2003). Prevalence and incidence of Roman Catholic clerical sex offenders. *Sexual Addiction & Compulsivity*, 10, 111–21.

McGlone, G. J. (2001). Sexually offending and non-offending Roman Catholic priests: Characterization and analysis. *Dissertation Abstracts International: Section B: The Sciences and Engineering*, 62 (1-B), 557.

Norris, D. M. (2003). Forensic consultation and the clergy sexual abuse crisis. *Journal of the American Academy of Psychiatry and the Law*, 31(2), 154–7.

Nunez, J. (2003). Outpatient treatment of the sexually compulsive ephebophile. *Sexual Addiction & Compulsivity*, 10(1), 23–51.

Paitich, D., Langevin R., Freeman R., Mann K., & Handy L. (1977). The Clarke SHQ: A clinical sex history questionnaire for males. *Archives in Sexual Behavior*, 6(5), 421–36.

Plante, T. G. (1999). *Bless me Father for I Have Sinned: Perspectives on Sexual Abuse Committed by Roman Catholic Priests*. Westport, CT: Praeger/Greenwood.

Plante, T. G. (1996). Catholic priests who sexually abuse minors: Why do we hear so much yet know so little? *Pastoral Psychology*, 44(5), 305–10.

Plante, T. G. (2003). Priests behaving badly: What do we know about priest sex offenders? *Sexual Addiction & Compulsivity*, 9, 93–7.

Plante, T. G. & Daniels C. (2004). The sexual abuse crisis in the Roman Catholic Church: What psychologists and counselors should know. *Pastoral Psychology*, 52(5), 381–93.

Plante, T. G., Manuel G., & Bryant C. (1996). Personality and cognitive functioning among hospitalized sexual offending Roman Catholic priests. *Pastoral Psychology*, 45(2), 129–39.

Regehr, C. & Glancy G. (2001). Empathy and its influence on sexual misconduct. *Trauma, Abuse and Violence*, 2(2), 142–54.

Robison, L. H. (2004). The abuse of power: A view of sexual misconduct in a systemic approach to pastoral care. *Pastoral Psychology*, 52(5), 394–404.

Rossetti, S. J. (1996). A *Tragic Grace: The Catholic Church and Child Sexual Abuse*. Collegeville, Minnesota, MN: The Liturgical Press.

Rossetti, S. J. & Anthony, P. (1996). Development and preliminary validation of the MMPI-II for same sex priest child molesters. *Sexual & Relationship Therapy. Special Cybersex*, 3(4), 341–56.

Rossetti, S. J., & Lothstein L. M. (1990). Myths of the child molester. In S. J. Rossetti (Ed.), *Slayer of the Soul: Child Sexual Abuse and the Catholic Church*, (pp. 9–18).

Ruzicjka, M. F. (1997). Predict of variables on clergy pedophiles. *Psychological Reports*, 81(2), 589–590.

Saradjian, A. & Nobus D. (2003). Cognitive distortions of religious professionals who sexually abuse children. *Journal of Interpersonal Violence*, 18(8), 905–23.

Scheper-Hughes, N. & Devine J. (2003). Priestly celibacy and child sexual abuse. *Sexuality*, 6(1), 15–40.

Seidman, B. T., Marshall W. L., & Hudson S. M. (1994). An examination of intimacy and loneliness in sex offenders. *Journal of Interpersonal Violence*, 9, 518–34.

Sheldon, J. P. & Parent S. L. (2002). Clergy's attitudes and attributions of blame toward female rape victims. *Violence Against Women*, 8(2), 233–56.

Sipe, A. R. (1999). The problem of prevention in clergy sexual abuse. In T. G. Plante (Ed.), *Bless me Father for I Have Sinned: Perspectives on Sexual Abuse Committed By Roman Catholic Priests*, (pp. 111–134).

Sipe, A. W. R. (1995). *Sex, Priests, and Power: Anatomy of a Crisis*. New York, NY: Brunner/Mazel.

Songy, D. G. (2003). Psychological and spiritual treatment of Roman Catholic clerical sex offenders. *Sexual Addiction & Compulsivity*, 10, 123–37.

Staff S. K. C. (1999). Aids and the Roman Catholic clergy. *The Kansas City Star*. Kansas City, MO.

Terry, K. J. & Tallon, J. (2004). *Child Sexual Abuse: A Review of the Literature*. The John Jay College Research Team. Accessed June 3, 2005. http://www.usccb.org/nrb/johnjaystudy/litreview.pdf.

Thoburn, J. W. & Balswick J. O. (1994). An evaluation of infidelity among male Protestant clergy. *Pastoral Psychology*, 42(4), 285–94.

Thomson, J. G., Marolla J. A., & Bromley D. G. (1998). Disclaimers and Accounts in Cases of Catholic Priests Accused of Pedophilia. In A. Shupe (Ed.), *Wolves Within the Fold: Religious Leadership and Abuses of Power*, (pp. 175–789). New Brunswick, NJ: Rutgers University Press.

United States Conference of Catholic Bishops. (2005). "Charter for the Protection of Children and Young People." United States Conference of Catholic Bishops, Washington, D.C. 20017. [online] Available at http://www.usccb.org/ocyp/charter.shtml

Wills, G. (2000). *Papal Sin*. New York, NY: Doubleday.

Wolfe, D. A., Jaffe P. G., Jetté J. L., & Poisson S. E. (2003). The impact of child abuse in community institutions and organizations: Advancing professional and scientific understanding. *Clinical Psychology: Science and Practice*, 10(2), 179–91.

Young, K. S., Eric G.-S., Al C., O'Mara J., & Buchanan J. (2000). Online infidelity: A new dimension in couple relationships with implications for evaluation and treatment. *Sexual Addiction & Compulsivity. Special Issue: Cybersex: The dark side of the force*, 7(1–2), 59–74.

Chapter 24

Manifestations of Sexual Sadism: Sexual Homicide, Sadistic Rape, and Necrophilia

Stephen J. Hucker

This chapter reviews a very wide range of sexually anomalous behavior that has been subsumed under the term *sexual sadism*. At the one end are individuals who engage in unusual but consensual sexual activities in private and commit no crime. Typically they do not regard themselves as either sexually deviant or criminal in any way. At the other end of the spectrum are behaviors that are criminally proscribed and viewed with revulsion by all but most of the offenders themselves.

The issue of where "normal" ends and the "pathological" begins is always contentious in the area of sexual anomalies or paraphilias and no more so than in the topics of sadism and masochism, known in some circles as "S & M" "bondage and domination" and similar terms. No position is taken here on that issue but rather they are treated as phenomena for observation and study. The extreme forms however justify medical or other professional concern and intervention and these are outlined.

HISTORY OF THE CONCEPT

History records possible examples of notorious criminals, whose crimes may have represented sexually sadistic behavior, including Gilles de Rais in the fifteenth century, who raped and murdered innumerable children, and Elizabeth Bathory, in the seventeenth century, who tortured young girls and drank their blood.

Richard von Krafft-Ebing is usually credited with the introduction of the term *sadism* from the name of the French nobleman, the Marquis de Sade, whose erotic novels clearly depict humiliation of women and cruelty towards them. *Psychopathia Sexualis* (Krafft-Ebing, 1886) contains descriptions of all manner of sexually sadistic behavior and has remained a classic account of the phenomenon. Before Krafft-Ebing's time, sexual behavior that would today be considered anomalous, was not considered within the purview of medicine but rather a matter of moral or criminal concern. As one of the leading psychiatrists of his day and, one who took part in the development of forensic psychiatry in Europe and testified regularly in court, he thus came to influence the perception of abnormal sexual behavior, including homosexuality, in a more humane way that could potentially benefit from medical understanding and intervention (Oosterhuis, 2000).

For Krafft-Ebing the cardinal feature sadism was,

the experience of sexual, pleasurable sensations (including orgasm) produced by acts of cruelty, bodily punishment afflicted on one's person or when witnessed by others, be they animals or human beings. It may also consist of an innate desire to humiliate, hurt, wound or even destroy others on order, thereby, to create sexual pleasure in oneself (Oosterhuis, 2000, p. 109).

The emphasis on infliction of pain was also central to the concept of "algolagnia" (literally "pain-craving") introduced by Schrenck-Notzing (1895) and which he subdivided into active (sadism) and passive (masochism) forms. Eulenberg (1911) included psychological pain in the form of humiliation in his conceptualization, as did Krafft-Ebing.

Further expansion of the concept occurred under the influence of psychodynamically oriented writers. Thus, Karpmann (1954, p. 10) observed that in the sadist, "the will to power is sexually accentuated . . . he revels in the fear, anger and the humiliation." Pain is not as important in itself but because it symbolizes power and control over the victim. Expanding on this idea, Fromm (1973) suggested that the

core of sadism . . . is the passion to have absolute and unrestricted control over living beings . . . whether an animal, child, a man or a woman. To force someone to endure pain or humiliation without being able to defend himself is one of the manifestations of absolute control, but it is by no means the only one. The person who has complete control over another living being makes this being into his thing, his property, while he becomes the other being's god (pp. 383–384).

This eroticization of feelings of power and control has also been emphasized by other writers (Brittain, 1970; MacCulloch, 1983; Myers, Burgess, Burgess, & Douglas, 1999).

The current official classification systems adopt a more limited view. Thus, ICD-10 (World Health Organization, 1992) defines sadism as the "preference for sexual activity that involves bondage or infliction of pain or humiliation" and the *Diagnostic and Statistical Manual of Mental Disorders* (DSM-IV; American Psychiatric Association) requires, inter alia, "psychological or physical suffering including humiliation" of the victim to cause sexual excitement in the sadist.

As will be discussed subsequently, however, experience has shown that these definitions have proven very difficult to apply in practice with the result that even experienced clinicians appear to employ criteria, whether "official" or idiosyncratic, quite inconsistently.

PREVALENCE

Given the problems of diagnostic consistency to be discussed presently, the data that have been offered in the literature on the frequency of sexual sadism have to be viewed with considerable skepticism, a point emphasized by Marshall with respect to offender populations (Marshall & Kennedy, 2002). Krafft-Ebing (1886) suggested that sadistic acts were more common among men and argued that subjugation of women was a natural propensity of men. It is therefore paradoxical that, in modern times, commercially produced sadomasochistic pornography commonly portrays women as the dominatrix (Weinberg, 1987) although typically these women are prostitutes catering to masochistic men (Breslow, Evans, & Langley, 1985, 303–317).

In their now classic study, Kinsey et al. (1953) reported that between 3% and 12% of women and 10% to 20% of men admitted to responding sexually to "sadomasochistic narratives." Crepault and Couture (1980) found that 14.9% of men in a sample from the general population reported fantasies of humiliating a woman and 10.7% of beating up a woman. While Arndt et al. (1985) also found that about a third of women and about 50% of men had sexual fantasies of tying up their partner, it does not seem likely that this represented their preferred sexual outlet but rather was simply part of their sexual repertoire.

Similarly, a survey of the covers of pornographic magazines (Dietz & Evans, 1982) noted that 10% to 20% of them illustrated bondage and discipline themes.

SADISM, MASOCHISM, AND OTHER PARAPHILIAS

Stekel's (1929) further elaborations of the concepts of sadism and masochism and their clinical features led to their increasingly wide acceptance of these terms among clinicians. However, as already noted, the varied definitions of the terms make it sometimes difficult to determine whether a case described by one author as a "sadist" would necessarily be accepted by another as qualifying for that term. Such problems aside, sadism and masochism have been regarded as complementary anomalies or separate poles of the same disorder (e.g., Karpmann, 1954). Supporting this idea is the finding that individuals who report masochistic fantasies are also likely to report sadistic fantasies as well (Arndt et al., 1985) and the survey by Spengler (1977) of self-identified sadomasochists found that 29% alternated between the two roles. Hucker and Blanchard (1992) noted also an association between asphyxiophilia (an expression of extreme masochism) and sadistic murder (Smith & Braun, 1978).

It is now well-recognized that paraphilic diagnoses tend to overlap in the same individual, with an average of two or three diagnoses being present. In one study, 18% of sadists were also masochistic, 46% had raped, 21% had exposed, 25% engaged in voyeurism and frottage, and a third in pedophilia (Abel, Becker, Cunningham-Rathner, Mittelman, & Rouleau, 1988). Similarly, other authors have noted particularly an overlap between sadism, masochism, fetishism, and transvestism (Gosselin & Wilson, 1980) in self-identified sadomasochists and among serious sadistic offenders, transvestism and fetishism is also strongly represented (Dietz et al., 1990; Prentky, Cohen, & Seghorn, 1985).

SADISTIC PERSONALITY DISORDER

Not all those who engage in cruelty, torture, and similar behavior are sexually aroused by the activity (Dietz et al., 1990). The type of person who deliberately behaves in this way but who derives no apparent sexual pleasure from it had received some attention in the psychiatric literature, notably from psychoanalytic writers (Kernberg, 1970; Schad-Somers, 1982), who delineated the central features of a sadistic personality disorder that became incorporated into DSM-III-R.

Berner et al. (2003) found a much greater number of individuals with the diagnosis of sadistic personality disorder in their forensic settings than in the general population. Also, using DSM-III criteria with a sample of 70 incarcerated sex offenders Berner et al. found that the diagnosis of sadistic personality disorder was made in 68% of sadists and 32% of nonsadists, those groups also being identified using strictly applied DSM-III criteria. They suggested a dimensional model for the diagnosis of sexual sadism may also be more appropriate.

However, it has been found that there is considerable overlap between sadistic personality disorder and with the narcissistic and antisocial personality disorders, in particular, and it did not appear in DSM-IV as a separate diagnostic category.

Types of Sexual Sadism

Krafft-Ebing himself described no less than eight subtypes of sexually sadistic behavior including lust murder (in which sexual arousal is intimately linked to the act of killing), necrophilia, injury of women by stabbing or flagellation, defilement of women, other types of assaults on women causing indirect harm (such as cutting off their hair), whipping of boys, sadism toward animals, and sadistic fantasies without any actual acts. Later, Hirschfeld (1956) made a simple distinction between "major" (including lust murder, necrophilia, and stabbing) and "minor" sadism (the rest of Krafft-Ebing's categories, as well as humiliation of a consenting partner using bondage, mild flagellation, submission, or degrading acts). Individuals who participate in voluntary, consenting acts of minor sadism, either as recipients or perpetrators, often refer to the activity as "bondage and discipline," "dominance and submission," or "sadomasochism" (Gosselin, 1987; Weinberg, 1987). The dominant partner places the submissive partner in a situation of helplessness and applies some form of discipline or punishment, typically accompanied by verbal degradation. Pain, humiliation, bondage are administered and there may also be whips, or fist insertion into the anus or vagina. Roles of master–slave, governess–pupil, and so on are used to ensure a tone of humiliation and debasement, along with cross-dressing, treating the submissive like an animal, sometimes urinating ("water sports") or defecating on his or her body. Further humiliation may be added by forcing the person to wear diapers or to lick the dominant's boots. Flagellation or flogging is applied typically to the buttocks while bindings, including gags or blindfolds, to render the submissive helpless and unable to move, are also frequently used. Enemas may be administered so that the submissive loses control of their bodily functions and their discomfort may be aggravated by forcing them to retain the enema for prolonged periods.

Although most large cities have networks of individuals with interests such as those just described, and there are specialized subcultures within homosexual communities catering to sadomasochistic partnerships, it is difficult to know how many such individuals progress to more serious "major" or "dangerous" sadistic activities though Freund suggested that this did occur (Freund, Seto, & Kuban, 1985). Certainly, early detection of major sadism can be difficult, though an obvious priority from the criminal justice perspective.

An early precursor of later rapists may include apparently nonsexual offenses, such as break and enters, during which a rape may occur (Revitch, 1978) and later manifest more obvious major sadistic behavior. In other cases, of course, the major sadism may have been present from the beginning but simply not disclosed or detected.

Major sadistic behavior includes "piqeurism" where the attacker stabs a female victim, usually in the buttocks or breast and then runs off (De River, 1958). The rare phenomenon of vampirism involves the letting of blood by cutting or biting, sometimes drinking it, accompanied by sexual arousal (Jaffe & DiCataldo, 1994). Some individuals will take their own blood for this purpose but, more importantly in the present context, vampirism is closely related to necrophilia and lust murder.

Necrophilia and Sadism

Although the term *necrophilia* appears to describe a fairly clear-cut sexual anomaly, like the term sexual sadism itself it has been used in a number of different ways by different authors including, some cases where there has been no contact with corpses at all, including "neurotic equivalents" of necrophilia based on material derived from psychoanalytic explorations of conscious and unconscious fantasy material (Calef & Weinshel, 1972).

Krafft-Ebing (1886) regarded necrophilia as a manifestation of sadism though Moll (1912) and Ellis (1936) observed that infliction of pain is not necessarily a feature. Krafft-Ebing was well aware of this and observed that, in some cases,

> When no other act of cruelty—cutting into pieces, etc.,—is practiced on the cadaver, it is probable that the lifeless condition itself, forms the stimulus for the perverse individual... the object of desire is seen to be capable of absolute subjugation, without possibility of resistance.

A strong fetishistic element is obvious in these cases (Ellis, 1936). Krafft-Ebing cited, from the original French literature, Bertrand, the Vampire of Paris, and Ardisson, the Vampire of Muy, as examples of these kinds of cases.

Like Krafft-Ebing, Hirschfeld (1956) divided necrophiliacs into those who violated a person who was already dead and those who sexually abused a person they had themselves murdered, "to possess and destroy her beyond death" (p. 425).

In an extensive review of previously reported and unreported cases Rosman and Resnick (1989) discriminated between "genuine" necrophilia, which fulfilled DSM-III-R criteria, from pseudonecrophilia. True to the formulae of the manual, they defined the former cases as those where during the preceding 6 months the individual reported recurrent, intense urges and sexually arousing fantasies involving corpses, which were either acted on or were markedly distressing. Conversely, "pseudonecrophilia" included "incidental" cases in which the subject had sex with the body without having had any preexisting fantasies of doing so, "necrophilic homicide" in which the murderer killed to obtain a body with which to engage in sexual activity, and "necrophilic fantasy" of activity with corpses without any actual activity with them.

Necrophilic behavior can vary from simply being in the presence of a corpse to kissing, fondling, performing sexual intercourse, or cunnilingus on the body (Hucker, 1990). In other cases, the behavior is even more grotesque and involves mutilation (Krafft-Ebing, 1886) or drinking the corpse's blood or urine (De River, 1958). Pseudo-necrophiles engage in mutilation and necrophagia (eating body parts) less commonly than genuine necrophiles (Rosman & Resnick, 1989).

Of particular concern are those who kill in order to obtain a body for subsequent violation and for whom the act of murder generates sexual frenzy (Brittain, 1970; Burgess, Hartman, Ressler, Douglas, &

McCormack, 1986). In an interesting anecdotal report (Smith & Braun, 1978, pp. 259–68) the subject needed to have complete control over his sexual partners and had them either simulate death or unconsciousness or strangled them himself. In the total sample collected by Rosman and Resnick (1989), 42% had committed homicide though these authors also note that sadism is not an intrinsic characteristic of true necrophilia.

Lust Murder and Sadistic Murder

Homicides in which the killer derives sexual pleasure from the act of killing are termed "lust murders" (Bartholomew, Milte, & Galbally, 1975, pp. 152–63) and sexual sadism generally appears to underlie the phenomenon (Brittain, 1970; Dietz et al., 1990; Ressler, Burgess, & Douglas, 1988). The killing itself may replace all other sexual activity (Podolsky, 1965).

Many authors have referred to Brittain's (1970) "profile" of the sadistic murderer though his observations have not been consistently supported (Langevin, Ben-Aron, Wright, Marchese, Handy, 1998). Brittain described the typical lust murderer as an overcontrolled, introverted, timid, and socially aloof individual who appeared to others as prudish and sanctimonious. Sexually inexperienced, though deeply deviant with vivid and violent sadistic fantasies, he is described as vain and egocentric but having a low self-esteem and his crimes enhance his feeling of superiority and power that he cannot otherwise attain. Grubin (1994) reported on 21 men who killed during a sexual attack and compared them with 121 rapists who did not kill their victims. Lifelong difficulties with heterosexual relationships and social isolation were typical of the sexual killers but Brittain's (1970) sadistic murderer profile was not more common among them.

MacCulloch and his colleagues (1983) also emphasized the importance of fantasy as a precursor to these offenses as have other workers (Burgess et al., 1986; Ressler et al., 1986; Prentky et al., 1985; Proulx, Blais, & Beauregard, 2005). Some offenders reveal their fantasies upon direct questioning whereas others reveal them indirectly in their drawings, writings, videotape collections, and libraries. It needs to be remembered that the kinds of imagery that appeals to sadists is not necessarily obviously pornographic to others. It has been noted that detective magazines, *Soldier of Fortune*, and similar publications may be preferred (Dietz, Harry, & Hazelwood, 1986, pp. 197–211).

The U.S. Federal Bureau of Investigation's Behavioral Science Unit has provided the material for some of the most detailed work on sexual sadists published so far, on the basis of their extensive, worldwide consultations (Dietz et al., 1990). Their 30 cases were all males, most were white, and almost half were married at the time of their crimes. Forty three percent had a history of homosexual experience, 20% crossdressed, and 20% had a history of other sexually anomalous behavior. Approximately half had parents with a history of marital infidelity or divorce. Twenty three percent reported they had been physically abused, and 205 reported that they had been sexually abused, as children. Half had had no previous criminal record and a number of them had a reputation in their communities as "solid citizens." Half tended to drive excessively with no clear goal and 30% were "police buffs" who collected police-related paraphernalia or modified their vehicles to resemble police cars. Most had carefully planned their offenses. Commonly they abducted their victims and held them captive for more than 24 hours, binding them up, blindfolding them, and gagging them. The typical activities were sexual bondage, rape, and forced fellatio though vaginal intercourse and insertion of foreign objects also occurred. All the victims were tortured and this characteristic was necessary for inclusion in the study and helped all subjects clearly fulfill DSM criteria. Seventy three percent of the victims were ultimately murdered. The subjects recorded their crimes in more than half the cases in diaries, audio- and videotapes, photographs, and drawings, and 40% kept mementoes of the victim. Dietz et al. (1990) also found that 50% had a history of drug abuse other than alcohol, and the group of Langevin et al. (1988) found that 75% abused nonmedical drugs and 50% were heavy drinkers.

Proulx et al. (2005) found that sadists were more likely than nonsadistic sexual offenders to have had a specific conflict with a woman during the 48 hours before the offense and to have had conflicts with women in general. They were also far angrier and sexually excited, and reported deviant sexual fantasies prior to their offenses. The sadists reported more often having planned their offense and deliberately selecting their victim than the nonsadistic offender controls.

Disturbed parentchild relationships and poor socialization are commonly noted (Dietz et al., 1990; Langevin, Ben-Aron, Wright, Marchese, & Handy,

1988) and 40% had antisocial personalities with a strong narcissistic element with a penchant for self-aggrandizement and media hunger (Brittain, 1970). Dietz et al. (1990) also highlighted the highly narcissistic personalities of these offenders. Proulx et al. (2005) also described personality features of their sexual sadists who, in comparison with a matched group of nonsadistic sexual offenders, showed more schizoid, schizotypal, histrionic, and avoidant personality features. Brittain (1970) observed an "effeminate tinge" in some sadistic murderers and Langevin et al. (1988) noted their strong tendency to crossdress and to experience gender dysphoria.

Dietz et al. (1990) reported that more than a third of their cases had an accomplice in their crimes. These partners are an interesting group as they illustrate the dominance of one individual over another. Hazelwood et al. (1993) reported on seven women who became involved with sexual sadists and who typically became subjected to a subtle process of seduction and transformation involving psychological, physical, and sexual abuse until they became "compliant appendages" of the sadistic man. In some cases the degree of compliance and time over which control was exerted were extraordinary. However, the extent of their apparent willingness to become involved in their partners' sadistic behavior has sometimes reflected on their own credibility during subsequent testimony against their former partners (e.g., Hill, 1995).

In a paper comparing the results of the FBI study with 29 sadistic and 28 nonsadistic sex offenders from their own facility, Gratzer and Bradford (1995) found a number of differences suggesting that the FBI-identified cases may not be representative of sexual sadists as a whole and constitute an extreme group. Indeed, as Marshall & Hucker (in press) point out comparison of several studies, including these and others done by Marshall in Canada (Marshall & Kennedy, 2003) show quite striking differences in certain respects suggesting, once again, that there are sometimes considerable differences in diagnostic practice that make comparison between studies somewhat confusing and perhaps less than meaningful.

There is some evidence of an occasional link between sexual murder and asphyxiophilia. Two men who practiced autoerotic asphyxia had also committed sexual murders or had fantasized committing a murder (Brittain, 1970; Hucker & Blanchard, 1992).

Sadistic Rape

It seems clear that rape is a multidetermined phenomenon and rapists do not constitute a homogeneous group (Marshall & Barbaree, 1990). It has been found that the degree of deviant sexual arousal, as determined by penile plethysmography, appears to be associated with the frequency and degree of violence in sexual assault (Abel, Barlow, Blanchard, & Guild, 1977; Becker, Blanchard, & Djenderedjian, 1978), suggesting that deviant arousal characterizes the most violent and habitual rapists. Moreover, as such people show a strong preference for sexually aggressive stimuli, it seems likely that they prefer such types of interaction that are sometimes referred to as the "preferential rape pattern" (Freund, Scher, & Hucker, 1983, 1984), "paraphilic coercive disorder" (Abel, 1989), or biastophilia" (Money, 1990). These men are sexually aroused by fantasies and urges of forcing themselves sexually on their victims.

While the preferential rapist is believed to not use greater force than is necessary to gain the victim's compliance, in contrast, the sexual sadist is aroused by the use of gratuitous violence (Abel, 1989), though the offender's estimate of how much force was required may, of course, be of dubious value. Preferential rape proneness may involve coercing the victim into fellatio or submitting to anal intercourse, behaviors typical of sexual sadists (Dietz et al., 1990). Also, targeting strangers occurs with both sadists and preferential rapists. That there may be an overlap between "courtship disorders" and sexual sadism is supported by the observation that, 9 out of 17 serial sexual murderers also showed evidence of voyeurism, telephone scatologia, or exhibitionism (Warren, Hazelwood & Dietz, 1996). However, "voyeurism" by such offenders may consist of prowling around in search of a victim to assault and, moreover, the simple dichotomy between sadistic and nonsadistic rape has not been supported by the researches of Knight and Prentky (1990, 1994).

Most researchers report that only 5% to 10% of their samples of rapists fulfill DSM criteria for sexual sadism (e.g., Abel et al., 1988) although some have reported figures much higher (Fedora, Reddon, Morrison, Fedora, Pascoe, & Yeudall, 1992; Hucker et al., 1988). It seems likely that these discrepancies reflect the fact that the subjects derived from very different populations, namely mental health versus correctional, although it is also likely that different researchers have used varying conceptualizations of sexual sadism despite apparent adherence to "official" criteria (see subsequent text for further discussion of this issue).

As a group, rapists show greater arousal to nonsexual violence than nonrapists (Barbaree, Marshall, & Lanthier, 1979; Quinsey, Lalumiere, & Seto, 1994; Seto & Kuban, 1996), and violent rapists tend to respond more strongly to depictions of sexual violence than do comparatively less violent rapists (Quinsey et al., 1994). However, the absolute value of these responses is, however, quite small. Moreover, rapists do not respond significantly more to nonviolence perpetrated by men against other men. These differential responses with respect to nonsexual violence between men and women appear to be due to implied sexual elements in the act, as opposed to an intrinsic response to aggression (Quinsey, Chaplin, & Upfold, 1984).

Complicating the matter further is the fact that 30% of "normal," noncriminal men admit to sexual fantasies of raping or tying up a woman (Crepault & Couture, 1980). In one study, 16% to 20% of those who did indicated they were highly aroused by sadomasochistic narratives (Malamuth, Haber, & Feshbach, 1980) and by those in which the victim is in pain (Malamuth & Check, 1983). Also, most young males appear to be aroused by depictions of women bound and in distress than by smiling, cooperative women (Heilbrun & Leif, 1988).

In another study, 45% of male college students stated that they would rape a woman if they would not be caught and 32% of women would enjoy being raped if no one were to know (Malamuth et al., 1980). Similar kinds of figures have been reported in a number of other studies (Malamuth & Malamuth, 1983; Malamuth, 1981; Koss, Gidycz, & Wisniewski, 1987). It appears that a degree of coercion in sexual relationships can lead to arousal and enjoyment in both sexes and plays a role in traditional courtship (Ellis, 1936). However, common though such themes may be in fantasy, such studies do not provide information on how frequently truly sadistic fantasies are acted upon or, more centrally, whether these themes represent the preferred method of sexual expression.

CURRENT ISSUES IN THE DIAGNOSIS OF SEXUAL SADISM

In a landmark review of studies of sexual sadism in sexual offenders Marshall and Kennedy (2003) found that although authors frequently indicated they had followed the criteria outlined in a relevant edition of the American Psychiatric Association's *Diagnostic and Statistical Manual of Mental Disorders* (DSM), the criteria that were actually used to identify the samples did not in fact correspond with DSM criteria. Several researchers (e.g., Brittain, 1970; Dietz, Hazelwood & Warren, 1990; Fromm, 1973; Gratzer & Bradford, 1995; Langevin, Ben-Aron, Wright, Marchese, & Handy, 1988; MacCulloch, Snowden, Wood, & Mills, 1983) regard the core feature of sexual sadism as the exercise of power and control over the victim, while other features (such as torture, humiliation, other forms of aggression) are seen as the means by which this end is achieved. Marshall and Kennedy also noted that some of these authors (e.g., Ressler, Burgess, & Douglas, 1988) also describe the expression of violence or aggression as the central feature of sexual sadism, as do Seto and Kuban, (1996), but, whatever characteristics are seen as diagnostic, sexual arousal by this feature is viewed as the necessary element.

The DSM-IV-TR (American Psychiatric Association, 2000) definition of sexual sadism requires the presence of "recurrent, intense sexually arousing fantasies, sexual urges, or behaviors involving acts (real, not simulated) in which the psychological or physical suffering (including humiliation) of the victim is sexually exciting to the person" (p. 574). Thus, the DSM requires that the psychological and physical suffering of the victim must be sexualized for the offender to meet criteria for sexual sadism. Unfortunately, this is a subjective feature that can only be confirmed by the offender. As few sexual offenders provide accurate self-reports, the clinician typically must infer this essential detail from other information such as details of the crime scene, reports by victims, the offender's life history, and the history of history. The DSM-III (American Psychiatric Association, 1980) acknowledged that the poor interdiagnostician reliability of earlier versions of DSM was the result of requiring diagnosticians to make inferences about a patient's motivations from unobservable processes. Consequently in DSM-III and subsequent editions, for almost all diagnoses except, regrettably, the paraphilias, it has been necessary to attempt to specify observable criteria.

Both from the point of view of research into the nature of sexual sadism and its characteristics, and in order to treat or manage the problems presented by sexually sadistic offenders, it is necessary to have a clear consensus definition of what constitutes sexual sadism. However, the DSM is intended to be the consensus document for researchers and clinicians attempting to study sexual sadism, as already noted. Marshall and Kennedy (2003) found that although almost all authors who claimed to adhere to DSM criteria, appeared not to do so in practice. Marshall and his colleagues then followed up their review of the literature with two studies to evaluate the reliability of the diagnosis of sexual sadism. Marshall et al. (2002) extracted from files in three Canadian federal prisons the psychiatric reports in which psychiatrists had conducted risk assessments of various types of sex offenders over a 10-year period. All of these sex offenders had previously identified as high risk to reoffend sexually using at least one actuarial risk assessment instrument. Fifty-nine evaluations were identified involving 41 cases where the offender was diagnosed as a sexual sadist ; the remaining 18 cases were given various other diagnoses. The 14 evaluators were all experienced forensic psychiatrists who reported using DSM-III-R or DSM-IV criteria. The offenders who were given a diagnosis of sexual sadism were compared with those who were not given this diagnosis on 20 offense characteristics extracted from extensive police and victim reports and from court records on the files, 10 sets of self-reported information, and 7 data sets derived from phallometric assessments of sexual interests. All this information was available to the psychiatrists performing the evaluations. It transpired that offenders who were not diagnosed as sexual sadists were significantly more likely to have beaten or tortured their victims than were those diagnosed as sexual sadists. Moreover, nonsadists showed greater sexual arousal to nonsexual violence and sadists displayed greater arousal to consenting sexual scenes. A composite sadism score was calculated from offense details but once again the nonsadists who scored higher than sadists. The only characteristic that predicted the psychiatrist's diagnosis was a prior psychiatric report giving that same diagnosis; none of the information provided by the researchers appeared to have any influence even when contradictory.

A subsequent study clearly showed that the findings of the earlier study cannot simply be dismissed as based on the idiosyncrasies of a small group of psychiatrists who were singled out by Marshall and his colleagues. Marshall et al. (2002) carefully extracted information from the files of 12 of the offenders in their first study, six of whom had been identified as being a sexual sadist while the other six had been given another diagnosis such as pedophilia or antisocial personality disorder. The information contained details of the offender's life history, crime scene details and other details of his offense(s), psychological and phallometric test results, and self-reported sexual interests and activities provided by the offenders themselves. All this information on each of the 12 offenders was provided to 15 internationally renowned forensic psychiatrists with experience, working with sexually sadistic offenders. These authorities were asked to complete several tasks, the most important of which was that they decide whether each offender was or was not a sexual sadist. Not only was the percent agreement among the experts quite low (75% agreement where chance agreement would be 53.3%), the *kappa* statistic revealed completely unsatisfactory interdiagnostician agreement (*kappa* = 0.14).

The two studies by Marshall et al. are not the only evidence of poor agreement between clinicians on the diagnosis of sexual sadism. Levenson (2004) assessed sex offenders for the application of a civil commitment as a Sexually Violent Predator (SVP) in Florida and compared the diagnoses identified by each of the two independent assessors. The resultant *kappa* coefficient for sexual sadism was only 0.3, again suggesting that clinicians cannot reach an acceptable standard of agreement on this diagnosis.

Despite this poor showing, most clinicians would argue that the studies indicate, as did the early studies of diagnostic disagreement over schizophrenia, a need to tighten up the criteria and exercise greater care in applying them. Also, the problem may lie in the DSM's requirement that the sadist must be sexually aroused by the suffering and humiliation of the victim. Since only the offender can know whether they were or were not so aroused, and their self-report is typically unreliable, the diagnosis requires the clinician to infer sexual motivation in the infliction of cruelty, torture, or degradation, thereby reducing diagnostic reliability.

Some authors have suggested that phallometric assessment can assist in increasing diagnostic reliability (Hollin, 1997; Hucker, 1997). However, a satisfactory stimulus set specifically for sadists has not yet been developed although several researchers have adapted available stimulus material for men who sexually assault adult females. Thus, Seto and Kuban (1996), used arousal to a description of a brutal rape as an index of sexual sadism. However, they found no differences between rapists they defined as *sadists* and *rapists* whom they determined were not sadists, a finding that replicated previous studies (Barbaree, Seto, Serin, Amos, & Preston, 1994; Langevin et al., 1985; Rice, Chaplin, Harris, & Coutts, 1994). Proulx, Blais, & Beauregard (in press) used a modification of their standard phallometric stimuli to include sets describing rapes that involved either extreme physical violence or had additional elements involving the humiliation of the victim. These stimulus sets are closer to the DSM criteria for sexual sadism than are any others currently available. Proulx et al. found that the sadistic rapists showed significantly greater arousal to both the physically violent and humiliating scenes than their nonsadistic rapists. These data suggest that specifically designed sadistic stimuli may reliably distinguish sadistic from nonsadistic sexual offenders. However, paradoxically, the sadists and nonsadists were differentiated as either sadistic or nonsadistic prior to the testing and yet the phallometric test was used to confirm or refute that diagnosis.

A PROPOSED SOLUTION

As an alternative to current diagnostic practices, Marshall & Hucker (in press) suggest that sexually sadistic behaviors may still usefully provide a basis for more accurately and more reliably identifying these problematic offenders. In the study by Marshall et al. (2002) where international experts were asked to identify sexual offenders as sadists or not, these experts were also asked to rate the importance for the diagnosis of sexual sadism of a variety of features of an offender's behavior. While the experts were not able to agree on the diagnosis, they nevertheless generally agreed on the features that are important in making the diagnosis.

Marshall & Hucker (submitted for publication) have developed a rating scale (see Table 24.1) derived from this study and based on the features weighted according to the values assigned by the experts in the Marshall et al. (2002) study. Inter-rater reliability studies are being conducted in several locations worldwide. It is hoped that this dimensional approach will prove more helpful than the categorical diagnosis has been and it is worth noting here that there have been other calls for the DSM to move to a more dimensional approach across all diagnoses (Widiger & Coker, 2003).

Treatment of sexual sadism is generally regarded as one of the most ominous paraphilias in terms of risk to potential victims. Consequently it is typically necessary to combine both psychological approaches and pharmacological treatments in order to minimize the possibility of a repeat offense.

Psychological approaches have been employed over the years with all types of sex offenders but met with little success until the advent of cognitive behavioral techniques. These have been demonstrated to have considerable effectiveness and form the mainstay of psychological treatments for sex offenders at the present time (Marshall, Anderson, & Fernandez, 1999). Much has been written on this topic and the specifics of the methodology are discussed elsewhere in this volume (see Chapter 9).

At this point in time, most medical specialists involved with treating sexual sadists, as well as other types of sex offenders, use a small range of pharmacological agents to suppress sexual drive as part of an overall treatment or management strategy in combination with cognitive therapy. These agents can be broadly grouped into hormonal agents and serotonergic drugs. Several authors have developed protocols for the use of these treatments (Reilly, Delva, & Hudson, 2000; Bradford, 2000). Bradford (2001), Briken, Nika, & Berner (2001), and Briken, Hill, & Berner (2003) have outlined algorithms to assist in the selection of the most appropriate medication based upon levels of severity of potential offenses. The use of serotonin reuptake inhibitors is recommended for the milder cases of sex offender or those with obsessive-compulsive features. Clearly, when sexual sadism is involved, the more potent hormonal agents such as leuprolide acetate, an LHRH agonist, will be required. Again this topic justifies extended coverage and is explored in more detail elsewhere in this book (see Chapters 9 and 14).

CONCLUSION

To this time, no research has demonstrated the effectiveness of treatment with sexual sadists although, as we have seen, there is evidence of their effectiveness with other sexual offenders. It will be difficult to evaluate treatment for these individuals because (fortunately) they constitute a small proportion of sexual offenders and thus there are rarely enough available to

TABLE 24.1 Rating Scale for Sexual Sadism

	Clearly Absent 1	Possibly Present 2	Present to Some Extent 3	Clearly Present 4	Clearly Dominant Feature 5
1. Offender is sexually aroused by sadistic acts					
2. Offender exercises power/control/domination over victim					
3. Offender humiliates or degrades the victim					
4. Offender tortures victim or engages in acts of cruelty on victim					
5. Offender mutilates sexual parts of victim's body					
6. Offender has history of choking consensual partners during sex					
7. Offender engages in gratuitous violence toward victim					
8. Offender has history of cruelty to other persons or animals					
9. Offender gratuitously wounds victim					
10. Offender attempts to, or succeeds in, strangling, choking, or otherwise asphyxiating victim					
11. Offender keeps trophies (e.g., hair, underwear, ID) of victim					
12. Offender keeps records (other than trophies) of offense					
13. Offender carefully preplans offense					
14. Offender mutilates nonsexual parts of victim's body					
15. Offender engages in bondage with consensual partners during sex					
16. Victim is abducted or confined					
17. Evidence of ritualism in offense					

From Marshall & Hucker, submitted.

justify an outcome study. In addition, quite a number of sexual sadists are incarcerated indefinitely, further reducing the number available for an outcome study.

References

Abel, G. G. (1989). Paraphilia. In H. Kaplan & B. Sadock (Eds.) *Comprehensive textbook of psychiatry* (Vol. 1, 5th Edition, pp. 1069–1085), Baltimore: Williams & Wilkins.

Abel, G., Barlow, D., Blanchard, E., & Guild, D. (1977). The components of rapists' sexual arousal. *Archives of General Psychiatry, 34,* 895–903.

Abel, G. G., Becker, J., Cunningham-Rathner, J., Mittelman, M., & Rouleau, J. (1988). Multiple paraphilic diagnoses among sex offenders. *Bulletin of the American Academy of Psychiatry & Law, 16,* 153–168.

Abel, G., Becker, J., Blanchard, E., & Djenderedjian, A. (1978). Differentiating sexual aggressives with penile measures. *Criminal Justice & Behavior, 5,* 315–322.

American Psychiatric Association. (1980). *Diagnostic and statistical manual of mental disorders, 3rd Edition.* Washington, D. C.: Author.

American Psychiatric Association. (2000). *Diagnostic and statistical manual of mental disorder,* 4th edition. Text revision. Washington, DC: Author.

Arndt, W., Foehl, J., & Good, F. (1985). Specific sexual fantasy themes: A multidimensional study. *Journal of Personality & Social Psychology, 48,* 472–480.

Barabaree, H., Marshall, W., & Lanthier, R. (1979). Deviant sexual arousal in rapists. *Behavior Research and Therapy, 17,* 215–222.

Barbaree, H. E., Seto, M. C., Serin, R. C., Amos, N. L., & Preston, D. L. (1994). Comparisons between sexual and nonsexual subtypes: Sexual arousal to rape, offense precursors, and offense characteristics. *Criminal Justice and Behavior*, 21, 94–114.

Bartholomew, A. A., Milte, K., & Galbally, A. (1975). Sexual murder: Psychopathology and psychiatric jurisprudential considerations. *Australia and New Zealand Journal of Criminology*, 8, 152–63.

Berner, W., Berger, P., & Hill, A. (2003). Sexual sadism. *International Journal of Offender Therapy & Comparative Criminology*, 47, 383–395.

Bradford, J. M. W. (2000). The treatment of sexual deviation using a pharmacological approach. *Journal of Sex Research*, 37, 248–257.

Bradford, J. M. W. (2001). The neurobiology, neuropharmacology, and pharmacological treatment of paraphilias and compulsive sexual behaviour. *Canadian Journal of Psychiatry*, 46, 26–34.

Breslow, N., Evans, L., & Langley, J. (1985). On the prevalence and roles of females in the sadomasochistic subculture: Report of an empirical study. *Archives of Sexual Behavior*, 14.4, 303–317.

Briken, P., Hill, A., & Berner, W. (2003). Pharmacotherapy of paraphilias with long-acting agonists of luteinizing hormone-releasing hormone: A systematic review. *Journal of Clinical Psychiatry*, 64, 890–897.

Brittain, R. (1970). The sadistic murderer. *Medicine, Science, and the Law*, 10, 198–207.

Burgess, A. W., Hartman, C. R., Ressler, R. K., Douglas, J. E., & McCormack, A. (1986). Sexual homicide: A motivational model. *Journal of Interpersonal Violence*, 1, 251–272.

Calef, V. & Weinshel, E. M. (1972). On certain neurotic equivalents of necrophilia. *International Journal of Psychoanalysis*, 53, 67–75.

Crepault, E. & Couture, M. (1980) Men's erotic fantasies. *Archives of Sexual Behavior*, 9, 565–581.

De River, P. (1958). Crime and the sexual psychopath. Springfield, Illinois: C.C. Thomas.

Dietz, P. & Evans, B. (1982). Pornographic imagery and prevalence of paraphilia. *American Journal of Psychiatry*, 139, 1493–1495.

Dietz, P. E., Harry, B., & Hazelwood, R. R. (1986). Detective magazines: Pornography for the sexual sadist? *Journal of Forensic Sciences*, 31.1, 197–211.

Dietz, P. E., Hazelwood, R. R., & Warren, J. (1990). The sexually sadistic criminal and his offenses. *Bulleting of the American Academy of Psychiatry and the Law*, 18, 163–178.

Ellis, H. (1936). *Studies in the psychology of sex*, (Vol. II). New York: Random House.

Eulenberg, A. von. (1911/1984). *Sadism and masochism*. New York: Bell.

Fedora, O., Reddon, J.R., Morrison, J., Fedora, S., Pascoe, H., & Yeudall, L. Sadism and other paraphilias in normal controls and aggressive and non-aggressive sex offenders. *Archives of Sexual Behavior*, 21, 1–15.

Freund, K., Scher, H., & Hucker, S. (1983). The courtship disorders. *Archives of Sexual Behavior*, 12, 369–379.

Freund, K., Scher, H., & Hucker, S. (1984). The courtship disorders: A further investigation. *Archives of Sexual Behavior*, 13, 133–139.

Freund, K., Seto, M., & Kuban, M. (1985). Masochism: A multiple case study. *Sexuologie*, 4(2), 313–324.

Freund, K., Scher, H., & Hucker, S. (1983). The courtship disorders. *Archives of Sexual Behavior*, 12, 369–379.

Freund, K., Scher, H., & Hucker, S., (1984). The courtship disorders: A further investigation. *Archives of sexual behavior*, 13, 133–139.

Fromm, E. (1973). *The anatomy of human destructiveness*. New York, NY: Holt.

Gosselin, C. C. (1987). The sado-masochistic contract. In G. D. Wilson (Ed.), *Variant sexuality: Research & theory* (pp. 229–257) Baltimore: Johns Hopkins University press.

Gosselin, C. C. & Wilson, G. D (1980). *Sexual variations*. London: Faber & Faber.

Gratzer, T. & Bradford, J. M. W. (1995). Offender and offense characteristics of sexual sadists: A comparative study. *Journal of Forensic Sciences*, 40, 450–455.

Grubin, D. (1994). Sexual murder. *British Journal of Psychiatry*, 165, 524–629.

Hazelwood, R., Warren, J., & Dietz, P., (1993). Compliant victims of the sexual sadist. *FBI Law Enforcement Bulletin*, 61, 12–20.

Heilbrun, A. & Leif, D. (1988). Autoerotic value of female distress in sexual explicit photographs. *Journal of Sex Research*, 24, 47–57.

Hill, B. (1995). *Double jeopardy*. New York, NY: William Morrow.

Hirschfeld, M. (1956). *Sexual anomalies*. New York, NY: Emerson.

Hucker, S. J. (1990). Necrophilia and other unusual philias. In R. Bluglass & P. Bowden (Eds.), *Principles and practice of forensic psychiatry* (pp. 723–728). London: Churchill Livingstone.

Hucker, S. J. & Blanchard, R. (1992). Death scene characteristics in 118 fatal cases of autoerotic asphyxia compared with suicidal asphyxia. *Behavioral sciences and the law*, 10, 509–523.

Hucker, S., Langevin, R., Wortzman, G., Dickey, R., Bain, J., Handy, L., Chambers, J., & Wright, P. (1988). Cerebral damage and dysfunction in sexually aggressive men. *Annals of Sex Research*, 1, 33–47.

Jaffe, P. & DeCataldo, F. (1994). Clinical vampirism: Blending myth and reality. *Bulletin of the American Academy of Psychiatry & the Law*, 22, 533–544.

Karpmann, B. (1954). The sex offender and his offenses. New York, NY: Julian Press.

Kernberg, O. (1970). A psychoanalytic classification of character pathology. *Journal of the American Psychoanalytic Association*, 18, 800–822.

Kinsey, A.C., Pomerory, W.B., Gebhard, P. H. (1953). *Sexual Behavior in the Human Female*. Philadelphia: W.B. Saunders.

Knight, R. & Prentky, R. (1990). Classifying sexual offenders: The development and corroboration of taxonomic models. In Marshal, W., Laws, R., & Barbaree, H. (Eds.), Handbook of sexual assault: Issues, theories, and treatment of the offender, (pp. 23–52). New York: Plenum Press.

Knight, R., Prenntky, R., & Cerce, D. (1994). The development, reliability, and validity, of an inventory for the multidimentional assessment of sex and aggression. Criminal Justice & Behavior, 21/1, 72–94.

Koss, M., Gidycz, C. & Wisniewski, N. (1987). The scope of rape: Incidence and prevalence of sexual aggression in a national sample of higher education students. Journal of Consulting and Clinical Psychology, 55, 162–170.

Krafft-Ebing, R. von (1886). Psychopathia sexualis. Philadelphia, FA: Davis.

Langevin, R., Bain, J., Ben-Aron, M. H., Coulthard, R., Day, D., Handy, L., et al. (1985). Sexual aggression: Constructing a predictive equation: A controlled pilot study. In R. Langevin (Ed.), Erotic preference, gender identity, and aggression in men: New research studies, (pp. 39–76). Hillsdale, NJ: Lawrence Erlbaum.

Langevin, R., Ben-Aron, M. H., Wright, P., Marchese, V., & Handy, L. (1988). The sex killer. Annals of Sex Research, 1, 263–301.

Levenson, J. S. (2004). Reliability of sexually violent predator civil commitment criteria. Law & Human Behavior, 28, 357–368.

MacCulloch, M., Snowden, P, Wood, P. & Mills, H. (1983). Sadistic fantasy, sadistic behaviour, and offending. British Journal of Psychiatry, 143, 20–29.

Malamuth, N.M., Rape Proclivity Among Males. Journal of Social Issues (1981), 37/4, 138–157.

Malamuth, N. & Check, J. (1983). Sexual arousal to rape depictions: Individual differences. Journal of Abnormal Psychology, 92, 55–67.

Malamuth, N., Haber, S., & Feshbach, S. (1980). Testing hypotheses regarding rape: Exposure to sexual violence, sex differences, and the normality of rapists. Journal of Research on Personality, 14, 121–137.

Malamuth, N., Heim, M., & Feshbach, S. (1980). Sexual responsiveness of college students to rape depictions: Inhibitory and disinhibitory effects. Journal of Personality and Social Psychology, 38, 399–408.

Marshall, W. L., Anderson, D., & Fernandez, Y. M. (1999). Cognitive behavioural treatment of sexual offenders. Chichester, UK: John Wiley & Sons.

Marshall, W. & Barbaree, H. (1990). An integrated theory of the etiology of sex offending. In : Marshall, W., Laws, R., & Barbaree, H. (Eds.) Handbook of sexual assault: Issues, theories and treatments of the offender. New York: Plenum.

Marshall, W. & Hucker, S. (2006). Issues in the diagnosis of sexual sadism. Sexual Offender Treatment, 1(2), Available at www.sexual-offender-treatment.org

Marshall, W. L. & Kennedy, P. (2003). Sexual sadism in sexual offenders: An elusive diagnosis. Aggression and Violent Behavior: A Review Journal, 8, 1–22.

Marshall, W. L., Kennedy, P., & Yates, P. (2002). Issues concerning the reliability and validity of the diagnosis of sexual sadism applied in prison settings. Sexual Abuse: A Journal of Research and Treatment, 14, 310–311.

Marshall, W. L., Kennedy, P., Yates, P., & Serran, G. A. (2002). Diagnosing sexual sadism in sexual offenders: Rehability across diagnosticians. International Journal of Offender Therapy and Comparative Criminology, 46, 668–676.

Moll, A. (1912). Handbuch de sexual wissenschaften. Leipzig: Vogel.

Money, J. (1990). Forensic sexology: Paraphilic serial rape (biastophilia) and lust murder (erotophonophilia), American Journal of Psychotherapy, 44, 1, 26–36.

Myers, W. C., Burgess, A. W., Burgess, A. G., & Douglas, J. E (1999). Serial murder and homicide. In V. Van Hasselt & M. E. Hersen (Eds.), Handbook of psychological approaches with violent offenders (pp. 153–172). New York, NY: Kluwer Academic/Plenum Publishers.

Oosterhuis, H. (2000). Stepchildren of nature: Krafft-Ebing, psychiatry, and the making of sexual identity. Chicago & London: University of Chicago Press.

Podolsky, E. (1965). The lust murderer. Medico-legal journal, 33, 174–178.

Prentky, R.A., Cohen, M.L., & Seghorn, T.K., (1985). Development of a rational taxonomy for the classification of sex offenders: Rapists. Bulletin of the American Academy of Psychiatry & the Law, 13, 39–70.

Proulx, J., Blais, E., & Beauregard, E. (2005). Sadistic sexual aggressors. In W. L. Marshall, Y. M. Fernandez, L. E. Marshall, & G. A. Serran (Eds.), Sexual offender treatment: Controversial issues (pp. 61–77). Chichester, UK: John Wiley & Sons.

Quinsey, V., Lalumière, M., & Seto, M. (1994). The current status of phallometric assessment. Violence Update, 4, 1–2, 4.

Quinsey, V., Chaplin, T., & Upfold, D. (1984). Sexual arousal to nonsexual violence and sadomasochistic themes among rapists and non-sex offenders. Journal of Consulting and Clinical Psychology, 52, 651–657.

Reilly, D., Delva, N., & Hudson, R. W. (2000). Protocols for the use of cyproterone, medroxyprogesterone and leuprolide in the treatment of paraphilia. Canadian Journal of Psychiatry, 45, 559–563.

Ressler, R. K., Burgess, A. W., & Douglas, J. E. (1988). Sexual homicide: Patterns and motives. New York, NY: Free Press.

Revitch, E. (1978). Sexually motivated burglaries. Bulletin of the American Academy of Psychiatry & the Law, 6, 277–283.

Rice, M. E., Chaplin, T. C., Harris, G. T., & Coutts, J. (1994). Empathy for the victim and sexual arousal among rapists and nonrapists. Journal of Interpersonal Violence, 9, 435–449.

Rosman, J. & Resnick, P. (1989). Necrophilia: An analysis of 122 cases involving necrophilic acts and fantasies. *Bulletin of the American Acvademy of Psychiatry & the Law*, 17(2), 153–163.

Schad-Somers, S. P. (1982). *Sadomasochism: Etiology and treatment*. New York: Human Sciences Press.

Schrenck-Notzing, A. von. (1895/1956). *The Use of Hypnosis in Psychopathia Sexualis*. New York: Julian Press.

Seto, M. C. & Kuban, M. (1996). Criterion-related validity of a phallometric test for paraphilic rape and sadism. *Behaviour Research and Therapy*, 34, 175–183.

Smith, S. M. & Braun, C. (1978). Necrophilia and lust murder: Report of a rare occurrence. *The Bulletin of the American Academy of Psychiatry and the Law*, 6.3, 259–268.

Spengler, A. (1977). Manifest sadomasochism in males: Results of an empirical study. *Archives of Sexual Behavior*, 6, 441–456.

Stekel, W. (1929). *Sadism and masochism: The psychology of hatred and cruelty* (Translation by L. Brink). New York: Horace Liveright.

Warren, J., Hazelwood, R., & Dietz, P. (1996). The sexually sadistic serial killer. *Journal of Forensic Sciences*, 41/6, 970–976.

Weinberg, T.S. (1987). Sadomasochism in the United States: A review of recent sociological literature. *Journal of Sex Research*, 23, 50–69.

Widiger, T. A. & Coker, L. A. (2003). Mental disorders as discrete clinical conditions: Dimensional versus categorical classification. In M. Hersen & S. M. Turner (Eds.), *Adult psychopathology and diagnosis* (4th edition. pp. 3–35). New York, NY: John Wiley & Sons.

World Health Organisation. (1992). *The ICD-10 Classification of Mental and Behavioural Disorders*: Clinical Descriptions and diagnostic guidelines. Geneva: World Health Organisation.

Chapter 25

Persons with Intellectual Disabilities Who Sexually Offend

Dorothy Griffiths and J. Paul Fedoroff

Persons with intellectual disabilities present many similar and some unique features that can contribute to the development of sexually offending behavior. This chapter will review: the history of sexuality of persons with intellectual disabilities, the prevalence of sexually offending behavior, methods of comprehensive assessment strategies to identify risk factors, vulnerabilities and central processing challenges, and methods to develop an integrated model of intervention.

While cognitive impairment can be caused by dementia, this chapter will deal only with global intellectual impairment secondary to intellectual disabilities present at birth or with pervasive developmental delay. Neither the criteria for sexual offense under the criminal code nor the diagnostic criteria for paraphilic sexual disorders currently explicitly include provisions for individuals with intellectual disabilities. Yet this group poses special challenges not only to the judicial system but also to those with the responsibility of providing for their care. There

are several reasons for this that will be expanded subsequently.

First, the criminal justice system requires that the accused understand the charges, the trial process, the consequences of being found guilty and that the accused be able to assist counsel in their own defense. By definition, accused with intellectual disabilities as a group are less likely to meet criteria for fitness to stand trial. However, intellectual disability by itself does not necessarily mean that a specific individual is unfit to stand trial.

Second, individuals with intellectual disability often live with less than normal degrees of privacy. They may have been raised and reside in group homes or even institutions. As a result, unconventional sexual behaviors are more likely to be detected.

Third, intellectual disability can manifest not only in academic deficiency but also, particularly in developmental delay syndromes like Asperger's disorder, in profound social skills impairment. Impairment in the development of normal social relations makes the expression of abnormal social relations more likely.

Intellectual disability, whatever its cause, often alters the presentation of comorbid medical and psychiatric disorders. Similarly, the presence of sexual problems often clouds the ability of care providers to evaluate complete differential diagnoses and treatment plans. The presence of an intellectual disability enlarges the differential diagnosis. The same is true for individuals who display unconventional sexual interests. Unfortunately, once a person has been diagnosed with intellectual disability or a sexual disorder, there is a tendency to attribute the cause of all problems to the intellectual disability or sexual disorder.

Embryologists often comment that ontogeny recapitulates phylogeny. By analogy, the perils and pitfalls faced by care providers of sex offenders with intellectual disabilities can be best understood by reviewing the perils and pitfalls that these men and women have historically faced themselves.

SOME HISTORICAL CONTEXT FOR UNDERSTANDING SEXUALITY OF PERSONS WITH INTELLECTUAL DISABILITIES

The sexuality of persons with intellectual disabilities largely led the direction of the field in the early part of the last century. Beliefs regarding the increased risk of sexual interest, promiscuity, impulsivity, and risk to children among the population of persons with disabilities fueled public policy. Early in the last century people with intellectual disabilities were considered to be sexually dangerous to society (Simmons, 1982). The agenda to control the sexuality of persons with disabilities was not promulgated solely on the concern to protect innocent individuals from sexual indiscretion or for moral reasons, but to control the potential sexual "by-products." The reproduction of a second generation of persons with genetic deficits was seen as a drain on society's resources. This social policy movement, known as Eugenics, resulted in large-scale identification, isolation, and segregation of persons with intellectual disabilities within Western society. Institutions were constructed to allow social control over the threat of future generations of persons with disabilities. Gender segregation, punishment of sexually active participants, and mass involuntary sterilization was enforced within institutions. These practices, subsumed under the rubric of "eugenics" were so well established in North America that they were studied and emulated by Hitler and the infamous Nazi regime. Although mass forced sterilization was discontinued in the 1970s, many of the premises of the eugenics movement continue to influence policy today. Although many individuals with disabilities now live in community care, they are still often denied routine sex education and their access to appropriate, loving relationships is often discouraged, restricted and even punished in both institutional and community settings.

Although sexual aggression by all persons, including those with developmental disabilities, is a significant concern in our society, it is erroneous to consider sexual aggression by persons with developmental disabilities as a direct product of the disability. The relationship between sexual aggression and persons with developmental disabilities has historically been grounded in myth. One of the most prevalent myths is the "eternal child" myth that states that mental age is a predictor of all aspects of the person's life rather than a description of functioning on a test of cognitive abilities. This results in people with disabilities being seen as children (Simmons, 1982) and as such their sexuality is ignored. A second yet contradictory myth is founded on the "dangerousness theory" of persons with disabilities and their sexuality. The "dangerousness" myth stems back to a very flawed study done at the beginning of the last century by Goddard (1912) who claimed to demonstrate that persons with intellectual disabilities were genetically linked to criminality, degeneracy, mental illness, and future generations of socially undesired offspring.

In fact, most people with intellectual disabilities, with the exception of those with certain genetic or endocrine abnormalities, develop secondary sexual characteristics at about the same rate as nondisabled people and the majority of disabling conditions are not genetic (Griffiths, 2003). For the most part they experience sexual feelings and respond sexually to the same stimuli as nondisabled persons do. They have the same variability in sex drive as others.

Like nondisabled people, persons with intellectual disabilities require normalized environments in which to be educated and experience social learning regarding personal, moral, social, and legal responsibility regarding sexuality. Individuals with disabilities also benefit from formal sociosexual education to gain sociosexual knowledge (Watson, Griffiths,

Richards, & Dykstra, 2003) and guidance necessary to learn responsibility about sexuality. It is also vital to learn appropriate sexual expression, and to reduce the vulnerability to abuse or be abused (Hard, 1986 as cited in Roeher Institute, 1988).

Moreover, there is no conclusive evidence that people with intellectual disabilities develop sexually inappropriate behavior more frequently than the general population if they have normal opportunities to learn about their sexuality. In fact, it may be less common than among people who are nondisabled (Day, 1994). As with nondisabled individuals, the development of sexually inappropriate behavior in persons with intellectual disabilities can be affected by many factors including lack of sexual education, deprivation of peer group interactions, family restrictions on activities, lack of social exposure, and even lack of motor coordination. The offenses committed by people with developmental disabilities are often less serious than offenses committed by nondisabled people (e.g., public exposure, masturbating in public, inappropriate touch).

PREVALENCE OF SEXUALLY OFFENDING BEHAVIOR AMONG THIS POPULATION

One other potentially misleading set of research regarding this population is based on prison statistics regarding sex offenders. Sex offenders with identified intellectual disabilities appear overrepresented in the charged and imprisoned population of sexual offenders. There is a great disparity in the reported incidence of sexually offending behavior of persons with intellectual disabilities; statistics range from 15% to 33% (Shapiro, 1986; Steiner, 1984). Day (1994) cautions that the prevalence rate may actually be higher because it does not account for those persons with intellectual disabilities who were not charged but diverted to residential care facilities. These rates appear alarming in relation to the 3% incidence of intellectual disability that exists in the general population until it is realized that the data were largely gathered from arrest and conviction rates.

There are two hypotheses that put perspective on the aforementioned statistics. First, overrepresentation of persons with disabilities within the offender population may not indicate a greater incidence of offense but an increased vulnerability

when persons with intellectual disabilities are within the judicial system. Second, because of the learning and environmental conditions posed to most persons with intellectual disabilities regarding their sexual life, many individuals may be deemed sexually inappropriate by virtue of their label or because of a lack of appropriate sociosexual conditions. Day (1997) argues that the high rates of sexual offense behavior committed by persons with developmental disabilities may be a reflection of the generally repressive and restrictive attitudes toward the sexuality of persons with disabilities (Day, 1997). Each of these hypotheses will be elaborated in the following sections.

Persons with intellectual disabilities and the judicial system: Griffiths et al. (2002) note that from arrest to trial, offenders who have cognitive disabilities are more likely to be disadvantaged. They are more likely to be arrested or waive their rights due to impaired understanding of caution and legal rights. To gain approval of authority figures they may false confessions or provide incriminating evidence, and fail to plea-bargain. They are also more likely to be jailed pretrial because of failure to meet bail or personal recognizance; offenders held pretrial are generally more likely to be convicted (Toberg, 1992). They are less likely to be able to afford or mount a solid legal defense and are more likely to be declared unfit to stand trial (Valenti-Heins & Schwartz, 1993) or convicted. In general their prison terms are longer than similar offenders without disabilities (Laski, 1992). However, if found unable to stand trial they are virtually denied due process in court, and typically institutionalized, presumably for rehabilitation or habilitation. The unfortunate outcome, however, is that often such services are not available and the individual ends up being confined for an indefinite period of time, without a process of redress (Fedoroff, Griffiths, Richards, & Marini, 2000).

Prevalence of sexually deviant versus inappropriate behavior caused by social conditions and learning: The full range of deviant sexual behavior (i.e., fetishes to pedophilia) similar to that of the nondisabled population have been noted in the population of persons with intellectual disabilities (Griffiths et al., 2007). The profile presented by this offender group is similar to that of nondisabled offenders (Day, 1997), with some exceptions. In general, sexual offenders with intellectual disabilities

- commit the same range of crime, including those of a sexual nature, as nondisabled persons (Luckasson, 1992). However, they are more likely to be the victims of sexual crime rather than victimizers (Griffiths, 2003);
- commit less serious assault offenses, but more inappropriate behaviors such as public masturbation, exhibitionism, and voyeurism (Gilby, Wolf, & Goldberg, 1989);
- have far fewer victims (Griffiths, Quinsey, & Hingsburger, 1989);
- have larger proportion of male victims, than the nondisabled population. The research varies as to whether the majority of their victims are female (Brown & Stein, 1997; Gilby et al., 1989; Murrey, Briggs, & Davis, 1992) or equivalent against males and females (Brown & Stein, 1997; Day, 1994; Griffiths, Hingsburger, & Christian, 1985; Griffiths et al., 1989);
- display more social skill deficits, are more sexually naive, lack interpersonal skills; and
- demonstrate increased difficulty interacting with the opposite sex (Tudiver, Broekstra, Josselyn, & Barbaree, 1997).

Day (1994) has proposed that there are two types of sexual offenders with intellectual disabilities. The first group commits only sexual offenses; this is a lower risk group that fits the aforementioned profile more closely. The second group presents with greater risk for violence and assault and commits not only sexual offenses but also a range of nonsexual offensive behaviors. This distinction represents a critical feature in this population.

The sexual offenders with intellectual disabilities who commit only sexual offenses present with a different profile and the nature of their offenses are typically less serious or persistent (Day, 1994). It may be argued that this group represents those described in the *Diagnostic and statistic manual of mental disorders* (4th Edition) (DSM-IV-TR) as those showing challenges in judgment, social skills, or impulse control that might result in sexual behavior that may be unusual but is diagnostically different than paraphilia (American Psychiatric Association [APA], 2000). Langevin & Curnoe (2003) suggest that sexual offense committed by persons with intellectual disabilities may not be a matter of paraphilia but of loneliness, lack of social skills, or even curiosity. Among persons with intellectual disabilities there is a higher experience of abuse (Griffiths et al., 1989; Gilby et al., 1989), poor self-esteem (Lackey & Knopp,

1989), lack of sociosexual knowledge and experience (Hingsburger, 1987), and poor social problem-solving skills (Hingsburger, 1987). All of the above may contribute to a false or counterfeit diagnosis of paraphilia. The latter, often referred to as counterfeit deviance, can be differentiated from paraphilia as these acts do not represent a person's preferred and recurring sexual behavior (APA, 2000).

"Counterfeit deviance" was illustrated in a series of case examples by Hingsburger et al. (1991), in which the sexually offensive behavior of persons with intellectual disabilities was the product of experiential, environmental, or medical factors, rather than a paraphilia. They demonstrated how lack of privacy (structural), modeling, inappropriate partner selection or courtship, lack of sexual knowledge or moral training, or a maladaptive learning history or medical or medication effects could present as paraphilia in this population (Hingsburger, Griffiths, & Quinsey, 1991).

The subgroup of offenders described previously differs significantly in profile from the subgroup of sexual offenders with intellectually disabled, who are at high risk of violence and reoffense. The latter group more closely resembles the nondisabled sexual offender. Day (1994) profiled this group as having a high incidence of sociopathic personality disorder, brain damage, family dysfunction, and who also engage in other nonsexual inappropriate behaviors. Day further found they had lengthy histories of antisocial behavior, were undersocialized, demonstrated poor impulse control, and were likely to commit serious sexual offenses. These high-risk sex offenders who are intellectually disabled have also been found to become more persistent sex offenders, and the nature of their crimes are more serious (Day, 1994). Day (1994) noted that the younger the age at first sexual offense and at first conviction, the more likely the individual would fall into this more serious group of offenders who are less sexually naïve and more specific and persistent in their sexual offenses.

Comprehensive clinical evaluation of the complex factors that could be influencing sexual aggression in persons with intellectual disabilities is required to distinguish paraphilia from sexually inappropriate behavior that may topographically look like paraphilia but lack the pathognomonic recurring and pathological use of sexual fantasies, urges or behavior. "A careful differential diagnosis, based on evaluation of the individual's environment, socio-sexual knowledge and attitudes, learning experiences, partner selection, courtship skills, and biomedical influences is required to differentiate paraphilia from counterfeit deviance" (Griffiths et al. 2007). The diagnostic distinction is important as it determines the nature of intervention.

CHALLENGES TO CLINICAL ASSESSMENT AND INTERVENTION (RISK FACTORS, VULNERABILITIES, AND CENTRAL PROCESSING CHALLENGES)

Griffiths (2002) summarized research from both the field of disability and the field of sex offender to illustrate the potential relationship between known risk factors for development of sexual offending behavior and the life experiences that have afforded most people with intellectual disabilities by virtue of nature or nurture.

Sex offender research shows an increased risk for sexual offense associated with certain neurological/biomedical abnormalities, mental illness, lack of attachment bonds, childhood sexual trauma, and a lack of empathy, skills and prosocial inhibition. These biomedical, psychological, and social risk factors or vulnerabilities are described in Table 25.1 with special reference to the increased vulnerabilities of persons with intellectual disabilities.

COMPREHENSIVE ASSESSMENT

Guidelines for the assessment and treatment of sex offenders generally have been developed by two organizations, the Association for the Treatment of Sexual Abusers (ATSA) and the International Association for the Treatment of Sexual Offenders (IATSO, Coleman et al., 1995). Neither organization has specifically addressed the issue of assessment and treatment of sexual offenders who are intellectually disabled (Langevin & Curnoe, 2002). While these guidelines are applicable to this population, there are some additional considerations. A careful differential diagnosis is based on evaluation of the relevant history, mental status examination, the context of the behavior, sociosexual knowledge and attitudes, partner preference and selection, and general risk.

Concern for Consent

There are two relevant areas of consent for consideration. Consent relative to assessing and determining consent issues involved in the events that prompted the assessment. Although these will be discussed briefly subsequently for expansion on these topics refer to Fedoroff et al. (2002) and Sheehan (2002) respectively.

First, the clinician needs to determine before proceeding to conduct an assessment if informed consent has been obtained to proceed, to gather background information, to speak with other parties, and in some cases to perform assessments such as phallometry or risk evaluations. There are some guiding questions that can aid the clinician in determining consent issues.

What is the benefit of the assessment for the person? If the assessment is to direct intervention or support, then the benefit for the individual appears clear. However, sometimes the assessment is requested for legal purposes, where the assessment may not only be not beneficial but damaging to the individual. Additionally the limits to confidentiality must be clearly discussed (Fedoroff et al., 2002).

Determining if the consent is informed differs depending on whether the person with intellectual disabilities is capable/competent to provide his/her own consent, or if substitute consent is required because of age or competency. Individuals with intellectual disabilities may feel undue pressure to agree to the assessment and to be reluctant to disappoint or anger staff or the clinician by refusing to participate. Persons with intellectual disabilities have been found to agree to persons in authority beyond the point where nondisabled persons would have begun resistance (Flynn, Reeves, Whelan, & Speake, 1985). Their history may have included formal or informal compliance training to authority figures that predispose concerns regarding compliance versus consent. Additionally, the learning challenges of persons with intellectual disabilities cause concern as to whether the consent is truly "informed." However, persons with intellectual disabilities are not ipso facto incompetent to make their own decisions or to provide informed consent for various treatments, activities, or personal/financial events. Legal incompetence based on intelligence is not absolute; a person may be legally incompetent to manage their finances but totally competent to make decisions within other areas.

TABLE 25.1 Biopsychosocial Risk Factors and Vulnerabilities Associated with Paraphilia Specific to Persons with Intellectual Disabilities

Risk Factors And Vulnerabilities	Association With Paraphilia	Risk Factors Specific To Persons With Intellectual Disabilities
Neurological/ Biomedical Abnormality	40% of sex offenders demonstrate neurological impairments (Hucker, Langevin, Wortzman, Bain, Handy, Cambers, & Wright, 1986; Hucker, Langevin & Bain, 1988); the nature of the sexual offense may correlate to the type of brain abnormality or endocrine disorder (Langevin, 1992). (i.e., sexually offensive behavior is frequently associated with temporal lobe abnormalities (Cummings, 1985; Hucker, Langevin, Dickey, Hardy, Chambers & Wright, 1986), with pedophiles and rapists being more likely to have left temporal dilation, whereas sadistic offenses are correlated with right temporal dilation (Langevin, Wortzman, Wright, & Hardy, 1988). The correlations although statistically significant are not perfect. In addition, endocrine disorders were apparent in 10% of sexual assault cases (Langevin, 1992), and most evident in cases involving pedophilia. Gaffney and Berlin (1984) demonstrated that pedophiles show hypersecretion of luteinizing hormone.	There is an overrepresentation of learning disability among persons who engage in exhibitionism and a greater likelihood of language-related problems, aphasia, and object identification problems in the pedophilia subgroup of offenders (Langevin, 1992). Among the offender group, pedophiles show the greatest cognitive challenge.
Mental Illness	Langevin (1992) has observed that one in ten cases of sexual offense involved a major mental illness. The DSM-IV-TR indicates that unusual sexual behavior may result from a manic episode, schizophrenia, or dementia (APA, 2000).	Twenty percent to thirty five percent of persons with intellectual disabilities will have a coexisting mental health problem (Nezu, Nezu, & Gill-Weiss, 1992), and among developmentally handicapped offenders this could be as high as 3047% (Steiner, 1984; White & Wood, 1988).
Lack of Attachment Bonds	Marshall et al. (1993) demonstrated a relationship between attachment bonds and paraphilia (conditioned link between the roles of domination and sexual satisfaction).	Persons with disabling conditions have been shown to have increased avoidance and disorganization in their attachment patterns (Goldberg, 1995).
Childhood Sexual Trauma (Traumagenic Experiences)	The relationship between childhood sexual or physical trauma and paraphilia has received much clinical attention (e.g., Money & Lamacz, 1989). Forty percent of child molesters and 25% of rapists had been abused as children. Between 20% and 75% of sex offenders grew up in families where violence was a way of life or where parents were alcoholic (Langevin, 1992). According to the traumagenic model, there is a correlation between the age of onset of fantasy-driven sexual aggression and the age of their own abuse, the duration of their abuse, and the level of invasiveness of the abuse (Pithers, 1993).	Sexual and physical abuse of persons with intellectual disabilities is extremely prevalent in our society. Eighty eight percent of persons with intellectual disabilities have been sexually exploited (Hill, 1987). Hard (1986, as cited in Roeher Institute, 1988), reported that 68% of females and 30% of males in his study of persons with intellectual disabilities were sexually abused before the age of 18 years. Although exact prevalence is difficult to determine due to differences in methodology used, Doucette (1986) suggested that persons with intellectual disabilities are at least one and one half times more at risk for sexual abuse than other members of society. Clinical reports of offenders have noted a high rate of abuse among individuals with disabilities who commit sexual offending behavior (Griffiths as cited in Roeher Institute, 1988; Hingsburger, 1987).

(continued)

TABLE 25.1 (Continued)

Risk Factors And Vulnerabilities	Association With Paraphilia	Risk Factors Specific To Persons With Intellectual Disabilities
Deficits in Skills of Empathy	Empathy is "capacity to cognitively perceive another's perspective, to recognize affective arousal within oneself, and to base compassionate behavioral responses on the motivation induced by these precepts." Barbaree and Serin (1993) suggest that the inhibition to sexual assault is a prosocial process, which is enhanced by positive attitudes toward others and sensitivity to another's pain and suffering. Some researchers have offered an "inhibition hypothesis" to explain sexual aggression (Barbaree, Marshal & Lanthier, 1979; Marshall & Barbaree, 1984).	Empathy requires an integration of cognition, affect, and behavior (Pithers, 1993). This difficulty in "compassionate understanding" may interfere with the individual's ability to take the perspective of their potential victim or of those who may influence the individual negatively in the commission of an offense (Pithers, 1993). Individuals with cognitive disabilities have increased difficulty in understanding the perspectives, feelings or thoughts of others. This perspective taking also has been identified as one of the underlying vulnerabilities of sex offenders (Pithers, 1993).
Skill Deficits	Sexual offenders may lack the necessary social skills, or sexual knowledge and experience to develop appropriate relationships (Abel, Rouleau, & Cunningham-Rathner, 1984). In addition, a sexual dysfunction, such as premature ejaculation, might be present which interferes with the aggressor's ability to engage in sexual activity that is socially accepted.	For persons with intellectual disabilities, thinking is very concrete and rooted in the here and now and more rigid and perseverative (McGee & Menolascino, 1992), leading to difficulty in interpreting relationships or contextual cues, such as private vs. public, and appropriate vs. inappropriate unless training is provided. Persons with intellectual disabilities often have difficulty acquiring social skills and in spontaneous generalization of skills outside the training environments unless training specifically focuses on developing these skills (Griffiths, Feldman & Tough, 1997). Most persons with intellectual disabilities are deficient in their knowledge of biological and social aspects of sexuality (Murphy, Coleman, & Haynes, 1983b), however are able to develop sexual knowledge if afforded the opportunity of education (i.e., Lindsay, Bellshaw, Culross, Staines & Michie, 1999).
Lack of prosocial inhibition	Sexual offenders justify their behaviors by distorting their belief system regarding the offending behavior; cognitive distortions are "self-statements made by offenders that allow them to deny, minimize, justify, and rationalize their behavior" (Murphy, 1990, p.332). This allows them to reduce the cognitive dissonance that might otherwise inhibit their behavior (Abel, 1984). Anger, alcohol, and intoxication can also act as to reduce prosocial inhibition and can contribute to sexually inappropriate behavior (MacDonald & Pithers, 1989; Pithers, Beal, Armstrong & Petty, 1989).	These distortions have been reported among offenders with intellectual disabilities (Murphy et al., 1983b). Additionally persons with intellectual disabilities have grown up in some cases in cultures where the typical social values were not present and the typical prosocial inhibitions were not developed (Griffiths et al., 1989). Tudiver et al. (1997) surveyed offenders who were developmentally disabled and found that although one-fifth of the group used alcohol and approximately 5% used other drugs, the consumption of alcohol and drugs played a role in only 3.5% of the sexual incidents.

The table indicates that individuals with intellectual disabilities may be at greater risk to develop sexually inappropriate sexual expressions not by virtue of their disability but because of the interplay of their learning challenges and the lack of appropriate sociosexual learning experiences typically afforded this population.

Adapted from Griffiths, 2002.

For an individual who is capable of making their own life decisions, informed consent may be and is likely possible. But it requires a rigorous procedure to ensure that it is truly informed and free of duress. Some ways to ensure this are to determine if the purpose and procedure for the assessment has been clearly explained and read to the individual to a point of understanding. For example, can the individual describe in his/her own words, what they will be asked to do, do they know who to talk to if they have questions, and do they clearly understand it is ok with everyone if they say they do not want to do this or continue? Probing questions can be helpful to ascertain this.

How can the clinician validate that the consent is informed and free of duress? The presence of an advocate of one's choosing or from an advocating agency, who knows the individual well, could cosign the consent to say they observed the process and believe the person to understand what was agreed to and the conditions of consent and their right to withdraw consent. It is often advisable to discern if the person has a history of overcompliance. Third party participants will know the compliance of the individual, however when in doubt the clinician could probe by asking some silly question to which the obvious answer would be "no." When the person is not able to consent, then third party or legal substitute consent is required for consent to be valid. Particularly in the case of forensic evaluations, consideration should be given to producing an independent record of the assessment by recording the assessment with audio or (preferably) videotape. This will not only provide a record of the assessment but also minimize the number of assessments the accused must undergo.

The consent or assent issues regarding the offending situation also need to be examined. The parties involved in the sexual act may have been in mutual agreement to the action that may indicate assent. However, legal consent requires a much more rigid criterion. Sheehan (2002) suggests legal consent should be based on evaluation of whether the individual has knowledge and understanding of (i) basic anatomy and physiology, such as that sex involves more than just penetration but the issues of pleasure (ii) privacy, (iii) of the risk of disease or pregnancy and that these can be prevented through safe sex measures, (iv) inappropriate partners, such as animals, children, immediate relatives or where money is exchanged, and that (v) consent can be withdrawn even if a person has consented before. She also suggests that the individual should be aware that some people believe that sex is only appropriate in a loving, respectful monogamous relationship.

The need to protect vulnerable individuals while still respecting their right to autonomy and right to make choices about their intimate lives makes generalizations difficult. DuVal (2002) recommends that determinations of capacity must be made within the context of a particular choice, rather than globally. Restrictions on choices must be reasonable and the least onerous, aimed at achieving specific protective purposes. DuVal summarizes the twin responsibilities, "While caregivers and families have an important obligation to advocate for and assist persons with developmental disabilities, they must be wary of infantilizing them or creating dependence in doing so" (p. 447). Although in some cases an individual may not be able to meet strict criteria for informed consent, the lack of informed consent should not be concluded to be sexual assault, but rather a lack of capacity to give legal consent. The other party may have assented to the action even though the strict legal definition was not met. Although the act is still nonconsenting and as such training is required to assist the person if possible to be able to learn what is required to give informed consent or teach the alleged offender about consent, the determination of "assenting" but "nonconsenting" action directs treatment in an entirely different way then if the action represented sexual assault.

Relevant History

The life experiences of the offender with intellectual disabilities can often reveal many clinically important facts. As with nondisabled offenders, the history of offense or offenses provides valuable information regarding the nature of the offense, the preferred target for the offense, and the conditions under which the offense occurred. Individuals with intellectual disabilities will often deny memory of the events to avoid punishment or ridicule, however many are also very poor historians of past events and as such may provide answers to questions they do not fully recall in an attempt to comply with the interviewer. The challenge in gaining the history from the individual with a disability is to attempt to differentiate issues of motivation to conceal from challenges in memory.

In the section that follows, Marinos and Griffiths (2006) provide generalized guidelines for interviewing offenders who are intellectually disabled. There are however 750 known genetic causes of intellectual disability and as such the reader should be aware that there may be great variation within the population and as such implement the generalizations with caution to individual differences.

Persons with intellectual disabilities are able to provide descriptions of past events but they will give less detail. In an interview, the person with an intellectual disability may need more time and support to provide adequate answers. The person may appear unresponsive to questioning; however it may actually be that the individual needs more time to process and respond. In some cases responses may come some time later in the conversation. When describing past events, persons with intellectual disabilities generally demonstrate difficulty recalling temporal order or duration because of challenges with time and date, for example a person may say they committed an offense last week but it was actually 2 years earlier.

Research has shown that individuals with intellectual disabilities are unable to recall events if subjected to unstructured questioning. They may also fabricate more on misleading short-answer questions and are more prone to errors on false leading specific and statement questions due to the demands of the situation and the desire to conform to the authority figure. If given a list of options the person with an intellectual disability is likely to choose the last one provided. They are also less able to correct information if given misleading recall questions or false leading specific and statement questions. They may be less accurate and less confident in recall if highly anxious; stress can create disassociation and suggestibility, especially when questions are posed to try to trip the person up.

Unfortunately, a secondary source of gathering data, client records, is similarly flawed.

Let us examine some examples:

Jon was identified as a high-risk offender based upon records from the institution. The records referred to several sexual assaults that he had committed before placement at the institution. He was denied community-access for many years until an interview with a family member revealed that the sexual assaults never happened. Jon had said that he wanted to be sexual with a girl and his concerned parents responded by placing him in the institution stating reason that "he was in danger because of his interest in girls." This was misinterpreted to mean that he was a sexual predator.

Roger was similarly labeled as a pedophile and was restricted from all activities where there were children. By going back into original sources, it was found that this 20-year restriction was on the basis of a report in his records that said that Roger had touched a 10-year-old girl on her genital area. What the report failed to indicate was that Roger was 11 at the time. Now 31 years of age, he had lived most of his life mislabeled as a pedophile.

Often the events surrounding a sexual misbehavior are not recorded accurately at the time or based on supposition rather than observations as in the situations described previously. However, at other times, events are recorded inaccurately. More often, events are not recorded because of concern regarding wrongful labeling. When events are recorded they are often written with bias or innuendo, for example "Paul should not be around children" or "John becomes bothered by children." Thus, although it is important to review the records for life history and sexual offense history, the records should be examined for inconsistencies and data should be verified where possible with interviews with family and longtime care providers.

The history of the individual can provide valuable information regarding the sociosexual learning experiences of the individual. A high percentage of individuals with intellectual disabilities have been sexually abused; the abuse is typically perpetrated by a caregiver, generally repetitive, and typically goes unidentified, unprosecuted, and without treatment for the victim (Sobsey, 1994; Sobsey & Doe, 1991; Sobsey & Varnhagen, 1991). Although some sex offenders within the general population may replay their own victimization in their subsequent offenses, the role of the victimization may be more currently salient for persons with intellectual disabilities because of a lack of opportunity for prosocial sociosexual education and experiences to replace the sexual abuse experiences. The abuse may have been their first or only sexual encounter before the event in question. If the individual has never experienced consenting sexual relationships, nor afforded education regarding these issues, then it may be that the behavior is motivated more out of ignorance than intent to violate. Lack of sex education has been demonstrated in some cases as a pivotal piece in "naïve offenders," however, it should not be assumed that all persons with intellectual disabilities lack knowledge about sex. Often the most dangerous offenders in this population are very knowledgeable.

Mental Status

Tests of intelligence: One of the common assessments conducted with persons with intellectual disabilities when they commit a sexual offense, is a test of intelligence. Unfortunately these test results are often misinterpreted as predictive of all aspects of the person's functioning rather then their ability to perform on a test that was designed to predict academic success. An evaluation of a cognitive ability is more than just an IQ score. An IQ score and the associated Mental Age (MA) are indicative of the person's performance at that point in time on a test of intelligence. However the IQ is not just a number but a continuum of skills that represent not only quantitative but qualitative differences in abilities, which results in a different developmental pattern, in both timing and degree (McGee & Menolascino, 1992). An individual with a developmental disability may be able to function fairly independently in society and may appear socially competent.

Marinos and Griffiths (2006) caution regarding the common use and misuse of the concept of MA in these cases. The MA refers to the number of questions a person can answer on the test compared to others of a certain age; it does not account in any way for the person's life experience or understanding of other aspects of life. For example, although an adult male may have an IQ that is described in terms of a MA of a child it does not mean that his thoughts, experiences, and general knowledge are that similar to a child. This man has lived an adult lifespan of experiences and physical maturation. Moreover because the predictive validity of most tests is less than accepted levels, caution must be used in applying the outcome of psychological tests to predict behavior (Aiken, 1994).

Intellectual disability refers to a permanent condition occurring before the 18th year that results in significantly below average intellectual functioning as measured on an individually administered test of test of intelligence (IQ less than 75) plus significant deficits in adaptive functioning (APA, 2000). An IQ measure may provide understanding about the method of central processing strategies the person uses and challenges to learning and as such may be of some benefit when designing a habilitative approach to teach alternative skills.

The American Association of Mental Retardation (AAMR) (1993) proposed additional criterion to the IQ measure that includes identification of the person's strengths and weaknesses, as well as the supports needed by the person to enhance functioning. A more accurate assessment of mental status therefore involves examining the adaptive functioning of the individual, including functional strengths as well as challenges.

Adaptive functioning: Assessment of adaptive functioning provides the clinician with information regarding issues such as personal strengths and habilitative needs that could be part of a package for building resiliency. This assessment might include lifestyle planning (such as domestic or vocational goals), basic functioning skills (such as communication), and also social goals (self-management strategies such as social skills, social problem solving, and anger management). The example of Bruce illustrates the value of understanding the person's functioning.

Bruce is an individual labeled with "low moderate" abilities. He can independently access his community; however, Bruce has difficulty with emotional regulation and communication. Bruce was accused of touching a child in the groin. He was arrested and charged. When the situation was reviewed, it became clear that Bruce did indeed point to the child's groin area and perhaps did touch it, but the motivation was not sexual but to point to the insignia that was on the child's pants in the groin area. Bruce had limited communication skills and typically communicated his thoughts to others by touching what interested him. The charges of sexual assault were dropped because the assessor was able to demonstrate that this behavior, although inappropriate communication, was nothing more then his attempt to communicate.

Mental health: Persons with intellectual disabilities are more likely than the general population to experience a coexisting mental health problem (Nezu, Nezu, & Gill-Weiss, 1992). Although Langevin (1992) noted that one in ten sex offenders have a coexisting mental illness, among offenders who have intellectual disabilities this could be as high as 30% to 47% (Steiner, 1984; White & Wood, 1988). In some cases the mental illness can be a cause or contributing condition to the sexual offense. For example, Jason has begun to touch individuals in a sexual manner at his school. He grabs at the private parts of young girls and the teacher. His behavior was considered "purpose-fully sexual" until the psychologist noted that along with this new behavior, Jason was constantly mov-ing, displaying very pressured speech patterns and had rapid flights of ideas. She investigated with his mother about his sleep patterns and found that he had not been sleeping. A referral to a psychiatrist resulted in a diagnosis of mania, which when treated resulted in the elimination of all symptoms including sexual touching.

Etiology of the disability: Some syndromes com-monly related to persons with intellectual disabili-ties (i.e., fetal alcohol syndrome, Tourette's disorder, and Asperger's disorder) have been associated with sexually inappropriate behavior (Griffiths, Richards, Fedoroff, & Watson, 2002). The expression of the inappropriate behavior therefore may be associated with the behavioral phenotype of the syndromes, respectively impulse control, tics, and social skill defi-cits. It should however be noted that Asperger's disor-der and Tourette's disorder do not necessarily imply intellectual disability, and indeed may present with normal or genius level intelligence. Nonetheless, these behavioral or central processing challenges present a risk that the individual may respond to arousing situations inappropriately. The offense to the victim remains unchanged; however, knowledge of the vulnerabilities that led up to the assault will alter treatment strategies.

It appears that certain types of brain damage may relate to how individuals centrally process informa-tion and may contribute, in some way, to the sexual offenses of persons with and without intellectual dis-abilities (i.e., impulse control) (see Langevin, 1992). Although direct application of this research to practice is still emerging, it has implications for neuropsycho-logical retraining and psychotherapy intervention.

Context

As stated earlier, appropriate sexual, sociosexual behavior was traditionally not taught to, made avail-able to, or permitted in social service agencies that support persons with intellectual disabilities. The learning environment of persons with intellectual dis-abilities can affect their sexual behavior in two ways. First, where sexual behavior has been so suppressed, controlled, or punished, individuals may develop "erotophobia," which may manifest itself as a negative reaction to anything sexual and denial, anger or self-punishment regarding one's sexuality (Hingsburger, 1992).

Second, the socioenvironmental context that is typically repressive and punishing may inadver-tently promote sociosexual behavior whose func-tion is driven primarily to gain sexual satisfaction while avoiding punishment and ridicule, rather then the engagement of sexual satisfaction in appropri-ate, consenting, and relationship driven contexts (Griffiths, 2003). The systems in which people with intellectual disabilities live can promote a "Catch 22" regarding the development of sexually appropri-ate behavior. Although persons with intellectual dis-abilities do not tend to demonstrate any more sexually inappropriate behavior than nondisabled persons if they are provided a normative learning experiences (Edgerton, 1973), the nature of the generally repres-sive and restrictive attitudes or conditions provided for persons with intellectual disabilities promotes a higher incidence of sexually inappropriate behavior (Day, 1997).

There are several contextual considerations to evaluating the sexual offense of a person with an intellectual disability:

First, if the person were not intellectually disabled would this be considered an offense?

The sexual behavior of an individual with an intellectual disability may be considered inappropri-ate because policy and procedure in the supporting agency dictate it to be so.

Second, the context in which the person lives may provide a basis for understanding if the sexually repressive or punitive nature of the environment is contributing to the expression of sexual behavior in an inappropriate manner.

Let us take a few examples:

John and Sean live in a group home where inti-macy, especially between the same sex is prohibited. After many reprisals in their group home for attempts at intimacy, they opt to seek privacy in the bushes in the park. Although the behavior resulted in the cou-ple being arrested for engaging in a public indecent act, the function of the behavior was not exhibition-ism but the desire for intimacy in a world that pro-vides them no respect for privacy. Thus knowledge of the supporting family attitudes or agency policy and procedures about sexual behavior may be an impor-tant consideration in the evaluation of the event.

Similarly, Peter masturbates openly in the living room of his group home. He is continually sent to his room, but comes out to the common area in just a few minutes and begins again. The staff members believe that his exposure is a paraphilia and believe that he may be at risk to display this behavior in the community. However, the assessment revealed that Peter engages in this behavior only in the presence of a few individuals, whom it appears he finds attractive. The initial impression was that he is engaging in this behavior to either shock or interest the women. However an alternative hypothesis is that the presence of an attractive woman is necessary for him to get an arousal and his home does not allow him any erotica for use in his bedroom. He was taken to a poster shop and helped to purchase of a poster of his choosing for his wall; he chose an attractive woman in bathing suit. He was then given a few instructions on privacy and private places to be sexual. From that moment on he stayed in his room to masturbate. This simple solution resolved the situation and allowed the clinician to evaluate that the apparent paraphilia was probably a by-product of the contextual restrictions combined with his disability. He was unable to use mental imagery of an attractive woman unless the stimuli was present, but because he had no access to arousing stimuli, because of policy and practice of the agency, and because he had not been taught the difference between public and private, he resorted to the public use of arousing stimuli (i.e., the presence of attractive women in the living room).

Sociosexual Knowledge and Attitudes

Sociosexual knowledge and attitudes are an important element in the assessment process for individuals with intellectual disabilities who sexually offend. Attitudes regarding sexual behavior are typically conducted with sexual offenders regarding attitudes toward women and cognitive distortions. However, in addition, a sociosexual knowledge and attitude assessment is recommended (Griffiths et al., 2007).

Attitudes and cognitive distortions: The Abel and Becker Cognition Scale (ABCS, Abel, Becker, & Cunningham-Rathner, 1984) was a measure designed for sexual offenders without disabilities. This was revised by Kolton et al. (2001) for use with persons with intellectual disabilities, however it does not have demonstrated validity for this population. The nature of the items may lead to individuals with intellectual disabilities giving responses that may be misleading

because the individual is responding to please the examiner.

Sociosexual knowledge and attitudes: Although not typical in a sexual evaluation for nondisabled persons, assessment of the sociosexual knowledge and attitudes of sexual offenders with intellectual disabilities provides valuable information in making a differential diagnosis of paraphilia. Adults with intellectual disabilities generally know less about their sexuality and sexual abuse than teenagers without disabilities (Murphy, 2003); sex education can make a significant difference in understanding and knowledge. Hingsburger et al. (1991) presented case examples of persons with intellectual disabilities for whom the treatment, for certain inappropriate sexual behaviors, was sex education alone. Other cases however represent more clinically complex intervention where sex education is often a critical vulnerability for the development of the inappropriate sexual expression and one of the main components of effective intervention (Griffiths, Quinsey, & Hingsburger, 1989; Griffiths, 2002).

The SocioSexual Knowledge and Attitudes Tool (SSKAAT-R) (Griffiths & Lunsky, 2003) and the Sexual Knowledge, Experience, Feelings and Needs Scale (SexKen-ID) (McCabe, 1994) represent two of the evaluative tools available that measure change in both knowledge and attitude. These measures provide an individually administered evaluation using a picture book, to which participants answer minimally verbally demanding questions. Although there are less complicated measures available (i.e., Timmers, Du Charne, & Jacob, 1981), the psychometric evaluation of the simpler measures is lacking (McCabe, Cummins, & Deeks, 1999).

The SSKAAT-R has been field-tested across North America and has excellent psychometric properties, including internal consistency, test-retest reliability, and content validity. This measure is particularly appropriate to identify the base of knowledge and attitudes that the individual has with regard to a range of sociosexual behaviors and as an aid in differential diagnosis of counterfeit deviance related to a lack of awareness of boundary issues. This measure includes the additional dimension of evaluating age and gender discrimination.

The Sex Ken-ID reports high levels of internal consistency for all subscales with the exception of the needs and feeling subscales (McCabe et al., 1999). Test–retest reliability data and validity data were less convincing. Whitehouse and McCabe (1997) state that future programmes need to consider the use of checklists and transcript analysis to cover both the more accurate but more limited assessment of sexual facts as well as the more complex analysis of feelings and attitudes. The Sex Ken-ID differs from the SSKAAT-R because it also requests information about experiences and as such would serve as a valuable tool in exploring experiences and feelings that may relate to sexual dysfunction.

PHALLOMETRY (PARTNER SELECTION AND PREFERENCE)

Diagnosis of paraphilia using sexual assessment procedures for this population should be undertaken cautiously. Typical sexual preference interviewing and testing procedures require adaptation and careful interpretation when used with this population. Individuals with intellectual disabilities may have difficulty providing self-report information; more concrete interview questions might be preferable (Murphy, Coleman, & Abel, 1983a). Although phallometric measures with this population have been reported to be accurate in determining sexual preference on both age and gender and useful for those who have committed a sexual offense (Murphy et al., 1983a), some individuals with intellectual disabilities may present with physical, communication, and behavioral challenges that can interfere with the evaluation and may not demonstrate the expected response to the testing situation. Murphy et al., (1983a) noted that common medications in this population can interfere with testing results. They further noted that some individuals were cognitively unable to focus on the visual test stimuli or had greater difficulty discriminating situations that were deviant. Griffiths et al. (1989) noted that some individuals had difficulty with age discrimination and suggested the use of a card sort test to assess if individuals could determine "who is like me?" and "who is it ok to have sex with?"

Phallometric testing is described in more detail elsewhere in this book (Fedoroff, Kuban & Bradford, 2006). Concerning phallometric testing of individuals with intellectual disabilities, it is most important to be aware that phallometric testing is not designed to determine guilt or innocence of an alleged crime. Its purpose is to objectively measure sexual arousal patterns in a controlled laboratory setting. Results of this testing can aid in the design of a comprehensive treatment plan but should never be relied upon in isolation.

Unfortunately, phallometric testing is underutilized in men with intellectual disabilities. This is due to a lack of suitably equipped facilities that are comfortable and experienced in dealing with this population. In addition, some care providers and agencies have a reluctance to agree to the testing due to an unproven belief that phallometric testing may somehow unleash deviant sexual interests. Likely this represents another manifestation of the "eternal child" myth described earlier in this chapter.

While there is no reason to consider the prescription of phallometric testing contraindicated in men with intellectual disability, special caution is needed. This is because abnormal test results can easily be misused by third party agencies to deny or delay appropriate treatment, housing, or enrollment in social and educational programs. Caution also needs to be exercised to ensure that collateral information from phallometric testing is not misused. For example, phallometric testing designed to investigate to presence or absence of sexual interest in children (pedophilia) will also reveal information about the subject's sexual orientation concerning adults. Regrettably, some care providers and agencies (officially or unofficially) treat homosexual clients differently than their heterosexual ones.

RISK ASSESSMENT

The research on differential evaluation procedures is largely unavailable for this population. Moreover, direct application of some testing procedures to this population may have potential challenges. For example, risk assessment in the general population of sex offenders is best evaluated using instruments like the Sex Offender Risk Appraisal Guide (SORAG) (Quinsey, Harris, Rice, & Cormier, 1998). However, persons with intellectual disabilities may score uniformly higher on various measures of the score by virtue of the experiences afforded them in life because of the disability label (Griffiths, Richards, & Fedoroff, 2002).

Researchers have now completed three studies that are relevant to this proposal. In the first study 18 male sex offenders with intellectual disability were case-matched on the basis of age and number of known victims to 18 male sex offenders with no intellectual disability (Fedoroff, Selhi, Smolewska, & Ng. 2001). They were scored on modified versions of the VRAG and SORAG in which Child and Adolescent Taxon (CAT) (Quinsey et al., 1998) scores were substituted for Hare Psychopathy Checklist scores. The data were analyzed retrospectively. The men with intellectual disability were scored significantly higher on both the VRAG and SORAG (VRAG mean scores: −0.11 vs. −5.5; $p = 0.01$ respectively) (SORAG mean scores: −0.11 vs. −5.3; $p = 0.04$ respectively). These results were interpreted as supportive of the hypothesis that some items on the VRAG and SORAG have different significance in men with intellectual disability. For example, the item "lived with both biological parents until age 16" was scored positively in significantly more men with intellectual disability than in the control group ($p = 0.0002$). Our group has speculated that the reasons that men without intellectual disability fail to live with their parents are different than those of men with intellectual disability. Since VRAG and SORAG scores are currently used to make treatment and disposition decisions in men with intellectual disability, it is vitally important that their validity be demonstrated in this group.

In a second study using a completely independent group of men, 38 men with chart diagnoses of intellectual disability who were accused of sexually offending against children were matched with 38 male child molesters without intellectual disability on the basis of age at the time of their index offense, and number and gender of their victims (Fedoroff, Curry, & Madrigrano, 2006). In this study VRAG and SORAG scores were based on scores that included Hare Psychopathy checklist scores but the item "Elementary school maladjustment" was scored as zero for all men since this information was not scored reliably in the database used. Again, this study involved retrospective analysis. In this study, although there were no significant differences between the two groups in VRAG or SORAG scores, the intellectually disabled group scored significantly lower than the nonintellectually disabled group on the Hare Psychopathy checklist (Hare, 1991)(16.38 vs. 20.80 respectively; $p < 0.05$). In addition, both groups had higher average VRAG and SORAG scores than in the previous study (mean VRAG score = 1.79; mean SORAG score = 2.41). Again, there were significant differences

on several individual items on both the VRAG and SORAG instruments (not all of which corresponded to the items identified in the first study). These findings support the hypothesis that individual items on the VRAG and SORAG have different significance in sex offenders with and without intellectual disability and raise the possibility that there may be other mediating factors. For example, it may be that VRAG and SORAG scores are falsely elevated in men with developmental delay who have low psychopathy scores but this difference may diminish in the sub-group of developmentally delayed sex offenders who have high levels of psychopathy. A study to investigate this possibility is currently under-way.

In a third study (Quinsey, personal communication) 58 men from institutions designed to house individuals with intellectual disabilities and serious histories of antisocial and aggressive behaviors were prospectively followed for an average of 16 months after discharge from their home institute. Items from two scales used to assess dynamic risk factors (the Problem Identification Checklist and Proximal Risk Factor scale (Quinsey, Coleman, Jones, & Altrows, 1997)) were subsequently selected if they exhibited a significant linear trend across previous, prior, and index months in which problematic incidents had occurred. The resulting instrument, the Short Dynamic Risk Scale was found to show significant linear trends for both nonviolent and violent incidents even when VRAG scores were statistically controlled. These results suggest that improved assessment instruments specifically designed for individuals with intellectual disability not only can but need to be developed and validated in this population.

INTEGRATED MODELS OF INTERVENTION

In the 1980's the first specialized treatment programs were developed for persons with intellectual disabilities who demonstrate sexually offensive behavior (i.e., Coleman & Murphy, 1980, Griffiths et al., 1989). Before the 1980s, persons with intellectual disabilities who engaged in sexual assault were managed by segregation and institutionalization (Griffiths et al., 1989), chemical arousal reduction (i.e., hormone therapy) or behavioral suppression (Foxx, Bittle, Bechel, & Livesay, 1986). It was common belief at that time that persons with intellectual disabilities would not benefit from traditional therapy or counselling. As a result it was uncommon for therapeutic interventions to be considered. However, in the 1980s, treatment programs began to emerge that promoted a therapeutic approach including training skills in sexual responsibility, sociosexual knowledge, coping skills, and control of deviant arousal through relapse prevention strategies (Griffiths et al., 1989; Haaven, Little & Petre-Miller, 1990; Lindsay, Marshall, Neilson, Quinn, & Smith, 1998; Nezu, Nezu, & Dudeck, 1998; Ward et al.,1992).

Habilitative Mental Health Model of Intervention

Griffiths et al. (1989) and Tudiver et al. (1997) recommend that treatment methods for developmentally delayed offenders be grounded on the same treatment approaches used for nondelayed offenders, but tailored to address the learning needs, and special issues of offenders with intellectual disabilities. The components identified by Griffiths et al. (1989) include social skills, sex education, responsibility training, relationship training, coping skills, and the control of deviance.

However, the general sexual offender treatment model is largely rehabilitative; rehabilitation implying the person receives treatment to return their sexual expression to a state of dignity. Persons with intellectual disabilities by virtue of their disability and life experiences have generally not been afforded the life experience or training to understand and experience their sexuality as normative. While this argument may be valid for some nondisabled sex offenders, sexual offenders with intellectual disabilities require an increased emphasis on "habilitation." Habilitation involves an active education and training component within a strong habilitatively supportive environment to set up the conditions by which the individual can assume, perhaps for the first time a sense of dignity and responsibility with regard to one's sexuality.

As noted in Table 25.1, multiple and co-occurring risk factors may increase the likelihood that persons with disabilities may experience challenges regarding their sexuality. The accumulation of risks or adversity over a lifespan can predispose an individual to act in a certain way. For example a lack of communication, social skills, or positive sex education, or the experience of victimization may alter how a person understands or responds to their sexuality.

Persons with intellectual disabilities are particularly disadvantaged in their life opportunities to develop adaptive and resilient lives that would allow them to respond positively to mental health challenges and risk factors. Resiliency is the developmental process that enables a person to adapt to adverse situations (Masten, 2001) in the absence of psychopathology or high-risk behavior related to a person's situation (Miller, 2002).

Multicomponent treatment is considered best practice in the field for persons with intellectual disabilities who commit a sexual offense (i.e., Griffiths et al., 1989 or Haaven et al., 1990; Nolley, Muccigrosso, & Zigman, 1996). Intervention typically includes development of a range of habilitative skills through individual and group therapy (such as sociosexual education, coping and anger management skills, and social communication and assertiveness skills).

However, habilitative intervention places strong emphasis on the role of the environment and coordination of a support network. Habilitation is based therefore on two primary and interacting intervention elements: development of habilitative strengths within the individual and exposure to the habilitatively appropriate environment by which the acquired habilitative strengths can become appropriated by the individual. Research would indicate that knowledge and skill is difficult to achieve with this population (Feldman, 1994) and dependent upon training in the natural environment or in settings that closely simulate real-life situations, using sufficient and relevant exemplars, and that is naturally trapped into the reinforcement conditions of the environment (Griffiths et al., 1997; Horner & Albin, 1988; Miltenberger et al., 1999; Neef, Lensbower, Hockersmith, & DePalma, 1990).

Habilitative Education

The critical difference in teaching persons with intellectual disabilities from teaching those who do not have disabilities is that they may not have ever developed the understanding or skills regarding normative sexual behavior. Granted some may argue, correctly, that the same could apply to some nondisabled offenders and conversely that some offenders with intellectual disabilities are all too knowledgeable about what is normative, but elect to act in a manner that is illegal and inappropriate (i.e., children and aggression). Both rival arguments are correct for some individuals.

However at the risk of overgeneralizing, most offenders with intellectual disabilities require training in appropriate sociosexual interactions and in the range of compensatory self-management skills necessary to provide prosocial responses in the presence of arousing events and the avoidance of same events.

Proactive strategies for managing sexually inappropriate responses: Knowledge of the instigating conditions for the behavior can suggest education approaches to (a) remove or reduce the contributing instigating conditions, (b) introduce instigating stimulus conditions to compete with the offensive behaviors, or (c) alter the individual's reaction to the instigating events.

This approach is based on education. For example a pedophile would be taught to (a) avoid situations that are considered high risk for repeated offense (i.e., babysitting, public parks, school yards, fairs) and/or (b) introduce instigating stimulus conditions that would compete with the possible offense such as the presence of others who will monitor the situation, and/or (c) alter the individual's reaction to the contributing conditions by teaching the individual new ways of coping with these events (i.e., walking away from a high risk situation where there is a child present). The latter is of course the most difficult proactive strategy.

Proactive strategies depend on solid behavioral analysis of the antecedents and setting events that precipitated previous events and that are related to the individual's arousal patterns as well as those antecedent conditions that tend to inhibit the presence of the offending behavior.

Teaching new skills: In addition to the proactive strategies, it is important to provide opportunity for the individual to learn new skills in dealing with these events. Skills in prosocial behavior such as sociosexual interactions and self-management/impulse control and anger management "training packages" for this population are available. Preset training packages however can fail to address the specific triggering conditions for an individual, and as such although an individual may have been deemed a graduate of "anger management" or "sociosexual education" programs, the training may be ineffective because it failed to address the specific anger or sociosexual factors that contribute or trigger the challenges for that individual. Thus although they represent an excellent starting point for habilitative skill development, these packages should be individualized to ensure they are meeting the needs of the individual.

Additionally, once skills are taught their use in the natural environment will depend on the value they have in the environment, as such the program should build in systematic recognition for the individual when the new skills are being effectively applied in previously challenging situations. However, sociosexual skills are complicated and as such ensuring their success in the real world can not always be predicted. The person may learn appropriate sociosexual interactions, choose an age appropriate partner but be rejected for reasons unknown. As a result, part of the educational process is that sexual attraction is unpredictable and that potential rejection is an expected behavior. Too often, persons with intellectual disabilities are taught the "appropriate behaviors" without being taught that the partner may or may not respond as scripted. Thus it is critical to review the contingencies and prepare alternative responses to the alternatives.

Developing a Supportive, Positive and Reinforcing Environment for the Treatment of Offenders

Many authors have described how the environment can influence the development of challenging behaviors in persons with intellectual disabilities (i.e., Gardner, 1996; Martens & Witt, 1988) and the role of the environment in treatment (i.e., Griffiths, Gardner, & Nugent, 1998), however few have discussed the nature of that environment for offenders with intellectual disabilities (i.e., Haaven et al., 1990; Griffiths et al., 1989).

Griffiths et al. (1998) suggest that the habilitatively appropriate environment should be as normalized as possible; normalized implies that "it promotes learning and use of those skills and behaviors that result in an enriched lifespace for the individual" (p.100). Unfortunately persons with intellectual disabilities who present with challenging behavior, such as sexual aggression, are typically provided physical conditions that are not normative, offered limited if any habilitatively appropriate programming, and given very limited, controlled, and sterile social conditions. Griffiths et al. (1998) suggest that such conditions combine with the preexisting challenges in coping, social, and related skills produce increased vulnerability to future challenges. The presence or absence of certain environmental events (i.e., availability of reinforcing experiences and associations, daily activities, material possessions, and valued relationships) as well as adaptations in the environment have been shown to influence the motivation and presentation of behavior (Gardner, Cole, Davidson, & Karan, 1986). Other environmental issues include clustering, size and space, and opportunity to access normative environments and interactions that can promote culturally appropriate expectations and learning and generalization opportunities (Griffiths et al., 1998).

The possibility of reoffense within programs is a particular concern that needs to be addressed in the treatment environment. Clear socially constructed expectations and standards of conduct function as guides for appropriate actions for both the individual and the care providers. Often individuals with disabilities have received inconsistent or poorly defined expectations; these conditions do not establish conditions for the development of prosocial inhibitions to impulses or stimulation present at the moment. As a result the individual does not learn to be concerned over the immediate or long-term consequences that may result.

Care providers also need guidance in how to provide respectful and consistent interactions with the individuals they support. Consistency among care providers shifts the emphasis in interactions from "testing the limits of each staff" to more developing constructive interactions. The respect element in the interactions allows for the promotion of increased social motivation, decreased aversive elements, and begins to provide, within the confine of the known expectations, the development of choice and prosocial problem-solving.

The role of the social environment is to ensure that the individual has the opportunity to develop, perhaps for the first time, the value of positive relationships with a variety of people, who become part of a person's life by mutual choice and maintain relationships because of mutual enjoyment. Another element to social habilitation is to develop a range of sustaining or stable relationships that provide potential opportunity for personal or, where appropriate, intimate relationships to develop.

A key factor in the long-term success and generalization of intervention may be the development of habilitatively appropriate social environments. Ultimately the outcome of the environment is to allow the person to experience success in social interactions and daily life, so that the person emerges with enhanced self-esteem awareness and control. The

"new identity" or "new me," as Haaven et al. (1990) describe it, is now based on these positive experience and the new strengths that have been developed. The person should emerge from the intervention with clear expectations for a new and improved quality of life within a life-space based upon an ongoing contingency plan, for both prosocial and inappropriate sexual expressions within the natural environment.

According to Renwick et al. (1994), quality of life is determined by three elements: first, a sense of meaning and physical/psychological health and wellbeing, second a sense of belonging in the community and with important others, and third a sense of engagement and growth in everyday life and of a future. The emphasis on building an improved quality of life for offenders is to shift the focus from hopelessness and a lack of control to a focus on hope and resiliency.

Factors such as trusting relationships, encouragement, personal strength and self-esteem, social and interpersonal skills, communication skills, as examples, are pivotal factors in building resilience (Masten, 2001). Additionally, certain qualities of the environment or the individual can compensate for or protect the individual in the face of risk. Applying a resiliency model of intervention to sex offenders with intellectually disabled offenders would suggest that recidivism could be enhanced by building a supportive, positive and reinforcing environment and the competencies to respond to risk factors.

Intervention Outcome—What Do We Want Them to Measure?

Sex offenders with intellectual disabilities, particularly those individuals who are labeled as mildly or moderately disabled, have been surprisingly responsive to treatment (Lackey & Knopp, 1989). Although the claims of success have generally not been followed up with strong empirical research; many studies lack pretreatment assessment or reliable direct observations in the generalizability of outcomes to the natural environment where the triggering events are naturally present and unrestricted.

In a proactive model of intervention, outcome evaluation goes beyond measuring the rate of offending behavior (recidivism). It includes evaluation of (a) the development and transfer of proactive skills to replace the sexually inappropriate behavior within the natural environment, (b) the ongoing system of support for the individual to ensure that the contingencies of reinforcement for prosocial behavior or for the inhibition of inappropriate behavior are maintained, and (c) evaluation of the outcome of an improved quality of life for the individual to ensure that resiliency has been developed.

Recidivism as an outcome measure: Commonly, recidivism is the only outcome measure employed. However, recidivism data relies on the person being caught and on reconviction rates, rather then actual offense rates. In reviewing five studies that reported recidivism as their treatment outcome data, rates ranged from 2% to 40% with follow up from 2 to 10 years post treatment (Demetral as cited in Nolley et al., 1996); Day, 1997; Lund, 1992; Haaven et al., 1990; Swanson & Garwick, 1990). The rate of recidivism reported was not related to the length of the follow up. In fact one of the largest rates of recidivism was reported in a study that had a 2.5-year follow-up (Swanson & Garwick, 1990). However, recidivism data may relate to treatment location (Nolley et al., 1996). For example, Demetral (as cited in Nolley et al., 1996) reported a recidivism rate of less than 2% within a community program; Haaven et al. (1990) indicated a rate of recidivism of 23% for their population of institutionalized offenders. Nolley et al. (1996) cautioned that these research findings may be interpreted in two ways. First one could assume that the populations differ or that the data from the community was less accurate.

However, Nolley and associates suggested that the better outcome data from the community programs were the result of highly qualified facilitators who provided increased social opportunities for persons with developmental disabilities, enlisted natural support systems, and ensured greater opportunity for learning about culturally acceptable ways of sexual expression. The aforementioned thesis, although still speculative, is consistent with the empirical understanding of generalization principles for teaching persons with intellectual disabilities (Griffiths et al., 1997) and with the clinical findings of Griffiths et al. (1989).

Direct observation as an outcome measure: The use of direct observation across individuals and settings in the natural environment provide increased levels of confidence in treatment effectiveness. Treatment outcomes are often measured in this population by use of the "Casper technique." This approach is used when the individual has demonstrated that they can meet set standards of competency in learning self-control and relapse skills in a "safe" environment. Once criteria within the safe environment are met, the individual is then given graduated opportunities to gain degrees of freedom to reduce supervision in the natural environment where previous triggering events may be present. For example the person may move from a direct escort on a low risk activity (e.g., walk to the corner store and back, or going on the bus to work, if those are deemed to be low-risk situations for the individual), to being allowed independent access but within a restricted time-frame (i.e., 15 minutes) and along a particular path (i.e., avoiding the school yard). Initially, however the degrees of freedom are provided with the person's knowledge that someone may be watching. A staff member that the individual does not know will be either shadowing the individual from a distance and recording if the individual employed his prosocial skills and showed inhibition of inappropriate behavior if the presence of potential triggers presented themselves (i.e., a child). The staff is therefore available to intervene should the individual not show the appropriate skills.

Initially a staff member would be watching each trip until a measure of confidence is gained that the individual is able to use the skills in different situations, with different people and in the proximity of potential relapse targets. This strategy provides three advantages. It begins to generalize the individuals learned skills from the safe environment to the natural community with graduated levels of supervision. Second, it provides an opportunity for the program to provide direct monitoring and evaluation of outcomes. Third, it enables the program to introduce generalization probes in a controlled manner that affords minimum risk to the community. Reduction of the supervision is carefully orchestrated to ensure changes reflect evidence that is based upon the outcome data and the individually determined degree of risk for various situations.

The "Casper" stage of intervention is developed in conjunction with the individual and explained as a way in which the person can gain confidence that their "new" skills are useful in allowing them to gain community opportunities in a manner that is safe for them to keep out of trouble. The cooperation and agreement of the participant is important; the motivation of the individual to ensure self and other safety is part of the process of change. The "Casper technique" has been used in many settings and appears to have both clinical and research applications.

BACKUP CONTINGENCIES: IF PROACTIVE APPROACHES ARE NOT EFFECTIVE

When proactive approaches are not effective, things can go wrong even in ideal practice environments. Usually it takes the form of a frantic telephone call saying: "there has been an incident." These calls often come from a front-line worker who is not the usual caretaker of the person in question. Typically, the usual frontline worker has gone on vacation, been transferred, or called in sick. This is because people with intellectual disability are upset by change in routine. A new worker can mean new problems.

The first response is to ascertain if anyone is hurt (physically or psychologically). If a sexual assault involving penetration is suspected the victim should be assessed by a rape crisis team at a medical facility as soon as possible.

Often the "incident" raises the question of whether the police need to be called. Almost always, the answer is "yes." Care providers and agencies are not detectives and it is vitally important that any investigations be done by a third party agency with experience in such matters. The police are the experts in deciding if a criminal charge is warranted.

Ideally, the agency involved will already have a working independent relationship with the hospital and the police. Assessment of victims with intellectual disability is a topic beyond the scope of this chapter. Similarly, the special procedures advised for police departments charged with the responsibility of investigating alleged sexual offenses committed by people with intellectual disabilities have been described in detail elsewhere (Richards, Watson, & Bleich, 2000).

If the accused is arrested and taken into custody, agency workers should be reminded that they have an obligation to respect the confidentiality rights of their clients. They should consult with their professional college if they are unsure of their obligations. In the event that they are requested to give statements to the investigating police, they should be clear about whether they are acting as a "fact" witness or as a professional.

If the accused is taken into custody, the agency and care providers normally suspend their treatment since this is now the obligation of the custodial facility. It is not uncommon however for the custodial facility to seek advice about how to manage the individual. There is no ethical problem in providing assistance to the accused provided the "assistance" does not devolve into an investigation of the alleged offense.

Once the individual is returned to the community either on bail or having been acquitted or found guilty, a full reassessment is required and appropriate treatment should be undertaken. These issues have been described in detail elsewhere (Fedoroff et al., 2002; Langevin & Curnoe, 2002). They can be summarized as follows:

1. Establish a comprehensive differential diagnosis.
2. Do not rely on the diagnosis of intellectual disability or a paraphilic disorder to explain everything. Is there a comorbid condition or environmental factors?
3. Treat the comorbid conditions.
4. Simultaneously treat the sexual problem(s).
5. For sexual problems, assess the severity/seriousness of the problem.
6. Present the treatment options including risks and benefits of not accepting treatment to the individual and/or substitute decision-maker.
7. Consider any treatment agreed upon as a trial that will be reevaluated regularly.

CONCLUSION

The history of persons with intellectual disabilities has been fraught with human rights violations, often because of concern regarding their sexuality. It is therefore not surprising that inappropriate sexual behavior was not addressed proactively or therapeutically until recently. In the past few decades, the forensic and disability fields have both begun to address treatment for this population.

Literature and research has begun to emerge that provides an increasing understanding of the similarity and differences in the etiology and treatment for sexual offense behavior in persons with intellectual disabilities compared to the nondisabled offender. This understanding will hopefully lead to improved assessment and intervention for those persons who are intellectually disabled and who offend sexually.

References

Abel, G. G., Becker, J. V., & Cunningham-Rathner, J. (1984). Compliance, consent and cognition in sex between children and adults. *International Journal of Law and Psychiatry*, 7, 89–103.

Abel, G. G., Rouleau, J., & Cunningham-Rathner, J. (1984). Sexually aggressive behavior. In W. Curran, A. L. McGarry, & S. A. Shah (Eds.), *Modern Legal Psychiatry and Psychology*. Philadelphia, FA: Davis Co.

Aiken, L. R. (1994). *Psychological testing and assessment 8th Edition*. Needham Heights, Mass: Allyn & Bacon.

American Association of Mental Retardation. (1993). *Mental retardation: Definition, classification, and system of support (9th Edition)*. Washington, D.C.: Author.

American Psychiatric Association. (2000). *Diagnostic and statistical manual of mental disorders, fourth edition, text revision*. Washington, D.C.: American Psychiatric Association.

Barbaree, H. E., Marshal, W. L., & Lanthier, R. (1979). Deviant sexual arousal in rapists. Behavior. *Research and Therapy*, 17, 215–202.

Barbaree, H. E. & Serin, R. C. (1993). The role of male sexual arousal during rape in various subtypes. In C. Hall, R. Hirschman, J. R. Graham, & M. A. Zaragoza (Eds.), *Sexual aggression: Issues in etiology and assessment, treatment and policy* (pp. 99–114). New York, NY: Hemisphere.

Brown, H. & Stein, J. (1997). Sexual abuse perpetrated by men with intellectual disabilities: A comparative study. *Journal of Intellectual Disabilities Research*, 41(Pt. 3), 215–224.

Coleman, E. M. & Murphy, W. D. (1980). A survey of sexual attitudes and sex education programs among facilities for the mentally retarded. *Applied Research in Mental Retardation*, 1, 269–279.

Coleman, E., Dwyer, S. M., Abel, G., Berner, W., Breiling, J., Hindman, J., et al. (1995). The treatment of adult sex offenders: Standards of care. *Journal of Offender Rehabilitation*, 23(3/4), 5–11.

Cummings, J. L. (1985). *Clinical neuropsychiatry*. New York, NY: Grune & Stratton Inc.

Day, K. (1994). Male mentally handicapped sex offenders. *British Journal of Psychiatry*, 165, 630–639.

Day, K. (1997). Clinical features and offence behavior of mentally retarded sex offenders: A review of research (pp. 95–99). In R. J. Fletcher & D. Griffiths (Eds.), *Congress Proceedings-International Congress II on the Dually Diagnosed*. New York: NADD.

Doucette, J. (1986). *Violent acts against disabled women*. Toronto: DAWN Canada.

DuVal, G. (2002). Summary of ethical issues. In D. Griffiths, D. Richards, P. Fedoroff, & S. Watson (Eds.), *Ethical dilemmas: Sexuality and developmental disabilities* (pp. 355–386). Kingston, NY: NADD Press.

Edgerton, R. (1973). Socio-cultural research considerations. In F. F. de la Cruz & G. G. La Veck (Eds.), *Human sexuality and the mentally retarded* (pp. 240–249). New York, NY: Brunner/Maze.

Fedoroff, P., Curry, S., Madrigrano, G., Cunningham, C., & Bradford, J. (2006). Comparison of Violence Risk Appraisal Guide and Sex Offender Risk Appraisal Guide Items in a sample of developmentally delayed sex offenders and non delayed sex offenders. American Psychiatric Association, 2006 Annual Meeting. Abstract, Toronto, Ontario Canada. p. 324.

Fedoroff, P., Fedoroff, B., & Peever, C. (2002). Consent to treatment issues in sex offenders with developmental delay. In D. Griffiths, D. Richards, P. Fedoroff, & S. Watson (Eds.), *Ethical dilemmas: Sexuality and developmental disabilities* (pp. 355–386). Kingston, NY: NADD Press.

Fedoroff, J. P., Griffiths, D., Marini, Z, & Richards, D. (2000). One of our clients has been arrested for sexual assault: Now what?—The interplay between developmental and legal delay. In Poindexter, (Ed.), Bridging the Gap—Proceedings 17th Annual NADD Conference. Kingston, (pp. 153–160). NY: NADD.

Fedoroff, J. P., Selhi, Z., Smolewska, K., & Ng, E. (2001). Risk assessment for men with paraphilias and developmental delay. Poster session presented at the twenty-seventh annual meeting of International Academy of Sex Research. Montreal.

Feldman, M. A. (1994). Parenting education for parents with intellectual disabilities: A review of outcome studies. *Research in Developmental Disabilities*, 15, 299–332

Flynn, M. C., Reeves, D., Whelan, E., & Speake, B. (1985). The development of a measure for determining the mentally handicapped adult's tolerance of rules and recognition of rights. *Journal of practical approaches to developmental handicap*, 9(2), 18–24.

Foxx, R. M., Bittle, R. G., Bechten, D. R., & Livesay, J. R. (1986). Behavioral treatment of the sexually deviant behavior of mentally retarded individuals. *International Review of Research in Mental Retardation*, 14, 291–317.

Gaffney, G. R. & Berlin, F. S. (1984). Is there hypothalamic-pituitary-gonadal dysfunction in pedophilia? A pilot study. *British Journal of Psychiatry*, 145, 657–660.

Gardner, W. I. (1996). Nonspecific behavioral symptoms in persons with a dual diagnosis: A psychological model for integrating biomedical and psychosocial diagnosis and interventions. *Psychologwy in Mental Retardation and Developmental Disabilities*, 21, 6–11.

Gardner, W. I., Cole, C. L., Davidson, D. P., & Karan, O. C. (1986). Reducing aggression in individuals with developmental disabilities: An expanded stimulus control assessment and intervention model. *Education and Training of the Mentally Retarded*, 21, 3–12.

Gilby, R., Wolf, L., & Golberg, B. (1989). Mentally retarded adolescent sex offenders: A survey and pilot study. *Canadian Journal of Psychiatry*, 34, 542–548.

Goddard, H. (1912). *The Kallikak family: A study in the heredity of feeblemindedness*. New York, NY: McMillan.

Goldberg, S. (1995). Attachment, parental behaviour, and early development in infants with medical problems. In K. Covell (Ed.), *Readings in child development* (pp. 89–128). Toronto: Nelson.

Griffiths, D. (2002). Sexual aggression. In Wm. I. Gardner (Ed.), *Aggression and other disruptive behavioral challenges: Biomedical and psychosocial assessment and treatmen* (pp. 525–398). New York, NY: National Association for Dual Diagnosis.

Griffiths, D. (2003). Sexuality and people with developmental disabilities: From myth to emerging practices. In I. Brown & M. Percy (Eds.), *Developmental disabilities in Ontario (2nd edition)* (pp. 677–690). Toronto, ON: Ontario Association on evelopmental disabilities.

Griffiths, D., Richards, D., Fedoroff, P., & Watson, S. (2002). Sexuality and mental health in persons with developmental disabilities. In D. Griffiths, C. Stavrakaki, & J. Summers (Eds.), *Dual diagnosis: An introduction to the mental health news of persons with developmental disabilities* (pp. 419–454). Sudbury, ON: Habilitative Mental Health Network.

Griffiths, D., Fedoroff, P., Richards, D., Cox-Lindenbaum, D., Langevin, R., Linsday, et al. (2007). Gender and sexual disorders. In R. Fletcher (Ed.), *DSM-IV TR modifications for persons with intellectual disabilities* (pp. 411–457). Washington, D. C.: American Psychiatric Association/NADD Press.

Griffiths, D., Gardner, W. I., & Nugent, J. (1998). *Individual centered behavioral interventions*. Kingston, NY: National Association for Dual Diagnosis.

Griffiths, D., Hingsburger, D., & Christian, R. (1985). Treating developmentally handicapped sexual offenders: The York Behaviour Management Treatment Program. *Psychiatric Aspects of Mental Retardation Reviews*, 4, 45–52.

Griffiths, D. & Lunsky, Y. (2003). *Socio-sexual knowledge and attitude assessment tool* (SSKAAT-R). Stoelting Company: Wood Dale, Illinois.

Griffiths, D. M., Quinsey, V. L., & Hingsburger, D. (1989). Changing inappropriate sexual behavior: A community based approach for persons with intellectual *disabilities*. Baltimore: Paul H. Brookes Publishing.

Griffiths, D., Richards, D., Fedoroff, P., & Watson, S. (2002). Sexuality and mental health issues. In D. Griffiths, C. Stavrakaki, & J. Summers (Eds). *Dual diagnosis: An introduction to the mental health needs of persons with developmental disabilities* (pp. 419454). Habilitative Mental Health Resource Network: Sudbury, Ontario.

Griffiths, D., Taillon-Wasmund, P., & Smith, D. (2002). Offenders who have a developmental disability. In D. Griffiths, C. Stavrakaki, & J. Summers (Eds.), *Dual diagnosis: An introduction to the mental health needs of persons with developmental disabilities*

(pp.387–418). Sudbury ON CA: Habilitative Mental Health Resource Network (NADD Ontario).

Haaven, J., Little, R., & Petre-Miller, D. (1990). *Treating intellectually disabled sex offenders: A model residential program*. Orwell, VT: Safer Society Press.

Hare, R. D. (1991). *The revised psychopathy checklist*. Toronto: Multi-Health Systems.

Hill, G. (1987) Sexual abuse and the mentally retarded. *Child Sexual Abuse Newsletter*, 6, 4.

Hingsburger, D. (1987). Sex counseling with the developmentally handicapped: The assessment and management of seven critical problems. *Psychiatric Aspects of Mental Retardation Reviews*, 6, 41–46.

Hingsburger, D. (1992). Erotophobic behavior in people with intellectual disabilities. *The Habilitative Mental Healthcare Newsletter*, 11, 31–34.

Hingsburger, D., Griffiths, D., & Quinsey, V. (1991). Detecting counterfeit deviance: Differentiating sexual deviance from sexual inappropriateness. *The Habilitative Mental Healthcare Newsletter*, 10, 5154.

Horner, R. H. & Albin, R. W. (1988). Research on general-case procedures for learners with severe disabilities. *Education & Treatment of Children*, 11, 375–388.

Hucker, S., Langevin, R., & Bain, J. (1988) A double blind trial of provera for pedophilia. *Annals of Sex Research*, 1, 227–242.

Hucker, S., Langevin, R., Dickey, R., Handy, L., Chambers, J., & Wright, S. (1988). Cerebral damage and dysfunction in sexually aggressive men. *Annals of Sex Research*, 1, 33–47.

Hucker, S., Langevin, R., Wortzman, G., Bain, J., Handy, L., Chambers, J., et al. (1986). Neuropsychological impairment in pedophiles. *Canadian Journal of Behavioural Science*, 18, 440–448.

Kolton, D. J. C., Boer, A., & Boer, D. P. (2001). A revision of the Abel and Becker Cognition Scale for intellectually disabled offenders. *Sexual Abuse*, 13, 217–220.

Lackey, L. B. & Knopp, F. H. (1989). A summary of selected notes from the working sessions of the First National Training Conference on the Assessment and Treatment of Intellectual Disabled Juvenile and Adult Sexual Offenders. In F. Knopp (Ed.), *Selected readings: Sexual offenders identified as intellectually Disabled*. Orwell, VT: Safer Society Press.

Langevin, R. (1992). A comparison of neuroendocrine abnormalities and genetic factors in homosexuality and in pedophila. *Annals of Sex Research*, 6, 67–76.

Langevin, R. & Curnoe, S. (2002). Assessment and treatment of sex offenders who have a developmental delay. In D. Griffiths, D. Richards, P. Fedoroff, & S. Watson (Eds.), *Ethical dilemmas: Sexuality and developmental disabilities* (pp. 387–416). Kingston, NY: NADD Press.

Langevin, R. & Watson, R. (1996). Major factors in the assessment of paraphilics and sex offenders. *Journal of Offender Therapy*, 23(4), 39–40.

Langevin, R., Wortzman, G., Wright, P., & Hardy, L. (1988). Studies of brain damage and dysfunction in sex offenders. *Annals of Sex Research*, 2, 163–179.

Laski, F. J. (1992). Sentencing the offender with mental retardation: Honoring the imperative for immediate punishments and probation. In R. W. Conley, R. Luckasson, & G. N. Bouthilet (Eds.), *The criminal justice system and mental retardation* (pp. 137–152). Baltimore: Brookes.

Lindsay, W. R., Marshall, I., Neilson, C., Quinn, K., & Smith, A. H. (1998). The treatment of men with a learning disability convicted of exhibitionism. *Research in Developmental Disabilities*, 19(4), 295–316.

Luckasson, R. (1992). People with a developmental disability as victims of crime. In R. W. Conley, R. Luckasson, & G. N. Bouthilet (Eds.), *The criminal justice system and mental retardation: Defendants and victims* (pp. 209–220). Baltimore: Paul H. Brookes.

Lund, C. A. (1992). Long-term treatment of sexual behavior in adolescent and adult developmentally disabled persons. *Annals of Sex Research*, 5, 5–21.

Marinos, V. & Griffiths, D. (2006). *Persons with intellectual disabilities and the courtroom experience.* National Judicial Institute: Ottawa, ON CA.

Marshall, W. L., Hudson, S. M, & Hodkinson, S. (1993). The importance of attachment bonds in the development of juvenile sex offending. In H. E. Barbaree, W. L. Marshall, & S. M. Hudson (Eds.), *The Juvenile Sex Offender* (pp. 164–181). New York, NY: Guilford Press.

Martens, B. K. & Witt, J. C. (1988). Ecological behavior analysis. In M. Hersen, R. M. Eisler, & P. M. Miller (Eds.), *Progress in behavior modification* (pp. 115–140). Newbury Park, CA: Sage.

Masten, A. S. (2001). Ordinary magic: Resilience processes in development. *American Psychologist*, 56, 227–238.

McCabe, M. P. (1994). *Sexual knowledge, experience, feelings and needs scale for people with intellectual disability, (Sex Ken-ID) (Fourth Edition).* Burwood, Australia: Deakin University.

McCabe, M. P., Cummins, R. A., & Deeks, A. A. (1999). Construction and psychometric properties of sexuality scales: Sex knowledge, experience, and needs scales for people with intellectual disabilities (SexKen-ID), people with physical disabilities (SexKen-PD), and the general population. *Research in Intellectual Disabilities*, 20, 241–254.

McGee, J. & Menolasino, F. J. (1992). The evaluation of defendants with mental retardation in the criminal justice system. In R. W. Conley, R. Luckasson, & G. N. Bouthilet (Eds.), *The criminal justice system and mental retardation: Defendants and victims* (pp. 55–78). Baltimore: Paul. H. Brookes.

Miller, M. (2002). Resilience elements in students with learning disabilities. *Journal of Clinical Psychology*, 58, 291–298.

Miltenberger, R. G., Roberts, J. A., Ellingson, S., Galenski, T., Rapp, J. T., Long, E. S., et al. (1999). Training and generalization of sexual abuse prevention skills for women with mental retardation. *Journal of Applied Behavior Analysis*, 32, 385–38.

Money, J. & Lamacz, M. (1989). *Vandalized lovemaps.* Buffalo, NY: Prometheus.

Murphy, W. D. (1990). Assessment and modification of cognitive distortions in sex offenders. In W. L. Marshall, D. R. Laws, & H. E. Barbarree (Eds.), *Handbook of sexual assault: Issues, theories and treatment of the offender* (pp. 331–342). New York, NY: Plenum.

Murphy, G. H. (2003). Capacity to consent to sexual relationships in adults with learning disabilities. *Journal of Family Planning and Reproductive Health Care*, 28(3), 148–149.

Murphy, W. D., Coleman, E. M., & Abel, G. G. (1983a). Human sexuality in the mentally retarded. In J. L. Matson & F. Andrasik (Eds.), *Treatment issues and innovations in mental retardation* (pp. 581–643). New York, NY: Plenum.

Murphy, W. D., Coleman, E. M., & Haynes, M. (1983b). Treatment and evaluation issues with the mentally retarded sex offender. In J. Greer & I. Stuart (Eds.), *The sexual aggressor: Current perspectives on treatment* (pp. 22–41). New York: Van Nostrand Reinhold.

Murrey, G. J., Briggs, D., & Davis, C. (1992). Psychopathic disordered, mentally ill, and mentally handicapped offenders: A comparative study. *Medical Law Science*, 32(4), 331–336.

Neef, N. A., Lensbower, J., Hockersmith, I., & DePalma, V. (1990). In vivo versus simulation training: An interactional analysis of range and type of training exemplars. *Journal of Applied Behavior Analysis*, 23, 447–458.

Nezu, C. M., Nezu, A. M., & Gill-Weiss, M. (1992). *Psychopathology in persons with mental retardation: Clinical guidelines for assessment and treatment.* Champaign, Il: Research Press.

Nezu, C. M., Nezu, A. M., & Dudek, J. A. (1998). A cognitive behavioral model of assessment and treatment for intellectually disabled sex offenders. *Cognitive and Behavioral Practice*, 5, 25–64.

Nolley, D., Muccigrosso, L., & Zigman, E. (1996). Treatment successes with mentally retarded sex offenders. In E. Coleman, M. Dwyer, & N. Pallone (Eds.), *Sex offenders treatment*: Biological dysfunctional, intrapsychic conflict, interpersonal violence (pp. 125–141). Hawthorn, UK: Hawthorn Press.

Pithers, W. D. (1993). Considerations in the treatment of rapist. In G. C. N. Hall, R. Hircshman, J. R. Graham, & M. S. Zaragosa (Eds.), Sexual aggression: Issues in etiology, assessment and treatment (pp. 167–196). Washington DC: Taylor & Francis.

Pithers, W. D., Beal, L. S., Armstrong, J., & Perry, J. (1989). Identification of risk factors through records analysis and clinical interview. In D. R. Laws (Ed.),

Relapse prevention with sex offenders (pp. 77–87). New York, NY: Guilford Press.

Quinsey, V. L., Coleman, G., Jones, B., & Altrows, I. (1997). Proximal antecedents of eloping and reoffending among mentally disordered offenders. *Journal of Interpersonal Violence*, 12, 794–813.

Quinsey, V. L., Harris, G. T., Rice, M. E., & Cormier, C. A. (1998). Violent offenders: Appraising and managing risk. Washington, D.C.: American Psychological Association.

Renwick, R., Brown, I., & Raphael, D. (1994). Quality of life: Linking a conceptual approach to service provision. *Journal on Developmental disabilities*, 3(2), 32–44.

Richards, D., Watson, S., & Bleich, R. (2000). Guidelines and practices for reporting a sexual assault for people who have a developmental disability. *Journal of Developmental Disabilities*, 7(1), 130–140.

Roeher Institute (1988). *Vulnerable: Sexual abuse and people with an intellectual handicap.* Downsview, ON: G. Allan Roeher Institute.

Shapiro, S. (1986). Delinquent and disturbed behavior within the field of mental deficiency. In A. V. S. deReuck & R. Porter (Eds.), *The mentally abnormal offender.* New York: Grune & Stratton.

Sheehan, S. (2004). Consent for sexual relations. In D. Griffiths, D. Richards, P. Fedoroff, & S. Watson (Eds.), *Ethical dilemmas: Sexuality and developmental disabilities* (pp. 133–174). Kingston, NY: NADD Press.

Simmons, H. G. (1982). *From asylum to welfare.* Toronto, ON: National Institute on Mental Retardation.

Sobsey, D. (1994). Violence and abuse in the lives of people with disabilities: The end of silent acceptance? Baltimore, MD: Paul H. Brookes.

Sobsey, D. & Doe, T. (1991). Patterns of Sexual Abuse and Assault. *Sexuality and Disability*, 9, 243–259.

Sobsey, D. & Varnhagen, C. (1991). Sexual abuse, assault, and exploitation of Canadians with disabilities. In C. Bagley & J. Thomlinson (Eds.), *Child sexual abuse: Critical perspectives on prevention, intervention, and treatment* (pp. 203–216). Toronto, ON: Wall & Emerson.

Steiner, J. (1984) Group counselling with retarded offenders. *Social Work*, 29, 181–182.

Swanson, C. K. & Garwick, F. B. (1990). Treatment for low functioning sex offenders: Group therapy and interagency cooperation. *Mental Retardation*, 28, 155–161.

Timmers, R. L., Du Charme, P. & Jacob, G. (1981). Sexual knowledge, attitudes and behavior of developmentally disabled adults living in a normalised apartment setting. *Sexuality and Disability*, 4, 27–39.

Toberg, M. A. (1992). *Pretrial release: A national evaluation of practice and outcomes.* McLean, VA: Lazar Institute.

Tudiver, J. Broekstra, S., Josselyn, S., & Barbaree, H. (1997). *Addressing the needs of developmentally delayed sex offenders: A guide.* Ottawa, Canada: Health Canada.

Valenti-Heins, D. C. & Schwartz L. D. (1993). Witness competency in people with mental retardation: Implications for prosecution of sexual abuse. *Sexuality and Disability*, 11, 287–294.

Ward, K. M., Heffern, S. J., Wilcox, D. A., McElwee, B. S., Dowrick, P., Brown, M. J., et al. (1992). *Managing inappropriate sexual behavior: Supporting individuals with developmental disabilities in the community.* Anchorage, AL: Alaska Specialized Training Services.

Watson, S., Griffiths, D., Richards D., & Dykstra, L. (2003). Sex education. In D. Griffiths, D. Richards, P. Fedoroff, & S. Watson (Eds.), *Ethical dilemmas: Sexuality and developmental disabilities* (pp. 387–416). Kingston, NY: NADD Press.

White, D. L. & Wood, H. (1988). Lancaster Counter MRO Program, In J. A. Stark, F. J. Menolascino, M. H. Albarelli, & C. C. Gray (Eds.), *Mental retardation/mental health: Classification, diagnosis, treatment, services.* New York, NY: Springer-Verlag.

Whitehouse, M. A. & McCabe, M. P. (1997). Sex education programs for people with Intellectual disability: How effective are they? *Education and Training in Mental Retardation and Intellectual Disabilities*, 32, 229–240.

Part VII

Forensics

Chapter 26

Forensic Considerations

Rusty Reeves and Richard Rosner

As described throughout this book, the identification, evaluation, and treatment of a sex offender requires specialized knowledge within the broader areas of forensic psychiatry and psychology. On the other hand, the forensic evaluation of a sex offender follows a principle common to all forensic evaluations. That is, all forensic psychiatric and psychological evaluations require the rational organization and analysis of data. A four-step method devised by Richard Rosner (2003) allows such rational organization and analysis. The four steps are issue, legal criteria, data, and reasoning.

Issue: What is the specific psychiatric—or psycholog-ical—legal issue?

Legal criteria: What are the legal criteria that will be used to resolve theissue?

Data: What are the data relevant to the legal criteria that will be used to resolve the issue?

Reasoning: How may the data be applied to the legal criteria to establish a rational psychiatric or psycho-logical opinion?

ISSUE

In any given forensic evaluation, whether a sex offender evaluation or not, numerous psychiatric—or psychological—legal issues may arise. The first step an evaluator takes is the identification of the specific legal issue or issues that the referring party wishes the evaluator to address. A judge, attorney, or mental health agency often will ask for a "psychiatric evalua-tion" of a defendant—and leave it at that. The evalua-tor is then left to identify the legal issue involved. Do not guess. The evaluator should instead contact the referring person and determine the precise legal issue or issues the referrer wishes the evaluator to address. If the evaluator fails to identify the correct issue or issues, the evaluator's report might address irrelevant issues, and thus prove not only useless to the legal system but also inimical to the evaluator's forensic career. Such mistakes are more common than one might think.

In a sex offender evaluation, for example, a judge might ask for just that—a "sex offender evaluation." The evaluator should clarify the issue or issues involved. The judge might want to know treatment options for an identified sex offender. Alternatively or in addition, the judge might want to know the nature of a sex offender's psychopathology, if any, and the risk of recidivism the offender poses. The issues might be more generic: competence to stand trial, legal insanity, and termination of parental rights are all issues that could arise in an evaluation of a sex offender. In jurisdictions with Sexually Violent Predator (SVP) statutes, the judge might wish to know whether a known sex offender is civilly committable under one of these statutes. In a typical forensic evaluation of a sex offender, several issues are involved. Each issue requires a separate evaluation according to the relevant legal criteria in the particular jurisdiction (see "Criteria" subsequently).

CRITERIA

There are numerous legal arenas in which a given forensic issue is relevant. Most legal systems are arranged hierarchically. For example, the United States has its federal, military, and 50 state jurisdictions plus the District of Columbia. A separate set of statutes (laws created by a legislature), case law (rulings made by judges), and administrative code (policies created by bureaucracies) govern each of these jurisdictions. Statutes, case law, and administrative code offer the legal criteria which define an issue. Thus, for the purposes of a forensic evaluation, statutes, case law, and administrative code all function as "law."

Numerous and diverse jurisdictions and their subdivisions ensure that the legal criteria defining an issue are themselves numerous and diverse. The forensic evaluator must be certain of the jurisdiction in which the evaluator is working, and then be certain of the legal criteria applicable to an issue within that jurisdiction. Such knowledge requires familiarity with the arrangement of the legal system within one's country. An evaluator also requires a means to

access the relevant criteria. Asking the referring attorney for the criteria is the most simple and most common means. The attorney should provide a written statement of the criteria. An oral report is unreliable. The attorney may be uncertain of the precise criteria. This circumstance is not uncommon, especially in SVP practice in which the law is evolving and is subject to constant challenge. The evaluator should either insist that the criteria be made available, or be independently certain of the criteria. If the criteria one uses in an evaluation are incorrect, one's opinion is logically unsupported. Subscriptions to legal publications (e.g., Westlaw) are an independent means for an evaluator to access the legal criteria. The Internet is tempting, tedious, and disappointing. Searches are slow, and the free information that is available (when it is available) is almost always incomplete.

Simply finding the criteria is insufficient. The criteria may be vague, and thus open to interpretation. For example, SVP statutes require, as a criterion for commitment, that an examinee exhibit a personality disorder or mental abnormality that makes one likely to commit acts of sexual violence. This ostensible single criterion actually contains within it terms that are themselves criteria (i.e., "mental abnormality," "personality disorder," "likely," and "acts of sexual violence"). An evaluator should not presume an understanding of these several criteria. For example, what does "likely" mean? Does it mean, as might seem intuitively obvious, 51% probability of recidivism? If so, over what period? Or does "likely" mean something else entirely?

In New Jersey, for example, "likely to engage in acts of sexual violence" is statutorily defined (NJSA [a]) to mean "the propensity of a person to commit acts of sexual violence is of such a degree as to pose a threat to the health or safety of others." If that definition is no less vague than the term it defines, New Jersey case law is equally unhelpful. The New Jersey Supreme Court construed the legislature's definition as requiring that a sex offender have "serious difficulty controlling his or her harmful sexual behavior such that it is highly likely that the person will not control his or her sexually violent behavior and will reoffend" (In re Commitment of W.Z). Thus we are back to "likely," again, but no further enlightened. One must peruse the court's dicta in the aforementioned case to learn that the court rejects the requirement that "likely" means a quantifiable standard, such as 51% chance of recidivism. In other words, "likely," in New Jersey means whatever amount and type of risk the judge considers unacceptable for the community to bear.

Although the term "likely" may be a definitional quagmire, not all criteria in SVP law are so troublesome. "Acts of sexual violence" are explicitly defined in the various SVP statutes, and typically include contact offenses (e.g., sexual assault) as opposed to noncontact offenses. (e.g., exhibitionism) However, even with this criterion there are wrinkles. In New Jersey, a sexual contact offense includes a perpetrator's sexual contact with himself (NJSA [b]). Therefore masturbation in the presence of a victim would be a sexually violent offense under New Jersey SVP law. Such peculiarities are common in other states as well, and demand close attention by the evaluator.

Then there are the terms "mental abnormality" and "personality disorder." These terms are so broad and ill-defined that an experienced practitioner in this area could be tempted to make an argument for a "mental abnormality" or a "personality disorder" in just about any sex offender. For example, antisocial personality disorder has been established in case law as a qualifying personality disorder under SVP statutes. Persons with antisocial personality disorder are at greater risk that those without the disorder to commit crimes of all sorts, *including* sex offenses. However, there is nothing about the *generic* antisocial personality disorder (at least as it is defined in the *Diagnostic and Statistical Manual of Mental Disorders—Fourth Edition, Text Revision* [DSM-IV-TR] [2000a]) that predisposes a person to commit sex offenses *in particular*. Yet courts accept this diagnosis with its limited albeit real association with sex offenses. An evaluator might also write that an offender's *particular manifestation* of his antisocial personality disorder includes sex offenses. Courts accept this argument also. However, this argument could be criticized for associating an offender's sex offenses too closely with the offender's antisocial personality disorder when perhaps it is some other mental condition—some as yet unidentified and unnamed mental state—that could better account for an offender's commission of sex offenses.

The situation is even more fraught with potential error when the qualifying diagnosis is "Personality Disorder NOS (Not otherwise specified)" or "Paraphilia NOS (Not otherwise specified)." In this situation, the evaluator is not constrained by established DSM-IV-TR personality disorder or paraphilic diagnoses and their criteria, but instead mixes and matches criteria from various personality disorder and paraphilic diagnoses, or creates diagnostic criteria de novo. One must be careful in this situation not to create a specious diagnosis simply to account for an offense. A common example of this situation is when an adult is attracted to, and engages in mutually voluntary sexual activity with postpubescent adolescents who are statutorily unable to provide consent (typically 14- and 15-year-olds.) Does this offender have a paraphilia? Is it a version of Pedophilia which is defined in DSM-IV-TR [2000b] as attraction to prepubescent children? Or is it something else? Does this person have any diagnosable mental disorder? That the offender broke the law is insufficient evidence, by itself, for the establishment of a psychiatric diagnosis. According to DSM-IV-TR (2000c), the key to whether such an offender exhibits a paraphilia is whether the offender's victims were able to give consent to the sexual activity. Simply because the law says an individual is unable to give consent, does not make it so within a psychiatric evaluation. Evidence suggests that many 14-year-olds have developed the decision-making capacities of adults (see summary of sources in Melton, Lyons, & Spaulding, 1998). If the offender's victims were able to give consent, the authors argue that such an offender does not have a paraphilia even if that offender commits socially objectionable acts.

On the other hand, under particular circumstances, the establishment of a qualifying diagnosis whose only evidence is the offenses themselves is entirely legitimate, and represents neither a tautology nor a capitulation to the prosecution. For example, an adult male who is convicted on four separate occasions of having sex with 8- to 10-year-old boys is a pedophile—whether that person admits to committing the acts or to experiencing pedophilic desires. Establishing a psychiatric diagnosis by behavior, including criminal behavior, is the nature of psychiatric and psychological practice. That is, we infer mental conditions from behavior, as we take as axiomatic a determinism in which all behavior arises from brain activity.

Although one can easily criticize the ambiguities in SVP law, the situation is not a free-for-all. The law does establish the rough boundaries of the issue. Even within the ambiguity of SVP law, an evaluator is unlikely to recommend, for example, commitment of a one-time incest offender with no diagnosis of Pedophilia and no other criminal history. Such an offender lacks a qualifying psychiatric diagnosis and (using actuarial instruments) most likely also represents a low risk for recidivism.

The foregoing paragraphs illustrate an essential problem in SVP law. That is, sexual recidivism in SVP statutes is keyed to psychiatric diagnoses when, as explained elsewhere in this book, recidivism is better predicted by things such as age of the offender, number of past offenses, and characteristics of the victims, rather than with psychiatric diagnoses. An evaluator performing SVP evaluations should keep this dilemma in mind, if only to clarify for oneself this messy mixing of psychiatry and law.

DATA

After the evaluator identifies the legal issue and the criteria defining the issue, the evaluator then gathers the data relevant to the criteria defining the issue. An old admonition bears repeating: forensic assessments are not confidential in the way that medical and therapeutic records are. The judges, attorneys, parole and probation officers, and other agencies requesting these evaluations use the same to render legal or administrative decisions that might benefit or hurt the examinee. Before a forensic evaluator conducts an evaluation, the evaluator must warn the subject about the purpose of the assessment, the lack of confidentiality, that the evaluator is not functioning as a therapist, and that the subject may choose not to participate (although the evaluator will complete the evaluation with or without the subject's participation.) Such a warning is required by the ethical guidelines of professional psychiatric and psychological societies (Weinstock, Leong, & Silva, 2003).

The consequences of sex offender evaluations are serious. Outcomes may involve a person's liberty, a person's reputation, and the stigma that will likely follow a person for the rest of the person's days. The subject of a sex offender evaluation has ample motivation to dissemble. Furthermore, many sex offenders are ambivalent about their offenses, and are defended against acknowledging both to themselves and to others the nature and extent of their crimes and passions. Such persons may require many years of confrontation and treatment before they even begin to acknowledge their thoughts and deeds. They may have been arrested many a time for sex offenses, and yet continue to offer superficially plausible and convincing

excuses for how they were framed by a jealous lover, mistakenly identified, caught in a sweep, and so on—the excuses are endless in their number and variety. Only when one steps back and regards, for example, the implausibility of three "unjustified" arrests for rape does one realize the skill with which offenders lie. Therefore, the forensic evaluator remains skeptical of any unsupported claim made by an examinee. A useful dialectic is, "Listen carefully, and never believe a word they say."

Pay close attention to the examinee's statements for contradictions, distortions, minimizations, and evasions. The examiner should persist in pursuing ostensibly closed lines of inquiry. These apparent dead ends may actually be the examinee's attempts to block disclosure through vagueness, circumlocution, distraction, and denial. The examiner compares the statements, behavior, and mental state of the examinee to what the examiner knows about genuine sex offender psychopathology and general psychopathology. A good evaluator is a good diagnostician. The evaluator should therefore maintain at least a part-time clinical practice.

Of equal or greater importance than the interview is the review of collateral information. Such a review is more useful than the interview itself when the issue is recidivism—as recidivism is currently predicted best by static factors such as number and type of sex offenses, age of the examinee, and type of victims. An evaluator does not require an interview to ascertain this historical information. Indeed the interview may actually prove counterproductive when assessing risk of recidivism. The examinee's statements about himself and his crimes may be wildly inaccurate. The evaluator might also be fooled by the examinee's intellectual understanding of his psychopathology and his apparent sincerity in avoiding reoffense.

Collateral information also allows the evaluator to investigate the truthfulness of the examinee's statements. An examinee's statements gain credibility if independent documentation supports the statements—and vice versa. Typical sources of historical information in a sex offender evaluation include criminal history, criminal complaints, police reports, records of institutional adjustment, actuarial assessments, general psychiatric records, statements from clinicians, and, of course, previous forensic evaluations.

At the same time that an evaluator is skeptical of an examinee's statements, the evaluator should also be skeptical of oral and written reports provided by the prosecution. Prosecutors are overworked. Their oral recounting of an offender's crimes may be inaccurate. Prosecutors are also, unsurprisingly, pro-prosecution. Their bias is toward conviction and incarceration. An evaluator does well to rely upon written reports rather than oral reports. However, even written reports contain errors. This is particularly true over time. Compared with original written reports, subsequent written reports referring to earlier reports invariably lose information, and sometimes even change information. The losses and changes may work for or against the examinee. Therefore, an evaluator should seek the earliest available documents.

If, in conducting an evaluation, the evaluator thinks that something is missing, then it is missing. The evaluator should seek the missing information. Such searches may involve securing a judge's order for release of information, and making numerous, unhelpful phone calls before one reaches the person who can actually answer the evaluator's question. These delays and hassles are a routine aspect of forensic work. The result, however, is a more accurate report. The evaluator also spares himself or herself the embarrassment of having a sedulous judge or attorney point out the missing information.

Normative tests and physiological arousal tests are additional diagnostic tools in sex offender evaluations. These tools are growing in number, diversity, and accuracy, and are slowly replacing unsupported and untested individual clinical opinion. A normative test is a test in which the distribution of results is known within a population. Such a test offers an established reliability and validity. A particular type of normative test, the actuarial assessment (discussed in Chapter 6), is now the standard of practice in assessing risk of sexual recidivism. Although an actuarial assessment is intended to remove clinical judgment from the evaluation, most actuarial assessments do require a modicum of professional judgment. More importantly, actuarial assessments require assiduous adherence to the coding rules of each particular instrument. The rules may seem intuitive, but they often are not. Conducting these assessments under time pressure, as deceptively simple as the assessment may seem, will result in errors that could have profound consequences. Furthermore, a given actuarial assessment may be inappropriate if the individual being evaluated differs from the members of population on which the test was developed. For

example, the Minnesota Sex Offender Screening Tool—Revised is explicitly contraindicated for incest offenders (Epperson et al. 1998).

Penile plethysmography is a useful independent measure of the object of a test-taker's sexual arousal. Sexual arousal to illicit objects (e.g., children) is, in turn, one of the strongest general predictors of sexual recidivism (Hanson & Morton-Bourgon, 2004.) Penile plethysmography is, unfortunately, and for various reasons described elsewhere in this book (Chapter 7), an underutilized diagnostic tool.

The support of normative testing and physiological arousal testing does not place one's final opinion beyond dispute, but does make one's opinion unlikely to be dismissed altogether as being unreliable, invalid, and obscure or idiosyncratic in its reasoning.

REASONING

After the evaluator gathers the data relevant to the legal criteria, the evaluator proceeds with what is arguably the most difficult part of the evaluation: the application of the data to the criteria to establish a rational opinion. The reasoning process requires not only logical thinking, but also logical thinking articulated on paper. The structure of a forensic opinion should follow the three steps of a syllogism. The first step is the assertion of a premise: All cheeses are curd separated from whey. The second step is the assertion of a minor premise or fact: Stilton is a cheese. The third step is a deductive inference or conclusion which follows from the premise and fact: Stilton is curd separated from whey.

In a forensic opinion, the premise is the legal criteria. The fact is the data relevant to the criteria. The conclusion is the final opinion. Take the generic SVP law, for example. A SVP is a person convicted of a sexually violent offense who suffers from a mental abnormality or a personality disorder that makes the person likely to engage in acts of sexual violence if not confined (the premise.) Mr. Smith is convicted of a sexually violent offense, suffers from Pedophilia, and has committed multiple pedophilic offenses even after numerous apprehensions (the fact). Therefore, Mr. Smith is an SVP (the conclusion).

Each step in a forensic opinion may be incorrect, and thus is open to refutation. The legal criteria may be incorrect—in a SVP evaluation, in a given jurisdiction, an evaluator might incorrectly assume that "likely to commit acts of sexual violence" means a 51% probability of recidivism over a lifetime. The data may not relate to the criteria: a mental status examination in the absence of a discussion of a person's sexual history neither supports nor refutes the question of whether an offender exhibits a mental abnormality or personality disorder associated with sexual offenses. The final opinion may have little or no relation to the criteria and data: a conclusion that a person requires antiandrogen treatment to reduce his risk of recidivism does not answer the question posed by an SVP evaluation of whether the person exhibits a mental abnormality or personality disorder that makes one likely to commit acts of sexual violence.

The forensic evaluator should assume that an intelligent and skeptical layperson will be reading the report. Jargon should be avoided unless it is subsequently explained. The evaluator should take time to explain clinical phenomena which the evaluator's experience has made obvious. Givens in therapeutic practice should be critically evaluated and supported with references in the scientific literature. Various contingent recommendations should be offered in anticipation of various judicial outcomes. Uncertainties—and uncertainties are the norm in this business—should be acknowledged. Such explanations are often more difficult to articulate than they might seem. In addition, the evaluator will routinely find that clinical assumptions the evaluator makes have little basis in the scientific literature.

For example, practitioners in sexual disorders know as a commonplace that incest offenders are, on average, at lower risk of recidivism than are extrafamilial offenders. However, a referring judge or agency may be entirely ignorant of this crucial distinction. An evaluator should make this distinction explicit, and should support the distinction with references to recidivism studies. On the other hand, the reason *why* incest offenders have a lower rate of recidivism is open to speculation. It might be that incest offenders exhibit better overall self-control than nonincest offenders. Or it might be that, with an exclusive incest offender, it is easy to remove and thus protect a single victim. Other explanations are also possible. The evaluator should explicitly state these limits of knowledge. Acknowledgement of uncertainty is not a reflection upon one's skill as a forensic evaluator. Rather, acknowledgement of uncertainty is a reflection of the primitiveness and difficulty of the science of prediction of human behavior. Normative data are simply unavailable to contribute to many assessments. Acknowledgement of uncertainty also adds to one's credibility as it reflects honesty. Finally, acknowledgment of uncertainty allows the trier of fact to place an opinion in perspective, and weight the opinion accordingly.

A forensic evaluation culminates in a written report. Courtroom testimony represents but a small fraction of forensic work. A well-written report may even render testimony superfluous. Thus the ability to write logically, comprehensively, and relevantly is an essential skill for the forensic practitioner. Although various formats for reports exist (Silva, Weinstock, & Leong, 2003), the following format is useful for most forensic reports, including sex offender evaluations:

I. *Identifying Data*—the name and date of birth of the examinee, the date of the evaluation, the date of the report, and the name of the evaluator

II. *Reason for referral*—the person or agency requesting the referral, the legal issue, and the legal criteria defining the issue

III. *Opinion*—following the convention of judicial opinion, the forensic evaluator's opinion should sit near the beginning of the report. The opinion should be stated in language meeting the legal standard for the issue at hand

IV. *Sources of information*—persons interviewed, dates of interviews, documents reviewed, and dates the documents were created

V. *Warning of lack of confidentiality*—a statement warning the examinee of the purpose of the evaluation and who will see the report, and an estimate of the examinee's comprehension of the warning

VI. *Relevant history*—the offense or incident that led to the referral with reports of the examinee and others, criminal history, psychiatric history, medical history, family history, and social and developmental history

VII. *Mental status examination*—appearance, attitude, movements, orientation, attention, memory, fund of knowledge, intelligence, speech, mood, range of emotional expression, perception, thought process, thought content, and insight into one's mental illness and/or circumstance precipitating the evaluation

VIII. *Test Results*—the results of normative testing (e.g., actuarial assessments)

IX. *Diagnostic Formulation*—an organization of the aforementioned data supporting a diagnosis, if any, including an acknowledgment of the diagnostic system and criteria that are used

X. *Forensic Formulation*—an organization of the aforementioned data which applies the data to the legal criteria and issue, and identifies the reasoning used to reach one's conclusion.

CONCLUSION

Rational organization and analysis in a forensic psychiatric or psychological report allows one to manage large amounts of complex data. Because forensic mental health issues rarely reach the level of scientific certainty that other areas of scientific inquiry do (e.g., as in DNA analysis), a common conceptual framework allows areas of uncertainty or disagreement to be highlighted and explained. A common framework also allows efficient communication among colleagues. Finally, rational organization and analysis is likely to make one's presentation more effective.

References

Diagnostic and statistical manual of mental disorders—fourth edition, text revision (p. 706). (2000a). Washington, D.C.: American Psychiatric Association.

Diagnostic and statistical manual of mental disorders—fourth edition, text revision (p. 572). (2000b). Washington, D.C.: American Psychiatric Association.

Diagnostic and statistical manual of mental disorders—fourth edition, text revision (p. 566). (2000c). Washington, D.C.: American Psychiatric Association.

Epperson, D. L., Kaul, J. D., & Hesselton, D. (1998). Final report on the development of the Minnesota Sex Offender Screening Tool—Revised (MnSOST-R). Paper presented at the 17th Annual Conference of the Association for the Treatment of Sexual Abusers. Vancouver, Canada.

Hanson, R. K. & Morton-Bourgon, K. (2004). Predictors of sexual recidivism: An updated meta-analysis 2004–02, Public Works and Government Services Canada, available at www.psepc-sppcc.gc.ca/publications/corrections/pdf/200402_e.pdf.

In re Commitment of W.Z., 339 N.J. Super. 549, 773 A.2d 97 [A.D. 2001], certification granted 169 N.J. 611, 782 A. 2d 428, affirmed as modified 173 N.J. 109, 801 A. 2d 205.

Melton, G., Lyons, P., & Spaulding, W. (1998). *No place to go—the civil commitment of minors* (p. 128). Lincoln, NE: University of Nebraska Press.

New Jersey Statutes Annotated (a) 30:4–27, et. seq., 2008.

New Jersey Statutes Annotated (b) 2C:14–1d., 2008.

Rosner, R. (2003) A conceptual framework for forensic psychiatry. In R. Rosner (Ed.), *Principles and practice of forensic psychiatry, 2nd edition* (pp. 3–6). London: Arnold.

Silva, J. A., Weinstock, R., & Leong, G. B. (2003). Forensic psychiatric report writing. In R. Rosner (Ed.), *Principles and practice of forensic psychiatry, 2nd edition* (pp. 31–36). London: Arnold.

Weinstock, R., Leong, G. B., & Silva, J. A. (2003). Defining forensic psychiatry: Roles and responsibilities. In R. Rosner (Ed.), *Principles and practice of forensic psychiatry, 2nd edition* (pp. 7–13). London: Arnold.

Chapter 27

Sexual Predator Laws
and their History

*Albert J. Grudzinskas, Jr., Daniel J. Brodsky,
Matt Zaitchik, J. Paul Fedoroff,
Frank DiCataldo, and Jonathan C. Clayfield*

For centuries, the criminal justice system has struggled to define the methodology of and the justifications for social control of sexual behavior that does not conform to community mores. This chapter will compare and contrast the historical and contemporary attempts in the United States and Canada to address the risk created by individuals who engage in behaviors broadly characterized as sexually deviant. It will consider the rationale for sentencing, and the earliest attempts to bring "treatment" into the criminal dispositional formula for sex offense based prosecution. It will also consider the impact that the choice of societal response has on risk assessment and evaluation in the two systems, including the assessment and commitment of juvenile offenders (for a more comprehensive discussion of risk assessment, see Chapter 5). The current United States practice of civil commitment for a person deemed to be a sexually violent predator (SVP) will be discussed beginning with the U.S. Supreme Court decision in *Kansas versus Hendricks*. This practice will then be compared and

contrasted with the Canadian approach of designating an offender as a dangerous offender (DO) or a long-term offender (LTO) under the criminal law. This chapter is intended as an overview of the law, as it exists, and not as a defense or a critique of any specific model.

COMMON LAW ORIGINS FOR CANADA AND THE UNITED STATES

Under English Common Law those offenses not specifically punishable at common law that involved matters of morality and family were assumed under the jurisdiction of the ecclesiastic courts. In 1558, the Court of High Commission was established by the English upper social classes. For a period until the middle of seventeenth century, crimes against morality (such as adultery, bigamy, incest, assault with intent to ravish, and blasphemy) were addressed by concurrent jurisdiction of the ecclesiastic courts and the Court of High Commission. An offender's economic and social rank often determined the venue. Penalties in the Court of High Commission actually proved to be more severe than those meted out by the ecclesiastic courts. Sanctions from both bodies however ignored the sentencing concept of proportionality and lacked connection to the prevalence of the acts or to the harmfulness of the offense. Although the ecclesiastic courts enjoyed a brief resurgence after the return of the monarchy in 1660, the common law eventually took control of matters of sexual aberration (Group for the Advancement of Psychiatry, GAP,[1] 1977).

The historical origin of the system, Parliament, enacted for protecting the public from mentally disordered individuals who pose a threat to the safety of others is also ancient and still evolving[2]. In fact, the present day legislative schemes in both Canada and the United States can be traced back through the writings of Sir Matthew Hale in the seventeenth century on the special verdict of "acquittal and enlargement," Sir Edward Coke in the sixteenth century and Brackton in the thirteenth century, and with rudimentary beginnings even earlier to Aristotle's fourth century bipartite division of knowing and acting. Before the invention of medicine, psychiatry, or psychology it was commonly believed that the only way to protect society was to keep mentally disordered offenders from places where they could cause harm.[3] Efforts to come to grips with the problem included the enactment of civil statutes such as the Vagrancy Act of 1744, but their use was informal and irregular. Under common law there was little difference if insanity was raised before the trial or as a defense because it was the question of "dangerousness" itself that informed detention status of the prisoner, as well as readiness for release even if the cause of the risk was unknown. There was no criminal sanction available to restrain insane acquittees and some considered it to be a problem that accused would "go at large" after a verdict (Keeton, 1961; MacDonald et al. v. Vapour Canada, 1977; R. v. LePage, 1994; Starnaman v. MHC-P, 1995; Walker, 1968; Winko v. British Columbia [Forensic Psychiatric Institute], 1999).

Early U.S. History

In the early colonial history of the United States, English common law principles prevailed in most jurisdictions. Sin and crime were often equated, and

treatment was tied to bodily punishment such as public flogging to prevent the "recurrence of individual sexual transgressors" (GAP, 1977, p. 847) and to serve as a deterrent to others. Enforcement of morals and religious values was seen as the purpose of the law. In fact the language of the Old Testament was incorporated into the language of statutes enacted by the colonies. In Massachusetts for example, since at least 1697, Sodomy and Buggery were defined as "abominable and detestable crimes against nature, either with mankind or with a beast" (MASS. GEN. LAW, c. 272, § 34 as quoted in GAP, 1977, 848–849). The definition remains the same in the 2007 edition of the statutes. The punishment, originally death in some jurisdictions, has been reduced to "imprisonment in the state prison for not more than twenty years."

The concept supporting punishment of the crime of rape has also evolved over time. Originally, rape of a "propertied virgin," was punishable by death and dismemberment, and included the severing of the tails of the offender's horse and dog (Bracton, 1968 as quoted in GAP, 1977, p. 850). As the colonies evolved into states, the common law evolved into criminal codes. Defenses made available for other criminal acts became available for sex crimes. "Some offenders were found incompetent to stand trial, others occasionally pled insanity when some major offense involving sexual violence occurred, and still others were handled civilly as being mentally ill and a final disposition was postponed indefinitely" (GAP, 1977, p. 851–852).

Early History in Canada

The contemporary Canadian model of preventative detention for noninsane offenders can be traced back to the Gladstone Committee Report in England (Gladstone Report, 1895) at the junction of two comparatively recent trends in modern British and American criminology: the expanding influence of the psychiatric interpretation of crime as symptomatic of mental disorder[4] and increasing confidence in the scientific method and empirical analysis to understand human behavior.[5] In 1895 the Report of the Departmental Committee on Prisons urged law reformers to exercise restraint when legal innovation in the name of science is based upon deduction or hypothesis, rather than empirical proof or proven guilt for acts committed, it is not unreasonable to acquiesce in the theory that criminality is a disease, and the result of physical imperfection...[and]...the time has come when the main principles and methods adopted by the Prison Acts should be seriously tested by the light of acquired experience and scientific research...(Gladstone Report, 1895, p. 5,8, and 34).

PRISON REFORM, OSCAR WILDE, AND THE GLADSTONE COMMITTEE

We punish and have always punished for many reasons including the accomemphatic demand by an alarmed public for severe reprisal or denunciation. By the late 1800s, a belief in punishment as the only object of sentencing and confidence in the prison system as a desirable and effective means of dealing with prisoners came increasingly into question (Hart, 1962). In 1841, Dorothea Dix exposed the terrible conditions under which Massachusetts housed inmates with mental illness at the East Cambridge jail. She began a crusade for prison reform and national legislation to provide for persons with mental illness who found themselves incarcerated. In January 1894, the London Daily Chronicle published a critical expose on London prisons that called into question the treatment of mentally disordered offenders. It also called into question the supposition that an insanity defense would always be sought if it were available; the assumption being that, trial counsel would recognize the issue and proceed accordingly. Other journals such as Truth, Pall Mall Gazette, and the Weekly Dispatch followed suit. The Liberal government considered it "a sweeping indictment" by the media "against the whole of the prison administration" including "the principles of prison treatment as prescribed by the Prison Acts." Home Secretary Herbert Asquith acted on June 5, 1894 by setting up a prison committee under Herbert John Gladstone to inquire to and report on the administration of prisons in England and the treatment of offenders, including juveniles, detained in them (Gladstone Report, 1895).

The Gladstone Committee's terms of reference were expanded on January 16, 1895 to include the prison treatment of "habitual criminals" and the classification of prisoners generally. The Prison Committee cited unchallenged evidence that, "as a criminal passes into the habitual class, prison life, subject to the sentences now given, loses its terrors and as familiarity with it increases."

The Committee was surprised to discover "that previous inquires have almost altogether overlooked this all important matter. The habitual criminals ..."

In examining the overlooked group of prisoners, the Committee noted that,

(i) Punishment for the particular offense in which the habitual offender was detected was almost useless because the real offense, it was thought, was the wilful persistence in the deliberately acquired habit of crime.

(ii) Habitual criminals were members of an undeterrable class because the prison regimen had little or no deterrent effect unless the offender was subjected to long periods of imprisonment and penal servitude.

(iii) While, the class of habitual offenders was generally orderly and easy to manage, they are seen as a most undesirable element in a mixed prison population. Therefore, it was proposed that habitual offenders should be kept segregated from other prisoners.

(iv) Most habitual criminals are not of the desperate order who run the risk of comparatively short sentences with comparative indifference.

The Committee would propose that a new form of sentence should be placed at the disposal of the judges involving long-term segregation, but they were not to be treated with the severity of first class hard labor or penal servitude and their forced work should be under less onerous conditions (Gladstone Report, 1895, p. a1–a2, 5, 7, 11–12, and 31).

After 2 months, one of the most infamous chapters in British legal history occurred and brought immense pressure on the uniquely situated Gladstone Investigative Committee.

On March 1, 1895, libel suit charging the Marques of Queensberry with publicly maligning Oscar Wilde as a sodomite brought the problem to the attention of the public. Oscar Wilde was enormously successful as a playwright, novelist, poet, short story writer, and beloved critic of literature and of society (Abrams, 1979; Hyde, 1948). Wilde was a 38-year-old married man when he met and established a homosexual relationship with the 22-year-old poet, Lord Alfred Douglas or "Boisie" as the young Lord was known. Boisie's father, the Marquis of Queensberry, did not approve of the relationship and he was persistent in a campaign to break up the relationship. Queensbury went to the Albermarle Club and told the porter to hand a card to Wilde. The Marquis' card read "Oscar Wilde posing as a Sodomite." Believing that the Marquis had gone too far and needed to be restrained, Wilde initiated a libel action. The trial proceeded before Collins J. at the Old Bailey. Queensberry argued; "isn't any father justified in endeavouring by all means possible to rescue a son from evil companionship?" So well-executed was the defence that Wilde elected to retire from the prosecution and the judge directed the jury to find that while the libel was in fact true, it was published for the protection of the community (Hyde, 1948, p. iv–v, 14–15, 17, 54–58, 102–104, 107–108, 173–176).

The evidence proffered during the aborted libel hearing lead to Wilde's arrest and charge with gross indecency. Wilde pleaded not guilty on April 26, 1895. The first trial proceeded before Charles J. at the Old Bailey and ended with a hung jury. The second trial proceeded before Wills J. but this time the jury returned a guilty verdict. Immediately thereafter, a sentence of 2 years at hard labor was imposed and he was taken to Wandsworth Prison and later to Reading Gaol. The Court would not permit Wilde to say anything on his own behalf before he was handed the maximum penalty permitted under English law. Wills J. had for many years presided over countless rape and murder trials declared Wilde's case to be "the worst" he had ever tried and that the defendant was deserving of the "severest" punishment. Justice Wills stated "In my judgment it [the sentence] is totally inadequate for a case such as this." (Hyde, 1948, p. 59–60, 63, 67, 93, 179–189, 265–266, 272, 336–339).

The iniquitous relationship with Queensberry's son sparked a massive public debate that informed the Gladstone Committee and propelled penal reform in England and abroad. The vexing questions included the following: Did Oscar Wilde show a failure to control his sexual impulses? Could he be cured? If he were at liberty, was Lord Alfred Douglas at risk? Was he likely to engage in homosexual acts with others thereby putting the public at risk? Was he insane or in danger of becoming insane? What could be done to convince him that his conduct was morally wrong? Should the sentence be indeterminate? If not, indeterminate, then what should the interval be

and under what conditions? If so, was treatment possible? How should the treatment be prescribed and monitored? (Hyde, 1948, p. ii–v, 365–366, 371–372).

Throughout the eighteenth century, Sodomy/Buggery was punishable by death[5]. The lesser offense of gross indecency was punishable pursuant to the *Criminal Law Amendment Act 1885* by a term of imprisonment not exceeding 2 years, with or without hard labor. The observations of U.S. Supreme Court Chief Justice Warren Berger in the case of *Bowers v. Hardwick* are apposite:

> the proscriptions against sodomy have very 'ancient roots'. Decisions of individuals relating to homosexual conduct have been subject to state intervention throughout the history of Western civilization. Condemnation of those practices is firmly rooted in Judeao-Christian moral and ethical standards. Homosexual sodomy was a capital crime under Roman law. See Code Theod. 9.7.6, Code Just. 9.9.31, (Bailey, 1975).

During the English Reformation when powers of the ecclesiastical courts were transferred to the King's Courts, the first English statute criminalizing sodomy was passed. 25 Hen. VIII, ch. 6. Blackstone described "the infamous crime against nature" as an offense of "deeper malignity" than rape, a heinous act "the very mention of which is a disgrace to human nature," and "a crime not fit to be named." (Tucker, Tucker, & Blackstone, 1996). The common law of England, including its prohibition of sodomy, became the received law of Georgia and the other Colonies.

The Gladstone Committee report was released on April 10, 1895, just 1 month before Oscar Wilde was committed to prison for 2 years of hard labor. Of course, the issues of Wilde's failed prosecution, arrest, incarceration, and presumptive risk informed the report and are inexorably entwined. The Prison Committee was highly critical of the administrative principles underpinning British prison life and it emphasized the pressing need for treatment in prison to take place alongside deterrence for the protection of the public (Gladstone Report, 1895, p. 5, 8–9, 45–47; Hyde, 1948, p. 103).

Oscar Wilde did not fare well in prison. In the first plea for clemency on July 2, 1896, Wilde argued that he was "rightly found guilty" of indecency, but forcefully argued that he should not be punished as a criminal, but treated as an unfortunate victim of sexual madness ("erotomania") which displayed itself in loathsome monstrous sexual perversions that could consume his entire nature and intellect. After 6 months, a second petition was filed, this time asking the Home Office implement the Gladstone Committee's recommendations to prevent his mental decompensation. Wilde's brilliance was self-defeating (Radzinowicz, & Hood, 1986). This time the petition was denied because it was "expressed in too lucid, orderly polished style to cause apprehension" (Hyde, 1948).

The Gladstone Committee's recommendations did result in legislative change. Indeed, before the Committee's recommendations were acted upon dangerous people were sentenced in England and Canada like all other offenders. Then in 1908 with the *Prevention of Crime Act, 1908*, the sentence of preventative detention and the "double-track system" became a part of the laws of England.[7] This new statute was enacted to put the Gladstone Committee's recommendations in play and thereby extend the reach of preventative detention to a group of incipient and persistent dangerous criminals engaged in the more serious forms of crime.[8] The statute was new, but the concept was familiar. Many years before the Inquisition would sometimes impose a sentence "for such time as seems expedient to the Church." The underlying concept was not even a uniquely British concept. For example, in 1787 Dr. Rush was invited to Benjamin Franklin's home in the United States where he read a pamphlet proposing that all criminals ought to be sentenced indeterminately and returned to the community with dispatch only after they have been rehabilitated. The new English law provided the authority for a court to impose a new form of sentence—an indefinite term of postsentence detention as relapse prevention. The beneficiary was to receive two sentences: the first punishment was fixed taking into account conventional sentencing principles including the moral culpability of the offender and the seriousness of the offense; the second was a special individuated measure. For offenders with three prior convictions, a sentence of preventive detention of not less than 5 years and not more than 10 years could be attached to the ordinary sentence (Hart, 1962; Morris, 1951; Pratt & Dickson, 1997; Radzinowicz, & Hood, 1986).

The minimum term was limited by the sentence imposed. The extended detention or second track was to be served under conditions less rigorous than penal servitude with enhanced opportunities for detainees to avail themselves of treatment. The offender would be unsure of how much time they would have to server, but s/he would be provided an opportunity to cut short the indeterminate sentence. Of course, this presupposed that criminal characteristics could be identified and modified through treatment. However, the sentence would be much longer for the "high needs" prisoner than s/he would get from a judge applying traditional sentencing principles including proportionality. For the treatment-resistant prisoner who managed to stay alive until the date of his or her release and suffered all the joy and fear of leaving the penitentiary, the news that the system claimed more years of detention must have been devastating. Herbert Lionel Hart, an eminent British legal philosopher, recognized that the offender's perspective might be somewhat at odds with this bifurcated sentence:

> Certainly the prisoner who after serving a three-year sentence is told that his punishment is over but that a seven year period of preventive detention awaits him and that this is a 'measure' of social protection, not a punishment, might think he was being tormented by a barren piece of conceptualistm though he might not express himself in that way (Hart, 1962).

The animating objective was to lay hold of two defined groups of lawbreakers and subject them to strong restraint and training where it was deemed expedient for reformation and the prevention of crime. The Committee found the following:

(i) As a consequence of "social conditions of the general population...Lads grow up predisposed to crime, and eventually fall into it." and

(ii) Most habitual criminals are "made" between the ages of 16–21

Consequently, to dam the headspring of recidivism, young offenders were prescribed indeterminate detention in juvenile reformatories with an emphasis on individual treatment and special arrangements for after care.[9] For, habitual offenders a new sentence was introduced to enable a deterrent sentence to be imposed that was longer than fixed principles would stand for to permit individual treatment during the custodial part and special arrangements for postsentence community after care (Fox, 1934; Gladstone

Report, 1895, p. 11–13, 31 & 34; Radzinowicz, & Hood, 1986, p. 465–489; Strange, 1996).

SEXUAL PSYCHOPATH LAWS IN THE UNITED STATES

Among the first to actually demonstrate a relationship between the law and psychiatry in terms of effect on social control efforts, Penrose (1939) described the "hydraulic model" of social control. He identified European countries where low numbers of persons committed to the mental health system corresponded to high numbers of persons committed to the prison system and vice versa (Penrose, 1939). Briefly, this theory suggests that the size of a jurisdiction's correctional and psychiatric institutional populations vary inversely, such that when the rate at which one of these social control agents is used declines, the utilization of the other will increase, thereby maintaining a kind of social control homeostasis.

Sutherland (1950) observed (p. 147) that "For a century or more two rival policies have been used in criminal justice. One is the punitive policy; the other is the treatment policy." Generally, the trend toward one and away from the other is based on cultural change in the society. Brakel and Cavanaugh (2000) considering changes in sex offender laws, observed that, "It is old news that the field of law known as mental health law is especially susceptible to these pendulum-like swings." The interdisciplinary character, the "vagaries of science...whose theories are not always easy to grasp by outsiders and whose relevance to legal methods and objectives is not always clear," may, according to Brakel (p. 70–71), lead to a "tendency to lurch from one positional extreme to the other." (See also: Grudzinskas, Clayfield, Fisher, Roy-Bujnowski, & Richardson Clayfield, 2005)

Considering the spreading of so-called "sexual psychopath" laws in the United States Sutherland observed (p. 147) that, "Treatment tends to be organized on the assumption that the criminal is a socially sick person." If a person is ill and that illness leads to or forms the basis for a behavior, then within acceptable bounds of public safety, we can feel justified in excusing the conduct. The concept of relief from responsibility for criminal conduct is premised on the idea that not only does a treatable psychiatric disorder exist, but that the disorder is directly related to the particular type of criminal behavior. Social control

turns to the medical model when we come to believe that advances in treatment will provide a reduction in crime. The growth of sexually violent person commitment laws seems premised on the idea that forcing a connection between the individual defendant and the treatment facility and then supervising that connection for a reasonable time period, the court can promote treatment. This treatment engagement is then expected to reduce criminal behaviors (Wolff, 2003).

In the United States, dangerous sexual offenders were dealt with by incarceration and punishment like all other offenders until the late 1930s when the first of two waves of civil legislation for the commitment of sexual offenders was initiated. Beginning in the 1930s, a handful of American States responded to anxiety in relation to sexual crimes, particularly those involving children, by passing laws with therapeutic intent targeting sexual psychopaths.[10] These statutes provided something of a moving target though because it was not consistently clear who the sexual psychopath was.[11] The varied and subjective thinking that is engendered by the term "sexual psychopath" is such that its application constituted a constantly shifting terrain for those accused and for counsel confronting it. Accordingly, there was no true recourse against the allegation that a person was a sexual psychopath other than by the accused indicating that in their own opinion they were not. The lack of a clear, objective and ascertainable standard in the legislation was caused by the false assumption that the target group was a consistent or homogeneous offender class and the fact that,

> Sexual psychopathy is not a psychiatric diagnosis. It is a term used with a variety of confusing meanings and applications but with no precise clinical meaning. Also, since sex psychopaths are defined in statutes, the term is therefore an established legal concept. Definitions of statutes of sex psychopaths which arose in the 1930s were taken from a confluence of sources. Legislative bodies drew on an amalgam of psychiatric and social concepts to encompass a heterogeneous group of individuals seen as dangerous with respect to control over their sexual behaviour but not seen as legally insane. (Brakel, & Rock, 1971, p. 341–359; Brakel, Parry, & Weiner, 1985; GAP, 1977, p. 840–841, 853, 861–867)

The idea was to identify as best as possible the group of habitual offenders at the time of sentence completion to send them to places of safekeeping until recovery was established. What informed this legislative initiative was an understanding that the habitual offender,

> would fail to control their sexual behavior or idiosyncrasies and that they could consequently be identified and segregated. In this sense, the grouping was analogous to that of individuals classified as possessing a certain propensity, such as drug addiction or alcoholism. They were to be dealt with even though they were not at present violating any law...They were viewed as alternatives to straight imprisonment for handling people who either had behaved sexually in a manner that got them into difficulties with the criminal law or who were seen as having the potential to do so. The 'sex statutes' were meant to be harbingers of a future in which all criminals would be 'treated' under similar provisions...Although the history of the sex statutes emphasizes dual goals—community safety and treatments-their origin appears more closely tied to desires of legislators to protect their constituents. The preservation of community safety is encompassed within the police power of the state, while any treatment measures are carried out under the *parens patriae* duty of the state to rehabilitate its wayward citizens (Brakel & Rock, 1971, p. 341–359).

Brakel and Rock (1971) identified 31 states as having sexual psychopath or sex offender statutes by 1971. The first rush to enact laws began in Michigan in 1937. This was followed in rapid succession by Illinois, California, and Minnesota by 1939. Vermont, Ohio, Massachusetts, Washington, Wisconsin, the District of Columbia, Indiana, New Hampshire, and New Jersey followed suit over the next 10 years (Sutherland, 1950). The pattern of enactment that he identified was eerily similar to the pattern in effect in recent years with the reemergence of sexually violent offender commitment laws in the United States. A state's fears are first aroused by a serious, often violent sex crime, frequently involving a child victim. A protracted manhunt for the offender adds to the fear. The fear is seldom related to the statistical evidence supporting risk of further offenses (see for example Chapters 1, 5, 16). This leads to the next step in the process, the agitation of community activity and the call for protective legislation. The third step is the appointment of a study group or task force to draft such legislation (the results of the group study are often ignored—in Massachusetts in 1948 the

study group recommended repeal of the law that had been passed before its study was complete, in favor of keeping sex criminals within the general correctional population [Massachusetts, 1948]). The final step is the presentation of the law as the most scientific and enlightened method of protecting society from dangerous sex criminals (Sutherland, 1950).

CANADA AND PREVENTIVE DETENTION

In 1936, the government of Canada announced the creation of a Royal Commission to Investigate the Penal System. Appointed as chairman of the Commission was Mr. Justice Joseph Archambault who considered it fundamental to the discharge of the Commission's mandate to examine local penal policy and the legislative changes that were taking place in England and the United States.

In January 1938 the Archambault Commission tabled its recommendations. While the Commission was impressed with various aspects of the English model, it thought improvements were possible. The Archambault Commission acknowledged the initial purpose of the British legislation as the reformation of professional or persistently dangerous criminals, but observed that this did not occur in the British practice. It noted however that,

> Notwithstanding the best methods of punishment and reformation that may be adopted, there will always remain a residue of the criminal class which is of incurable criminal tendencies and which will be unaffected by reformative efforts. These become hardened criminals for whom 'iron bars' and 'prison walls' have no terrors, and in whom no hope or desire for reformation, if it ever existed, remains (*Report of the Royal Commission*, Archambault, 1938).

Recognizing that the nature of a prisoner's confinement to a behavior modification unit is for treatment, the Commission recommended that legislation be enacted to mark this residual class of offenders and to provide for their indeterminate detention in a special prison(s) because they "with few exceptions, [they] should never be set at liberty." However, "preventative detention should be less rigorous than penal servitude" and modeled after the approach taken in New York State in "a special prison that is neither punitive nor reformative but primarily segregation from society" (Brakel & Rock, 1971, p. 358–359; *R vs. Lyons*, 1987, p. 16–23).

By March 1939 a new *Penitentiary Act* had been drafted. However, with the outbreak of war in Europe and with Canada entering the war on September 10, 1939, attention to issues of domestic crime and punishment were diverted.

August 15, 1945 marked the end of the World War II and just 4 months later, in December 1945, Parliament finally enacted the *Penitentiary Act* that had been drafted years earlier. In 1947, Canada enacted its first preventative detention legislation. Speaking in the House of Commons on July 3, 1947 John Diefenbaker urged the Canadian Parliament to move quickly on criminal law reform because,

> psychological and penological advances have been made which in considerable measure necessitate an early alternation in the law with respect to insanity and also with respect to the principles applicable to responsibility.[12]

It was not a particularly infamous offender or shocking crime that brought the problem of violent recidivism to the forefront of public attention again to spur legislative action. The postwar world just seemed to be a more dangerous place as the troops returned home and increasingly attention was redirected to issues of public safety on the home front.

This postwar trepidation led to a backlash in the spring of 1947 that began the Canadian Dangerous Offender provisions of the *Criminal Code*. Canada's first Commissioner of Penitentiaries, General Ralph Burgess Gibson, who appointed by the Minister of Justice pursuant to the terms of reference contained in s. 4(a) of the 1945 *Penitentiary Act* to "Consider and report on the several recommendations made by the Archambault Committee before the war." On February 5, 1947, General Gibson reported to the Minister of Justice that it would be advisable if most of the prewar Archambault Commission recommendations were acted upon. He took no position on habitual offender legislation or indeterminate sentences (*Act to amend the Criminal Code* S.C. 1947, c. 55, s.18; *House of Commons Debates*, 1947, p. 4685, 5029–5031, 5065; Pratt, & Dickson, 1997, p. 371; *Report of the Royal Commission*, Archambault, 1938; *Report of the Special Commissioner*, Gibson, 1947, p. 1; Sutherland, 1950, p. 142–143, p. 10–11, 218–219. 224).

It was against this backdrop on June 26, 1947 that the Minister of Justice, James Ilsley, introduced legislation proposed by the Conference of Commissioners on Uniformity of Legislation in Canada (now called the *Uniform Law Conference of Canada*) to give recognition to the habitual offender as a distinct criminal class to be indeterminately segregated and flagged for intensive treatment. It was thought, especially for young offenders, that rehabilitation would be "ever so much easier" this way. The habitual offender statute to incapacitate the risk posed by the new criminal class was enacted on July 3, 1947. The new law also purported to give judges the power to order convicts admitted to specially designed treatment facilities that could really offer tailor made treatments that held out the best prospect of rehabilitation. (The term of imprisonment was not indefinite; rather, it was indeterminate and the term commonly referred to as "The Bitch" and the designation as the "feet first only exit designation.") One MP, Frank Jaenicke, underscored the relationship between the new class of offender and the not criminally responsible,

> I would consider an incurable criminal on par with a mentally incompetent person. Criminals who persist in committing crimes, in spite of their previous punishments are, in my opinion, mentally defective as compared with ordinary law abiding citizens who accept our moral code, which is reflected in our criminal law as reasonable and necessary…the state of mind of a habitual criminal is somewhat equal to a defective mind (*House of Commons Debates*, 1947, p. 5030–5035).

The Canadian habitual offender law only superficially emulated British law introduced in 1908,[13] but it was far more onerous because, among other things, it

(i) conferred discretionary jurisdiction on judges to impose either determinate or indeterminate sentences;

(ii) made the legislation apply to young persons 18 years of age or more;

(iii) took away the right to state funded counsel.

(*Act to amend the Criminal Code* S.C. 1947, c. 55, s.18; Brakel, Parry, & Weiner, 1985, p. 739; *House of Commons Debates*, 1947, p. 4685, 5029–5031, 5037, 5065; Pratt, & Dickson, 1997, p. 371; *Report of the*

Royal Commission, Archambault, 1938, p. 10–11, 218–219, 224).

The prerequisite for habitual offender designation was that the offender had been convicted of three or more indictable offenses and could be shown to be "persistently leading a criminal life."

Canada expanded its definition to include Criminal Sexual Psychopaths on June 14, 1948 in a move to bring the law more in line with the American habitual offender classification.

> John Diefenbaker: Legislation similar to this exists in eight states of the American Union… Where does the minister get the definition of 'criminal sexual psychopath'?
>
> James Iseley: From Massachusetts.[12]

The amendment gave discretion to the court in determining whether an accused should be found to be a "criminal sexual psychopath" in section 1054A which read in part "the court, before passing sentence, may hear evidence as to whether the offender is a criminal sexual psychopath" and "such other evidence as it may deem necessary" in addition to the mandated evidence of at least two psychiatrists. The power was not only a discretionary one but could also be exercised by the Court on its own motion without application by counsel for the prosecution or for the prisoner, and the exercise of the power did not depend in any way upon the consent of counsel.[14] In *R. v. Carey*, Laidlaw J. pointed out (p. 29) that

> during the argument of the appeal, attention was directed to s. 1054A of the Cr. Code, enacted by 1948, c. 39, s. 43. That section empowers the Court before passing sentence to hear evidence as to whether the offender is a criminal sexual psychopath. The power so given to the Court is a discretionary one. It may be exercised by the Court on its own motion without application by counsel for the prosecution or for the prisoner, and the exercise of the power does not depend in any way upon the consent of counsel (*Act to amend the Criminal Code* S.C. 1948, c. 39, s. 43; *House of Commons Debates*, 1948, p. 5195–5199, 5203).

In December 1953, a *Department of Justice* committee to inquire into the principles and procedures followed by the Remission Service was established and Mr. Justice Gerald Fauteux was appointed chairman of the Commission. Its report was released in the spring of 1956 (Fauteux Committee, 1956).

In 1954, the *Criminal Code* was revised after some 27 years. The preventive detention provisions were now all contained in Part XXI of the Criminal Code and had new section numbers. Section 660 dealt with the application to find an offender a "habitual criminal" and section 661 dealt with the application to find an offender a "criminal sexual psychopath." Under section 661 the court was now given a discretion "upon application" to hear evidence as to whether the accused was a criminal sexual psychopath and to hear "any evidence it considers necessary" as to whether the accused was a sexual psychopath (*Act to amend the Criminal Code* S.C. 1954, c. 51).

The legislation remained unchanged until amendments were made in 1961 which changed the terminology from "criminal sexual psychopath" to "dangerous sexual offender," the timing of the application and the language associated with the court's mandate to hear that type of application. With respect to the new designation of "dangerous sexual offenders" the court was now mandated to hear "any relevant evidence" upon application being made (S.C. 1960–61, c. 43, s. 34). Section 660 continued to relate to "habitual criminals" and section 661 now related to "dangerous sexual offenders." Dangerous Sexual Offender would now replace the older term, Criminal Sexual Psychopath (*Act to amend the Criminal Code* S.C. 1960–1961, c. 43, s. 32).

Accordingly sentences of preventive detention could be imposed if an offender was found to either be a habitual criminal, criminal sexual psychopath or a dangerous sexual offender (DSO):

(i) Habitual Criminals

Individuals who, since attaining the age of 18 years, had, on at least three separate occasions, been convicted of an indictable offense for which s/he was liable to imprisonment for 5 years or more and was leading a persistently criminal life (repealed October 15, 1977).

Legislation at this time allowed the following options:

- convicted, not sentenced and then found to be a habitual criminal for which an indeterminate sentence would be imposed; or,
- convicted, sentenced and then found to be a habitual criminal with the indeterminate sentence replacing the original sentence imposed.

(ii) Criminal Sexual Psychopaths

Persons who, by a course of misconduct in sexual matters, have shown a lack of power to control their sexual impulses and who, as a result, are likely to attack or otherwise inflict injury, pain, or other evil on any person (repealed 1960–1961 and replaced with "dangerous sexual offender" provisions).

(iii) Dangerous Sex Offenders (DSO)

Persons who, by their conduct in any sexual matter, have shown a failure to control their sexual impulses and, who are likely to cause injury, pain, or other evil to any person, through failure in the future to control their sexual impulses (repealed October 15, 1977).

KANSAS VERSUS HENDRICKS AND MODERN SEXUAL PREDATOR LAWS

At the time of this writing, the United States has 21 jurisdictions with post-criminal sentence civil commitment laws for sexually violent predators. This new wave began in the state of Washington with the 1990 enactment of the Community Protection Act. Following the pattern identified by Sutherland, the law came about after considerable public outcry when a 7-year-old boy was abducted, raped, mutilated, and left for dead (he survived) by a recidivist sex offender who had been released from prison some 2 years earlier. Washington first formed a commission (The Task Force on Community Protection). The Task Force issued its report, and called for a scheme of proportional sentences for sex crimes. Rather than alter the mental health commitment law, the Task Force recommended a narrowly drawn sex offender commitment statute. The Washington Legislature enacted the recommendations (Wash. Rev. Code Ann., 2008b). The statute served as the nearly identical model for the Kansas statute that served as the basis for the United States Supreme Court decision that redefined the field.

In 1994, the Kansas Legislature facing issues similar to those in Washington, borrowed on the Washington experience and enacted its own "sexually violent predator" law. In the Act's preamble, the Legislature found that the "treatment need of this population are very long term and the treatment modalities for this population are very different that the traditional treatment modalities for people appropriate for commitment under the general involuntary civil commitment statute" (Kan. Stat. Ann., 1995).

Leroy Hendricks had served 10 years of his sentence for a conviction for taking "indecent liberties" with two 13-year-old boys. The Kansas Act went into effect shortly before his release. The state moved to commit Hendricks. At his commitment hearing he testified that when he "get[s] stressed out," he "cannot control the urge" to molest children. The state also presented testimony from a licensed clinical social worker that Hendricks had a diagnosis of personality trait disturbance, passive-aggressive personality, and pedophilia. The chief psychologist at the facility holding him after his release from a halfway house testified that Hendricks suffered from pedophilia and that he would likely commit offenses against children if not confined. He further opined that pedophilia met the statutory definition of "mental abnormality." Hendricks defense offered testimony from a forensic psychiatrist that it was not possible to predict future dangerousness with any degree of accuracy. The jury found beyond a reasonable doubt that he was a sexually violent predator. The Court committed him to the custody of the Kansas Secretary of Social and Rehabilitation Services. Hendricks appealed. The Kansas Supreme Court found that to commit a person, a state is required by substantive due process to prove by clear and convincing evidence that a person is both mentally ill and dangerous to himself or others. (*In re Hendricks*, 1996) The United States Supreme Court reversed the Kansas Court (*Kansas v. Hendricks*, 1997). The Constitutional legal arguments raised are not relevant to this discussion (see Grudzinskas, & Henry, 1997). The issues that are relevant relate to the underlying justification for commitment. The Court noted that some additional factor beyond dangerousness, such as mental illness, must be coupled with the dangerousness. Justice Thomas writing for the majority explained that the Court had upheld Kentucky's commitment of "mentally ill" or "mentally retarded" individuals. (Citing *Heller v. Doe*, 1993) The Court had also upheld Minnesota's commitment of persons with a "psychopathic personality" (Citing *Minnesota ex rel. Pearson v. Probate Court of Ramsey Cty.* 1940). According to the decision, the term "mental illness" does not carry any "talismanic significance" (*Kansas v. Hendricks*, 1997, p. 359). Justice Thomas noted that the definition of terms of a medical nature that have legal significance has traditionally been left to legislators. He concluded that,

> ...it would be of little value to require treatment as a precondition for civil confinement of the dangerously insane when no acceptable treatment existed. To conclude otherwise would obligate a State to release certain confined individuals who were both mentally ill and dangerous simply because they

could not be successfully treated for their afflictions. Cf. *Greenwood v. United States*, (1956).

"The fact that at present there may be little likelihood of recovery does not defeat federal power to make this initial commitment of the petitioner" *O'Connor v. Donaldson*, 422 U.S. 563, 584 (1975) Burger, C. J., concurring; "It remains a stubborn fact that there are many forms of mental illness which are not understood, some which are untreatable in the sense that no effective therapy has yet been discovered for them, and that rates of 'cure' are generally low" *Kansas v. Hendricks*, 1997, p. 366).

Once the Supreme Court approved the process, a flood of state statutes followed. At this writing, Arizona, California (2006) (Greenwood v. United States, 1956), Florida (1998), Illinois (2008), Iowa (2008), Kansas, Massachusetts (2007, 2008), Minnesota, Missouri, Nebraska (2007), New Hampshire (2008), New Jersey (2008), New York (2008), North Dakota (2008), Pennsylvania (2003), South Carolina (2007), Texas (2007), Virginia (2008), Washington (2008a, 2008b), Wisconsin (2007), and the District of Columbia (2008) all have civil commitment statutes to commit sex offenders (nytimes.com, 2007).

The early Sexual Psychopath laws in the United States have generally become known as sexually dangerous person (SDP) laws and survive today in some states alongside the new SVP laws. Essentially the key difference between a SDP and a SVP civil commitment proceeding is the matter of timing. Generally, the prosecution had the ability to invoke the old law even if the dangerous person was not in prison at the time. The new law may only be invoked if the violent predator is imprisoned but nearing sentence completion. Treatment potential is relevant only to the issue of whether a SDP or SVP can be discharged, it is not relevant in determining whether a person does or does not meet the statutory criteria.

What marks the SVP acts as distinctive legislation are the following central features: (1) their stated purpose is to detain, in fact, to continue to detain, sex offenders who are already in custody and who are likely to reoffend if set free; and (2) their continued detention objective is accomplished via civil commitment to a treatment facility. The acts are different from the old sex offender (psychopath) laws to the extent that the latter prescribed treatment instead of incarceration…the population targeted for its treatment mandates is, by

most conventional standards, neither mentally ill nor treatable *(Kansas v. Hendricks*, 1997, p. 361. See also Brakel & Cavanaugh, 2000, p. 77–78, 82–87; *Minnesota ex rel. Pearson v. Probate Court of Ramsey Cty.*, 1940, p. 271–272).

Although the organizational structure and facility operations in each state vary, the key fundamentals of SVP laws are similar and have survived court challenges. This system to segregate convicted criminal offenders (in this case pursuant to Washington Revised Code 7 1.09.020(1) deemed likely to reoffend was approved by the Supreme Court in *Kansas v. Hendricks*, but the Court underscored that civil commitment on a finding of dangerousness standing alone is generally not a sufficient ground upon which to justify indefinite involuntary commitment. Proof of more than a predisposition to violence is necessary and past acts of sexual violence that resulted in convictions must be reasonably linked to a diagnosed mental disorder that predisposes the person to commit criminal sexual acts and a likelihood of the past repeating itself. The Supreme Court clarified that the SVP Accused must have a history of criminal sexual behavior, and must meet two other criteria for SVP commitment: a mental disorder or personality disorder predisposing the individual to sexual violence as a result of the abnormality and a likelihood of future sexually violent behavior without appropriate treatment and custody. The Court explained that civil commitment statutes are lawful because,

they have coupled proof of dangerousness with the proof of some additional factor, such as a 'mental illness' or 'mental abnormality'…These added statutory requirements serve to limit involuntary civil confinement to those who suffer from a volitional impairment rendering them dangerous beyond their control (*Addington vs. Texas*, 441 U.S. 418, 432–33, 1979; *Baxstrom vs. Herold*, 383 U.S. 107, 1966; *Kansas vs. Hendricks*, 521 U.S. 346, 1997 at 357–358, 369; *Seling vs. Young* 531 U.S. 250, 2001).

In clarifying the volitional impairment qualification, the Supreme Court ruled in *Kansas v. Crane* (2002), 534 US 407 (2002) that while the inability to control sexual behavior need not be absolute when viewed in light of such features of the case as the nature of the psychiatric diagnosis and the severity of the mental abnormality itself. The loss of volitional control must however be sufficient to distinguish the dangerous sexual offender whose serious mental illness, abnormality, or disorder subjected the offender to civil commitment, from the dangerous but typical sexual recidivist convicted in an ordinary criminal case (pp. 409–413).

CANADA'S PREVENTIVE DETENTION SCHEME AFTER AUGUST 1, 1997

The DO legislation was amended again on August 1, 1997, limiting the judge's discretion to sentence by requiring that a sentence of detention in a penitentiary for an indeterminate period be imposed upon finding an offender to be a dangerous offender. Although the new law applied to all offenders, in practice most people so designated are under custody for sexual offenses.

Effective August 1, 1997, Part XXIV of the *Code* was substantially amended.[15] First, section 753.1 was added to the *Code* thereby creating long-term offender designation:

753.1(1) The court may, on application made under this Part following the filing of an assessment report under subsection 752.1(2), find an offender to be a long-term offender if it is satisfied that

(a) it would be appropriate to impose a sentence of imprisonment of 2 years or more for the offense for which the offender has been convicted;

(b) there is a substantial risk that the offender will reoffend; and

(c) there is a reasonable possibility of eventual control of the risk in the community.

(2) The court shall be satisfied that there is a substantial risk that the offender will reoffend if

(a) the offender has been convicted of an offense under section 151 (sexual interference), 152 (invitation to sexual touching) or 153 (sexual exploitation), subsection 173(2) (exposure) or section 271 (sexual assault), 272 (sexual assault with a weapon) or 273 (aggravated sexual assault), or has engaged in serious conduct of a sexual nature in the commission of another offense of which the offender has been convicted; and

(b) the offender

(i) has shown a pattern of repetitive behavior, of which the offense for which he or she has been convicted forms a part, that shows a likelihood of the offender's

causing death or injury to other persons or inflicting severe psychological damage on other persons,[16] or

(ii) by conduct in any sexual matter including that involved in the commission of the offense for which the offender has been convicted, has shown a likelihood of causing injury, pain or other evil to other persons in the future through similar offenses.[17]

(3) Subject to subsections (3.1), (4) and (5), if the court finds an offender to be a long-term offender, it shall

(a) impose a sentence for the offense for which the offender has been convicted, which sentence must be a minimum punishment of imprisonment for a term of 2 years; and

(b) order the offender to be supervised in the community, for a period not exceeding 10 years, in accordance with section 753.2 and the *Corrections and Conditional Release Act*.

Second, the dangerous offender provisions were amended to take away the trial judge's discretion to grant a determinate sentence to those who are found to be dangerous offenders. Under the new provisions, the Court was required to impose an indeterminate sentence following a dangerous offender designation.

Finally, subsection 753(5) was added to the *Code* which provides as follows:

753(5) If the court does not find an offender to be a dangerous offender,

(a) the court may treat the application as an application to find the offender to be a long-term offender, section 753.1 applies to the application and the court may either find that the offender is a long-term offender or hold another hearing for that purpose; or

(b) the court may impose sentence for the offense for which the offender has been convicted.

A 1995 report on high-risk offenders described the purpose of the long-term offender legislation:

Currently in Canada community supervision generally is imposed by means of probation or it may be the eventual result of a custodial sentence and the grant of parole or the operation of Statutory Release...The current probation scheme would not be generally adequate for the purpose of long term supervision because...

the maximum duration of a probation order, 3 years, is not sufficient for those offenders who can be managed in the community but who require an extended period of supervision and treatment to be stabilized,

probation cannot be attached to sentences of 2 years or more, leaving lacunae in two ways:

more serious offenders, that is, those who receive penitentiary length sentences, cannot receive the support of extended community supervision other than through parole as a result of the imposition of a long custodial sentence

on dangerous offender applications, the court currently has only the alternative of indefinite detention at one extreme, and a definite sentence at the other.

Long-term supervision (LTS) should have as its objective the enhanced safety of the public through targeting those offenders who could be effectively controlled in the community, based on the best scientific and clinical expertise available. Such control may be the most effective approach in helping to reduce violent criminal acts, fostering and maintaining prosocial behavior, and reducing the adverse impact of incarceration. Supervision under such a scheme should be designed to avoid long-term or indefinite incarceration: the focus should be, instead, to exert all possible effort, short of incarceration, to stabilizing the offender in the community, with particular attention to any precursors to reoffending that may be identified. LTS is based on the assumption that there are identifiable classes of offenders for whom the risk of reoffending may be managed in the community with appropriate, focused supervision and intervention, including treatment.

A sentencing option providing for long-term supervision would be aimed at cases where an established offense cycle with observable cues is present, and where a long term relapse prevention approach may be indicated (Victoria, 1995, pp. 18–19).

At the same time the *Criminal Code* was amended to create the long-term offender provisions, the *Corrections and Conditional Release Act* was also amended. Under s. 134.1 of the *CCRA*, individuals released on a long-term supervision order are subject to the same conditions as attach to any parole order as well as any condition that the Parole Board considers "reasonable and necessary to protect society and to facilitate the successful reintegration into society of the offender." (*Corrections and Conditional Release Act*, s. 134.1; Corrections and Conditional Release Regulations, s. 161).

The new legislation was introduced to replace legislation dealing with habitual offenders. The dangerous offender provisions in s. 753 of the *Code* allow courts to remove so-called dangerous offenders from society on the basis of a future prediction (not punishment for a past crime) and impose an indeterminate sentence of preventive detention[18.] Pursuant to s. 753.1 of the *Criminal Code*, if a high-risk/high-needs offender is found to be a long-term offender, the court is required to impose a sentence of not less than 2 years for the offense committed plus an order that the offender be supervised in the community for a period not exceeding 10 years. Many NCR Accused, DO and LTOs are habitual criminals (*R vs. P.H.*, 2005 in para. 21–24).

After the implementation of *Bill C-55* on August 1, 1997, an accused designated a dangerous offender automatically receives an indeterminate penitentiary sentence and no statutory release date is set (*Corrections and Conditional Release Act*, s. 127, 134.1, s. 134.1). The parole eligibility date (PED) was increased to seven (7) years from the date of arrest relative to the offense for which the offender received the indeterminate sentence to bring this parallel with the eligibility restrictions for offenders serving sentencs of life imprisonment *An Act to amend the Criminal Code (high risk offenders)*, S.C. 1997, c. 5 *Department of the Solicitor General Act*, S.C. 1997, c. 17, s. 4–8. The day parole eligibility date (DPED) received a coincident increase to three (3) years before the PED as pursuant to s. 761(1) of the Code.

The legislative objectives serve both punitive and preventive purposes and resemble the case-law criteria for imposing a life sentences that are primarily imposed for the same purposes (Victoria, 1995). In *R. v. Hill*, Jessup J. noted that,

When an accused has been convicted of a serious crime in itself calling for a substantial sentence and when he suffers from some mental or personality disorder rendering him a danger to the community but not subjecting him to confinement in a mental institution and when it is uncertain when, if ever, the accused will be cured of his affliction, in my opinion the appropriate sentence is one of life. Such a sentence, in such circumstances, amounts to an indefinite sentence under which the parole board can release him to the community when it is satisfied, upon adequate psychiatric examination, it is in the interests of the accused and of the community for him to return to society. (*R. v. Hill*, 1974, pp. 147–148; *R. v. Kempton*, 1980, p. 191–192).

Chief Justice McLachlin in delivering the judgment of The Supreme Court of Canada in the *Charkaoui* case highlighted the punitive component of preventative indeterminate detention (PID):

> It is thus clear that while the IRPA in principle imposes detention only pending deportation, it may in fact permit lengthy and indeterminate detention or lengthy periods subject to onerous release conditions. The next question is whether this violates s. 7 or s. 12 based on the applicable legal principles.

This Court has previously considered the possibility of indefinite detention in the criminal context. In Lyons, a majority of the Court held that "dangerous offender" legislation allowing for indefinite detention did not constitute cruel and unusual treatment or punishment within the meaning of s. 12 of the Charter because the statutory scheme includes a parole process that "ensures that incarceration is imposed for only as long as the circumstances of the individual case require" (in p. 341, per La Forest J.). It is true that a judge can impose the dangerous offender designation only on a person who has been convicted of a serious personal injury offense; this Court indicated that a sentence of indeterminate detention, applied with respect to a future crime or a crime that had already been punished, would violate s. 7 of the Charter (in pp. 327–28, per La Forest J.). But the use in criminal law of indeterminate detention as a tool of sentencing—serving both a punitive and a preventive function—does not establish the constitutionality of preventive detention measures in the immigration context.

The principles underlying Lyons must be adapted in the case at bar to the immigration context, which requires a period of time for review of the named person's right to remain in Canada. Drawing on them, I conclude that the s. 7 principles of fundamental justice and the s. 12 guarantee of freedom from cruel and unusual treatment require that, where a person is detained or is subject to onerous conditions of release for an extended period under immigration law, the detention or the conditions must be accompanied by a meaningful process of ongoing review that takes into account the context and circumstances of the individual case. Such persons must have meaningful opportunities to challenge their continued detention or the conditions of their release.

The type of process required has been explored in cases involving analogous situations. In Sahin, Rothstein J. had occasion to examine a situation of ongoing detention (for reasons unrelated to national security) under the Immigration Act. He concluded that "what amounts to an indefinite detention for a lengthy period of time may, in an appropriate case, constitute a deprivation of liberty that is not in accordance with the principles of fundamental justice" (p. 229) (*Charkaoui v. Canada (Citizenship and Immigration)*, 2007, p. 105–110).

For a DO in Canada the chances of the National Parole Board granting parole are remote. However, if parole is granted monitoring of the DO in the community will be for the rest of his or her life. The DPED will be the longer of

- parole eligibility date, as determined in accordance with section 761(1), less 3 years.
  In other words DPED = [PED of 7 years–3 years]; and,
- parole eligibility date, as determined in accordance with subsection 120.2(2) of the *Corrections and Conditional Release (CCRA)*, less 3 years. However,
- in the case of a combination of life and indeterminate sentences, the sentence which produces the longest parole eligibility date will govern what the parole eligibility date will be; and,
- if an offender is in custody when s/he commits an offense for which another indeterminate sentence is imposed, the date of arrest in these circumstances is considered to be the date the offender was charged with the new offense.

Should an offender receive additional determinate sentences any time while lawfully or unlawfully does not count as part of the parole ineligibility period and the date of each sentence will determine the eligibility rules to be followed (An Act to amend the Criminal Code (high risk offenders), S.C. 1997, c. 5).

Of course, once a dangerous offender designation is made under the new provisions, the trial judge must impose an indeterminate sentence. Despite the enactment of the amendment to Part XXIV of the *Criminal Code*, many dangerous offender hearings still proceeded on the basis of the old provisions and little seemed to change after August 1, 1997. If both the old and new provisions were available sentencing alternatives, the prevailing view was that, because of the mandatory indeterminate sentence provisions, the new provisions did not create a "lesser penalty" for purposes of the *Charter* (*R. v. Gibbon*, 1998).

The creation of the long-term offender designation did raise a new issue of whether judges were vested with a residual discretion to consider the long-term offender provisions in section 753.1 on applications under section 753 and if so, under what circumstances. As set out previously, s. 753(5), which was added to the *Code* in the 1997 amendments stated that if the Court does not find an offender to be dangerous, the Court may treat the application as an application to have the offender designated as a long-term offender. The plain language of s. 753(5) of the *Code* seemed to suggest that the long-term offender provisions were only available at a dangerous offender hearing if the dangerous offender criteria were not met.

Prior to the touchstone decision of the Supreme Court of Canada in *R. v. Johnson* in September 2003 (*R. v. Johnson*, 2003) there were few guiding cases on the relationship between long-term offender and dangerous offender laws.

For example, in *R. v. C.M.M.*, dated November 7, 1997, the Court held that the application of the long-term offender provisions only arose if the offender was found not to be a dangerous offender. In that case, the Court found that the Crown had met the burden in section 753(b) beyond a reasonable doubt. The judge therefore declined to consider the long-term offender provisions (*R. v. C.M.M.*, 1997, in para. 14, 61, 64, 66).

Similarly, in *R. v. Gibbon*, a British Columbia judge held that the amendments did not apply retro-actively. Indeed, the trial judge observed that section 753.1 is only available where the accused is not found to be a dangerous offender:

I might be attracted to the defence argument if I were to find that the accused is not a dangerous offender. However, the evidence is overwhelming that he is a dangerous offender. Under the new s. 753(5), the Court can treat the Crown's dangerous offender application as a long-term offender application under s. 753.1, only if it does not find the accused to be a dangerous offender. *Since I find the accused to be a dangerous offender, the option of finding him a long-term offender does not arise.* (*R. v. Gibbon*, 1998 at para. 814).

Several questions remained. For example, could a trial judge consider and apply the long-term offender provisions during a hearing commenced under the dangerous offender provisions? Could a trial judge consider the prospect of positive therapeutic intervention when determining whether the offender met the test under s. 753 of the *Criminal Code*? These issues remained unresolved until the Supreme Court decided the *Johnson* case (*R. v. Johnson*, 2003).

Courts in Canada were slow to address the issue whether, and under what conditions, a long-term offender designation could be imposed in the course of deciding a dangerous offender application. In *R. v. Turley* the accused was convicted of a number of sexual offenses. Mr. Turley was found to be dangerous offender under the pre-1997 provisions and given a determinate sentence of 10 years. He appealed the dangerous offender designation and the prosecution appealed the determinate sentence. In granting the appeal and substituting a long-term offender designation the British Columbia Court of Appeal observed thatSince the conclusion of the dangerous offender proceedings and the imposition of the previously noted sentence, there have been significant *Code* amendments concerning dangerous offenders. The dangerous offender category remains and the new amended provisions now make mandatory an indeterminate sentence "[i]f the court finds an offender to be a dangerous offender" (s. 753(4)). The other major change, aside from some evidentiary provisions, is that a new class or category has been created, namely, the designation of "long-term offender." As I see it, the long-term offender category might be analogized to finding of a lesser included offence on a dangerous offender application (*R. vs. Turley*, 1999).

The state of the law in this regard remained unsettled (*R. vs. F.W.M.*, 2001 in paras. 74–75) while the *Johnson* case worked it's way through the courts.[19]

On October 16, 1998, Jeremiah Johnson was found to be a dangerous offender and given an indeterminate period of incarceration. In his reasons for judgment, the trial judge made no reference at all to the long-term offender provisions. (*R. v. Johnson*, 1998 per Tysoe J.)

Mr. Johnson appealed and argued that the trial judge erred in failing to consider the application of the long-term offender provisions during his dangerous offender hearing. Mr. Johnson was granted a new hearing at which he was entitled to call evidence and make submissions on whether he ought to be designated a long-term offender rather than a dangerous offender and on September 26, 2003, the Supreme Court of Canada released its decision which clarified many of the unsettled issues surrounding the 1997 amendments to the dangerous offender regime (*R. v. Johnson*, 2001 in para. 80, 98 and 104; *R. v. Johnson*, 2003).

First, the Court confirmed that the sentencing judge retains the discretion *not* to impose a dangerous offender designation even if the accused meets all the statutory requirements:

[N]either the purpose of the dangerous offenders regime, nor the principle of sentencing, nor the principles of statutory interpretation suggest that a sentencing judge must designate an offender dangerous if the statutory criteria in s. 753(1)(a) or (b) have been met. On the contrary, each of these factors indicates that a sentencing judge retains the discretion not to declare an offender dangerous even if the statutory criteria are met. This is particularly true now that it is clear that offenders declared dangerous must be given an indeterminate sentence.

The Court went on to explain the rationale for maintaining this discretion:

The proposition that a court is under a duty to declare an offender dangerous in each circumstance in which the statutory criteria are satisfied is in direct conflict with the underlying principle that the sentence must be appropriate in the circumstance of the individual case.[20] A rigid rule that each offender who satisfies the statutory criteria in s. 753(1) must be declared dangerous and sentenced to an indeterminate period of detention undermines a sentencing judge's capacity to fashion a sentence that fits the individual circumstances of a given case (*R. v. Johnson*, 2003 at para. 18, 25).

Second, the Court held that sentencing judges *must* consider treatment *and* management prospects independently and reject both before imposing a dangerous offender designation. This is especially important since treatment may prove to be more promised than delivered (*R. v. Johnson*, 2003, in para. 35–36; Webster, Dickens, & Addario, 1985, p. 47–48, 144–145).

Finally, the Supreme Court finally ruled on the relationship between the dangerous offender and the long-term offender provisions:

In those instances where both the dangerous and long-term offender provisions are satisfied, it may be that the sentencing sanctions available under the long-term offender provisions are capable of reducing the threat to the life, safety or physical or mental well-being of other persons to an acceptable level... If the public threat can be reduced to an acceptable level through either a determinate period of detention or a determinate period of detention followed by a long-term supervision order, a sentencing judge cannot properly declare an offender dangerous and sentence him or her to an indeterminate period of detention.

Later in the judgment, the Court summarized its decision as follows:

As we have discussed, a sentencing judge should declare the offender dangerous and impose an indeterminate period of detention if, and only if, an indeterminate sentence is the least restrictive means by which to reduce the public threat posed by the offender to an acceptable level (*R. v. Johnson*, 2003, in para. 32, 37, 44).

The *Johnson* decision resolved several issues that had arisen since the 1997 amendment to the *Criminal Code*. Principally, that an individual who meet the criteria for designation as both a dangerous and a long-term offender has the right pursuant to s. 11(i) of the *Charter of Rights and Freedoms* to be designated a long-term offender and given a determinate sentence followed by a long-term supervision order:

[A] sentencing judge should declare the offender dangerous and impose an indeterminate period of detention if, and only if, an indeterminate sentence is the least restrictive means by which to reduce the public threat posed by the offender to an acceptable level. The introduction of the long-term offender provisions expands the range of sentencing options available to a sentencing judge who is satisfied that the dangerous offender criteria have been met. Under the current regime, a sentencing judge is no longer faced with the stark choice between an indeterminate and a determinate sentence. Rather, a sentencing judge may consider the additional possibility that a determinate sentence followed by a period of supervision in the community might adequately protect the public. The result is that some offender who may have been declared dangerous under the former provisions could benefit from the long-term offender designation available under the current provisions (*R. v. Johnson* (2003), 177 C.C.C. (3d) 97 (S.C.C.), at 119–120).

RISK ASSESSMENT APPROACHES IN THE UNITED STATES

There is no uniform standard in the United States regarding SDP cases. However, for an individual to be committed as a sexually violent/dangerous person, the majority of states require that the offender be convicted of (or incompetent to stand trial for) a sexual offense and that they have a "mental disorder," "mental abnormality," or "behavioral disorder" that leads to dyscontrol of sexual urges and behaviors. Forensic evaluations of sexual predators, therefore, focus on an understanding of the offender's psychopathology (broadly defined) as well as factors that lead to increased risk of sexual reoffense.

Mental Abnormality/Disorder

The terms "mental abnormality" or "disorder" are legal constructs in the context of SDP laws, not necessarily clinical diagnoses. Ultimately, whether the condition in question meets commitment standards is decided by the trier of fact. Many mental health professionals, however, refer to personality disorders or paraphilias listed in the DSM-IV (American Psychiatric Association, 2000) in reaching their opinion, and leave it to the Court to determine if the legal threshold of "mental abnormality" is reached.

The most common disorders found in sex offenders are substance abuse disorders, paraphilias, and personality disorders (Conroy, 2003). These diagnoses are determined primarily by behaviors that are overt and measurable. It has been argued that many such disorders are not mental illnesses but, rather, determined solely by patterns of behavior (Harris, Rice, & Quinsey, 1998) and that these disorders (especially personality disorders) are not amenable to treatment. The Kansas statute, challenged in *Kansas v. Hendricks* (1997) acknowledges that most SDPs meet *diagnostic* criteria for antisocial personality disorder (APD), that APD is not a "mental illness," and that such individuals are not amenable to treatment (Conroy, 2003;

Cornwell, 1998). Hendricks argued that without legitimate treatment for his disorder, civil commitment would, "amount(s) to little more than disguised punishment," but the Supreme Court disagreed.

Clinicians, then, are faced with a dilemma. They are required to give an opinion about the presence or absence of a statutorily defined "*disorder*" for which treatment may not exist; yet, they are also required to provide an opinion as to whether commitment to a treatment facility is appropriate. In his seminal monograph on risk assessment, John Monahan (1981) posed the following question to clinicians asked to complete an evaluation of violence risk: "Are any issues of personal or professional ethics involved in this case?" (p. 103). This question is relevant regarding risk assessments of sexual dangerousness. Clinicians must address the question in deciding whether to proceed with an evaluation. They must be comfortable with presenting the court with legally-relevant data regarding the offender's pathology and letting the trier of fact determine whether the legal standard is met.

In addressing the issue of "mental disorder" the clinician should proceed, as in all forensic evaluations, by collecting data from multiple sources including collateral document review, interview, and psychological testing. Particular attention should be paid to historical patterns that suggest repetitive and compulsive criminal/antisocial behaviors, life-long maladaptive personality characteristics, lack of stable adult relationships, and a pattern of impulsivity. Interview characteristics of note include failure to take responsibility for offending behavior or antisocial acts, antisocial attitudes, lack of empathy, and lack of remorse. Psychological tests, such as the Millon Clinical Multiaxial Inventory-III (MCMI-III; Millon, 1994), which assess personality style, the presence of specific symptoms, and the presence of major metal illnesses, may also be useful. The MMCI-III validity scales also evaluate the attitude with which the offender answered the test questions (Heilbrun, Marczyk, & DeMatteo, 2002). Some clinicians focus on the offender's impulsivity as an index of dyscontrol. The Barratt Impulsivity Scale (BIS; Barratt, 1985; Stanford & Barratt, 1995) may be a test that is considered for this purpose.

Risk Assessment

Assessments of future risk of violence are difficult and controversial. Assessments of future risk of sexual violence are even more so, yet "dangerousness is...the unambiguous justification for the civil commitment of sex offenders" (Prentky, Janus, Barbaree, Schwartz, & Kafka, 2006, p. 371). Historically, "dangerousness assessments" were based on clinical judgments unguided by empirical data or empirically validated risk assessment instruments. Such clinical assessments are particularly prone to false-positive predictions, even when general criminal recidivism or violence are to be predicted (Cocozza & Steadman, 1978; Monahan, 1981). Clinical assessments refer to relatively unstructured evaluations in which clinicians rely on their own experience and clinical expertise. They, therefore, tend to be idiosyncratic and unreliable and may include clinical interview, a review of records, observation of the subject, and the use of psychological tests that are not specifically designed for the assessment of sex offenders. These assessments ultimately rest upon the arbitrary judgment of the clinician and they lack explicit parameters that define what factors are relevant and what relative weight they are given (Conroy, 2003; Prentky et al., 2006; Witt & Schneider, 2005). The advantage of the clinical approach to risk assessment is that, because it is unstructured, it allows for broader, individualized assessment of the subject as opposed to seeking specific nomothetic factors and applying them to the individual. Due to problems with reliability and validity, however, purely clinical assessments are not recommended. Nonetheless, courts have continued to allow testimony from mental health professionals based solely on clinical judgment (Conroy, 2003). As the limitations of clinical assessment became more apparent to the scientific community, research began to identify actuarial predictors of recidivism.

As individual risk factors were identified, instruments were developed to predict recidivism with the goal of removing evaluator bias. Risk variables can be divided into *static* (historical, unchanging) and *dynamic* (variable, amenable to intervention). Actuarial assessment instruments initially focused on static, historical risk factors predictive of sexual recidivism. Monahan had noted that "If there is one finding that overshadows all others in the area of prediction; it is that the probability of future crime increases with each prior criminal act" (1981, p. 71). The static risk factors found to be predictive of sexual recidivism were not identical to those predictive of general criminal recidivism (Conroy, 2003; Hanson & Bussiere, 1998). Measures such as the RRASOR (Rapid Risk

Assessment for Sex Offense Recidivism) (Hanson, 1997) and the Static-99 (Hanson, & Thornton, 1999) focused on risk factors such as history of antisocial behavior, history of sexual offending, characteristics of the victims (e.g., gender; relationship to perpetrator), and age of first offense. Static risk factors are gathered from archival data, such as court, educational and psychological treatment documents and a clinical interview is not required. In general, scholars have concluded that actuarial assessment is superior to clinical assessment of risk (Monahan et al., 2001; Prentky et al., 2006). Yet, actuarial assessment also has its limitations. None of the current actuarial instruments, for example, accounts sufficiently for dynamic risk factors of reoffense (Hanson, 1998). Also, instruments developed for one group of sexual offenders are, typically, inappropriate for use with another group. For example, an instrument developed for use with adult male offenders may not be appropriate for use with female offenders or adolescent offenders (Prentky et al., 2006). Since the underlying justification for commitment, identified in the *Hendricks* decision is treatment (even if it is currently ineffective), assessments that fail to consider change over time do not measure the variable the legislatures and courts are requesting the evaluator to consider. There is no purpose to a reevaluation if the result will always be the same.

Some scholars suggest that pure actuarial assessment should always be used in evaluating risk of sexual recidivism (e.g., Quinsey, Harris, Rice, & Cormier, 1998). Others, noting the limitations of pure actuarial methods, have suggested some combination of clinical judgment and empirically-derived actuarial risk assessment. Hanson (1998) noted that actuarial instruments lack "comprehensiveness." Not only do they fail to address dynamic risk factors, they also "cannot even claim to address all relevant static risk factors" (p. 65). Hanson suggested an adjusted actuarial approach that "begins with actuarial predictions and then adjusts these assessments on the basis of other compelling evidence" (p. 65). Others have suggested a "guided clinical approach" or "structured professional judgment" approach (Douglas, & Kropp, 2002; Hanson, 1998). In this approach relevant clinical data are collected from multiple sources, including clinical interview, and then this information is informed by empirically-identified risk factors. This approach allows for flexibility in weighing risk factors guided by idiographic information. The guided clinical approach allows for professional judgment and discretion (Chapter 5). As Hanson (1998) pointed out, however, "[a]n inherent problem with the guided clinical approach is that there is no explicit method of translating combinations of individual risk factors into overall recidivism probabilities" (p. 62).

Each approach to sex offender risk assessment has its limitations. Recently, however, researchers have focused on the importance of dynamic risk factors in assessment (e.g., Hanson, 2000; Hanson, & Harris, 2000; Witt, & Schneider, 2005). Areas of interest include: antisocial lifestyle and attitudes, poor social supports, substance abuse, age, participation in psychotherapy, and sexual deviance. Because of the importance of dynamic risk factors, many mental health professionals in the U.S. utilize a guided clinical approach or adjusted actuarial approach to risk assessment. This is especially true in *reassessments* of risk, when a civilly committed sex offender's ongoing risk must be reviewed.

Although there is substantial research on static risk factors and these factors have been shown to be useful for identifying long-term risk of sexual reoffending, these factors "provide no information concerning when offenders are likely to reoffend or how to intervene to reduce the potential for recidivism" (Hanson, 2000, p. 108). Of particular concern is that relatively little is known about dynamic risk factors, especially the effects of psychotherapy on mitigating recidivism risk. Hanson (2002) found that participation in treatment was associated with lower rates of sexual recidivism, and recent studies have addressed the effects of psychotherapy, community supervision, age, and self-regulation on recidivism (Barbaree, Blanchard, & Langton, 2003; Doren, 2006; Langton, Barbaree, & Harkins, 2006; Witt, & Schneider, 2005), but considerably more research is needed to fully understand dynamic risk factors.

THE CIVIL COMMITMENT OF JUVENILES AS SEXUALLY DANGEROUS OR VIOLENT PERSONS IN THE UNITED STATES

It seems unlikely that juvenile sex offenders were primarily on the minds of state legislatures when they enacted their respective civil commitment laws for sexual violent persons and predators. They more than

likely were thinking of the Leroy Hendricks of the world, adult repetitive pedophiles, and adult repetitive violent rapists when they passed these legislative schemes. This has not prevented juvenile sex offenders or, more likely, adults whose only sex offense occurred when they were juveniles from being captured within these civil commitment proceedings (For a comparative Canadian case see R. *vs.* Lyons [1987] 2 S.C.R. 309). There is no systematic national data maintained about how many adolescents are subjected to civil commitment procedures as SDPs. Likewise, there is no national data available about how many of the total population of individuals civilly committed as SDPs committed their only known sexual offense or offenses as adolescents, never having sexually offended as adults. Moreover, there has been little empirical research generally regarding the application of SDP and SVP laws to juvenile sex offenders or about the criminal or clinical characteristics of involuntarily committed juvenile sex offenders or adults whose only known sex offense occurred when they were adolescents.

In the state of Washington—the only state that has made available data about the civil commitment of juvenile sexual offenders—the SVP statute allows for the commitment of adults and juveniles. Since the enactment of the law in 1990 to the end of 2003, a total of 35 referrals (31 individuals) for juveniles aging out of the juvenile justice system were identified as likely meeting the statutory criteria for involuntary civil commitment, representing only approximately 1% of the total juvenile sex offenders paroled during this 13 year period (Milloy, 2006). The state declined to file a petition on 23 (a total of 21 individuals) or approximately two-thirds of these referrals. In the case of the other 12 referrals, a petition was filed resulting in six commitments, two dismissals and four were still awaiting an outcome. Follow-up data through December 2005 on the 21 juveniles for whom a petition was not filed revealed that 15% or 71% were convicted of a new offense and eight or approximately a third were convicted of a new felony or misdemeanor sex offense.

A necessary condition for the application of any of the civil commitment procedure for sexual offenders is the prior conviction for a sexual offense. Those without a prior conviction are not subject to its reach and scope. Conviction as the outcome of a criminal trial or hearing is not a term historically in use in juvenile court proceedings, however. The juvenile court, on the basis of its foundation in rehabilitation and treatment as opposed to retribution and punishment, has eschewed many of the traditional terms and phrases of the criminal court. In an attempt to avoid the potential negative effects associated with the application of terms and labels used for adult felons, the juvenile court has developed its own lexicon for juvenile offenders. Instead of "criminal convictions" it has substituted "delinquency adjudications."

Many state legislatures in their SDP laws circumvent the problem posed by the requirement of a prior "conviction" for a sexual offense by specifically declaring that delinquency adjudications for a sexual offense constitutes a conviction for the purpose of civil commitment proceedings as sexual dangerous persons. For example, Arizona defines a conviction to "include any finding of guilt at any time for a sexually violent offense or an order of the juvenile court adjudicating the person delinquent for any sexually violent offense." (Ariz. Rev. Stat.§§ 36–3701). This elastic use of delinquency adjudications to serve as the functional equivalent of criminal convictions raises very important procedural questions, however, such as whether juveniles have been properly informed about the potential collateral use of their delinquency adjudications, many of which are undoubtedly delinquent pleas without the benefit of trial.

The presence of some requisite mental condition, defined within most states as a "mental abnormality and some other personality disorder" is a second necessary criteria for civil commitment. The presence of a mental disorder or abnormality is especially critical according to the majority in *Hendricks* because these laws can only be credibly considered civil in nature if they are applied to a distinct subpopulation of sexual offenders who are defined as being dangerous because of a mental disorder or abnormality. If they are being preventively detained merely because they are dangerous and nothing more, then the procedure is revealed as starkly retributional and thereby unconstitutional. If, however, the state moves against the liberty of the individual because they are sexually dangerous by means of some underlying abnormal mental condition, then the process can be neatly folded into the long standing precedent of depriving the liberty rights of the mentally ill who have some impaired control over their dangerous behavior.

The two mental conditions that are typically diagnosed among civilly committed sexual offenders are the Paraphilias and APD (Doren, 2002). A problem

immediately emerges, however, when the application of the paraphilias and the personality disorders are considered in the case of juveniles facing possible civil commitment as sexual offenders. It is unclear to what extent juveniles, particularly early aged ones, are eligible for such qualifying diagnoses.

According to DSM-IV, to be diagnosed with Pedophilia, adolescents must be at least 16 years old and must be at least 5 years older than the child or children victims. This requirement is in addition to the presence of Criterion A: "Over the course of at least 6 months, recurrent, intense sexually arousing fantasies, sexual urges or sexual behaviors involving sexual activity with a prepubescent child or children (generally 13 years or younger)." (DSM-IV-TR, 2000, p. 572). The DSM-IV additionally rules out the case of a late adolescent involved in an ongoing relationship with a 12- or 13-year-old. Using DSM-IV criteria as a strict guide to the diagnosis of pedophilia, a juvenile adjudicated delinquent at age 15, for instance, for the sexual abuse of a 9-year-old and 10-year-old female victim separated in time by less than 6 months could not be diagnosed with pedophilia absent any further evidence of continued deviant urges, fantasies or desires for similar aged victims when he is age 16 or beyond. This evidence may be hard to come by if the juvenile has been confined in a secure treatment program without access to younger female children.

The problem with the use of such diagnostic categories as Antisocial Personality Disorder and Conduct Disorder in juveniles facing civil commitment as sexual offenders is whether such categories, which describe general patterns of problematic behavior, can be used to identify specific problems of sexual deviance and volitional impairments. According to *In re to the Care and Treatment of Michael T. Crane* (2000), to satisfy the volitional impairment criterion a total or complete lack of control is not necessary but only serious difficulty controlling ones deviant sexual urges. What is not settled in either *Hendricks* or *Crane*, however, is how these standards or objectives are to be applied to adolescents. What is the meaning of the terms mental abnormality and personality disorder for a juvenile? Are these manifested in a similar manner for adolescents as they are for adults? Do adolescents have similar volitional capacities as adults when it comes to controlling their sexual urges? Do we hold adolescents to the same standard of serious difficulty controlling sexual urges as adults? Or does their immature status require that we think about these capacities differently? What is the predictive value of a sexual offense committed by an adolescent to their later risk of committing sexual offenses as an adult?

The formulation of a generalized link between a mental disorder and a volitional impairment is more easily established for pedophilia, a diagnostic category which by definition provides a ready-made link to a volitional impairment and risk. Conduct disorder, for instance, bears no specific relationship with sexual recidivism. A conduct disorder or APD in conjunction with prior delinquency adjudication for a sexual offense along with the testimony of expert witnesses who concluded that the individual's conduct disorder or APD in his particular case predisposed him to violent sexual acts may provide the necessary nexus between a mental disorder and the predisposition for violent sexual acts. But such a line of clinical reasoning opens the door for potential tautological thinking: A person has an APD because he has prior acts of sexual violence and his prior acts of sexual violence provide the necessary evidence that his particular form of APD results in a volitional impairment to control such acts from occurring in the future.

The demonstration that the individual facing potential civil commitment poses a substantial risk of committing future acts of sexual violence is often another criterion required for involuntary commitment as a sexual offender. The problem with this criterion in the context of the civil commitment of juveniles or the commitment of adults whose only sexual offense occurred while they were juveniles is that the research literature has consistently reported a low sexual recidivism rate for juvenile sexual offenders, lower than for adult sexual offenders and very much lower than for general delinquency for juveniles (Caldwell, 2002; Righthand, & Welch, 2001; Weinrott, 1996; Worling, & Langstrom, 2006; Zimring, 2004). Two related issues emerge regarding the prediction of sexual recidivism for juveniles and for adults whose only offense occurred while they were juveniles. First, given that the base rate of sexual recidivism is relatively low can an argument be credibly made that a particular juvenile's risk to commit future sexual acts of violence when the recidivism rate is so low for the aggregate of juvenile sexual offenders? Second, should juveniles or for that matter adults whose only sexual offense occurred when they were juveniles be assessed with actuarial prediction instruments that were developed and normed on adult sexual offenders?

Problems emerge when juvenile sex offenders or adults whose only sexual offense occurred when they were juveniles are assessed on the number of actuarial assessment instruments that have been developed for adult sexual offenders (Maurutto & Hannah-Moffat, 2007). For instance, the Minnesota Sex Offender Screening Tool-Revised (MnSOST-R; Epperson, Kaul, Huot, Hesselton, Alexander, & Goldman, 1999) does not provide criteria for how to score the case of a person who has been incarcerated since age 15 and may have been a full-time student at the time of his initial detainment on the employment history item. An item on the Static-99 (Hanson, & Thornton, 1999) asks if the offender ever lived with a lover for at least 2 years. But how is such an item to be scored in the case of a dependent adolescent who still lived with his parents at the time of his arrest?

There have been a number of actuarial risk assessment instruments developed specifically for juvenile sex offenders in the past decade such as the Juvenile Sex Offender Assessment Protocol-II (J-SOAP-II; Prentky & Righthand, 2003), the Estimated Risk of Adolescent Sex Offender Risk (ERASOR; Worling, 2004; Worling, & Curwen, 2001), and the Sexual Offense Recidivism Risk Assessment Tool-II (JSORRAT-II; Epperson, Ralston, Fowers, & Gore, 2006). Overall, these risk assessment instruments which assess various combinations of static and dynamic factors of sexual recidivism risk have established good reliability and to some extent concurrent validity with other established measures and external criterion but have not as yet been able to report any predictive validity data. The problem uniformly across them has been the apparently insurmountable issue of the consistently low sexual recidivism rate of juvenile sexual offenders which has prevented these test authors from establishing the predictive validity of their instruments, a vital psychometric characteristic allowing for their use in contexts like civil commitment proceedings where the validity of such predictions will be a central issue.

There is no national data currently about how many juvenile sexual offenders or how many adults whose only sexual offense was committed as a juvenile have been civilly committed as sexually dangerous or violent persons. The direct interface of the juvenile justice system and SDP proceedings unveils some potentially unanticipated fault lines such as whether juveniles have been properly informed of the collateral use of their delinquent pleas in SDP hearings before their tendering such pleas.

The requisite presence of a mental abnormality or personality disorder is deeply problematized in the case of juvenile sexual offenders. First, it is unclear if young adolescents are able to be diagnosed with a paraphilia, particularly pedophilia, before the age 16. Also other frequent diagnoses such as APD and Conduct Disorder do not provide a specific nexus to a volitional impairment or risk for future sexual offending. It is necessary that evidence for the nexus be established in the specific case through the presence of prior sexual offending which opens the door to potential tautological reasoning: Their prior sexual offense is used to support the presence of a mental disorder and the nexus of their mental disorder to a volitional impairment is the presence of a prior history of sexual offending. Finally, problems emerge when attempts are made to establish their future risk of sexually violent acts. First, juvenile sexual offenders have an empirically established lower recidivism than adult sexual offenders, making the argument about their future risk more difficult to establish. Second, it is unclear that the actuarial assessment instruments in wide use with adult sexual offenders can be employed with juvenile sexual offenders or even with adults whose only sexual offense occurred when they were juveniles. Lastly, there has been a number of actuarial assessment instruments developed over the past decade designed and normed specifically on juvenile sexual offenders. However, these instruments have yet to establish sufficient predictive validity, mostly due to the low base rates of sexual recidivism for juveniles that have posed difficult, even insurmountable, problems for the test developer.

Notes

1. The Group for the Advancement of Psychiatry (GAP) was founded in 1946 by a group of physicians under the leadership of William Menninger. GAP advocates for greater public awareness of the need for new programs in mental health and analyzes significant data in psychiatry and human relations, reevaluates old concepts, develops new ones, and applies this knowledge for the advancement of mental health.

2. For our purposes, since treatment is the justification for civil commitment of sex offenders, and since the concepts of mental illness and sexual offending are often confounded within the law, the origins of treatment rationales are relevant.

3. Up until a few decades into the nineteenth century the medical profession knew little about mental disorder and believed insanity to be incurable. The treatments that were attempted, such as those involving leeches to remove "tainted" blood from the insane were futile.

4. Such illness, disability, or disorder is not understood to be freely chosen although susceptibility or recovery is linked in part to choices offenders have made or can potentially make. It is hypothesized that this "sickness" can be "cured" by proper classification, segregation, training, education, and supervision.

5. It is important to understand that the strength of a conclusion is a function of both the *quality* of the evidence provided in its support and the *a priori* reliability of the claim being supported.

6. Canada enacted its first *Criminal Code in 1892 and s.145 made the "Unnatural Offence" punishable by penal servitude up to life.*

7. Transportation from Britain ended officially in 1868. In theory it should have been the perfect solution to the problem. It has been tried and abandoned by England, France, Russia, Portugal, Spain, Italy, Holland, Denmark, and others, it has been a complete failure every time.

8. The ambitious new law embodied the Gladstone Committee's finding that, "There but few prisoners other than those who are in a hopeless state through physical or mental deficiencies who are irreconcilable. Even in the case of habitual criminals there appears to come a time when repeated imprisonments or the gradual awakening of better feelings wean them from habitual crime." (Gladstone Report, 1895; See also Leon Radzinowicz and Roger Hood, The Emergence of Penal Policy in Victorian and Edwardian England in A History of English Criminal Law and its Administration from 1750, Vol. 5 (London, 1986) at 231–397).

9. In 1900, a small group of boys in London were drawn together and separated from adult prisoners in Bedford prison and carefully selected according to their likely ability to respond to specialized vocational training and ability to be managed on discharge from prison. Later, in 1902 a wing of the convict prison at Borstal, now Rochester Borstal was taken over for a similar purpose. These beginnings formed the basis of the Borstal system by which boys would be carefully chosen, made subject to strict discipline, expected to work hard, and given special supervision on discharge through the Borstal Association. The model for habitual offenders emulated the Borstal experiment. Regrettably, the impetus to expand well-funded training facilities for young offenders and habitual offenders was undermined by resources shortages.

10. Psychopathy is a term derived from the Greek *psyche* (mind) and *pathos* (suffering) and was once used to denote any form of mental illness. It is now regarded as a personality syndrome or constellation of affective, interpersonal, and behavioral characteristics, including egocentricity; impulsivity; irresponsibility; shallow emotions; lack of empathy, guilt, or remorse; lying; manipulativeness; and the persistent violation of social norms and expectations.

11. It is hardly surprising that the views of the public, mental health professionals, and the legal profession were divergent as to what criterion defines the sexual psychopath. The consequence was the indeterminate civil commitment of offenders who deviated from sexual

norms, but did not present a significant threat of future sexual violence.

12. Transcript in the authors' possession, copy provided upon request.

13. The British social experiment was faltering and the dual-track system was abandoned by 1948. Then the English *Criminal Justice Act. 1948* was enacted providing that "if the court is satisfied that it is expedient for the protection of the public, [the dangerous offender] should be detained for a substantial period of time." The statute made no mention of the types of offenses for which a person could be subjected to an indefinite sentence for and consequently, many property offenders were deemed dangerous by the courts. By the 1960s, however, the scope of dangerous offender provisions had narrowed to focus primarily on sex offenders.

14. Two years later in 1950, the Criminal Code was amended to require that the notice of an application to find a person to be a "criminal sexual psychopath" must be in writing and filed with the court, but nothing further (*An Act to amend the Criminal Code* S.C. 1950, c. 11, s. 19).

15. The Applicant's primary focus in this case is not upon the purported "behaviour by an offender, associated with the offense for which he or she has been convicted, that is of such a brutal nature as to compel the conclusion that the offender's behavior in the future is unlikely to be inhibited by normal standards of behavioral restraint" pursuant to s. 753(1) (iii) of the *Criminal Code*.

16. The elements of s. 753.1(1) (a) and 753.1(2) (i) are (1) a pattern of repetitive behavior, (2) but the predicate offenses must form only a part of that pattern, (3) the predicate offenses must be such that a 2-year sentence of imprisonment will be imposed, and (4) the pattern must be proof of a likelihood of the offender's causing death or injury to other persons or inflicting severe psychological damage on other persons. With the exception of the 2-year sentence precondition, the elements are the same as those required by s.753 (1) (a) (i).

17. Section 753.1(2) (ii) is similar to the single incident/nonpattern analysis in section 753 (a) (iii). However, there are two important differences: (1) The LTO provision is limited to conduct in sexual matters and (2) the DO enactment requires compelling proof of only one conclusion in section while the LTO enactment requires only proof of a likelihood of causing injury, pain, or other evil to other persons in the future through similar offenses.

18. The preventative measures of Part XXIV of the *Criminal Code* have not been evaluated on the basis of how successful they are at actually reducing recidivism.

19. See also *R. vs. M.B.*, decided May 4, 2000 where Knazan J. (at para. 245–246, 280–303) found that the accused met the definition for a dangerous offender but that a determinate sentence was appropriate refusing to adopt the reasoning of the British Columbia Court of Appeal in the Turley case. In *R. v. Ferguson*, [2000] O.J. No. 3008 (Ont. S.C.) at para. 97& 99) and *R. v. Payne*, [2001], O.J. No. 146 (S.C.J.) at para. 107–116) where

Hill J. held that the long-term offender provisions were still available where it can be established that there remains a reasonable possibility of eventual control in the community. *In R. v. Mason* (2001), 156 C.C.C. (3d) 97 (Ont. C.A.) the Court of Appeal for Ontario declined, in *R. v. Mason*, to settle the law in Ontario. Rosenberg J.A. (at para. 29) held that because Mr. Mason had not tendered sufficient evidence to show that there was a reasonable possibility of eventual control of the risk in the community, the Court did not have to consider the "the relationship between the dangerous offender and long-term offender provisions and whether the new provisions give the judge a discretion not to make a finding that the accused is a dangerous offender because he or she meets the long-term offender pre-requisites."

20. There is no sentence a Judge can typically impose that will fully assuage the feelings of the victim, her family, and the community at large in a sex offender case. Every sex offender leaves in his or her wake varying amounts of sorrow, grief, anger, fear, and frustration. In many cases lives are shattered or ruined and families are devastated and torn apart. It's a normal public sentiment to wish the perpetrator to be locked up forever, tortured, and even killed. The imposition of sentence, however, is governed by statute and fixed principle, not by emotional reaction. It does not measure the value of the victims either in absolute or in relative terms and it is not revenge. The principles of sentencing dictate that a sentencing court must impose a fit sentence; no more—no less. It is not justifiable to then further encumber a defendant's liberty and justify the special restraint on the basis of fear. Fear that those who are charged with the responsibility of sentence implementation will fail. A sentence enhanced on that basis would be is unfit. Further, the failure of governments to provide reasonable treatment and infrastructure cannot justify indeterminate detention (*R. v. Nikolovski*, [2002] O.J. No. 5026 (S.C.J.) at para. 263–269; Aff'd (2005), 194 O.A.C. 258 (Ont. C.A.). See also *R. v. Nault* (2002), 59 O.R. (3d) 388 (C.A.) at 391).

21. Christopher Webster, Bernard Dickens and Susan Addario, Constructing Dangerousness: Scientific, Legal and Policy Implications (Toronto, 1985) at 47–48, 144–145.

References

Act to amend the Criminal Code S.C. (1947), c. 55.

Act to Amend the Criminal Code S.C. (1950), c. 11, s. 19.

Act to amend the Criminal Code S.C. 1954, c. 51.

Act to amend the Criminal Code S.C. 1960–1961, c. 43, s. 32.

American Psychiatric Association. (2000). *Diagnostic and Statistical Manual For Mental Disorders. Fourth Edition. Text Revision.* Washington, D.C: American Psychiatric Association.

An Act to amend the Criminal Code (high risk offenders), S.C. 1997, c. 5.

Arizona: Ariz. Rev. Stat. Ann. §§ 13–4601 et seq.

Ariz. Rev. Stat. §§ 36–3701.

Bailey, D. (1975). *Homosexuality and the western Christian tradition* (pp. 70–81). North Haven, CT: Archon Books, The Shoe String Press, Inc.

Barbaree, H. E., Blanchard, R., & Langton, C. M. (2003). The development of sexual aggression through the life span: The effect of age on sexual arousal and recidivism among sex offenders. *Annals of the New York Academy of Sciences*, 989, 59–71.

Barratt, E. S. (1985). Impulsiveness subtraits: Arousal and information processing. In J. T. Spence & C. E. Izard (Eds.), *Motivation, emotion, and personality*. North-Holland: Elsevier Science.

Bowers v. Hardwick, 478 U.S. 186 (1986) at 196–197.

Henry of Bracton. (1968). Bracton on the Laws and Customs of England. Latin Text edited by George E. Woodbine. Translated, with revisions and notes by Samuel E. Cambridge, MA: Thorne Belknap Press of Harvard.

Brakel, S. J., & Cavanaugh, J. L. (2000). Of psychopaths and pendulums: Legal and psychiatric treatment of sex offenders in the United States. *New Mexico Law Review*, 30, 69–94.

Brakel, S. J., & Rock, R. S. (1971). *The mentally disabled and the law*. Chicago: University Press.

Brakel, S. J., Parry, J., & Weiner, B. (1985). *The mentally disabled and the law* (pp. 741–742). Chicago, IL: American Bar Foundation.

Caldwell, M. F. (2002). What we do not know about juvenile sex reoffense risk. *Child Maltreatment*, 7(4), 291–302.

California: Cal. Welf. & Instit. Code §§ 6600 et seq. (2006).

Charkaoui v. Canada (*Citizenship and Immigration*), S.C.J. No. 9 (2007).

Cocozza, J. L., & Steadman, H. J. (1978). Prediction in psychiatry: An example of misplaced confidence in experts. *Social Problems*, 25(3), 265–276.

CODE THEOD. 9.7.6.

Conroy, M. A. (2003). Evaluation of sexual predators. In I. B. Weiner (Series Ed.) & A. M. Goldstein (Volume Ed.), *Handbook of psychology: Vol. 11. Forensic psychology* (pp. 463–484). Hoboken, NJ: Wiley.

Cornwell, J. K. (1998). Understanding the role of the police and *parens patriae* powers in involuntary commitment before and after *Hendricks*. *Psychology, Public Policy, and Law*, 4, 377–413.

Corrections and Conditional Release Act, s. 134.1. (1997).

Corrections and Conditional Release Act, s. 127, 134.1, s. 134.1. (1997).

Corrections and Conditional Release Regulations, s. 161. (1997).

Department of the Solicitor General Act, S.C. 1997, c. 17 s. 4–8.

Diagnostic and Statistical Manual of Mental Disorders DSM-IV-TR Fourth Edition (Text Revision). (2000). Arlington, VA: American Psychiatric Publishing, Inc.

District of Columbia: D.C. Code § 16–801 and D.C. Code § 22–3808 et seq. (2008).

Doren, D. (2002). *Evaluating sex offenders: A manual for civil commitments and beyond*. Thousand Oaks, CA: Sage Publications.

Doren, D. M. (2006). What do we know about the effect of aging on recidivism risk for sexual offenders? *Sexual Abuse: Journal of Research and Treatment*, 18(2), 137–157.

Douglas, K. S., & Kropp, P. R. (2002). A prevention-based paradigm for violence risk assessment: Clinical and research applications. *Criminal Justice and Behavior*, 29(5), 617–658.

Epperson, D.L., Kaul, J.D., Huot, S.J., Hesselton, D., Alexander, W., & Goldman, R. (1999). *Minnesota Sex Offender Screening Tool-Revised (MnSOST-R): Development, performance, and recommended risk level cut scores*. Retrieved from http://www. psychology.iastate.edu/faculty/epperson/ publications. Last visited: Oct 10, 2008.

Epperson, D. L., Ralston, M. S., Fowers, D., DeWitt, J., & Gore, M. S. (2006). Actuarial risk assessment with juveniles who offend sexually: Development of the Juvenile Sexual Offense Recidivism Risk Assessment Tool-II (JSORRAT-II). In D. Prescott (Ed.), *Risk assessment of youth who have sexually abused: Theory, controversy, and emerging strategies*. Oklahoma City, OK: Woods 'N' Barnes.

Fauteux Committee. (1956). Report of a committee (Chair: Gérald Fauteux) appointed to inquire into the principles and procedures followed in the remission service of the Department of Justice of Canada.Ottawa.

Florida: Fla. Laws ch. 98–64 (1998).

Fox, L. (1934). *The modern English prison* (p. 168). London: George Routledge & Sons.

Gladstone Report. (1895). Prisons Committee (Chair: Hebert John Gladstone), Report from the Departmental Committee on Prisons. London.

Greenblatt, S., Abrams, M. H., Simpson, J. (9179). Oscar Wilde in The Norton Anthology of English Literature 5th edition (Vol. 2) (pp. 1675–1677). New York.

Greenwood v. United States, 350 U.S. 366 (1956).

Group for the Advancement of Psychiatry (GAP), Committee on Psychiatry and the Law (1977). Psychiatry and the sex psychopath legislation: The 30's to the 80's, vol. 9. American Psychiatric Association, No. 98, 845–846.

Grudzinskas, A. J., Clayfield, J. C., Fisher, W. H., Roy-Bujnowski, K., & Richardson, M. H. (2005). Integration of mental health treatment and criminal justice involvement: the worcester experience. *Behavioral Science and the Law*, 23(2), 277–293.

Grudzinskas, A. J. & Henry, M. G. (1997). Analysis and commentary, Kansas v. Hendricks. *Journal of the American Academy of Psychiatry and the Law*, 25, 607–612.

Hanson, R. K. (1997). The development of a brief actuarial risk scale for sexual offense recidivism. (User Report No. 1997–04). Ottawa, Ontario, Canada: Department of the Solicitor General of Canada.

Hanson, R. K. (1998). What do we know about sex offender risk assessment? *Psychology, Public Policy, and Law.* 4, 50–72.

Hanson, R. K. (2000). Will they do it again? Predicting sex-offense recidivism. *Current Directions in Psychological Science,* 9(3), 106–109.

Hanson, R. K. (2002). Recidivism and age: Follow-up data form 4, 673 sexual offenders. *Journal of Interpersonal Violence,* 17(10), 1046–1062.

Hanson, R. K., & Harris, A. J. (2000). Where should we intervene? Dynamic predictors of sexual assault recidivism. *Criminal Justice and Behavior,* 27(1), 6–35.

Hanson, R. K., & Thornton, D. (1999). Static-99: Improving actuarial risk assessments for sex offenders (User Report 1999–02). Ottawa, Ontario, Canada: Department of the Solicitor General of Canada.

Harris, G. T., Rice, M. E., & Quinsey, V. L. (1998). Appraisal and management of risk in sexual aggressors: Implications for criminal justice policy. *Psychology, Public Policy, and Law,* 4, 73–115.

Hart, H. L. (1962). *Punishment and the Elimination of Responsibility* (pp. 859–860). London: Oxford University Press.

Heller v. Doe, 509 U.S. 312 (1993).

Heilbrun, K., Marczyk, G. R., & DeMatteo, D. (2002). *Forensic mental health assessment: A casebook.* New York, NY: Oxford University Press.

House of Commons Debates, (1947) Vol. V, 3rd Sess., 20th Parl. 11 George IV, at 5030–5035.

House of Commons Debates, (1947) Vol. V, 3rd Sess., 20th Parl. 11 George IV, at 4685, 5029–5031, 5065.

Hyde, H. M. (1948) *The Trials of Oscar Wilde.* London.

Illinois: 725 Ill. Comp. Stat. §§ 205 et seq.

In re Care and Treatment of Michael T. Crane. 7 P.3d 285 (2000).

In re Hendricks, 912 P.2d 129 (Kan. 1996).

Iowa Code §§ 229A et seq.

Kansas v. Crane, 534 US 407 (2002).

Kansas v. Hendricks, 117 S. Ct. 2072 (1997).

Kansas v. Hendricks, 521 U.S. 346 (1997).

Kansas: Kan. Stat. Ann. §§ 59–29a01 et seq.

Keeton,G. (1961). *Guilty but insane* (pp.14–15). *London.*

Langton, C. M., Barbaree, H. E., & Harkins, L. (2006). Sex offenders' response to treatment and its association with recidivism as a function of psychopathy. *Sexual Abuse: Journal of Research and Treatment,* 18(1), 99–120.

MASS. GEN. LAW c. 272 § 34 (2007).

MASS. GEN. LAW c. 6 §178 C–Q et seq. (2008).

MASS. GEN. LAW c. 127 § 133D.

Massachusetts. (1948) Report of the Commission for Investigation of the Prevalence of Sex Crimes, House Reports, Nos. 1169 and 2169 (as cited in Sutherland 1950).

Maurutto, P., & Hannah-Moffat, K. (2007). Understanding risk in the context of the youth criminal justice act (Canada), *Canadian Journal of Criminology,* 49(4), 465–491.

MacDonald et al. v. Vapour Canada (1977) 2 S.C.R. 134.

Millon, T. (1994). *Millon clinical multiaxial inventory-III: Manual.* Minneapolis, MN: Interpretive Scoring Systems.

Milloy, C. (2006). Juvenile sex offenders recommended for commitment under Washington's Sexually Violent Predator Law, where no petition was filed. Washington State Institute for Public Policy. Retrieved from www.wsipp.wa.gov October 10, 2008.

Minnesota ex rel. Pearson v. Probate Court of Ramsey Cty., 309 U.S. 270 (1940).

Minnesota: *Minn.Stat.* § 253B.02, subd.18b et seq. (2008)

Missouri: Mo. Rev. Stat §§ 632–480 et seq.

Monahan, J. (1981). *Predicting violent behavior: an assessment of clinical techniques.* Troy, NY: Sage Press.

Morris, N. (1951). *The habitual offender* (pp. 20–23). Connecticut.

Nebraska: R.R.S. Neb. §§ 29–2922–2934 et seq. (2007).

New Hampshire: N.H. Rev. Stat. Annot. ch. 135–E et seq. (2008).

New Jersey: N.J. Rev. Stat. § 30:4–82.4 et seq. (2008).

New York: Mental Hygiene Law (MHL) Article 10 et seq. (2008).

New York: NY CLS Correc. § 168–h, et seq. (2007).

North Dakota: N.D. Cent. Code §§ 25–03.3 et seq. (2008).

O'Connor v. Donaldson, 422 U.S. 563, 584, (1975) Burger, C. J., concurring.

Pennsylvania: 42 Pa.C.S. § 6401 et seq. (2003).

Penrose, L. S. (1939). Mental disease and crime: Outline of a comparative study of European statistics. *British Journal of Medical Psychology,* 18, 1–15.

Pratt, J. & Dickson, M. (1997). *Dangerous, inadequate, invisible, out: Episodes in the criminological career of habitual criminals,* (pp. 364–366). Theoretical Criminology, Vol. 1, No. 3, 363–384.

Prentky, R. A., Janus, E., Barbaree, H., Schwartz, B. K., & Kafka, M. P. (2006). Sexually violent predators in the courtroom. *Psychology, Public Policy, and Law,* 12(4), 357–393.

Prentky, R. A. & Righthand, S. C. (2003). *Juvenile sex offender Assessment protocol-II: Manual.* Retrieved from www.csom.org. October 10, 2008.

Prevention of Crime Act, 1908, 8 Edw. 7, c. 59

Quinsey, V. L., Harris, G. T., Rice, M. E., & Cormier, C. A. (1998). *Violent offenders: Appraising and managing risk.* Washington D.C.: American Psychological Association.

R. v. Carey, (1951) 102 C.C.C. 25 (Ont. C.A.).

R. v. C.M.M., (1997) S.J. No. 860 (Sask. Ct. Q.B.).

R. v. Ferguson, (2000) O.J. No. 3008 (Ont. S.C.).

R. v. F.W.M., (2001) O.J. No. 4591 (S.C.J.).

R. v. Gibbon, (1998) B.C.J. No. 3210 (S.C.).

R. v. Hill, (1974) 15 C.C.C. (2d) 145 (Ont. C.A.).

R. v. Johnson, (1998) B.C.J. No. 3216 (S.C.).

R. v. Johnson (2003) 177 C.C.C. (3d) 97 (S.C.C.).

R. v. Kempton, (1980) 53 C.C.C. (2d) 176 at (Alta. C.A.).

R. v. LePage, (1994) O.J. No. 1305 at para. 65.

R. v. Lyons, (1987) 37 C.C.C. (3d) 1 (S.C.C.) at 24–25.

R. v. Mason (2001) 156 C.C.C. (3d) 97 (Ont. C.A.).

R. v. *M.B.*, (2000) O.J. No. 2135 (Ont. C.J.).

R. v. Payne (2001) O.J. No. 146 (S.C.J.).

R v. P.H., (2005) O.J. No. 5698 (S.C.J.).

R. v. Turley, (1999) 136 C.C.C. (3d) 426 (B.C.C.A.).

Radzinowicz, L., & Hood, R. (1986). *The Emergence of penal policy in Victorian and Edwardian England in a history of English Criminal Law and its administration from 1750*, (Vol. 5, pp. 588–591). London, Oxford: Clarendon, (out of print.

Report of the Royal Commission (Chair: Joseph Archambault) to Investigate the Penal System of Canada (Ottawa, 1938) at 4, 7–9, 220–223, 355–356.

Report of the Special Commissioner (Chair: General Ralph Burgess Gibson) to Consider the Several Recommendations Contained in the Report of the Royal Commission to Investigate the Penal System of Canada, April 4, 1938 (Ottawa, 1947) at 1 House of Commons Debates, Vol. V, 3rd Sess., 20th Parl. 11 George IV, 1947 at 4685, 5029–5031, 5065.

Righthand, S., & Welch, C. (2001). *Juveniles who have sexually offended: A review of the professional literature.* Washington, D.C: Office of Juvenile Justice and Delinquency Prevention.

S.C. Code Ann §§ 44–48 et seq. (1998).

Seling v. Young, 531 U.S. 250 (2001)

Stanford, M. S., & Barratt, E. S. (1995). Factor structure of the Barratt Impulsiveness Scale. *Journal of Clinical Psychology*, 51(6), 768–774.

Starnaman v. MHC-P (1995), 24 O.R. (3d) 701 (Ont. C.A.).

Strange, C. *Qualities of Mercy: Justice Punishment and Discretion*, Vancouver, 1996 quoted in Devereaux, S: *In Place Of Death: Transportation, Penal Practices, and The English State, 1770–1830.*

Sutherland, E. H. (1950). The diffusion of sexual psychopath laws. *American Journal of Sociology*, 56, 147.

Sutherland, E. H. (1950). The diffusion of sexual psychopath laws. *American Journal of Sociology*, 56, 142–148.

Texas: Tex. Health & Safety Code § 841.003 et seq.

Tucker, G., Tucker, S. G., & Blackstone, W. (1996). *Blackstone's commentaries: with notes of reference to the Constitution and Laws, of the Federal Government of the United States, and of the Commonwealth of Virginia : In five volumes.* Accessed at: http://www.lonang.com/exlibris/tucker/index.html Last accessed: October 10, 2008.

Vagrancy Act of 1744, 17 George II, c.5.

Victoria: Department of Justice: (1995) *Federal/Provincial/Territorial Task Force on High Risk Violent Offenders: Strategies for Managing High Risk Offenders.*

Virginia: Va. Code Ann. § 37.2–903 et seq.

Walker, N. (1968). *Crime and insanity in England* (vol. 1, pp. 84–85). Edinburgh: Edinburgh University Press.

Wash. Rev. Code Ann. § 4.24.550 et seq.

Wash. Rev. Code Ann. §§ 71.09 et seq. (1997).

Webster, C., Dickens, B., & Addario, S. (1985). *Constructing dangerousness: Scientific, legal and policy implications* (pp. 47–48, 144–145). Toronto: University of Toronto, Centre of Criminology.

Weinrott, M. R. (1996). *Juvenile sexual aggression: A critical review.* Boulder, CO:University of Colorado, Center for the Study and Prevention of Violence.

Winko v. British Columbia (Forensic Psychiatric Institute), (1999) 2 S.C.R. 625, at para.17–43.

Wisconsin: Wis. Stat. § 980.01 et seq.

Witt, P. H., & Schneider, J. (2005). Managing sex offenders by assessing dynamic risk factors. *Sex Offender Law Report*, 6, pp. 49, 54–57.

Wolff, N. (2003). Courting the court: courts as agents for treatment and justice. In W.H. Fisher (Ed.), *Community-based interventions for criminal offenders with severe mental illness* (pp. 143–197) Kidlington, Oxford UK: Elsevier Science.

Worling, J. R. (2004). *The Estimate of Risk of Adolescent Sexual Offense Recidivism (ERASOR)*: Preliminary psychometric data. *Sexual Abuse: A Journal of Research and Treatment*, 16, 965–982.

Worling, J. R., & Curwen, T. (2001). Estimate of risk of adolescent sexual offense Recidivism (The ERASOR: Version 2.0). Available from the author, j.worling@ ican.net.

Worling, J. R., & Langstrom, N. (2006). Risk of sexual recidivism in adolescents whooffend sexually: Correlates and assessment. In H. E. Barbaree & W. L. Marshall (Eds.), *The Juvenile sex Offender, Second Edition.* New York, NY: The Guildford Press.

Zimring, F. (2004). *An American travesty: Legal responses to adolescent sexual offending.* Chicago: University of Chicago Press.

Chapter 28

Community-Based Management of Sex Offenders: An Examination of Sex Offender Registries and Community Notification in the United States and Canada

Lisa Murphy, Daniel J. Brodsky, S. Jan Brakel, Michael Petrunik, J. Paul Fedoroff, and Albert J. Grudzinskas, Jr.

In Western societies, there is "no victim more sacred than a child and no offender more profane than one who spoils the innocence of children" (Petrunik, 2003, p. 352). During the 1980s and 1990s, sexual abuse of children emerged as a major social problem with high-profile incidents in the United States, Canada, and Europe arousing shock and anger among community members and acting as a catalyst for legislative innovation (Petrunik, 2005; Petrunik & Weisman, 2005; Jenkins, 2001). In addition to high-profile incidents, research began to be published showing the prevalence of sexual abuse was far higher than it had been previously thought to be. In the United States, one estimate is that as many as one in five children are sexually abused before the age of 18 years (Freeman-Longo, 1996). In Canada, a national victimization survey found just over one in two adult females and nearly one in three adult males reported being the victim of at least one unwanted sexual act over the course of their lifetime with over 80% of these acts occurring before the age of 18 years

(Committee on Sexual Offences Against Children and Youth, 1984).

In the late twentieth century a broad spectrum of sex offender policies were introduced across North America, Britain, Australia, New Zealand, and parts of continental Europe in response to an emerging perception of sex offending as a serious social problem. Their underpinnings can be traced to the junction of two trends in modern criminology: the expanding influence of the psychiatric interpretation of crime as symptomatic of mental disorder and increasing confidence in the scientific method and empirical analysis to understand human behavior. The innovation in the name of science was the community protection model justifying preventive legal action based upon deduction or hypothesis, rather than empirical proof or proven guilt for acts committed (Grant, 1998; Jackson, 1982; Krueger, 2007; Leggatt, 1984; Ouimet, 1969).

The community protection model also reflects the concerns of victim rights groups, crime prevention advocates, and the general public that sex offending, especially against children, is a serious problem necessitating strict and comprehensive measures of control (Jenkins, 2001; Petrunik, 2002; Petrunik & Deutschmann, 2008). According to this model, the best approach to the management of the high-risk sex offenders is a combination of social controls including longer sentences and stricter limits on parole, intensive community supervision, sex offender registration, community notification, orders restricting freedom of movement and association, mandatory antiandrogen treatment as a parole or probation condition, and criminal and civil statutes providing for indeterminate confinement based on findings of dangerousness and severe personality disorder (Petrunik, 1994, 2002, 2003, 2005).

The emergence and maintenance of two dominant forms of community-based risk management for sexual offenders within the United States and Canada are examined in this chapter: sex offender registries (SORs) and community notification of a previously confined sex offender's release. It will examine the rationale behind the use of these mechanisms for offender risk management and the events that led to the emergence of these legislative approaches, discuss how the policies work in practice, and identify some of their problematic consequences.

UNDERSTANDING THE RATIONALE BEHIND SEX OFFENDER REGISTRIES AND PUBLIC NOTIFICATION

Sex offender registries (SORs) require that convicted sex offenders or those found not criminally responsible or individuals designated as "sexually violent predators (SVPs)" when released from psychiatric institutions register with local police, provide personal details about themselves, and report future changes in their life circumstances (e.g., change in address). In Canada, these offenses may include sexual interference, invitation to sexual touching, sexual exploitation, sexual assault, the creation, possession and distribution of child pornography, and bestiality (Ministry of Community Safety and Correctional Services, 2004). In the United States, these offenses may include felony offenses such as rape, indecent assault and battery on a child under 14 years, indecent assault and battery on a mentally retarded person, rape of a child under 16 with force, rape and abuse of a child under 16, and drugging persons for sexual

intercourse. They may also include such crimes as: open and gross lewdness and lascivious behavior and accosting or annoying persons of the opposite sex and lewd, wanton and lascivious speech or behavior, and "any attempt to commit any of the aforementioned crimes or a like violation of the laws of another state, the United States or a military, territorial or Indian tribal authority any other offense, the facts of which, under the totality of the circumstances, manifest a sexual motivation or pattern of conduct or series of acts of sexually-motivated offenses" (Mass. Gen'l Law, ch. 123 § 1).

SORs are based on the hypothesis that having current reliable data about convicted sex offenders, particularly where they live, can reduce the risk of their reoffending and help police identify and apprehend suspects (Brodsky, 2006; Cole & Petrunik, 2006, 2007; Hudson, 2005).

According to Matravers (2003), persistent attention to sex offenders is based on the construct of the "predatory pedophile," who while neither normal nor insane, is a high-risk threat to the safety of children. Reports by commercial media often sensationalize high-profile cases resulting in facilitation of the "spectre of an invisible stranger in our midst, preying on the vulnerable young" (Matravers, 2003, p. 110). The image of predators sharing common characteristics lurking behind bushes waiting to pounce on unsuspecting victims is not rooted in reality. The vast majority of sexual offenses are committed by someone who is well-known to the victim (Greenfield, 1997). This is particularly true for child victims. A recent review of research (McAlinden, 2007) found that 80% to 98% of child sexual abuse victims are abused by someone known to them. If most offenders are already known to their victims, one may question whether SORs and public notification add significant protection (Freeman-Longo, 1996).

In Canada, access to the National SOR and Ontario's SOR is restricted to specific designated criminal justice officials. In the United States, SORs are more publically accessible, in most states via the Internet (please see discussion of the *Walsh Act* herein), and are directly linked with systems of community notification that disclose various amounts and kinds of information about convicted sex offenders residing in the community (Matson & Lieb, 1996). The use of public notification works from the assumption that registration alone inadequately protects community members from known sex offenders.

Notification is thought to help prevent further sexual offenses by alerting communities to the arrival of individuals with histories of criminal sexual behavior. The idea or hope is that public safety is enhanced as parents warn their children about allegedly dangerous members of the community and report suspicious behavior to the authorities (Petrosino & Petrosino, 1999). The concomitant belief is that potential reoffenders may be deterred from seeking new victims (Freeman-Longo, 1996).

While most jurisdictions in the United States mandate formal community notification to some degree, in the case of all registered sex offenders, community notification in Canada is not linked to the registration process and occurs only in some provinces under the auspices of provincial community safety legislation and even there, only rarely (Petrunik, 2003). Despite variation in the specifics of SOR and notification systems, there are some common principles. Decisions regarding who warrants a community notification and which communities are informed are typically based on estimates of the offender's risk to the community. In determining whether to initiate a public notification, criminal justice officials must work to achieve a balance between the safety of the public and the offender's right to privacy.

In the United States, notification decisions in most states are based on a three-tier model which ranks individuals at a high-, moderate-, or low-risk to reoffend and provides information accordingly. Generally, the more dangerous the offender is deemed to be the wider the range of entities to be notified. Typically, there is an independent board which makes an individual risk assessment and then determines how much of a danger the offender poses upon release. In the case of individuals designated as low-risk only local law enforcement agencies will be informed. Examples of low-risk offenders could include a man convicted of incest who is deemed unlikely to offend again against a family member or anyone outside of his immediate family or an adolescent convicted of statutory rape for having sex with a girlfriend who is a few years younger. For those designated as moderate risk a broader spectrum of community organizations may be notified including schools and recreational organizations. Those deemed high-risk require notification of the general public or all those living within a certain radius of the offender's residence (Center for Sex Offender Management, 1997; Kabat, 1998; Matson & Lieb, 1996).

Photographs and maps showing where registered offenders reside may also be provided on state-run web sites (Kabat, 1998; Matson & Lieb, 1996; Petrunik, 2005). In some states, sex offenders placed on probation or convicted for failure to register may be required to wear a global positioning device (GPS) monitored by local law enforcement and/or probation officials (See Mass. Gen'l Law, ch. 6 §178 C-Q; c. 127 § 133D, 2006).

In Canada, formal public notification does not occur with all or even most sex offenders and is not limited just to sex offenders. Formal notification is used by police and local offender risk-assessment committees only in the case of offenders considered to pose an immediate and serious risk of a violent offense or sexual offense. Generally, formal notification is rare although there are some frequency variations among municipalities with certain local police forces electing to use provincial community safety legislation more than others.

When looking at these tools it is important to examine the historical development which led to the implementation of such measurements for the community management of sexual offenders and how these mechanisms work.

LEGISLATIVE DEVELOPMENTS WITHIN THE UNITED STATES

A key event sparking the emergence of the community protection approach in the United States was the 1989 abduction, sexual assault, and mutilation of a 7-year-old boy in the state of Washington by Earl Shriner, a mentally disordered offender with a long history of sexual violence. Public outrage ensued when it was learned that, although Shriner's residence was on a street used by many children to go to school, school officials had allegedly not been informed of Shriner's presence nearby because of constraints posed by state privacy legislation. The subsequent aggressive lobbying by the victim's mother and various victim advocacy groups led to the appointment of a Community Protection Task Force (CPTF). On the basis of the recommendations of the task force, the Washington Senate passed the *Community Protection Act (CPA)*. This included a set of measures that allowed for post-sentence civil commitment of individuals who met the criteria for the newly created category of "SVP," the implementation of a statewide sex offender registry

(SOR) and a three-tiered approach to community notification (Petrunik, 2003; State of Washington, 1989) (See Table 28.1).

At about the same time, victim rights organizations across the United States began to lobby for child protection legislation and following the lead of Washington, many other states enacted laws for the community-based management of sexual offenders. The legislation was often named after the victims of sex crimes. This was the case of the federal *Jacob Wetterling Law* mandating states to set up sex offender registration systems, the federal and the state of New Jersey's *Megan's Law* mandating community notification, and *Zachary's Law* in Indiana which created the first online SOR to allow the public to access specific sexual offender information via the internet. Currently, there are over 30 states that allow for the online access to SORs (Petrunik, 2003).

The 1994 *"Jacob Wetterling Crimes against Children and Sexually Violent Offender Registration Act"* or JWA required all states to set up a functioning SOR within 3 years or receive a penalty consisting of a 10% cut in state federal funding for criminal justice initiatives (Lewis, 1996). The law required that the Registry include at a minimum the names, identifying features such as scars or tattoos, residence information, offenses, and treatment histories of released sex offenders (Jacob Wetterling Crimes Against Children and Sexually Violent Offender Registration Act, 1994). Currently, every state in the United States requires some form of sex offender registration (Petrunik, 2005).

While the specific characteristics of SORs tend to vary by jurisdiction, most share a set of common features. Across the United States, registries tend to be run by state agencies that delegate law enforcement officials to collect offender information including photos, fingerprints, social security numbers, places of employment, and vehicle registrations. A smaller number of states also collect blood samples for DNA identification (Finn, 1997).

The time frame for initial registration can vary from before release, to immediately upon release and up to 1 year post release. The most common time is

TABLE 28.1 U.S. Legislative Developments for SORs and Community Notification

Year	Legislative Change	Location	Implications
June 1989	Community Protection Task Force (CPTF)	Washington	Governor sets up force to deal with intense community reaction over abduction of a young boy by Earl Shriner
February 1990	Community Protection Act (CPA)	Washington	Based on recommendations by CPTF, policy is implemented for civil commitment of SVPs, state-wide SOR and approach to public notification
June 1994	Zachary's Law	Indiana	Sets up first online SOR
July–October 1994	Megan's Law	New Jersey	Modeled after Washington's CPA. Passed within 89 days
September 1994	Jacob Wetterling Act (JWA)	National	Requires all states to set up a SOR within 3 years or receive a criminal justice funding cut
May 1996	Megan's Law	National	Amendments to JWA. All states required to set up community notification process within 3 years or receive criminal justice funding cut
October 1996	Pam Lychner Sex Offender tracking & Identification Act	National	FBI mandated to establish National SOR and requires lifetime registration for sex offenders with victims under 12
July 2006	Adam Walsh Child Protection Act	National	National SOR based on three-tiered system; requires unified system of criteria for online SOR; makes failure to comply a felony

within 30 days of the offender's release. This is logical as the defendant has 30 days to file a notice of appeal. For most of the states the required duration of registration is a minimum of 10 years. In some cases, registration can be for life, at least for the most serious tier of offenders. It is possible for an offender to challenge their classification and time on the registry. It is possible to make this challenge even after initially being placed on the registry. The time designated to be on a SOR is typically influenced by offense type, sentence length, and age and number of victims (Finn, 1997).

In 1996, an amendment to the federal JWA known as *Megan's Law* (there is also a New Jersey law by that name after Megan Kanka who was assaulted and murdered by a sex offender in that state) required all states to implement mechanisms, based on federal standards, to provide members of the community with specific information on registered sex offenders deemed relevant to protect the public (notably, place of residence). States not complying within 3 years faced criminal justice funding cutbacks similar to those outlined under the JWA (Brakel & Cavanaugh, 2000). By the end of 1996, 32 states had initiated notification policies which enabled individuals to submit requests for offender information or to require law enforcement agencies to disseminate offender information upon their release within the community (Finn, 1997). Currently, all states in the United States provide formal community notification of the whereabouts and characteristics of registered sex offenders (Petrunik, 2005).

In about half the states that have notification legislation, law enforcement officials have discretion to determine the extent to which community agencies and members of the public need to be notified about the presence of a given sex offender. The privacy rights of both victims and offenders come into play, particularly in the case of intrafamilial offenses where the risk of recidivism may be low and notification could be harmful to healing and reconciliation between and among family members (Kabat, 1998).

Under a subsequent amendment to the JWA known as the *Pam Lychner Sexual Offender Tracking and Identification Act of 1996* the Federal Bureau of Investigation was required to establish a National SOR which linked individual state databases to enable officials to track sex offenders across state lines. Additionally, this law required lifetime registration for sexual offenders whose victims were below 12 years of age. All states were also required to make

failure to register at least a misdemeanor (Wetterling Act at § 1407[d]).

In 2006, the United States Congress repealed the Wetterling Act and replaced it with the *Walsh Act* (18 USCS § 2250 and 42 USCS § 16901), which organizes offenders according to a three-tiered system: 15-year registration for tier I offenders; 25 years for tier II; and lifetime for tier III. States are to follow a unified set of criteria for posting offender information on internet accessible SORs taking into account designations of offender risk level. Failure to comply by an offender is a felony offense. Other elements provided for within the Act include registration before release from custody, or within 3 days thereof for all levels of sex offenders, including juveniles 14 years or older if convicted of aggravated sexual abuse (as federally defined) and a requirement on the part of authorities to obtain a DNA sample from each offender. Information must also be disseminated to law enforcement, social service agencies, volunteer agencies, and other organizations in the community where the person lives, works, and attends school. Again, states failing to comply face the loss of specific federal "crime-fighting funds."

LEGISLATIVE DEVELOPMENTS IN THE CANADIAN CONTEXT

Compared to the rapid development of American sexual offender laws and policies, Canadian developments generally came at a slower pace (Petrunik, 2003) (see Table 28.2). Indeed, it was not a particularly infamous offender or shocking crime that initially brought the problem of violent sexual recidivism to the forefront of public attention in Canada to spur legislative action. The post-war world just seemed to be a more dangerous place as the troops returned home and attention was increasingly redirected to issues of public safety on the home front. In particular, Canadians were sensitized by popular American media portrayals of sex offenders driven by uncontrollable perverted lust (Chenier, 2008). Later, in the late 1980s and 1990s the community containment approach in Canada, as in the United States, escalated in response to the sensational media coverage of a high-profile sexual offender, the victims left behind and the demands of an alarmed public.

The widely publicized abduction, sexual assault, and murder of Christopher Stephenson by Joseph

TABLE 28.2 Canadian Legislative Development for SORs and Community Notification

Year	Legislative Change	Location	Implications
March 1992	Bill C-36 under Corrections and Conditional Release Act	National	Allows for correctional officials to provide information to the police pertaining to the release of an offender where there is reasonable grounds to believe that the offender will pose a significant threat to persons in the community
September 1992–Janruary 1993	Coroner's Inquest into death of Christopher Stephenson	Ontario	Releases recommendation for the adoption of a SOR, a law modeled after Washington's SVP statute, 10 years of probation (postsentence) for high-risk offenders and changes to CPIC to allow better data on high-risk offenders
February 1995	Community safety Legislation	Manitoba	First to introduce community notification protocol allowing police to notify public about presence of high-risk offenders in community. Other provinces quickly follow suit
March 2001	Canadian Alliance Party advocates NSOR	National	House of Commons unanimously supports creation of NSOR. But Solicitor General states Canadian Police Information Centre (CPIC) can function as SOR
April 2001	Bill 31 creates Christopher's Law	Ontario	Implements Canada's first provincial SOR in memory of Christopher Stephenson. Other provinces and territories begin to follow
May 2001	Plans for Provincial interlinking SORs to create NSOR	Provincial	Provinces provide political pressure by announcing plans to develop provincially interlinking SORs to create NSOR
December 2004	Bill C-23 creates Sex Offender Information Registration Act (SOIRA)	National	Creation of NSOR

Fredericks in 1988 acted as a catalyst for change and set the stage for Canadian legislative reform. Fredericks was a convicted pedophile and diagnosed psychopath who had spent over two decades in a high security psychiatric hospital and had been out of prison on federal statutory release for only a few months when he murdered his victim. Christopher's parents began a highly public attempt to understand how and why such a predator with a lifelong history of sexual violence had been released to the community. As a result of their efforts, in 1992 a Coroner's Inquest was initiated into the circumstances of Christopher's death and the evident failure of the criminal justice and mental health system to protect the public (Petrunik & Weisman, 2005).

One of the recommendations flowing from the Inquest was for the creation of a National Sex Offender Registry (NSOR) which required such offenders to register with their local police station. It was suggested that this SOR be modeled after Washington's 1990 CPA (Petrunik & Weisman, 2005). The recommendations reflected the perceived need for policy that allowed for more comprehensive monitoring of sexual offenders within the community. Initially, neither the federal nor provincial governments responded to the recommendations to enact a SOR but, in 1999, Ontario acted on its own to become the first jurisdiction in Canada to set up a SOR. With the public support of the Stephenson family, law enforcement organizations and victims' rights groups, the Ontario legislature made the registry a reality when it proclaimed Christopher's Law in April of 2001 (Ministry of Community Safety and Correctional Services, 2004).

The Ontario Sex Offender Registry is maintained by the Ontario Provincial Police (OPP) on behalf of the Ministry of Community Safety and Correctional Services. Under Christopher's Law, all Ontario residents convicted of a sexual offense (as defined by the legislation since the policy's implementation) and any resident serving a sentence for a sexual offense on the day that the policy came into force, are subject to registration. Also required to register are individuals found not criminally responsible by reason of mental disorder of a designated sex offense and juvenile offenders convicted of a designated sex offense and sentenced as adults. All individuals meeting at least one of these criteria are automatically placed on the Ontario SOR.

Anyone convicted of a designated sex offense must report in person to a specified police station or detachment within 15 days of being released from custody if incarcerated, after a conviction if not given a custodial sentence, after a change in address, after becoming an Ontario resident, or after ceasing to be an Ontario resident. Individuals meeting these criteria are also required to register annually within the 11th and 12th month of the last reporting period. The designated reporting period is either 10 years or life, depending on the maximum length of the sentence and the number of criteria offenses committed. A person may be put on the registry for 10 years if the maximum sentence for the offense for which he was convicted is less than 10 years. If the maximum sentence is more than 10 years and/or the person has committed more than one designated sex offense registration may be for life. Information that appears on the registry includes the offender's name, date of birth, current address, a photograph, and the sex offense(s) for which they have been convicted (Christopher's Law, 2000).

Failure to comply with registration requirements can result in significant penalties. A first conviction of failure to register can result in a fine of no more than $25,000, a term of imprisonment for no more than 1 year, or both. All subsequent offenses of failure to comply warrant a fine of $25,000, a term of imprisonment of no more than 2 years less, a day, or both. Currently, the only way to have one's name removed from the Registry is to obtain a formal pardon. Unlike U.S. SORs, those in Canada are not open to the public. While the national sex offender database in Canada is maintained by the Royal Canadian Mounted Police (RCMP), it may be searched by any police agency across the country to investigate crimes of a sexual nature. Ontario's database cannot be used for the purposes of public notification under provincial legislation (Christopher's Law, 2000).

Upon the implementation of the Ontario SOR, several other provinces indicated they would follow suit. However, Canada's national government was initially quite resistant to the pressures to implement a NSOR similar to the United States. Rather than responding swiftly, the federal officials created a federal, provincial, and territorial task force to address the issue. As a result of proceeding so cautiously, legislative reforms that were established within a few years in the United States took well over a decade to emerge within the Canadian context. It was not until other provinces besides Ontario announced plans to independently establish a system of interlinked registries across Canada that the national government announced plans to take action (Petrunik, 2003).

The Sex Offender Information Registration Act (SOIRA) came into force on December 15, 2004. The RCMP is responsible for the administration and maintenance of the NSOR. It is accessible to police agencies in every province and territory across Canada. SOIRA works to ensure that only specific individuals are able to access the information on the registry. This includes law enforcement personnel who are investigating a crime in which there is reasonable grounds to suspect that the offense is of a sexual nature. There is substantial controversy over this issue. During abduction investigations, time is of the essence and unless investigators provide reasonable grounds that an offense is of a "sexual nature," they are unable to access the National database. This is one of the main differences between the NSOR and the Ontario SOR, since Christopher's Law contains no such restriction (Ministry of Community Safety and Correctional Services, 2004).

Other individuals who are permitted to access the registry include employees at the registration centre who maintain the database and those who ensure that offenders are complying with the established requirements. Also, individuals who have been retained by the Commissioner to conduct research under the act are permitted access (Sex Offender Information Registration Act, 2005).

The SOIRA amends the *Criminal Code* by allowing prosecutors to make a formal request to the court for the offender's inclusion on the NSOR (Sex Offender Information Registration Act, 2005). Unlike the Ontario SOR where the sex offenders are placed on the registry automatically, a sexual offender is placed on the NSOR only if a formal request is made at the time of sentencing. The SOIRA makes it an offense to fail to comply with the order or to report false information (Sex Offender Information Registration Act, 2005). The NSOR is not retroactive; so an offender who completed his or her sentence before the date the legislation became law is not registered. However, all sex offenders who were under sentence for a designated offense on the date the legislation became law were served a Notice of Obligation to Comply with SOIRA and be registered. From December 15, 2004 onward prosecutors may apply to a Judge for an order to comply with the SOIRA after the sentencing of an offender for a designated sex offense. After an order is granted, the offender will be registered on the database.

Under the SOIRA a sex offender may be required to report for a period of 10 years, 20 years or life, depending on the maximum length of the sentence. The Act requires that all registrants report on an annual basis and 15 days before a change in residence or legal name. The information required by the NSOR is more extensive than is the case with the Ontario SOR. It includes the offender's name and aliases, date of birth, height, weight, distinguishing marks, finger prints, residential address, telephone number(s), place of work, paid or volunteer, or educational institution, type, date and place of offense(s), age and gender of victim(s), and the duration of registration required by the statute (Sex Offender Information Registration Act, 2005).

If the registrant does not comply or provides false information, as a first offense he is subject to a fine of $10,000, a sentence of 6 months, or both. On subsequent offenses the penalty increases to a fine of $10,000, a sentence of 2 years, less a day, or both. Similar to the Ontario SOR, the NSOR is not retroactive, meaning individuals will be placed on the NSOR only if they are convicted of a designated sexual offense after the implementation of the SOIRA, or were serving a sentence for a designated offense on the day that the act came into effect (Sex Offender Information Registration Act, 2005).

Although the use of SORs and the process of community notification have been directly linked across the United States, both Canada and the United Kingdom have resisted legislation requiring notification of the community about the location of registered sex offenders and their identifying characteristics.

The reason for this resistance is the belief that notification has more negative consequences than benefits. In particular, there is a concern that public notification has the effect of decreasing SOR compliance. This notion is supported by data indicating that in the United States compliance rates though varying are overall much lower than the over 95% compliance rates reported in Canada and the United Kingdom (Cole & Petrunik, 2006, 2007).

Subsection 25(3) of the 1992 Corrections and Conditional Release Act requires correctional officials to inform local police of the release from custody of all offenders detained to warrant expiry or on temporary absence, parole, or mandatory supervision. In the case of offenders released on warrant expiry who are considered to poses a significant threat to persons in the community, correctional officials are required to provide the police with all information within their control pertaining to the perceived threat posed by the released offender (Corrections and Conditional Release Act, 1992). The decision to make a community notification about the release of a sexual offender into the community takes place under provincial community safety legislation and is decided by the police and sometimes involves high-risk offender committees.

In February 1995, Manitoba became the first province to enact a specific protocol for community notification which authorized police agencies to disclose information to the public regarding the release of a high-risk sex offender (Sutherland, 1999). Once the dam was broken in Manitoba other provinces followed. In 1998 Ontario created its own notification protocol with the enactment of Bill 102, the *Community Safety Act* (Petrunik, 2003).

Most of the offenders who are subject to notification are judged to be at such a high risk that they are kept to warrant expiry; that is, to the end of their sentence when the criminal justice system no longer has any controls over the offender. This also means, however, that at that point the offender is free to go into the community irrespective of his lingering risk to recidivate. The law includes guidance points for municipal police on the release of information on high-risk sex offenders (National Joint Committee, 2006).

While the Canadian SORs, in contrast to those of the United States, do not allow community notification, such notification may occur under separate provincial community legislation in specific cases. Currently, there is no single method of notifying the community under provincial legislation; the approaches are diverse. Methods include holding community forums, notifying particular institutions such as schools or recreation centers, creating bulletin boards, and issuing press releases (Brodsky, 2006). At least one province (Alberta) has an Internet site providing information on offenders for whom public notification is appropriate under provincial community safety legislation (Petrunik, 2003).

LIMITATIONS AND CHALLENGES TO SORS AND PUBLIC NOTIFICATION

Sex offender registration and public notification are controversial concepts and have been subject to considerable litigation across the United States and Canada. Opponents of SORs and public notification have drawn attention to a number of problematic issues with regard to fundamental human rights. These critics argue that it is not fair to impose additional measures on sex offenders after the completion of their sentence on the ground that they have already paid their debt to society and should not be burdened with additional scrutiny from which "normal" offenders would be immune.

Because legislators have designated sex offenders to be a greater risk to community safety than other kinds of offenders those who have committed sex crimes have been subject to extensive monitoring and restrictions on their freedom of movement and association even after the completion of sentence. This can be challenged on several grounds. First, sex offenders as a general category do not have higher rates of recorded new offenses than the categories of nonsexual violent offender and nonviolent offender (Hanson & Bussiere, 1998). Second, sexual offenders are not a homogenous group. Different types of offenders vary greatly in their risk of future offending and their amenability to treatment.

Meta-analysis of 61 studies by Hanson and Bussiere (1998), that followed up sex offenders for 4 to 5 years after release from prison found that the average rate of conviction for a subsequent offense was 13.4%. A comprehensive study by Quinsey et al. (1998) found that among a population of convicted child molesters, intrafamilial (incest) offenders with opposite sex victims posed a much lower risk of being detected, apprehended and convicted in the commission of subsequent sexual offenses than did extrafamilial offenders whose victims were of the same sex or of both sexes. Pedophiles with boy victims have the highest rates of apprehension and conviction for new offenses.

Many sex offenders only commit a single, situational sexual offense that is not part of any broader pattern of offending. By virtue of the generic label of "sexual offender," this one-time offender is grouped within the same category as a predatory, multiple-victim offender. Insult is added to injury so to speak when criminal justice agencies use investigative and assessment methods that do not distinguish between risk levels for specific offender types.

The aforementioned becomes more problematic yet when SORs are publiclly accessible via the Internet. Although the mechanism of notification is supposed to elicit a process of support and supervision by the community, it often also creates feelings of anger and increases the danger of vigilantism (Brodsky, 2006). There have already been incidents of serious violence associated with notification and online access to offender information in the United States. In the state of Washington, following a notification an angry mob from the community surrounded the house of a known sex offender and burned it down. In New Jersey, an innocent man was mistaken for a sex offender and assaulted (Freeman-Longo, 1996). A 20-year-old man from New Brunswick Canada shot and killed two individuals whose name, photo, and home address appeared on the neighbouring State of Maine's online SOR, and then took his own life. One of the individuals killed had been convicted of a statutory offense after having sexual intercourse with his girlfriend who was only a few years younger than he was but legally a minor (Ranalli & Heinz, 2006).

Encouragement to take personal action against sex offenders has increased with groups such as *Perverted Justice*, which has a website spreading fear and resentment against "sexual predators." This group consists of private citizens who work together against sexual victimization and they have hinted at the use of force in some instances. The group, which claims to be a nonprofit organization, seeks to portray sex offenders as an uncontrollable group and encourages site visitors to join forces in the protest movement designed to instil a "chilling effect" within the network of sexual offenders (see perverted-justice.com).

An additional consequence of notification concerns the privacy of the victims and their families. In instances where the case has been publicized and the victim is known to the community, notification often draws unwanted attention to the victim. Although victims' names do not appear directly on SORs, when the authorities notify the public there is a risk of exposing the identities of victims of offenses. This issue is a particular concern in cases where a child was a victim of an incest offense. Notification can stigmatize victims and other family members and impede efforts to achieve healing and reconciliation. Research in New Jersey has found that incidents of incest offenses are not being reported as victims fear a variety of negative consequences as a result of notification. This problem is especially acute when the victim is living with the offender (Freeman-Longo, 1996).

Other concerns arise in connection with the use of these community containment techniques as a mechanism for general social control. Because the majority of sexual offenses are not committed by strangers but by someone known to the victim, public notification provides a false sense of security for the community (Freeman-Longo, 1996). Furthermore, even if SORs and community notification provide members of the public with a general feeling of safety, such feelings may be illusory. Indeed, some research has shown that widespread community notification without effectively utilizing public education tends to heighten general fear of victimization (Brodsky, 2006; Zevitz & Farkas, 2000a).

The cost to implement and successfully maintain state or provincial as well as National SORs and notification systems is high. Many of the criticisms about SORs focus on the costs of keeping information in the databases accurate and up to date. Since sex offenders are required to register from periods of 10 years up until life, it is foreseeable that maintenance costs will continue to increase substantially, as there is currently no set or ready way for most offenders to get off of the Registry.

Various cases across the United States and Canada have challenged the laws based on the offenders' rights to privacy. Many courts have deferred rulings in anticipation of changes in legislation or have had their decisions rendered moot with the enactment of newer legislation. However, some cases have proved to be an exception to this scenario.

Challenges which claim that the law is an imposition of a new or second penalty and therefore violates constitutional prohibitions against ex post facto laws and double jeopardy have met with little success. Basically, courts in the United States have held that the Eight Amendment (which prohibits "cruel and unusual punishment") or the Fifth Amendment (which contains the double jeopardy prohibition) do not apply to registration since it is a civil process whose manifest intention is to regulate future behavior and not punish someone for a past offense. However, the imposition of enhanced penalties (lifetime community parole) for violating the registration requirement before the law's enactment has prompted at least one court to declare that the enhanced penalties are permitted only for violations committed after the statute went into effect (*Commonwealth v. Talbot*, 2005).

Governmental privacy invasions may under some circumstances be permitted but they must be supported by adequate, if not compelling, justification and must be minimally impairing. At least one New Jersey case has held that the SOR and community notification are not in violation of the offender's constitutional right to privacy (*Doe v. Poritz*, 1995). However, a later (2001) New Jersey decision held that giving complete public access to all sex offender information is unconstitutional and ordered that the home address of sex offenders must be withdrawn from the state's online notification system (*A.A. v. New Jersey*, 2001).

In Ontario, if it is found that the requirement for an individual to register as a sex offender is a grossly disproportionate violation of the offender's rights to privacy under the Canadian Charter of Rights and Freedoms then that individual can be exempted from registering (*R. v. Burke*, 2005). However, in *R. v. Ayoob* (2005) the court did not find that there was a grossly disproportionate violation of the offender's privacy rights and he was not exempt from the process. The outcome in these cases ultimately turned on the extent of the offender's criminal record and the relative seriousness of the offense violation. In the case of *R. v. Dyck*, in December of 2005, the Ontario Superior Court of Justice ruled in favor of the Ontario SOR stating that being placed on the Registry was not in violation of offender's constitutional rights under the Charter.

Now that SORs and public notification are established mechanisms, research should consider the effectiveness of such community management tools.

RESEARCH ON REGISTRATION AND NOTIFICATION

The literature on SORs and public notification tends to be classified into four broad types: statistical profiles of registrant's demographics, evaluations of the effect on recidivism, assessments of the accuracy of reported information, and examinations of the collateral consequences of the process of registration (Mustaine, Tewksbury, & Stengel, 2006).

Since a fundamental goal of the utilization of SORs and public notification systems is to decrease recidivism and victimization, research to establish how effective they are should arguably play a pivotal role in justifying the use of such tools. However, there currently exists no research that demonstrates the effectiveness of registration and notification in decreasing recidivism. A study by Schram and Milloy (1995) examined the impact of notification on subsequent recidivism in a group of Washington sex offender who received notifications as compared to a group of sex offenders who did not receive notification. The results were measured over a 4.5 year follow-up and showed no statistically significant difference in the overall levels of general recidivism and for sexual recidivism the rates differed insignificantly. The main difference between the two groups was that the offender's subject to notification requirements tended to be rearrested sooner than those without notification.

A study conducted in Iowa assessed the impact of SORs on recidivism and found "mixed effects" on the rates of reoffending (Adkins, Huff, & Stageberg, 2000). Such research indicates that overall SORs and notification have little, if any, effectiveness in reducing sex offenders' propensity to commit new crimes.

Research shows that results in terms of level of compliance are disappointing. Criminal investigators in Iowa estimate that 40% of sex offenders who are supposed to be registered actually are not so registered (Scholle, 2000). In 2003, California's SOR system reported it had "lost track" of 33,296 registrants. These were sex offenders who had, at one point, been properly registered and then were just forgotten about. Most likely these are individuals who were registered but failed to report a change of address and it was never noticed. This means that California lost contact with a staggering 44% of all registrants across the state (Cohen & Jeglic, 2007). Canada has demonstrated compliance rates of about 95% showing significant difference in compliance rates of Canadian and U.S. sex offenders.

Another area of interest is the potential collateral consequences experienced by the sex offenders

subject to registration and notification. Insight into this area is provided by interviews with registered sex offenders who experienced community notification. Results show that the most common problems reported by sex offenders are difficulties obtaining employment and securing housing, being ostracized and harassed by the community, and financial loss. Many offenders also explained that it caused emotional issues for their family and as a result some family members ostracized the offender (Pogrebin, Dodge, & Katsampes, 2001; Zevitz & Farkas, 2000b). According to Tewksbury (2005) differences in patterns across groups reveal that registrants in nonmetropolitan communities are subject to more social consequences as a result of registration.

This research suggests that the process of registration and notification sets the stage for many potentially negative social consequences for the offender. When the public learns that a sex offender resides within their community they may become more fearful and harass, discriminate against, or even victimize the registered offender. As a result, the offender may experience an increase in stress and frustration whereby the offender may become more isolated. Such events could act as a possible antecedent to a relapse. Thus, aggressive responses of the community to registered sex offenders may heighten stress levels which may indirectly contribute to subsequent reoffending (Zevitz & Farkas, 2000b).

Surprisingly, postrelease sex offenders may be less opposed to SORs then generally assumed. Some say the requirement to register yearly is no more onerous than renewing their driver's license. Others even claim that being on an SOR has decreased the number of times they are interviewed by police when a new unsolved sex offense occurs since they can be ruled out more quickly (P. Fedoroff, personal communication). What offenders do object to is any measure that increases their visibility in the community. Measures such as police checks by officers in unmarked cars and in plain clothes create less chance of stigmatization. In contrast, postrelease offenders who are publicly identified are much more likely to lose their jobs, their social supports, and their accommodations. Paradoxically, in these cases, public notification may actually increase risk to the community by destabilizing the offender and interfering with his ability to seek treatment.

CONCLUSION

The process of maintaining a balance between protection of the public and individuals' rights to privacy becomes increasingly difficult when the offender is considered dangerous or "morally tainted." Mechanisms such as SORs and community notification have been implemented as a political response to highly publicized cases of sexual victimization. Supporters of these interventions claim that such supervisory methods will deter sexual offenders from reoffending while providing information on which the public may act to protect its children and others who may be vulnerable and at the same time giving an investigative tool with which police can more efficiently "solve" sexual offenses.

In contrast, opponents of SORs and community notification stress concerns about a discriminatory aspect to the regulations that specifically targets sex offenders when there is an absence of evidence that sex offenders, as a general category, are at a greater risk to reoffend than other categories of offenders. Additionally, critics have raised concerns about the ethics or legality of infringing on the rights of a segment of the population whose targets have already served their sentence and paid the penalty for their misconduct. These contending positions make clear that the underlying value and utility of SORs and community notification need to be realigned with the stated goals of these mechanisms, while eliminating to the extent possible the unintended negative costs and consequences.

References

A.A. v. New Jersey, 176 F. Supp. 2d 274 (2001).

Adkins, G., Huff, D., & Stageberg, P. (2000). *The Iowa sex offender registry and recidivism*. Des Moines: Iowa Department of Human Rights.

Berliner, L. (1998). *Sex offenders: Policy and practice*, 92 Nw. U. L. Rev. 92(4) 1203–1204.

Brakel, S. J. & Cavanaugh, J. (2000). *Of psychopaths and pendulums: Legal and psychiatric treatment of sex offenders in the Unites States*, 30 N.M.L. Rev. 69.

Brodsky, D. (2006). *The 'predator' next door: Risk management at the community interface*. 37th Annual AAPL meeting. Chicago, USA.

Center for Sex Offender Management. (1997). *An overview of sex offender community notification practices: Policy implications and promising approaches*. Silver Spring, MD: Center for Sex Offender Management.

Chenier, E. (2008) *Strangers in our midst: Sexual deviancy in postwar* Ontario, Toronto: University of Toronto Press.

Christopher's Law (Sex Offender Registry), 2000, S.O. 2000, c.1

Cohen, M. & Jeglic, E. (2007). Sex offender legislation in the United States: What do we know? *International Journal of Offender Therapy and Comparative Criminology*, 51(4), 369–383.

Cole, M. & Petrunik, M. (2006). Sex offender registration and privacy rights. *Criminal Justice Reports*, 21(3), 30–33.

Cole, M. & Petrunik, M. (2007). Sex offender registries. In W. Staples (Ed.), Encyclopedia of privacy, (Vol. 2, pp. 493–496). Westport, CT: Greenwood Press.

Committee on Sexual Offences Against Children and Youths. (1984). Sexual Offences Against Children and Youth (Vol. 1) Ottawa: Supply and Services Canada.

Commonwealth v. Talbot, 444 Mass. 586, 597 (2005).

Corrections and Conditional Release Act, S.C. 1992, c. 20.

Doe v. Poritz, 142 N.J. 1; 662 A.2d 367 (1995).

Finn, P. (1997). *Sex offender community notification*. U.S. Department of Justice Office of Justice Programs, National Institute of Justice.

Freeman-Longo, R. (1996). *Feel good legislation: Prevention or calamity. Journal of Child Abuse & Neglect*, 20(2), 95–101.

Grant, I. (1998). *Legislating public safety: The business of risk. Canadian Criminal Law Review*, 3(2), 177–142.

Greenfield, L. (1997). *Sex offenses and offenders: An analysis of data on rape and sexual assault*. Washington, D.C.: U.S. Department of Justice.

Hanson, R. K. & Bussiere, M. T. (1998). Predicting relapse: A meta-analysis of sexual offender recidivism studies. *Journal of Consulting and Clinical Psychology*, 60, 348–362.

Hudson, K. (2005). *Offending identities: Sex offenders' perspectives on their treatment and management*. Portland, OR: Willan Publishing.

Jackson, M. (1982). *Sentences that never end: The report on the habitual criminal study*. Vancouver, Canada: University of British Columbia.

Jacob Wetterling Crimes Against Children and Sexually Violent Offender Registration Act. (1994). Public law 103–322. 42 U.S.C. §§ 14071 et seq.

Jenkins, P. (2001). How Europe discovered its sex offender crisis. In J. Best (Ed.), *How claims spread: Cross-national diffusion of social problems* (pp. 147–167). Hawthorne, New York, NY: Aldine de Gruyter.

Kabat, A. (1998). Scarlet letter sex offender databases and community notification: Sacrificing personal privacy for a symbol's sake. American Criminal Law Review, 35, 333.

Krueger, R. (2007, March 11). *The new American witch hunt, The Los Angeles Times*, 2.

Leggatt, S. (1984). *Report of the inquiry into habitual criminals in Canada*. Ottawa, Canada.

Lewis, C. (1996). The Jacob Wetterling Crimes against Children and Sexually Violent Offenders registration Act: An unconstitutional deprivation of the right to privacy and substantive due process. *Harvard Civil Rights and Civil Liberties Law Review.* 39, 89–118.

Mass. Gen'l Law, ch. 6 §178 C-Q; (1996, c. 239, § 1).

Mass. Gen'l Law, c. 127 § 133D, 2006.

Mass. Gen. Law, ch. 123§ 1 et seq. (1970, c.888, § 4).

Matravers, A. (2003). *Sex offenders in the community: Managing and reducing the risks.* Portland, OR: Willan Publishing.

Matson, S. & Lieb, R. (1996). *Sex offender community notification: A review of laws in 32 states.* Washington State Institute for Public Policy.

Ministry of Community Safety and Correctional Services. (2004). *Sex offender registry- Christpoher's Law: A bold measure in community safety.* Ottawa; ON: Queens Printer for Ontario.

McAlinden, A. M. (2007). *The shaming of sex offenders: Risk, retribution and reinteg*ration. Portland OR: Hart Publishing.

McAllister, S. R. (1998). "Neighbors Beware": The Constitutionality of State Sex Offender Registration and Community Notification Laws.29 *Texas Tech Law Review,* 97–136.

Mustaine, E., Tewksbury, R., & Stengel, K. (2006). Social disorganization and residential locations of registered sex offenders: Is this a collateral consequence? *Deviant Behavior,* 27(3), 329–350.

National Joint Committee. (2006). Enhancing community protection in the release of the detained offender: Inter-jurisdictional & inter-agency issues and resolutions. International Centre for Criminal Law Reform and Criminal Justice Policy. Final Report on the International Meeting of Experts. Vancouver, BC.

Ouimet, R. (1969). *Toward unity: Criminal justice and corrections report* (pp. 502–505). Ottawa, Canada: Community Protection Policies of the Canadian Committee on Corrections.

Pam Lychner Sexual Offender Tracking and Identification Act of 1996, 42 U.S.C. 14072 et seq.

Petrosino, A. & Petrosino, C. (1999). The public safety potential of Megan's Law in Massachusetts: An assessment from a sample of criminal sexual psychopaths. *Crime and Delinquency,* 45(1), 140–158.

Petrunik, M. (1994). *Models of dangerousness: A cross jurisdictional review review of dangerousness legislation and practice.* The Ministry of the Solicitor General of Canada.

Petrunik, M. (2003). *The hare and the tortoise: Dangerousness and sex offender policy in the United States and Canada. The Canadian Journal of Criminology and Criminal Justice,* 45(4) 43–72.

Petrunik, M. (2002). Managing unacceptable risk: Sex offenders, community response and social policy in the United States and Canada. *International Journal of Offender Therapy and Comparative Criminology,* 46(4), 483–511.

Petrunik, M. (2005). Dangerousness and its discontents: A discourse on the socio-politics of dangerousness. In S. Burns (Ed.), *Ethnographies of law and social control. The sociology of law, deviance and social control,* (Vol. 6, pp. 49–74). New York, NY: Elsevier, JAI.

Petrunik M. & Weisman, R. (2005). Constructing Joseph Fredericks: Competing narratives of a child sex murderer. *International Journal of Law and Psychiatry,* 28, 75–96.

Petrunik, M. & Deutschmann, L. (2008). The exclusion-inclusion spectrum in state and community responses to sex offenders in Anglo-American and European jurisdictions. *International Journal of offender Therapy and Comparative Criminology,* 52 (5), 499–519.

Pogrebin, M., Dodge, M., & Katsampes, P. (2001). The collateral costs of short-term jail incarceration: The long-term social and economic disruptions. *Corrections Management Quarterly,* 5(4), 64–69.

Quinsey, V., Harris, G. Rice, M., & Cormier, C. (1998). *Violent offenders: Appraising and managing risk.* Washington, D.C.: American Psychological Association.

Ranalli, R. & Heinz, H. (2006, April 17). Man tied to 2 deaths kills self aboard bus: Canadian was person of interest in Maine slayings. *Boston Globe.*

R. v. Ayoob, (2005) O.J. No. 4874 (S.C.J.).

R. v. Burke, (2005) O.J. No. 4267 (S.C.J.).

R. v. Dyck, (2005) O.J. No. 47771 (S.C.J.).

Scholle, A. D. (2000). *Sex offender registration. FBI Law Enforcement Bulletin,* 69(7), 18–24.

Schram, D. & Milloy, C. (1995). *Community notification: A study of offender characteristics and recidivism.* Olympia, WA: Washington Institute for Public Policy.

Sex Offender Information Registration Act (SOIRA), 2004, c.10.

State of Washington. (1989). *Task force on community protection: Final report.* Olympia, WA: Department of Health and Social services.

Sutherland, L. (1999). *Parental response to community notification: A school based response.* Ottawa, Canada: National Library of Canada.

Tewksbury, R. (2005). Collateral consequences of sex offender registration. *Journal of Contemporary Criminal Justice,* 21(1), 67–81.

Walsh Act, 18 USCS § 2250 and 42 USCS § 16901 et seq.

Zevitz, R. G. & Farkas, M. (2000a). Sex offender community notification: Assessing the impact in Wisconsin. Washington, DC: National Institute of Justice.

Zevitz, R. & Farkas, M. (2000b). Sex offender community notification: Examining the importance of neighborhood meetings. *Behavioral Sciences and the Law,* 18(2–3), 393–408.

Chapter 29

Ethical Issues in the Treatment of Sex Offenders

Howard Zonana and Alec Buchanan

The evaluation, treatment, and lack of treatment of sex offenders are fraught with many ethical questions and pitfalls. A common thread underlying the unique rules applying to sex offenders is that there is a "special depravity" associated with sexually related crimes, to the extent that sex offenders are perceived as "especially vile and loathsome people who really do not deserve to be treated like defendants in other crimes" (Lanyon, 1997). Many of these dilemmas have become more prominent since the passage of the sexually violent predator (SVP) commitment statutes and the developing of sex offender treatment programs both within and outside of prisons. Some treatment programs raise questions regarding the ability to obtain meaningful consent from prisoners, as participating in treatment is tied to conditions of release or parole. Forensic evaluations required by the SVP statutes have also posed other difficult questions relating to the psychiatrist's ability to predict future dangerousness. Actuarial risk assessment instruments, touted as more accurate than clinically based evaluations are not applicable or well validated for the specific questions asked in SVP statutes. Some are based on different populations than the individual who is being evaluated. How should the lack of a personal examination, because of refusals to participate by the inmate, be handled and what is the impact upon the conclusions that can be drawn? Issues of permissible intrusiveness have been raised by the use of polygraph testing or monitoring, and penile plethysmography. This chapter will attempt to review some of the major issues.

ISSUES AROUND TRIAL

Pretrial Evaluations for Defense Attorneys

Sex crimes are defined by both federal law and individual states. At the present time downloading a single pornographic picture of a minor is a federal crime.[1] These crimes are being actively prosecuted in the United States and Canada. The profiles of individuals who are engaged in this activity are very broad—from college students competing with each other to see who can download the most pornography, to men who are schizoid, socially isolated, and have major impairments in their ability to socially relate to others. There are also aggressive pedophiles who use the Internet to arrange trysts with minors or have them perform sexual activities using webcams online (Eichenwald, 2005). Because of the increasingly severe penalties and mandatory minimum sentences of imprisonment meted out to sex offenders, defense attorneys have sought out psychiatric and psychological evaluations of defendants very early in the criminal process. Such requests may be made before the individual has been arrested, but after he has become aware that an investigation is ongoing and has hired an attorney. At this point the attorney is looking for information that might be useful in convincing the prosecutor to reduce the possible charges from the outset or to negotiate an acceptable plea bargain. This strategy has become increasingly utilized by defense attorneys at every stage of a criminal proceeding before trial and then later during post-conviction proceedings such as parole hearings and appeals.

One of the problems that has emerged during the course of these evaluations (and apply to other evaluations of sex offenders as well) is that during the course of a comprehensive evaluation, including a careful longitudinal history of the defendant's sexual development and history, the defendant/evaluee may reveal information that is sufficiently detailed about other crimes or activities that bring into play mandatory child abuse reporting statutes. All 50 states have such statutes and the laws of Canada create equivalent obligations. These statutes often have no time limits on the obligation to report. They also designate psychiatrists as mandated reporters. When this information is included in reports additional investigations will ensue and further charges may be laid. Canada does not have a statute of limitations and historic sex crimes are prosecuted with vigor. In the United States, the statutes of limitations on sexual crimes against minors have been extended in many states in the wake of reports of clergy abuse and repressed memory research.[2] We have also heard of threatened

prosecution or licensure board referral of the expert for not making child abuse reports for such events when they were included in their report but not reported to the state agency responsible for Child Protective Services. This has led to recognizing the importance of warning evaluees, at the outset of the evaluation, regarding their reporting of information that would make a prior, heretofore unknown, young victim identifiable, and thus trigger reporting requirements even though the forensic evaluation was generally protected under attorney–client privilege.

Other possible exceptions exist, such as Tarasoff obligations, if specific threats are disclosed during the course of a forensic evaluation. In one case, a defendant who fire bombed his therapists home causing the death of her husband and severe burns to the therapist, made further threats to kill the therapist's brother as well as his former wife's employer. He stated he could accomplish this while in jail by hiring another inmate who was about to be released. After an in-camera hearing at the first penalty trial, the trial court ruled that an exception to the psycho-therapist–patient privilege permitted disclosure of the defendant's threats to kill. The defendant also argued that since it was a forensic evaluation it was covered by the attorney–client privilege and should not have been disclosed. The California Supreme Court did not definitively resolve the attorney–client issue but said, in this case, that "even if erroneously admitted, the evidence was not prejudicial."[3]

The Canadian Supreme Court did create a specific exception to the solicitor–client privilege in 1999.[4] In this case a man awaiting trial for aggravated sexual assault on a prostitute told the evaluating psychiatrist that he had intended to kill her and was still going to the same area. The majority noted that

despite its importance, the (solicitor–client) privilege is not absolute and remains subject to limited exceptions, including the public safety exception. While only a compelling public interest can justify setting aside solicitor-client privilege, danger to public safety can, in appropriate circumstances, provide such a justification.

They felt the following three factors needed to be taken into consideration in assessing the public safety considerations: "(1) Is there a clear risk to an identifiable person or group of persons? (2) Is there a risk of serious bodily harm or death? (3) Is the danger imminent?" They concluded the solicitor–client privilege must be set aside for the public protection. In this case he defendant was diagnosed with multiple paraphilias, in particular sexual sadism and the group of victims—prostitutes in a specific area—was deemed sufficiently specific. He also had detailed plans for the attack which were to result in death and violated his bail conditions by returning to the area after his arrest while awaiting sentencing which the court felt was sufficient to see the threat as imminent. The court also noted that "so long as the psychological harm substantially interferes with the health or well-being of the complainant, it properly comes within the scope of the phrase 'serious bodily harm.'" There can be no doubt that psychological harm may often be more pervasive and permanent in its effect than any physical harm. In Canada both the psychiatrist and the attorney can be obligated to warn or take other appropriate steps to protect.

If the overall summary of the clinical findings indicate that it would not be useful to the legal representation of the case, reports to protective services are still required even if the attorney does not want a formal written report. It is also important to remember that reports to Protective Services may only require sufficient information to document the basis for the reporting but not every detail of the offense known to the evaluator (*State v. Andring*). There remains some tension between the reporting requirements and the physician–patient privilege. Reporting statutes generally override patient privilege but the subsequent use of additional data the physician possesses, to convict the person, may be more protected. Because of the consequence of possible new criminal charges it is important to review such obligations with the defense attorney before beginning the evaluation.

Another consequence of the aggressive prosecution policy regarding the downloading of child pornography to personal computers is the increased risk for suicide by these defendants (*Los Angeles Times*, 2004). Many of these individuals fear the consequences of public disclosure which will have a substantial detrimental impact on their jobs careers as well as on family relationships. An important part of the forensic assessment when it occurs before arrest or arraignment is to explore the potential consequences of having the charges become public for the individual as well as making sure that appropriate treatment or hospitalization, if necessary, is obtained.

Because many psychiatrists do not treat sex offenders, they are frequently unaware of the reactions that may be precipitated or the difficulty that some offenders have in stopping the downloading in spite of the fact that they are being prosecuted. They are also unaware of appropriate medications that might be used to decrease the sexual drive. In some cases, it has become difficult to maintain clear boundaries for the forensic evaluation when clinical issues become severe enough to warrant emergency treatment or hospitalization. Even after hospitalization, we have seen evaluees who do not tell their therapists they have guns at home and continue to harbor strong suicidal impulses but are willing to tell that information to the forensic evaluator consulting to their attorney. Concerns about splitting may make it imperative to have the evaluee's permission to confer with their treatment team about information derived from the forensic evaluation.

Presentence Reports

Probation and parole services are generally involved in the preparation of presentence and postsentence reports following a conviction and may also be monitoring the offender following release from prison if there is a supervised probationary or parole period. Collaboration in careful demarcation of boundaries can be an important aid in treatment planning and providing incentives to participate in treatment. Historically many treatment programs were unwilling to work with "law enforcement" personnel or lawyers but experience with substance abusers and sex offenders have changed that opinion especially when treatment is a condition of probation or parole. It is important to have a clear contract about what information will be shared and what remains confidential at the outset of the relationship. For example, attendance and remaining in good standing in treatment are often factors that are reported. This permits programs to develop guidelines that do not require the reporting of every dirty urine test unless specifically required as a condition of probation (to remain in good standing many programs require more than three dirty urines in a defined time period). Likewise, mere appearance for treatment but not participation in the process, for example, remaining mute for an hour, is not fulfilling the minimum requirements of being in treatment. The details of the contract should be clear to the probationer. We have seen some boundary issues where probation officers become treatment providers as well as trying to maintain their probation role.

TREATMENT AND COERCION

Treatment in Prison

Treatment of prisoners within the correctional institution poses a number of problems that differ from treatment in mental health settings. There are special problems relating to maintaining the confidentiality of medical/psychiatric records from custodial staff as well as obligations which require the reporting of potential escape plans. Mental health records are frequently requested by parole boards as part of their consideration of early release. Some prison conditions may deter sex offender treatment in correctional settings. First, there is stigmatization by other inmates if the treatment itself becomes public knowledge. Pedophiles are often at the bottom of the "pecking order" in prisons and many will avoid treatment to maintain a degree of deniability. In addition, a recent U.S. Supreme Court case illustrates some additional complexities in different jurisdictions (*McKune v. Lile*).

In 1982, Robert Lile lured a high school student into his car as she was returning home from school. At gunpoint, he forced the victim to perform oral sodomy on him and then drove to a field where he raped her. After the sexual assault, the victim went to her school, where, crying and upset, she reported the crime. The police arrested Lile and recovered on his person the weapon he used to facilitate the crime (*State v. Lile*).

Although Lile maintained that the sexual intercourse was consensual, a jury convicted him of rape, aggravated sodomy, and aggravated kidnapping. Both the Kansas Supreme Court and a Federal District Court concluded that the evidence was sufficient to sustain conviction on all charges.

In 1994, a few years before he was scheduled to be released, prison officials ordered him to participate in a Sexual Abuse Treatment Program (SATP). The program requires participating inmates to complete and sign an "Admission of Responsibility" form, in which they discuss and accept responsibility for the crime for which they have been sentenced. They also are required to complete a sexual history form, which details all prior sexual activities, regardless of

whether such activities constitute uncharged criminal offenses. A polygraph examination is used to verify the accuracy and completeness of the offender's sexual history.

While such information is felt to enhance treatment and rehabilitative goals, the information is not privileged. Kansas leaves open the possibility that new evidence might be used against sex offenders in future criminal proceedings. In addition, Kansas law requires the SATP staff to report any uncharged sexual offenses involving minors to law enforcement authorities. According to Kansas authorities, no inmate has ever been charged or prosecuted for any offense based on information disclosed during treatment. At the Supreme Court, there was no contention that the program was a mere subterfuge for the conduct of a criminal investigation. The possibility of prosecution, however, remains.

Prison officials informed Mr. Lile that if he refused to participate in the SATP, his privilege status would be reduced back from Level III to Level I. As part of this reduction, respondent's visitation rights, earnings, work opportunities, ability to send money to family, canteen expenditures, access to a personal television, and other privileges automatically would be curtailed. In addition, he would be transferred back to a maximum-security unit, where his movement would be more limited, he would be moved from a two-person to a four-person cell, and he would be in a potentially more dangerous environment.

Lile refused to participate in the SATP on the ground that the required disclosures of his criminal history would violate his Fifth Amendment privilege against self-incrimination. He brought an action under 42 U.S.C. §1983 against the warden and the secretary of the Department, seeking an injunction to prevent them from withdrawing his prison privileges and transferring him to a different housing unit. The trial and appellate courts granted him relief feeling that the state had other alternatives and that the consequences were quite severe. The Supreme Court in a narrow 5–4 decision reversed the trial and appellate courts. The majority gave more discretion to the program with their review standard.

Determining what constitutes unconstitutional compulsion involves a question of judgment: Courts must decide whether the consequences of an inmate's choice to remain silent are closer to the physical torture against which the Constitution clearly protects or the de minimis harms against which it does not (536 US 24 at 41).

The majority noted

> Although no program participant has ever been prosecuted or penalized based on information revealed during the SATP, the potential for additional punishment reinforces the gravity of the participants' offenses and thereby aids in their rehabilitation. If inmates know society will not punish them for their past offenses, they may be left with the false impression that society does not consider those crimes to be serious ones. The practical effect of guaranteed immunity for SATP participants would be to absolve many sex offenders of any and all cost for their earlier crimes. This is the precise opposite of the rehabilitative objective.

Another case cited by the Court of Appeals (1st Cir.) (*Ainsworth v. Risley*) noted that some program conditions requiring disclosure might not meet constitutional standards.

> A treatment program that conditioned participation on incriminating admissions might violate the Fifth Amendment if that program was in turn a condition of probation or of maintaining parole, but a program that conditioned participation on incriminating admissions as a condition of obtaining release on parole does not. Case law recognizes this distinction. Some courts have found Fifth Amendment violations where sex offenders were required to disclose past misconduct for treatment programs that were a condition of probation or a court-suspended sentence.

Some states address the incrimination dilemma posed by sex offender treatment programs by asking inmates seeking treatment only to admit to misconduct of which law enforcement officials are already aware (*Neal v. Shimoda*).[5]

A grant of limited use immunity need not conflict with public safety, since it allows the state to prosecute the recipient "for any crime of which he may be guilty…provided only that his own compelled testimony is not used to convict him" (see *Lefkowitz v. Cunningham*, comparing use immunity to broader transactional immunity which immunizes witnesses from prosecution for any transaction about which they testify). Granting use immunity may in fact

further the state's goal of rehabilitation by encouraging inmates to admit their sex offenses, thus removing an obstacle to treatment. Use immunity is the solution proposed by commentators concerned about the tension between an inmate's right against self-incrimination and the state's interest in pressing sex offenders to admit past misconduct as a first step toward effective treatment.

In a strongly worded dissent written by Justice Stevens and joined by Souter, Ginsberg, and Breyer they argued:

> No one could possibly disagree with the plurality's statement that "offering inmates minimal incentives to participate [in a rehabilitation program] does not amount to compelled self-incrimination prohibited by the Fifth Amendment." The question that this case presents, however, is whether the State may punish an inmate's assertion of his Fifth Amendment privilege with the same mandatory sanction that follows a disciplinary conviction for an offense such as theft, sodomy, riot arson, or assault. Until today the Court has never characterized a threatened harm as "a minimal incentive." Nor have we ever held that a person who has made a valid assertion of the privilege may nevertheless be ordered to incriminate himself and sanctioned for disobeying such an order. This is truly a watershed case (*McKune vs. Lile at 54*).

They emphasized that because he had testified at trial that his sexual intercourse with the victim before driving her back to her car was consensual, the District Court found that a written admission on this form would subject respondent to a possible charge of perjury (24 F. Supp. 2d 1152, 1157 (Kan. 1998)). In addition, the SATP requires participants to

> generate a written sexual history which includes all prior sexual activities, regardless of whether such activities constitute uncharged criminal offenses (ibid. at 1155). The District Court found that the form clearly seeks information that could incriminate the prisoner and subject him to further criminal charges (ibid. at 1157).
>
> Through its treatment program, Kansas seeks to achieve the admirable goal of reducing recidivism among sex offenders. In the process, however, the State demands an impermissible and unwarranted sacrifice from the participants. No matter what the goal, inmates should not be compelled to forfeit the privilege against self-incrimination simply

because the ends are legitimate or because they have been convicted of sex offenses. Particularly in a case like this one, in which respondent has protested his innocence all along and is being compelled to confess to a crime that he still insists he did not commit, we ought to ask ourselves—what if this is one of those rare cases in which the jury made a mistake and he is actually innocent? And in answering that question, we should consider that even members of the Star Chamber thought they were pursuing righteous ends (*McKune v. Lile at 70*).

While this is an interpretation of Kansas law, it is clear that states and the federal system have chosen different procedures and guidelines for their sex offender treatment programs. Any treater within a correctional setting should be acquainted with the appropriate standards under which they are operating and be clear with prospective patients about the requirements and consequences of electing to participate in sex offender treatment. As the preceding discussion illustrates, these guidelines can be quite intricate and complicated. Thus, consultation with knowledgeable staff or attorneys may be necessary. Kansas and other states, as noted, may use polygraph testing, plethysmography or other tests to monitor treatment. These protocols are more akin to treatment and monitoring of substance abusers than usual psychotherapy or group therapy modalities.

Consent and Castration

A good example of a treatment which raises some interesting ethical questions of consent involve the use of chemical or surgical castration for offenders who are seeking favorable parole or probation consideration. As a means to control sex offender recidivism, nine states have passed legislation since 1996, authorizing the use of chemical or physical castration. In many of these statutes, release back to the community is predicated on the acceptance of mandated hormonal therapy. The states that have passed such laws include California, Florida, Georgia, Iowa, Louisiana, Montana, Oregon, Texas, and Wisconsin (Scott & Holmberg, 2003).

Montana's statute is a good example.[6] The statutes vary as to whether a medical evaluation is statutorily required. While not explicit in Montana the statute does specify that the treatment be "medically safe drug treatment" and the person must be informed

regarding side effects. Some states provide explicit immunity for prescribing physicians but Montana does not. There is also no required therapy in addition to the medication. Texas offers the opportunity only for surgical castration. They, however, ask the Medical Board to appoint a monitor in addition to the physician who obtains consent to be sure that the consent is not coerced.

The antiandrogen treatments are generally mandated until either the defendant or the state Departments of Correction (or Correctional Service of Canada [CSC]) determines that it is no longer necessary. These statutorily prescribed treatments may pose a number of ethical concerns for psychiatrists including the adequacy of the consent, the capacity to give consent, the adequacy of the overall treatment program as well as appropriate continued monitoring. One of the more difficult issues will be when a person requests the medication as an aid in obtaining parole but continues to deny doing the original crime and the history of paraphilia is marginal or nonexistent. Is the medication "medically indicated" under these circumstances or is it being prescribed to facilitate release? Or are antiandrogens medically indicated for the antisocial rapist with no paraphilia? These cases do not have any scientific literature to guide decision-making.

SEXUALLY VIOLENT PREDATOR EVALUATIONS

The Content of the Statutes

In 1997 Canada enacted criminal law that permits trial judges to label convicts as dangerous offenders and thereafter impose a sentence of detention in a penitentiary for an indeterminate period in lieu of any other sentence that might be imposed for the offense for which the defendant had been convicted (Part XXIV of the Canadian Criminal Code). In the United States, after several decades during which "sexual psychopath" laws had fallen into disuse, the state of Washington passed legislation permitting the detention of sexual offenders beyond the end of their prison sentences in 1990 (Fitch & Hammen, 2003). Seventeen U.S. states have since adopted "sexually violent predator" (SVP) statutes. The American statutes provide for the control and supervision of people found by a judge or jury to pose a continued risk of sexual offending. The administration of the laws and the treatment of those subject to them vary. Texas, for instance, requires outpatient treatment while other states require confinement.

California requires that an SVP have two or more victims while most states require only one offense (Lieb, 2003). Under all of the U.S. statutes confinement depends on an SVP suffering from some form of mental abnormality. The name given to the abnormality varies. The laws of Florida and New Jersey state that personality disorders qualify. Those of Iowa and Kansas do not. While all of the statutes refer to a risk of future offending the nature of this offending varies also. Thus while Texas and Washington have statutes that refer to "predatory sexual violence", Arizona's refers to "sexual violence" and that of Minnesota only to "harmful sexual conduct" (Lieb, 2003). The level of risk required for detention ranges from "likely" (Arizona) to "substantially probable" (Illinois and Wisconsin) and "more likely than not" (Missouri).

General Issues Raised by the Statutes

The Problem of Operationally Defining Legal Language

A medical witness in a legal forum faces questions that are couched in legal terms. SVP statutes require assessors to testify to some legally derived qualities that have no direct clinical equivalents. SVP detention requires "volitional impairment" (*Kansas v. Crane*). The absence of a meaningful clinical distinction between a recidivist with a "volitional impairment" and one without, however, caused both the American Psychiatric Association (APA) and the American Bar Association to oppose the inclusion of a volitional limb in the insanity defense (American Bar Association, 1989; American Psychiatric Association, 1984). The consequent difficulty for medical and psychological witnesses is made more acute by a tendency on the part of courts to accept whatever operational definition a witness has adopted (Doren, 2002).

The Presentation of Evidence

Experts who are concerned to present their evidence to minimize the chances of its being used improperly face two difficulties in SVP hearings. The first is the possibility that evidence will be treated as "conclusory" on the ultimate issue. A clinician can seek to avoid providing an opinion on whether the assessed person should be made subject to the SVP statute. But it is difficult to see how he or she can avoid answering questions such as, "does he suffer from a mental abnormality" and, "does he present a substantial risk", the answers to which, taken together, amount to much the same thing.

The second difficulty concerns the effect on a court of an expert's assessment of dangerousness. Even reviews that are otherwise supportive of lay people's abilities to make complicated decisions in legal settings acknowledge that juries find evidence relating to probabilities particularly difficult (Jacobs, 1993). One way clinicians have been advised to maximize the accuracy of their predictions is to use actuarial scales. Actuarial scales, however, seem particularly prone to the hazards of what Tribe (1971, p.1360) called *"the overpowering number"*: an illusion of precision arising from the use of statistical terms. Similar concerns have been expressed by reviewers more recently (Grisso, 2000).

Psychiatry and Preventive Detention

SVP statutes are a form of preventive detention (Doren, 2002). To describe them otherwise, for instance as a means of providing necessary treatment, seems to ignore the timing of SVP legislation (in the wake of publicized atrocities), the (limited) degree to which psychiatric services have previously provided treatment to this group, and the (seemingly slim) likelihood of treatment leading to release for many of those detained. Preventive detention has been criticized by English (*Everett v. Ribbands*) and American courts. "It is…difficult to reconcile with traditional American law", wrote the United States Court of Appeals, "the jailing of persons by the courts because of anticipated but as yet uncommitted crimes" (*Williamson v. United States at* 282).

Preventive detention in criminal law, however, has also had its authoritative supporters (Blackstone, 1783, p. 251; Holmes, 1881, p. 43). The U.S. Supreme Court has been offered the chance to declare preventive detention unconstitutional and has declined to do so (Dershowitz, 1973). The Supreme Court has also found psychiatric evidence on the likelihood of future offending to be admissible at the sentencing stage of criminal trials (*Barefoot v. Estelle*). Civil detention in a psychiatric hospital itself seems to involve an element of preventive detention. Taken alone, the fact that a statute legislates for preventive detention seems not to preclude clinical involvement.

SVP laws represent a particular form of preventive detention, however. First, and while rates of sexual offending are particularly difficult to measure, the laws are targeted at a group that does not appear to have a higher recidivism rate than many other groups of offenders (Hanson, 2003; U.S. Department of Justice, 2005). The selection of this group for special legislation seems, instead, to relate to the revulsion that sexual offenses arouse (see introduction to this chapter). Second, while SVP statutes make provision for regular reassessment, most of those detained seem likely to remain incarcerated for long periods. As of December 2004, of 3493 people held for evaluation or committed under the statutes, only 12% had been released (Washington State Institute for Public Policy, 2005). This may reflect the fact that the most valid predictors of future offending in this group do not change with time or treatment (Hanson, 2003).

Third, when psychiatrists contribute to preventive detention by recommending civil commitment there is a "therapeutic justification." A patient is receiving care and treatment that they need and that they would not otherwise receive. The care and treatment provided under SVP statutes is likely to differ substantially from that which psychiatrists are used to providing, not least because the psychiatric conditions that are being treated are also different. To the extent that clinicians see the provision of necessary care and treatment as one justification for compulsory admission to a psychiatric hospital, SVP statutes require them to consider the extent to which the same justification applies to this new group.

The passing of the SVP statutes in the United States and similar legislation in other jurisdictions has presented new challenges to the use of diagnoses in court. In civil commitment hearings, as in psychiatric practice generally, diagnoses help clinicians to describe their patient's mental disorder, the treatments available and, sometimes, the likely response. The diagnosis is seldom required to act as a "gatekeeper" to detention: the history and mental state usually suffice to demonstrate that a mental disorder of some kind is present. When detention in hospital is proposed, the court can then concentrate on whether the risk is sufficient to justify this.

In SVP hearings, on the other hand, the risk is frequently obvious. The question that then determines whether the person will be detained is whether he suffers from the required mental condition or not. Using diagnosis in this way seems to run counter to the injunctions in diagnostic manuals that they not be used to reach legal conclusions (American Psychiatric Association, 1994). Because they have been designed to serve purposes that are largely descriptive, modern psychiatric diagnoses are ill suited to act as justifications for detention (Buchanan, 2005).

"Risk" Under the Statutes

Actuarial and Clinical Aspects of the Assessment of Risk

All SVP Statutes make detention dependent on risk. The approaches that mental health professionals use to assess risk are usually divided into the "actuarial" and the "clinical." Most actuarial approaches use instruments that were initially developed to predict all forms of violent recidivism, sometimes referred to as "generic" instruments (Janus & Prentky, 2003). The degree to which they are appropriate for use in assessing the risk of sexual recidivism is controversial (Conroy, 2003; Harris, Rice, & Quinsey, 1998; Rogers & Jackson, 2005) and probably varies from one instrument to another (Doren, 2002, Rice & Harris, 1997).

The appropriateness of a scale that has been developed for use in one setting for use in a different situation is sometimes referred to as the "fit" of a scale. Two aspects of fit seem to be particularly relevant to the use of actuarial instruments in SVP hearings. First, the person being assessed may not resemble those on whom the predictive accuracy of the scale was measured. Second, different behaviors are predicted with different levels of accuracy by the same scale (Sjöstedt & Grann, 2002) and the behavior that the scale was developed to assess may not be the behavior that the SVP statute requires experts to predict (Rogers & Jackson, 2005). Some SVP statutes, for instance, require the expert to assess the risk of offending in the presence of supervision (Janus & Prentky, 2003).

The period since the passing of Washington's SVP statute has also, however, seen the development of specialized instruments for the estimation of recidivism in sex offenders. These include the "SORAG," (Quinsey, Rice, & Harris, 1995) the "Static-99" (Hanson & Thornton, 1999) and the "RRASOR" (Hanson, 1998). The accuracy of these specialized scales has now been shown to be on par with that of instruments for the prediction of all kinds of violence (Harris, Rice, Quinsey, Lalumière, Boer, & Lang, 2003). Inevitably, however, the newer instruments are less extensively cross-validated and less fully described (for instance, in terms of their standard error rates), leading some to argue that their use in court cannot yet be justified (Janus & Prentky, 2003).

Actuarial instruments nevertheless seem to offer a number of advantages over "unstructured" clinical judgment. They can help to ensure that evaluations are impartial, systematic and thorough (Mossman, 2002). They are by nature "transparent": those not practiced in their use can see what is being scored and why. In a field where forensic psychologists who can successfully predict "general" violence sometimes perform no better than chance with respect to sexual violence (Jackson, Rogers, & Shuman, 2004) they offer a means whereby specialist expertise can be disseminated. Finally, assessors can minimize the impact of the idiosyncrasies of particular instruments by using multiple actuarial approaches simultaneously (Grisso, 2000).

The disadvantages of actuarial instruments include the difficulty of adapting them for use in different circumstances without generating a need for further testing. Doubts over the applicability of actuarial instruments have contributed to their being excluded from hearings (Rogers & Schuman, 2005). The Static-99 and RRASOR were both held by the Illinois courts to fail the Frye, or "general acceptance" test of admissibility (In re Detention of Jeffrey Hargett). More often, however, courts seem to have been willing to admit evidence based on the use of actuarial scales (*People v. Ward*). The scales are now in widespread use in SVP evaluations (Doren, 2002).

Potential assessors contemplating a purely clinical approach to the assessment of risk will note also that most reviews have found actuarial approaches to be more accurate, particularly when the predictions sought cover periods longer than a few weeks (Quinsey, Harris, Rice, & Cormier, 1998; but see also Litwack, 2001). Many of the strongest reasons to doubt the accuracy of actuarial predictions, such as the status of the information on which the prediction is based, apply equally to clinical approaches. Actuarial methods seem at least to be potential "starting points" in the light of which other factors, such as the person's past response to treatment and current intentions can be considered (Mossman, 2002).

Limits to the Accuracy of Risk Assessment

Predictive accuracy can be described in terms of the area under the Receiver Operating Characteristic (ROC) curve. An area under the ROC curve (AUC) of 1 reflects perfect prediction and an AUC of 0.5 reflects an accuracy that is no better than chance. Mossman's review suggested an area under the ROC curve (AUC) for all violence prediction techniques of 0.78. This fell to 0.71 and 0.67 for validated actuarial and clinical approaches respectively (Mossman, 1994). Subsequent reviews of actuarial instruments suggest similar levels of accuracy (Buchanan & Leese, 2001). Validation of the most recent actuarial approach, an "iterative classification tree," generates an AUC of 0.63 (Monahan et al., 2005).

The ROC curve has the advantage of making a description of predictive accuracy that is independent of the base rate of violence in the sample in which the instrument was tested. It seems unlikely, however, that courts will always understand what the practical implications are. One way of describing those implications uses a different statistic, the "number needed to detain." Used on a population where the base rate of violence is 9.5% and where detaining 10 people at random could therefore be expected to prevent one offense, modern approaches to risk assessment would require the detention of 6 people to achieve the same end (Buchanan & Leese, 2001).

No one knows what the base rates of offending are in those assessed for detention under SVP legislation. Three problems follow. First, the accuracy of actuarial risk assessments is greatest when they are used on a population where the base rate of violence is similar to the base rate in population in which the instrument was tested. Deviation from that base rate reduces the accuracy of predictions. The degree to which this happens depends on the difference between the two base rates. If this difference is not known, the accuracy of the procedure cannot be assessed. Second, when the base rate is not known it becomes difficult for an assessor to describe the accuracy of the procedure that he or she is using. Without knowledge of the base rate, for instance, no assessor can say how many false positives and false negatives there are likely to be.

Finally, the "number needed to detain" changes with the base rate. When the base rate is lower it becomes more difficult to identify accurately people who will act violently because the proportion of the time that the assessor is right by chance is lower also. The U.S. Department of Justice gives a 3-year rearrest rate for sex crimes among male sex offenders released from prisons in 1994 of 5.3% (U.S. Department of Justice, 2005). Applied to a population where the base rate is 5%, modern actuarial instruments would result in the detention of 14 people to prevent one unwanted event (Buchanan & Leese, 2001). Any failure to obtain all of the information on which to base an assessment of risk will further decrease the accuracy of any assessment.

Conclusions Regarding the Ethical Issues Raised by SVP Statutes

SVP statutes have survived the legal challenges of *Kansas v. Hendricks*. As others have pointed out, however, this does not make giving testimony in SVP proceedings ethical (Grisso, 2000). In the absence of directives from the usual professional organizations, practitioners facing a choice over whether and how to participate are likely to be influenced by what they see.

Some will note the difficulties inherent in operationally defining qualities such as volitional impairment, in presenting evidence so that it will not be used inappropriately and in accurately assessing the type of risk defined by each statute and decide not to undertake SVP assessments. Others are likely to make the same choice because they question the appropriateness of using psychiatric categories to authorize the preventive detention of a group whose status as psychiatric patients, newly conferred by statute, seems arbitrary.

Clinicians choosing whether to participate will also be influenced by the extent to which they think that they can communicate to a court not only their conclusions regarding diagnosis and risk but also their level of confidence in those conclusions. One ethical requirement must be for candor but candor is only possible if a witness is capable of describing the approach, its reliability, and its predictive validity in terms that the court will understand.

Finally, clinicians choosing whether to participate will be influenced by local conditions. Those who see an arbitrary process where no guidelines are provided to help prosecutors decide who will be assessed for detention, where practitioners are discouraged from discussing what they do, where public defenders work with inadequate resources, and where prosecutors

go "shopping" for psychiatric opinions that support continued detention (Mansnerus, 2003) will presumably not become involved. Those who see a system that provides detention in humane conditions, where effective treatment is provided and where there is the realistic prospect of release if treatment is successful may reach different conclusions.

What seems clear is that technology is not about to resolve the clinician's dilemma. There will, presumably, be some further improvement in the accuracy of generic predictions of violence and further progress in applying these improvements to scales designed specifically to predict sexual recidivism. The research gives little reason to suppose, however, that these developments will soon produce instruments that perform substantially better than those that require, at a base rate of 5%, the detention of approximately 15 people to prevent one unwanted event.

These error rates (and worse) have been accepted in psychiatry for many years. They have not led to the abandonment of civil detention, presumably because a number of additional factors help to justify the compulsory hospitalization of some psychiatric patients. These additional factors include the provision of nursing care and psychiatric treatment to people who are mentally unwell and whose psychiatric condition impairs their ability to choose such things for themselves. It is the absence of these additional factors that is likely to mean that the current generation of SVP statutes will remain ethically problematic for many clinicians.

ETHICAL ASPECTS OF OBTAINING INFORMATION

Offering Opinions without Examination

A part of the SVP evaluation process permits or requires a personal examination of the inmate by a mental health professional. In a significant number of cases the person potentially subject to commitment refuses to participate in the evaluation. When this occurs the psychiatrist will usually feel some unease as the APA ethical guidelines appears to say that it is unethical to offer a diagnostic opinion. Section 7 (3) of the Guidelines states

On occasion psychiatrists are asked for an opinion about an individual who is in the light of public attention or who has disclosed information about himself/herself through public media. In such circumstances, a psychiatrist may share with the public his or her expertise about psychiatric issues in general. However, it is unethical for a psychiatrist to offer a professional opinion unless he or she has conducted an examination and has been granted proper authorization for such a statement (American Psychiatric Association, 2001).

This statement was developed in the context of a FACT magazine poll asking if psychiatrists thought that Barry Goldwater was psychologically fit to be President of the United States. Many psychiatrists filled out the questionnaire, offering what appeared to be a professional opinion. This guideline has remained very questionable as to its scope and application as it would seem to preclude not only SVP evaluation conclusions without an interview but also any book or article discussing psychological profiles of public figures, world leaders or developing profiles of historical figures based on documents or even medical records.

Other professional organizations have developed guidelines for this contingency; for example, the Ethical Guidelines from the American Psychological Association leave room for reports without a personal examination.[7] The Ethical Guidelines developed by the American Academy of Psychiatry and the Law also takes a more pragmatic approach and states

> Honesty, objectivity and the adequacy of the clinical evaluation may be called into question when an expert opinion is offered without a personal examination. For certain evaluations (such as record reviews for malpractice cases), a personal examination is not required. In all other forensic evaluations, if, after appropriate effort, it is not feasible to conduct a personal examination, an opinion may nonetheless be rendered on the basis of other information. Under these circumstances, it is the responsibility of psychiatrists to make earnest efforts to ensure that their statements, opinions and any reports or testimony based on those opinions, clearly state that there was no personal examination and note any resulting limitations to their opinions (American Academy of Psychiatry and the Law, 2005).

This latter approach recognizes that some conclusions can be drawn in the absence of a personal examination but some appraisal of the information is necessary. If, for example there is a 20-year history of multiple hospitalizations and a consistent diagnosis of Chronic Paranoid Schizophrenia with well documented symptoms it would be within reasonable practice criteria to say the diagnosis was reasonably well established. This does not mean that the individual could not have other diagnoses of relevance that have been of more recent origin. Data which would require a personal examination might be the assessment of the effects of treatment, if there were not a good paper record or the availability of prior treaters.

In addition, not all information found in records is necessarily accurate. An interview permits further exploration of details or discrepancies which can be further evaluated, if necessary. In some states the evaluations are court ordered so that full informed consent may not be a formal legal requirement, but, from an ethical standpoint, notice to the evaluee should be provided. This should minimally include the purpose of the evaluation and lack of confidentiality of the evaluation.

Interviews with Victims

Another potentially thorny ethical issue involves the use of collateral interviews from victims. Victims who have been traumatized by the original crime can be retraumatized as a result of an interview that reviews the details of the original assault. Yet victims often are concerned about the potential release of offenders and are often willing to appear to testify at parole hearings. Sensitivity to this can be shown by talking first with the states attorney who has had prior contact and experience with the victim. They can be aware of the victim's attitudes and wishes and may also be in a better position to make the initial contact.

ETHICAL ISSUES IN THE USE OF USUAL COMMITMENT STATUTES

During the last half of 2005, the Governors of New York State and Rhode Island have publicly expressed dismay at the release of sex offenders from prisons at the end of their sentences. These concerns were precipitated by horrendous crimes committed by recently released felons with histories of prior sexual offenses. They have taken an unusual step in attempting to use the regular civil commitment statutes to keep these offenders confined.

New York has subsequently passed a commitment statutes.

Most general civil commitment statutes generally require, or have been interpreted to require, a recent predicate act indicating dangerousness in addition to the presence of a mental disorder. Thus, it came as a surprise to many mental health professionals to see Governors attempt to use these statutes and to be able to find psychiatrists willing to find such individuals certifiable.

The two governors requested psychiatrists within correctional facilities to review the sex offenders who were about to be released and to use the usual civil commitment statutes for those who were felt to be mentally ill and dangerous to have them transferred to mental health facilities rather than permitting them to be released into the community. In New York, 12 individuals were recently committed to Department of Mental Health facilities and they immediately challenged their confinement. The initial court rulings were that the proper procedures had not been followed, since independent physicians had not been appointed and a judge had not made the necessary findings before the transfer, as required following the US Supreme Court decision in *Vitek v. Jones*. As of mid 2008, these procedures have been clarified and approximately 180 individuals have been committed in New York State under the new SVP statute.

One individual was admitted "voluntarily" to the State hospital in Rhode Island under questionable legal proceedings. When this occurred, the Superintendent of the facility resigned in protest. Rhode Island's civil commitment statute contains an interesting caveat *"If a patient has been incarcerated, or institutionalized, or in a controlled environment of any kind, the court may give great weight to such prior acts, diagnosis, words, or thoughts."*[8]

These events have raised many questions. One is a question of what disorders can be used as a basis for civil commitment. Hendricks and the predator statutes clearly changed the ground rules as the legislature began defining "mental abnormality" very broadly to include those that they wanted hospitalized. Even the DSM-IV has a caveat, stating that "the clinical and scientific considerations involved in categorization of these conditions as mental disorders may not be wholly relevant to legal judgments."

It may be difficult to understand how psychiatry can be excluded from the decision-making process in an area in which psychiatric input has usually been dispositive. Organized psychiatry has not wanted to be overly restricted by diagnostic categories and saw no need to answer it as long as physicians were making the decision to hospitalize patients that they felt required hospitalization. For many years, most civil commitment statutes were, and many continue to be, written in very broad language. For example, in Connecticut, for the first two-thirds of the last century the commitment criteria required the presence of a mental illness, which was defined "as a mental or emotional condition which has substantial adverse effects upon his or her ability to function and who requires care and treatment," as well as a finding that the person was "a fit subject for confinement." This was the legislature's way of giving physicians broad discretion in hospitalizing the mentally ill, with the implicit message that physicians knew who should be hospitalized and could be trusted to use that authority appropriately with the protection of judicial review. With the civil rights revolution, this broad trust was narrowed and "dangerousness" and/or "grave disability" became required minimal criteria, not only in Connecticut, but also in all states.

However, the definitions of mental disorders have remained quite broad. This has opened the door for some pressure to be placed on physicians in prisons to think about petitioning to commit more individuals who are emerging from prison. The DSM-IV is the psychiatric compendium of mental disorders which now includes over 250 such disorders. The manual makes no list of disorders which qualify for use as a basis for civil commitment and those that do not. The "model civil commitment statute" developed by the APA talks about "serious" mental disorders that suggest psychoses but leave much flexibility. Most psychiatrists would not want to exclude personality disorders per se as an inappropriate basis for civil commitment, for example, many individuals with borderline personality disorders can become seriously suicidal, have significant impairments in reality testing and require hospitalization. Pedophilia is an Axis I diagnosis but had not been widely used in the past as a basis for commitment, since there was no formal thought disorder and most individuals had sufficient control so as not to be seen detainable on that basis. The inclusion of antisocial personality disorder (APD) as the only mental abnormality, however, has generally not been seen by physicians, in this country, as a sufficient predicate to justify involuntary commitment.

The U.S. Supreme Court has also acknowledged that there must be some way to distinguish the typical prison felon with APD from the individual whose commitment is being sought in these special circumstances.

> And we recognize that in cases where lack of control is at issue, 'inability to control behavior' will not be demonstrable with mathematical precision. It is enough to say that there must be proof of serious difficulty in controlling behavior. And this, when viewed in light of such features of the case as the nature of the psychiatric diagnosis, and the severity of the mental abnormality itself, must be sufficient to distinguish the dangerous sexual offender whose serious mental illness, abnormality, or disorder subjects him to civil commitment from the dangerous but typical recidivist convicted in an ordinary criminal case (Kansan v. Crane).

Governors and the public do not have these compunctions and thus it is interesting to see how this will play out once the procedural issues get resolved and more substantive questions arise in the courts.

The Rhode Island case raises different questions. The individual involved there was diagnosed with schizophrenia as well as being a sexual offender. Here, the Superintendent had concluded that the schizophrenia was not a contributing factor in the sexual offenses, and that the individual was adequately treated for his schizophrenia; and on that basis did not require hospitalization. Presumably, if he felt the schizophrenia was a contributing factor and was not adequately treated he would not have objected. These distinctions are not easily drawn and good treatment plans should include appropriate treatments for the paraphilia as well. The Rhode Island civil commitment statutes have an interesting provision that have not been seen in many others:

> (ii) In determining whether there exists a likelihood of serious harm the physician and the court may consider previous acts, diagnosis, words or thoughts of the patient. If a patient has been incarcerated, or institutionalized, or in a controlled environment of any kind, the court may give great weight to such prior acts, diagnosis, words, or thoughts.

This may broadens the basis for civil commitment in Rhode Island and may be so interpreted by the courts.

Thus, we may see more use of ordinary civil commitment statutes or efforts to amend them.

The courts have not agreed with organized psychiatry's view that the SVP commitment redefines sexual criminal behavior as a mental illness for the purpose of allowing continued preventive detention—an unacceptable medicalization of deviance. While most of us would agree that hospitals are not appropriate for most, if not all, antisocial rapists, the paraphilias do represent a different cluster of disorders which also offer significant treatment prospects. I believe most of us would admit a pedophile requesting admission because he was fearful of reoffending and wanted to obtain treatment. The challenge remains how to avoid becoming a warehouse/prison for individuals who are indistinguishable from "ordinary criminals" and yet be open to those needing treatment. Our civil commitment statutes should not become so flimsy as to make a mockery of mental disorders so as to accomplish preventive detention for individuals who are not seriously ill. The ethical dilemma for psychiatrists working in correctional facilities will be how to apply these broad definitions of mental disorder usually found in civil commitment statutes to individuals who are to be released in the face of political pressures and the absence of clear professional guidelines. This will be easier in states where the statutes require recent evidence of dangerousness. In addition, once committed, the decision to release is totally in the physician's discretion and generally has not been challenged by the state.

THE PROBLEM OF TREATMENT AVAILABILITY

While an ethical problem only in the abstract sense, it is noteworthy that treating sex offenders has not been an area of large interest for most psychiatrists. Many do not read the research literature and few have experience with the use of antiandrogens or other hormonal treatments. While there are legitimate arguments about the misuse of psychiatry by "civilly committing" convicted felons with the sole diagnosis of antisocial personality at the end of their sentences, this does not deal with the effects of paraphilic disorders that can take over and destroy people's lives. How much of this a legacy of the last century's classification of homosexuality as a mental disorder or fears of being held responsible for relapses if new offenses occur while someone is in treatment is not possible to discern. We remain at a primitive level of understanding of sexual object choice and arousal patterns. Our current treatments are presently directed at correcting cognitive distortions, decreasing the intensity of a person's sexual drive, and offering social supports.

Even in states that do not have SVP laws the growing numbers of patients who are listed on sex offender registries make this a group that cannot be ignored. Risk assessment demands by community agencies and treatment plans that address these issues are growing needs. Our Canadian colleagues seem to have developed a more positive attitude and approach to treating these patients and report gratifying results. Even the older literature shows some positive benefits of treatment. Of course, the public expectation of 0% recidivism as the only acceptable standard is unrealistic, but this is an area of great public health need and research.

CONCLUSION

Clinicians who assess and treat offenders sometimes become aware of criminal activity not known to the police. The expectation that an assessment conducted at the request of the defense attorney will be confidential can conflict with the need to communicate worrying information with treating clinicians. Treating psychiatrists can find that their understanding of what they are, and are not, expected to regard as confidential is different from that of the probation service staff. Treatment in prison raises issues of confidentiality. Making treatment a condition of release raises the question of the extent to which that treatment is voluntary.

None of these ethical questions are unique to the treatment of sex offenders. Treatment of this group, however, does present familiar problems in new guises. The relative newness of SVP legislation, in particular, means that many important questions, including whether treatment can lead to release and the meaning of volitional impairment, as yet have no answers. Some of the answers will be provided by empirical research. Other answers, however, can only be provided by the response of the health professions to the challenge that a group, previously peripheral to the concern of most psychiatric services, can now more readily be detained and treated by psychiatric services.

Notes

1. "Any person who…knowingly possesses any book, magazine, periodical, film, videotape, computer disk, or any other material that contains an image of child pornography that has been mailed, or shipped or transported in interstate or foreign commerce by any means, including by computer, or that was produced using materials that have been mailed, or shipped or transported in interstate or foreign commerce by any means, including by computer…shall be punished…." 18 U.S.C. 2252A (a)(5)(B). Every person who transmits, makes available, distributes, sells, advertises, imports, exports, accesses, possesses any child pornography is guilty and liable to a minimum punishment of imprisonment. See also Section 163.1 of the Criminal Code of Canada.

2. See Connecticut General Statutes '52–577d. Limitation of action for damages to minor caused by sexual abuse, exploitation, or assault. Notwithstanding the provisions of section 52–577, no action to recover damages for personal injury to a minor, including emotional distress, caused by sexual abuse, sexual exploitation, or sexual assault may be brought by such person later than 30 years from the date such person attains the age of majority.

3. People v. Clark 789 P.2d 127 (Cal 1990).

4. James Jones v. John Smith, [1999] 1 S.C. R. 455; 1999 s.C.R. LEXIS 13.

5. In Neal v. Shimoda, the court referred to a sex offender consent that stated, "I understand that I am not required to provide information about crimes that no one knows about"; see also, Russell v. Eaves. Courts have also suggested that states grant use immunity to sex offenders before requiring them to disclose past misconduct during the course of treatment. See Lile v. McKune; Montana v. Imlay; Mace v. Amnesty; State v. Fuller.

6. Mont. Code Anno., Э 45-5-512 (2005) 45-5-512 Chemical treatment of sex offenders. (1) A person convicted of a first offense under 45-5-502(3), 45-5-503(3), or 45-5-507(4) may, in addition to the sentence imposed under those sections, be sentenced to undergo medically safe medroxyprogesterone acetate treatment or its chemical equivalent or other medically safe drug treatment that reduces sexual fantasies, sex drive, or both, administered by the department of corrections or its agent pursuant to subsection (4). (2) A person convicted of a second or subsequent offense under 45-5-502(3), 45-5-503, or 45-5-507 may, in addition to the sentence imposed under those sections, be sentenced to undergo medically safe medroxyprogesterone acetate treatment or its chemical equivalent or other medically safe drug treatment that reduces sexual fantasies, sex drive, or both, administered by the department of corrections or its agent pursuant to subsection (4). (3) A person convicted of a first or subsequent offense under 45-5-502, 45-5-503, or 45-5-507 who is not sentenced to undergo medically safe medroxyprogesterone acetate treatment or its chemical equivalent or other medically safe drug treatment that reduces sexual fantasies, sex drive, or

both, may voluntarily undergo such treatment, which must be administered by the department of corrections or its agent and paid for by the department of corrections. (4) Treatment under subsection (1) or (2) must begin 1 week before release from confinement and must continue until the department of corrections determines that the treatment is no longer necessary. Failure to continue treatment as ordered by the department of corrections constitutes a criminal contempt of court for failure to comply with the sentence, for which the sentencing court shall impose a term of incarceration without possibility of parole of not less than 10 years or more than 100 years. (5) Before chemical treatment under this section, the person must be fully medically informed of its effects. (6) A state employee who is a professional medical person may not be compelled against the employee's wishes to administer chemical treatment under this section.

7. American Psychological Association (2002) states the following 9.01 Bases for Assessments (a) Psychologists base the opinions contained in their recommendations, reports, and diagnostic or evaluative statements, including forensic testimony, on information and techniques sufficient to substantiate their findings (See also Standard 2.04, *Bases for Scientific and Professional Judgments*).(b) Except as noted in 9.01c psychologists provide opinions of the psychological characteristics of individuals only after they have conducted an examination of the individuals adequate to support their statements or conclusions. When, despite reasonable efforts, such an examination is not practical, psychologists document the efforts they made and the result of those efforts, clarify the probable impact of their limited information on the reliability and validity of their opinions, and appropriately limit the nature and extent of their conclusions or recommendations (See also Standards 2.01, Boundaries of Competence, and 9.06, Interpreting Assessment Results).(c) When psychologists conduct a record review or provide consultation or supervision and an individual examination is not warranted or necessary for the opinion, psychologists explain this and the sources of information on which they based their conclusions and recommendations.

8. R.I. Gen. Laws § 40.1–5–2.

References

Ainsworth v. Risley, 244 F.3d 209 (2001).

American Academy of Psychiatry and the Law. (2005). *Ethical guidelines for the practice of forensic psychiatry*. Bloomfield, CT: American Academy of Psychiatry and the Law.

American Bar Association. (1989). ABA criminal justice mental health standards. Washington, D.C.: American Bar Association, Criminal Justice Standards Committee.

American Psychiatric Association. (1984). *Issues in Forensic Psychiatry*. Washington, D.C.: American Psychiatric Press.

American Psychiatric Association. (1994). *Diagnostic and statistical manual of mental disorders: DSM-IV*. Washington, D.C.: American Psychiatric Association.

American Psychiatric Association. (2001). *The principles of medical ethics, with annotations especially applicable to psychiatry, 2001* (includes Nov. 2003 amendments) *Edition*. Washington, D.C.: American Psychiatric Association.

American Psychological Association. (2002). Ethical principles of psychologists and code of conduct. Washington, D.C.: *US American Psychologist*, 57(12), 1060–1073.

Barefoot v. Estelle 463 U.S. 880 (1983).

Blackstone, W. (1783). *Commentaries on the Laws of England*. Book IV. London and Oxford: Strachan, Cadell and Prince.

Buchanan, A. (2005). Descriptive diagnosis, personality disorder and detention. *Journal of Forensic Psychiatry and Psychology*, 16, 538–551.

Buchanan, A. & Leese, M. (2001). Detention of people with dangerous severe personality disorders: A systematic review. *Lancet*, 358, 1955–1959.

Conroy, M. (2003). Evaluation of sexual predators. In A. Goldstein & I. Weiner (Eds.), *Handbook of Psychology. Forensic Psychology* (Vol. 11 pp. 463–84). New York, NY: Wiley.

Dershowitz, A. (1973). Preventive confinement: A suggested framework for constitutional analysis. *Texas Law Review*, 51, 1277–1324.

Doren, D. (2002). *Evaluating sex offenders*. Thousand Oaks, CA: Sage.

Eichenwald, K. (2005, December 19). Through his webcam, a boy joins a sordid online world. *New York Times*, A1.

Everett v. Ribbands 2 Q.B. 198 (1952).

Fitch, W. & Hammen, D. (2003). The new generation of sex offender commitment laws: Which states have them and how do they work? In B. Winnick & J. LaFond (Eds.), *Protecting society from sexually dangerous offenders* (pp. 27–39). Washington, D.C.: American Psychological Association.

Grisso, T. (2000). Ethical issues in evaluations for sex offender re-offending. Invited address to Sinclair Seminars seminar in Madison, Wisconsin. On file with editors.

Hanson, R. (1998). What do we know about sex offender risk assessment? *Psychology, Public Policy and Law*, 4, 50–72.

Hanson, R. (2003). Who is dangerous and when are they safe? Risk assessment with sexual offenders. In B. Winnick & J. LaFond (Eds.), *Protecting society from sexually dangerous offenders* (pp. 63–74). Washington, D.C: American Psychological Association.

Hanson, R. & Thornton, D. (1999). Static-99: Improving actuarial risk assessments for sex offenders. User Report 99–02. Department of the Solicitor General of Canada: Ottawa.

Harris, G., Rice, M., Quinsey, V., Lalumière, M., Boer, D., & Lang, C. (2003). A multisite comparison of actuarial risk instruments for sex offenders. *Psychological Assessment* 15, 413–425.

Harris, G., Rice M., & Quinsey, V. (1998). Appraisal and management of risk in sexual aggressors: Implications for criminal justice policy. *Psychology, Public Policy, and Law* 4, 73–115.

Holmes, O. (1881). *The common law.* Boston: Little, Brown.

In re Detention of Jeffrey Hargett 338 Ill. App. 3rd 669 (2003).

Jackson, R., Rogers, R., & Shuman, D. (2004). The adequacy and accuracy of sexually violent predator evaluations: Contextualized risk assessment in clinical practice. *International Journal of Forensic Mental Health*, 3, 115–129.

Jacobs, M. (1993). Testing the assumptions underlying the debate about scientific evidence: A closer look at jury "incompetence" and scientific "objectivity". *Connecticut Law Review*, 25, 1083–1115.

Janus, E. & Prentky, R. (2003). Forensic use of actuarial risk assessment with sex offenders: Accuracy, admissibility and accountability. *American Criminal Law Review*, 40, 1443–1449.

Kansas v. Crane 534 US 407 (2002).

Kansas v. Hendricks 521 US 346 (1997).

L.A. Times. (2004, June 26) Man facing child porn trial is found hanged. B6.

Lanyon, R. (1997). Scientific status of the concept of continuing emotional propensity for sexually aberrant acts. *Journal of American Academy of Psychiatry and the Law*, 25, 59–60.

Lefkowitz v. Cunningham, 431 U.S. 801, at 809 (1977).

Lieb, R. (2003). State policy perspectives on sexual predator laws. In B. Winnick & J. LaFond (Eds.), *Protecting society from sexually dangerous offenders* (pp. 41–59). Washington, D.C.:American Psychological Association.

Lile v. McKune, 24 F. Supp. 2d 1152 (1998).

Litwack, T. (2001). Actuarial versus clinical assessments of dangerousness. *Psychology, Public Policy and Law*, 7, 409–443.

Mace v. Amnesty, 765 F. Supp. 847 (1991).

Mansnerus, L. (2003, November 17). Questions rise over imprisoning sex offenders past their terms. *New York Times*, p. A1.

McKune v. Lile, 536 U.S. 24 (2002).

Monahan, J., Steadman, H., Robbins, P., Appelbaum, P., Banks, S., Grisso, T., et al. (2005). An actuarial model of violence risk assessment for persons with mental disorders. *Psychiatric Services*, 56, 810–815.

Montana v. Imlay, 506 U.S. 5 (1992).

Mossman, D. (1994). Assessing predictions of violence: Being accurate about accuracy. *Journal of Consulting and Clinical Psychology*, 62, 783–792.

Mossman, D. (2004). Understanding prediction instruments. In R. Simon & L. Gold (Eds.), *Textbook of forensic psychiatry* (pp. 501–523). Washington, D.C.: American Psychological Association.

Neal v. Shimoda, 131 F.3d 818, 832, 833 (9th Cir. 1997).

People v. Ward 71 Cal. App. 4th 368 (1999).

Quinsey, V., Harris, G., Rice, M., & Cormier, C. (1998). Violent offenders: Appraising and managing risk. Washington, D.C.: American Psychological Association.

Quinsey, V., Rice, M., & Harris, G. (1995). Actuarial prediction of sexual recidivism. *Journal of Interpersonal Violence*, 10, 85–105.

Rice, M. & Harris, G. (1997) Cross validation and extension of the Violence Risk Appraisal Guide for child molesters and rapists. *Law and Human Behavior*, 21, 231–241.

Rogers, R. & Jackson, R. (2005). Sexually violent predators: The risky enterprise of risk assessment. *Journal of the American Academy of Psychiatry and the Law*, 33, 523–528.

Rogers, R. & Shuman, D. (2005). *Fundamentals of forensic practice. Mental health and criminal law.* New York, NY: Springer.

Russell v. Eaves, 722 F. Supp. 558, 560 (E.D. Mo. 1989).

Scott, C. & Holmberg, T. (2003). Castration of sex offenders: Prisoners rights versus public safety. *Journal of American Academy of Psychiatry and the Law*, 31, 502–09.

Sjöstedt, G. & Grann, M. (2002). Risk assessment: What is being predicted by actuarial prediction instruments? *International Journal of Forensic Mental Health*, 1, 179–83.

State v. Andring 342 NW. 2d 128 (1984) LEXIS 1199.

State v. Fuller, 915 P.2d 816 (1996).

State v. Lile 237 Kan. 210, 211–212, 699 P.2d 456, 457–458 (1985).

Tribe, L. (1971). Trial by mathematics. *Harvard Law Review*, 84, 1329–1393.

U.S. Department of Justice. (2005). *Criminal offenders statistics.* Washington, D.C.: Bureau of Justice Statistics.

Washington State Institute for Public Policy. (2005). Involuntary commitment of sexually violent predators: Comparing state laws. Olympia, WA: Washington State Institute for Public Policy.

Williamson v. United States 184 F.2d 280 (1950).

Chapter 30

Commentary

James C. Beck

One of the editors was kind enough to offer me the opportunity to write this comment, and I was honored to accept. I say "kind enough" because I began by reading the book—a valuable experience I would not have had otherwise. This is an excellent compendium of what we know as well as what we do not know about sex offenders: identification, risk assessment, treatment, and legal issues.

The editor has chosen a commentator with extensive forensic experience but not someone who would hold himself out as an expert on sex offenders. Once I get beyond a factual summary of what the book concerns, my commentary will necessarily reflect who I am and my experience. Since this is a book that is addressed to a wide audience, not just to the fellow experts in the field, perhaps the editor has made a sensible choice in asking a nonexpert for commentary. In any case, in fairness to the reader, here is a summary of what you need to know about me to judge the relevance of my commentary to your own experience.

My clinical experience includes 17 years as a court clinic psychiatrist, and in that role I evaluated all types of criminal defendants. In my private practice I have evaluated and treated several dozen clinicians and patients who were involved in a sexual relationship. I was one of the earlier psychiatrists who tried to bring this problem into sharper focus for the profession—a profession unfortunately that took longer than it should have to acknowledge its own transgressions and to adopt a code of ethics that recognized that sex with patients is never ok. I have seen enough psychiatrists, and heard enough from their former patients to have some clinical sense of what drove these men. I have also evaluated half a dozen men who were sexually abused by catholic clergy. I have a very clear idea of what this experience has done to the victims.

I think it is safe to say that sex offenders stir up stronger feelings than almost any other perpetrators of violence. Incest, child sexual abuse, rape, necrophilia, and violation of fiduciary duties to patients, clients or parishioners arouse strong feelings of anger, revulsion, and disgust, mixed perhaps with some degree of sympathy for the perpetrator if or when we happen to know enough about him so that we get beyond the offense to the person. In my clinical practice I have a reputation, which I believe is accurate, for being more civil libertarian than most psychiatrists. My threshold for involuntary hospitalization is higher than that of my colleagues. For that reason it is surprising to me that I find myself uncomfortable enough with the idea of, for example, pedophiles running loose in the community that my idea of "least restrictive alternative" treatment for these men is quite restrictive indeed.

With that introduction, I turn to the book. What I propose to do in this commentary is to summarize the contents and add my own comments where I have opinions based solidly on my professional experience. There are four editors—two psychiatrists and two attorneys. The psychiatrists have substantial experience in the legal context and the attorneys have exercised their legal expertise in relation to a wide range of clinical problems. The four editors represent an enormous amount of relevant expertise packed into a small group of people. How efficient.

This is an excellent book, and will serve as a valuable reference or introduction to the subject for a wide range of people in the clinical and legal fields. Because it is so comprehensive, it can serve on the one hand as an introduction for people who know nothing about the field—for example, students in a college course on abnormal psychology, for medical students or residents, or law students taking a course in criminal law. For the more experienced clinician or attorney who has any need to know more about any of the topics in this book, this is an excellent place to start. The editors have clearly instructed their contributors to include a comprehensive literature review and the contributors have met that obligation. In the areas I know well—forensic assessment, competency to consent to evaluation, risk assessment, and sexual abuse by fiduciaries—I am impressed that the authors have covered their piece of the waterfront thoroughly.

Paul Appelbaum's foreward begins with a review of the current social climate—a climate in which society inposes punitive legal sanctions for sex offenders. He makes the important point, as do several following chapters, that sex offenders are not a homogeneous group, either in what they do or in who they are. To the extent that we understand it, the developmental path to incest is different from the path toward rape.

The author goes on to say, "the only hope for escaping the legal, ethical, and political tangle associated with sex offenders is the development of effective treatment," and here we come to the first statement of what I see as a serious problem. Treatment in its usual meaning is medical, or more broadly, clinical. I question whether it is realistic to hope for effective treatment, if by treatment we mean some degree of voluntary engagement with a clinician as distinct from forced compliance. There are incest perpetrators who know that what they are doing is wrong, and are deeply conflicted about it. For them, treatment is an option. The mental health professions have treatment for people like these.

By contrast there are sex offenders who believe that what they are doing is right, that society is wrong in criminalizing it, and they will do whatever they can in order to continue offending. It is hard for me to see that "treatment" for these people is a reasonable goal. Management of their risk or even control may be a reasonable goal, but not treatment.

The second aspect of the problem is that it is difficult, and at times impossible, to assess the effectiveness of any proposed treatment, or for that matter, any proposed method of control. The reason is simple. Accurate assessment of treatment efficacy depends ultimately on truthful reporting by the subject of his behavior. When truthful reporting leads to rearrest and likely incarceration, truth takes a pass.

The book is organized in seven parts: An introduction provides a perspective on what we understand by normality as relating to sexual behavior. The second chapter describes paraphilia in careful detail, and introduces the concept of "lovemap." As far as I could see "lovemap" refers in common parlance to what turns you on, but does not carry us any further into understanding why some people are turned on by paraphilic fantasies.

The second part presents what we know about the neuropsychology and neurobiology of these disorders. What was true here, as I read it, was true consistently throughout the book: we have good data describing antecedents of offending and good data on associated conditions. These antecedents and these associated conditions are both associated with sex offending and with various other mental disorders and behavioral difficulties in adulthood. What we do not appear to have at present is sufficient understanding of why some men with these risk factors go on to become sex offenders and other men do not.

Men (the offenders are almost always men; there is one chapter on women) who offend are more likely to be substance abusers, to have attention-deficit hyperactivity disorder (ADHD), or to have other evidence of neuropsychological impairment. But we appear to know essentially nothing about why some men with these conditions go on to become sex offenders and others do not. Later chapters will document the association between early childhood abuse or other maltreatment or neglect and various types of sexual offending, but again, with no knowledge of why some children who have these tragic experiences go on to offend sexually and others do not.

The third part is on diagnosis and assessment. There is an excellent review of risk assessment for violence in relation to mental disorder generally followed by a chapter applying what we know about risk assessment to sexual offending. The authors conclude that assessment tools cannot estimate the probability of future sexual offending in the individual case, and they suggest supplementing the actuarial tool with structured professional judgment. Buchanan et al. (2008) reached a similar conclusion for risk assessment generally, and this approach makes the most sense to me also (Beck, 2008). Estimated recidivism rates quoted as high as 52% for child molesters and 39% for rapists highlight the importance of improving our capacity to predict and control the behavior of these offenders. The quoted fact that one-third of prisoners in some states are sex offenders, speaks of the importance of not just improved prediction but for developing improved methods for behavior control in the community.

Two chapters on laboratory methods of assessment are followed by chapters on mental disorder; psychopathy, and personality disorders generally in relation to sex offending. These chapters summarize what we know, and also what we do not. The chapters on assessment will be of interest primarily to specialists. The descriptive chapters following are relevant to any clinical or legal professional who evaluates sex offenders.

The fourth part on treatment begins with a chapter on psychosocial treatment that has an excellent summary of the relevant history. In particular, the authors note that relapse prevention therapy continues to be employed in spite of evidence in a controlled study by the man who invented it that it may actually be ineffective. Two studies showed that therapists who were empathic, warm, rewarding, and somewhat directive produced maximal results with these patients. Only "somewhat directive" distinguishes these therapists from the maximally effective therapist for any other patient. There is an excellent discussion of the risks and benefits of manually driven versus more individually tailored therapy.

The chapter on orchiectomy is of largely historical interest. The discussion of pharmacological treatments by Saleh is useful for an understanding of how to manage and mitigate a paraphilic sex offender's risk for sexual recidivism.

The fifth part on juveniles covers forensic assessment; epidemiology, risk assessment and treatment; and intervention and treatment in three excellent chapters. They should serve as cautionary reading for any clinician who imagines that adult clinical training is sufficient to engage with juveniles either in the legal or clinical setting. The discussion of forensic assessment makes very clear just how different this assessment is for juveniles as opposed to adults. The chapter on epidemiology presents epidemiologic data on offenders who are apprehended—as with adults we have far less accurate data on the incidence and prevalence of these behaviors in the community. Both this chapter and that following make the important point that adolescents are not fixed either in development or in behavior in a way that adults are, and that therefore their prognosis is potentially better. As with adults, we know little about what distinguishes juvenile sex offenders from juvenile offenders generally. For example, data are quoted showing that these adolescents have higher rates of neuropsychological difficulties. We found the same for a sample of unincarcerated delinquents (Robbins, Beck, Pries, Cage, & Smith, 1983). Again, we have no idea why some adolescents with neuropsychological impairments become sex offenders and others become delinquent.

Part six focuses on special populations.

Chapter 18 presents data, no surprise, that substance abuse is associated with increased risk for sexual offending. Chapter 19 presents the sparse data on female sexual offenders. Only 1% of sentenced sex offenders are women. The relative lack of data pertaining to female offenders is clearly one impediment to learning more about them.

The chapter on professionals who are accused of sexual boundary violations reviews a subject that for far too long was tolerated by psychiatry. The authors discuss boundary violations, ethical obligations, social response to perpetrators, and their program for evaluating physicians who have had sexual relations with patients. Missing was any discussion of who these physicians are. In my experience there has been a dramatic shift in who commits these violations. In the 1960s when I trained it was commonly thought by the residents that more than one of our supervisors had been involved sexually with patients. I have personally evaluated several dozen women who gave credible accounts of sexual relationships—in the most egregious of these cases I spoke with five women who reported sex with one psychiatrist and five others who reported sex with a different psychiatrist. These relationships went on because for many years the women found that if they complained they were called "*borderline*," the allegations of a sexual relationship were denied; and the perpetrator continued unchecked.

As society has imposed sanctions and as the profession has taken a firm stand condemning this behavior the few psychiatrists I have seen recently are what have been described as "love sick therapists." These are typically men who are in bad marriages, angry at their wives but unable for characterological reasons to express the anger, who become involved with patients who have dependent needs of their own. The patient wants the therapist to care for her. He is empathic and feels her need. He does not feel his own less conscious need for a new relationship. He responds to the patient who then asks him to hug her. He does hug her; once, and then repeatedly. Over time, biology asserts itself and the cases we see have ended with an angry, badly damaged patient who makes a complaint to the appropriate authorities.

If the profession is going to be more successful in reducing the incidence of these regrettable events we must do more than publish appropriate ethical guidelines. We need to teach our trainees and our peers how to recognize the psychosocial states that create a potential risk of ethical violations with patients.

This part also contains chapters on stalking, Internet child pornography, clergy sex abuse, sexual sadism, and intellectual disabilities.

The last part is on forensic issues. The first chapter on forensic considerations gives a clear and complete outline of what is involved in a forensic examination. Then they apply their general paradigm to the forensic evaluation of; sexual offenders. If a general psychiatrist were somehow put in a position to do a forensic assessment, or a forensic psychiatrist to do an assessment of a sex offender, following this outline would

get them through admirably. The chapter on sexual predator laws and their history should be required reading for any judge or other legal or clinical professional involved with these cases. I have lived long enough to have practiced under the various systems employed. They may be summarized as follows: either treatment is provided, or it is not. If it is provided either it is only for those who ask for it, or it is mandatory for all offenders. Confinement is either for a fixed or an indeterminate period. It may be in prison or in a hospital or in a "treatment center." All combinations of the treatment and confinement variables have been tried. There are no data sufficient to inform the choice. As a practical matter, the choices are made on sociopolitical grounds. At present in the United States we come down on the side of incarcerating people for long periods with or without something called treatment that may or may not exist, or if it exists, have any evidence base of support. When we release people to the community, we impose conditions that make their lives almost impossible. Civil libertarians are appropriately troubled. If parents are troubled, I suspect it is because the offenders have been released at all. The last chapter reviews current case and statute law in the United States and Canada, and addresses the ethical questions musrarise when the question of self-disclosure of illegal activities is posed. Their discussion of ethical issues involved in certifying a person as a sexually violent predator for purposes of indefinite commitment and "treatment" is particularly apt. There are no easy answers to these, or indeed, any of the questions raised by the assessment and management of men who commit these crimes.

In this context, I offer my own suggestion for potentially adequate control of recalcitrant sex offenders in the community. I base this proposal on my own experience providing "psychiatric probation" through a court clinic on mentally ill violent offenders who had less than no interest in seeing me. My impression was that the experience of having a responsible person consistently inquiring into their situation and behavior served to help these men behave themselves. I adapt this experience here.

First, determinate sentences appropriate to the crime as the government sees fit. This confinement would be followed by extremely close supervision in the community. It costs, per recent estimates I have seen, $40,000 per year to house a prisoner. This fact provides a comparative financial basis on which to argue that intensive community supervision can be delivered in a less costly way that hopefully provides a better balance between risk to the community and the civil rights of the offenders.

Suppose we conceive of specially trained probation officers whom we teach what we know clinically and what we understand practically about probationary supervision. If we pay these men and women $100 K to 120 K per year including fringe and we assign each officer six offenders to supervise, the state will save roughly 50% of what it costs now. Lastly, as part of the team we would include investigators who would be charged to make random surveillance of the probationers. Extremely close supervision would be mandatory, and it would last for many years.

Conviction for reoffending would lead to indefinite institutionalization. These conditions are severe, but not as severe as incarceration. Some long-incarcerated men have learned to prefer the institution to the street. These offenders could be given a choice after they maxed out of indefinite commitment or this kind of probation.

References

Beck, J. C. (2008). Ch. 12. Outpatient settings. In R. I. Simon & K. Tardiff (Eds.), *Textbook of violence assessment and management* (pp. 237–257). Washington, D. C.: American Psychiatric Publishing.

Buchanan, A. (2008). Risk of violence by psychiatric patients: Beyond the "actuarial versus clinical" assessment debate. *Psychiatric Services* (Washington, D.C.), 59(2), 184–90.

Robbins, D., Beck, J. C., Pries, R., Cage, D. J., & Smith, C. (1983). Learning disability and neuropsychological impairment in adjudicated, unincarcerated male delinquents. *Journal of the American Academy of Child Psychiatry*, 22, 40–46.

Index

Note: Page numbers in *italics* refer to figures and tables.